Cosmeceuticals and Active Cosmetics

COSMETIC SCIENCE AND TECHNOLOGY

Series Editor
ERIC JUNGERMANN
*Jungermann Associates, Inc.
Phoenix, Arizona*

1. Cosmetic and Drug Preservation: Principles and Practice, *edited by Jon J. Kabara*
2. The Cosmetic Industry: Scientific and Regulatory Foundations, *edited by Norman F. Estrin*
3. Cosmetic Product Testing: A Modern Psychophysical Approach, *Howard R. Moskowitz*
4. Cosmetic Analysis: Selective Methods and Techniques, *edited by P. Boré*
5. Cosmetic Safety: A Primer for Cosmetic Scientists, *edited by James H. Whittam*
6. Oral Hygiene Products and Practice, *Morton Pader*
7. Antiperspirants and Deodorants, *edited by Karl Laden and Carl B. Felger*
8. Clinical Safety and Efficacy Testing of Cosmetics, *edited by William C. Waggoner*
9. Methods for Cutaneous Investigation, *edited by Robert L. Rietschel and Thomas S. Spencer*
10. Sunscreens: Development, Evaluation, and Regulatory Aspects, *edited by Nicholas J. Lowe and Nadim A. Shaath*
11. Glycerine: A Key Cosmetic Ingredient, *edited by Eric Jungermann and Norman O. V. Sonntag*
12. Handbook of Cosmetic Microbiology, *Donald S. Orth*
13. Rheological Properties of Cosmetics and Toiletries, *edited by Dennis Laba*
14. Consumer Testing and Evaluation of Personal Care Products, *Howard R. Moskowitz*
15. Sunscreens: Development, Evaluation, and Regulatory Aspects. Second Edition, Revised and Expanded, *edited by Nicholas J. Lowe, Nadim A. Shaath, and Madhu A. Pathak*

16. Preservative-Free and Self-Preserving Cosmetics and Drugs: Principles and Practice, *edited by Jon J. Kabara and Donald S. Orth*
17. Hair and Hair Care, *edited by Dale H. Johnson*
18. Cosmetic Claims Substantiation, *edited by Louise B. Aust*
19. Novel Cosmetic Delivery Systems, *edited by Shlomo Magdassi and Elka Touitou*
20. Antiperspirants and Deodorants: Second Edition, Revised and Expanded, *edited by Karl Laden*
21. Conditioning Agents for Hair and Skin, *edited by Randy Schueller and Perry Romanowski*
22. Principles of Polymer Science and Technology in Cosmetics and Personal Care, *edited by E. Desmond Goddard and James V. Gruber*
23. Cosmeceuticals: Drugs vs. Cosmetics, *edited by Peter Elsner and Howard I. Maibach*
24. Cosmetic Lipids and the Skin Barrier, *edited by Thomas Förster*
25. Skin Moisturization, *edited by James J. Leyden and Anthony V. Rawlings*
26. Multifunctional Cosmetics, *edited by Randy Schueller and Perry Romanowski*
27. Cosmeceuticals and Active Cosmetics: Drugs Versus Cosmetics, Second Edition, *edited by Peter Elsner and Howard I. Maibach*

Cosmeceuticals and Active Cosmetics

Drugs Versus Cosmetics

Second Edition

edited by

Peter Elsner
*University of Jena
Jena, Germany*

Howard I. Maibach
*University of California
San Francisco, California, U.S.A.*

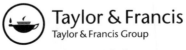

Taylor & Francis
Taylor & Francis Group

Boca Raton   London   New York   Singapore

Published in 2005 by
Taylor & Francis Group
6000 Broken Sound Parkway NW
Boca Raton, FL 33487-2742

© 2005 by Taylor & Francis Group

No claim to original U.S. Government works
Printed in the United States of America on acid-free paper
10 9 8 7 6 5 4 3 2 1

International Standard Book Number-10: 0-8247-5943-5 (Hardcover)
International Standard Book Number-13: 978-0-8247-5943-8 (Hardcover)
Library of Congress Card Number: 2004063459

This book contains information obtained from authentic and highly regarded sources. Reprinted material is quoted with permission, and sources are indicated. A wide variety of references are listed. Reasonable efforts have been made to publish reliable data and information, but the author and the publisher cannot assume responsibility for the validity of all materials or for the consequences of their use.

No part of this book may be reprinted, reproduced, transmitted, or utilized in any form by any electronic mechanical, or other means, now known or hereafter invented, including photocopying, microfilming, and recording, or in any information storage or retrieval system, without written permission from the publishers.

For permission to photocopy or use material electronically from this work, please access www.copyright.com (http://www.copyright.com/) or contact the Copyright Clearance Center, Inc. (CCC) 222 Rosewood Drive, Danvers, MA 01923, 978-750-8400. CCC is a not-for-profit organization that provides licenses and registration for a variety of users. For organizations that have been granted a photocopy license by the CCC, a separate system of payment has been arranged.

Trademark Notice: Product or corporate names may be trademarks or registered trademarks, and are used only for identification and explanation without intent to infringe.

Library of Congress Cataloging-in-Publication Data

Cosmeceuticals and active cosmetics : drugs versus cosmetics / edited by Peter Elsner, Howard I. Maibach.-- 2nd ed.
   p. cm. -- (Cosmetic science and technology series)
  First ed. published in 2000 under title: Cosmeceuticals.
  Includes bibliographical references and index.
  ISBN 0-8247-5943-5 (alk. paper)
  1. Dermatologic agents. 2. Cosmetics. I. Elsner, Peter, 1955-
II. Maibach, Howard I. III. Cosmeceuticals. IV. Title. V. Series.
  RL801.C67 2005
  615'.778--dc22

                         2004063459

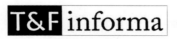

Taylor & Francis Group
is the Academic Division of T&F Informa plc.

Visit the Taylor & Francis Web site at
http://www.taylorandfrancis.com

About the Series

The Cosmetic Science and Technology series was conceived to permit discussion of a broad range of current knowledge and theories of cosmetic science and technology. The series is composed of books written by one or two authors and edited volumes with a number of contributors. Authorities from industry, academia, and the government participate in writing these books.

The aim of the series is to cover the many facets of cosmetic science and technology. Topics are drawn from a wide spectrum of disciplines ranging from chemistry, physics, biochemistry, and dermatology to consumer evaluations, safety issues, efficacy, toxicity, and regulatory questions. Organic, inorganic, physical, analytical, and polymer chemistry, microbiology, emulsion, and lipid technology all play important roles in cosmetic science.

There is little commonality in the scientific methods, processes, and formulations required for the wide variety of toiletries and cosmetics in the market. Product categories range from hair, skin, and oral care products to lipsticks, nail polishes, deodorants, body powders, and aerosols to cosmeceuticals, which are quasi-pharmaceutical over-the-counter products such as antiperspirants, dandruff shampoos, wrinkle reducers, antimicrobial soaps, acne treatments, and sunscreen products.

Cosmetics and toiletries represent a highly diversified field involving many subsections of science and "art." Even in these days of high technology, art and intuition continue to play an important part in the development of formulations, their evaluation, selection of raw materials, and, perhaps most importantly, the successful marketing of new products. Fragrance, color, and packaging selections can often be as important to the success of a new product introduction as delivering the promised (implied) performance. The application of more sophisticated scientific methodologies to the evaluation of cosmetics that began in the 1980s has continued and has greatly impacted such areas as claim substantiation, safety testing, product testing, and development of "organic" raw materials, the last resulting in the emergence of a new market of "organic" cosmetics.

Emphasis in the Cosmetic Science and Technology series is placed on reporting the current status of cosmetic science and technology, the ever changing regulatory climate, and historical reviews. The series has now grown to 27 books dealing with the constantly changing trends in the cosmetic industry, including globalization. Several of the books have been translated into Japanese and Chinese. Contributions range from highly sophisticated and scientific treaties to primers and presentations of practical applications. Authors are encouraged to present their own concepts as well as established theories. Contributors have been asked not to shy away from fields that are in a state of transition or somewhat controversial, and not to hesitate to present detailed discussions of their own work. Altogether, we intend to develop in this series a collection of critical surveys and ideas covering the diverse phases of the cosmetic industry.

The current volume is the second edition of *Cosmeceuticals* first published in 2000. The field has expanded tremendously since that time. In the U.S. alone, the market has continued to grow at a 7% rate and reached an annual volume of $6.4 billion in 2004. The second edition mirrors this growth: the number of chapters in the book has grown from 20 chapters in the first edition to the current 38. The number of contributors to the second edition has more than doubled to 70, representing a virtual *Who's Who* of experts from all over the globe. The chapters have been separated into categories such as classes of cosmeceuticals, raw materials (substances), toxicology, product development, regulatory, and an industry overview. Scientifically tremendous changes have occurred and many new products have appeared in the market place, sometimes making extravagant claims. Cosmeceuticals, that is, products marketed as cosmetics that contain biologically active ingredients, can be confusing to consumers overwhelmed by massive promotional campaigns appealing to the youth-obsessed generation of baby boomers with promises of eternal youth. In the process, the lines between medicine, specifically dermatology, and cosmetology can become somewhat blurred. Dermatology is the medical specialty concerned with skin diseases, but it has become as much involved with improving appearance by medical means, with physicians dispensing botox and hyaluronic acid (Restylane) shots, chemical peels, laser treatments, and other special formulations, as it has on the treatment of serious skin disorders. On the other hand, cosmetologists are concerned with improving appearance and appealing to vanity the old-fashioned way.

It is only fitting that the first chapter of the book is written by Professor Albert Kligman, who can be considered the father of cosmeceuticals. In the 1970s, he coined the term "cosmeceutical" to describe cosmetic products with quasi-pharmaceutical properties. This led to the foundation for a host of new product categories and new marketing opportunities, as well as to global controversy on how to regulate and classify these products. There are legal definitions for cosmetics and drugs, and there are lay perceptions of these materials. Implicit

About the Series

in the definition of cosmetics is the concept that they are inert substances used for adornment and beautification. But, as physics teaches us, for every action there is an equal and opposite reaction. There is little that is applied to skin that does not evoke an equal and opposite reaction. Even innocuous materials, such as water and Vaseline, can under some circumstances alter the structure of the skin (moisturize). At what point do such changes merit classification as a drug? Has the 1938 Act of Congress that defines drugs as articles *intended to affect the stricture and function of the body (including skin and hair)* become outdated?

I want to thank all contributors for participating in this project and the editors, Dr. Peter Elsner and Howard I. Maibach, for expanding, organizing, and coordinating this edition. On a private note, publication of this book culminates a rewarding 40-year personal friendship and professional relationship with Howard that has significantly influenced my own career. Finally, I want to thank Marcel Dekker and the many people in his organization, particularly Sandra Beberman, with whom I have worked since the inception of this series, for their support and help. Adieu!

Eric Jungermann, Ph.D.
Series Editor

Preface

The term "cosmeceuticals", coined by Albert Kligman 20 years ago, has rightfully provoked discussions among scientists, the industry, and regulating authorities. Basically, the controversy may be reduced to the question of whether there are any substances applied to the skin that do not modify its structure and function. Since scientific evidence shows that even purportedly "inert" substances such as water may profoundly change the structure and function of the skin, this condition does not seem helpful to differentiate cosmetics from drugs. Indeed, this is a problem of legal definition of cosmetics in the US, but not in other major countries such as Europe and Japan, as evidenced by the contributions in this book.

In Europe, the Council Directive 76/768/EEC of July 27, 1976, as amended by six directives, defines cosmetic products in Article 1: "A cosmetic product means any substance or preparation intended for placing into contact with the various parts of the human body (epidermis, hair system, nails, lips and external genital organs) or with the teeth and mucous membranes of the oral cavity with a view exclusively or principally to cleaning them, perfuming them or protecting them, in order to keep them in good condition, change their appearance or correct body odours."

Thus, a cosmetic is defined by its way of application and by the intention with which it is used. While cosmetics are used on normal or nearly normal skin, drugs are defined as preparations to be used for the treatment of diseased skin. Obviously, there remains a gray zone between what is still to be considered as normal skin and what is already a skin disease. The perceived border between healthy and diseased may vary depending on the individual, the society, and over time. In this situation, Article 2 of the Council Directive is helpful. It states that "A cosmetic product put on the market within the Community must not cause damage to human health when applied under normal or reasonably foreseeable conditions of use". Therefore, consumer safety is an absolute goal of highest importance in cosmetics, while safety is a relative issue in drugs where a balanced benefit–risk assessment has to be made, depending on the severity of the disease.

The first edition of this book, published in 2000, received wide interest, and it contributed, as we had hoped, to a sincere discussion on the status of "cosmeceuticals", that is, products that are intended for a cosmetic use, but contain active substances. Regulatory aspects have changed little since, but new data have been published for known substances and an astounding array of new compounds, rightfully labeled cosmeceuticals, have entered the field. Therefore, it seemed worthwhile to rewrite chapters and add new ones. We hope this will be useful reading for cosmetic scientists, pharmacists, dermatologists, and regulators alike.

We finally take the opportunity to thank the contributors to this book, all experts in their fields, who devoted time and effort to their chapters. We are also indebted to Sandra Beberman and Kerry Doyle of Marcel Dekker, who were more than helpful in the editorial process.

Peter Elsner
Howard I. Maibach

Contributors

Gurpreet S. Ahluwalia *Gillette Advanced Technology Center, Needham, Massachusetts, USA.*

Yohini Appa *Neurogena Corporation, Los Angeles, California, USA.*

Kumi Arakane *Research & Development Division, KOSE Corporation, Tokyo, Japan.*

Saqib J. Bashir *Department of Dermatology, University of California, San Francisco, California, USA.*

Eric Bauza *Vincience Research Center, Sophia Antipolis, France.*

C. Bayerl *Department of Dermatology, Venerology and Allergology, Mannheim University Clinic, Mannheim, Germany.*

Cynthia A. Berge *The Procter & Gamble Company, Miami Valley Laboratories, Cincinnati, Ohio, USA.*

Christiane Bertin *Johnson & Johnson Consumer Products Co., Skillman, New Jersey, USA and Issy les Moulineaux, France.*

Sulochana Bhandarkar *Department of Dermatology, University of California, San Francisco School of Medicine, San Francisco, California, USA.*

Kimberly A. Biedermann *The Procter & Gamble Company, Miami Valley Laboratories, Cincinnati, Ohio, USA.*

Donald L. Bissett *The Procter & Gamble Company, Miami Valley Laboratories, Cincinnati, Ohio, USA.*

C. Bouillon *R&D, Cosmetic Scientist and Senior R&D Consultant, Soisy-sous-Montmorency, France.*

Ratan K. Chaudhuri *EMD Chemicals, Inc., Hawthorne, New York, New York, USA.*

Ai-Lean Chew *Department of Dermatology, University of California, San Francisco, California, USA.*

William J. Cunningham *CU-Tech, LLC., Mountain Lakes, New Jersey, USA*

Nouha Domloge *Vincience Research Center, Sophia Antipolis, France.*

Frank Dreher *Department of Dermatology, University of California, San Francisco, California, USA and TOPALIX, Topical Product Development, San Francisco, California, USA.*

Tamotsu Ebihara *Saiseikai Central Hospital, Tokyo, Japan.*

Peter Elsner *Department of Dermatology and Allergology, Friedrich-Schiller University, Jena, Germany.*

Jan Faergemann *Department of Dermatology, Sahlgrenska University Hospital, Gothenburg, Sweden.*

Claude Dal Farra *Vincience Research Center, Sophia Antipolis, France.*

Mary Beth Finkey *Neurogena Corporation, Los Angeles, California, USA.*

Tobias W. Fischer *Department of Dermatology and Allergology, Friedrich-Schiller University, Jena, Germany.*

Richard E. Fitzpatrick *Dermatology Associates of San Diego County, Inc., Encinitas, California, USA.*

J. W. Fluhr *Department of Dermatology, Friedrich-Schiller University, Jena, Germany.*

Rachel Grossman *Johnson & Johnson Consumer Products Co., Skillman, New Jersey, USA and Issy les Moulineaux, France.*

Philip G. Hewitt *Merck kGaA, Darmstadt, Germany.*

Peter Barton Hutt *Covington & Burling, Washington, DC, USA.*

Nathalie Issachar *Johnson & Johnson Consumer Products Co., Skillman, New Jersey, USA and Issy les Moulineaux, France.*

Tsuneo Jinnai *Sansho Pharmaceutical Company, Fukuoka, Japan.*

Alain Khaiat *Johnson & Johnson Asia Pacific, Singapore.*

Albert M. Kligman *University of Pennsylvania School of Medicine, Philadelphia, Pennsylvania, USA.*

François Lamy *Sederma, Paris, France.*

Cheryl Levin University of California—San Francisco Medical Center, San Francisco, California, USA.

Stanley B. Levy University of North Carolina School of Medicine, Chapel Hill, North Carolina, USA.

Karl Lintner Sederma, Paris, France.

Marie Lodén ACO Hud AB, Upplands Väsby, Sweden.

Howard I. Maibach Department of Dermatology, University of California—San Francisco Medical Center, San Francisco, California, USA.

Claire Mas-Chamberlin Sederma, Paris, France.

Mitsuteru Masuda Lion Corporation, Tokyo, Japan.

Bozena B. Michniak New Jersey Center for Biomaterials, New Jersey, USA.

Philippe Mondon Sederma, Paris, France.

Joseph P. Morton Morton Associates Inc., Silver Spring, Maryland, USA.

Hideo Nakayama Nakayama Dermatology Clinic, Tokyo, Japan.

Birgit A. Neudecker University of California, San Francisco, California, USA.

Kenkichi Oba Lion Corporation, Tokyo, Japan.

John E. Oblong The Procter & Gamble Company, Miami Valley Laboratories, Cincinnati, Ohio, USA.

Olivier Peschard Sederma, Paris, France.

L. Petit Department of Dermatopathology, University Medical Center Sart Tilman, Liège, Belgium.

G. E. Piérard Department of Dermatopathology, University Medical Center Sart Tilman, Liège, Belgium.

C. Piérard-Franchimont Department of Dermatopathology, University Medical Center Sart Tilman, Liège, Belgium.

J. Praessler Department of Dermatology, Friedrich-Schiller University, Jena, Germany.

Kazutami Sakamoto Ajinomoto Co., Tokyo, Japan.

Noriko Satoh Yanagihara Hospital, Tokyo, Japan.

Abel Saud The Procter & Gamble Company, Miami Valley Laboratories, Cincinnati, Ohio, USA.

Frank Schönlau University of Münster, Münster, Germany.

Mitchell L. Schlossman Kobo Products, Inc., South Plainfield, New Jersey, USA.

Dörte Segger Skin Investigation and Technology, Hamburg, Germany.

Douglas Shander Gillette Advanced Technology Center/US, Needham, Massachusetts, USA.

Robert Stern University of California, San Francisco, California, USA.

Koji Takada Biological Science Research Center, Research & Technology Headquarters, Lion Corporation, Odawara, Japan.

Kazuyuki Takagi Mizuho Industrial Co., Ltd., Osaka, Japan.

Yoshimasa Tanaka Biological Science Research Center, Research & Technology Headquarters, Lion Corporation, Odawara, Japan.

Jens J. Thiele Department of Dermatology, Northwestern University, Chicago, Illinois, USA.

Amy V. Trejo The Procter & Gamble Company, Miami Valley Laboratories, Cincinnati, Ohio, USA.

E. Uhoda Department of Dermatopathology, University Medical Center Sart Tilman, Liège, Belgium.

Bert Jan Vermeer Leiden University Medical Center, Leiden, The Netherlands.

F. Verrière Pierre Fabre Dermo-Cosmétique, Lavaur, France.

Philip W. Wertz Dows Institute, University of Iowa, Iowa City, Iowa, USA.

Chu Zhu The Procter & Gamble Company, Miami Valley Laboratories, Cincinnati, Ohio, USA.

Contents

About the Series iii
Preface vii
Contributors ix

1. Cosmeceuticals: A Broad-Spectrum Category between
   Cosmetics and Drugs 1
   Albert M. Kligman

2. Definition 11
   Bert Jan Vermeer

Classes

3. Amino Acids and Derivatives 17
   Kazutami Sakamoto

4. Antioxidant Defense Systems in Skin 37
   Jens J. Thiele and Frank Dreher

5. Botanical Extracts 89
   Alain Khaiat

6. Cutaneous Barrier Repair 99
   Karl Lintner, Claire Mas-Chamberlin, Philippe Mondon,
   François Lamy, and Olivier Peschard

7. Seborrheic Dermatitis (Dandruff) 129
   Jan Faergemann

8.	Decorative Products Mitchell L. Schlossman	137
9.	Depigmentation Agents Hideo Nakayama, Tamotsu Ebihara, Noriko Satoh, and Tsuneo Jinnai	185
10.	Hydroxyacids E. Uhoda, C. Piérard-Franchimont, L. Petit, and G. E. Piérard	207
11.	Moisturizers Marie Lodén	219
12.	Alternative Drugs in Dermatology: An Overview Cheryl Levin and Howard I. Maibach	247
13.	Cosmeceuticals in Photoaging William J. Cunningham	261
14.	Phytosterols C. Bayerl	279
15.	Protective Creams J. W. Fluhr, J. Praessler, and Peter Elsner	293
16.	Sebum Philip W. Wertz and Bozena B. Michniak	307
17.	Topical Retinoids Ai-Lean Chew, Saqib J. Bashir, and Howard I. Maibach	319
18.	UV Care Kumi Arakane	333
19.	Use of Growth Factors in Cosmeceuticals Richard E. Fitzpatrick	349

Substances

20.	Dimethylaminoethanol Rachel Grossman, Christiane Bertin, and Nathalie Issachar	365

21.	Hyaluronan: The Natural Skin Moisturizer .... Birgit A. Neudecker, Howard I. Maibach, and Robert Stern	373
22.	Kinetin .... Stanley B. Levy	407
23.	Melatonin: A Hormone, Drug, or Cosmeceutical .... Tobias W. Fischer and Peter Elsner	413
24.	Topical Niacinamide Provides Skin Aging Appearance Benefits while Enhancing Barrier Function .... Donald L. Bissett, John E. Oblong, Abel Saud, Cynthia A. Berge, Amy V. Trejo, and Kimberly A. Biedermann	421
25.	Topical Retinyl Propionate Achieves Skin Benefits with Favorable Irritation Profile .... John E. Oblong, Abel Saud, Donald L. Bissett, and Chu Zhu	441
26.	*Phyllanthus* Tannins .... Ratan K. Chaudhuri	465
27.	Management of Unwanted Facial Hair by Topical Application of Eflornithine .... Douglas Shander, Gurpreet S. Ahluwalia, and Joseph P. Morton	489
28.	Ellagic Acid .... Koji Takada and Yoshimasa Tanaka	511
29.	Heat Shock Proteins for Cosmeceuticals .... Claude Dal Farra, Eric Bauza, and Nouha Domloge	523
30.	Evelle® Supplementation .... Dörte Segger and Frank Schönlau	537
31.	Retinaldehyde: A New Compound in Topical Retinoids .... F. Verrière	545
32.	Copper Peptide and Skin .... Mary Beth Finkey, Yohini Appa, and Sulochana Bhandarkar	549

Toxicology

33. Dermatotoxicology Overview 567
    Philip G. Hewitt and Howard I. Maibach

34. Contact Urticaria Syndrome and Claims Support 587
    Saqib J. Bashir and Howard I. Maibach

Product Development

35. Process Engineering in Cosmetics to Utilize
    Active Ingredients 603
    Kazuyuki Takagi

The Industry View

36. Cosmeceuticals or Not? The Industry View: Europe 615
    C. Bouillon

Regulatory

37. The Legal Distinction in USA between Cosmetic
    and Drug 625
    Peter Barton Hutt

38. Drugs versus Cosmetics: Cosmeceuticals? 643
    Kenkichi Oba and Mitsuteru Masuda

Index 655

1

Cosmeceuticals: A Broad-Spectrum Category between Cosmetics and Drugs

Albert M. Kligman
*University of Pennsylvania School of Medicine,
Philadelphia, Pennsylvania, USA*

The Origin of the Cosmeceutical Concept	3
Enter Cosmeceuticals	4
The International Scene	6
Cosmeceuticals: A Diversity of Opinions	7
References	8

I introduced the term "cosmeceuticals" almost 20 years ago at a meeting of the Society of Cosmetic Chemists. I thought this neologism was both timely and useful, as it would reconcile archaic legal statutes with modern science. I defined cosmeceuticals as topical formulations which were neither pure cosmetics, like lipstick or rouge, nor pure drugs, like corticosteroids. They lay between these poles, constituting a broad-spectrum intermediate group. Some were closer to drugs, such as the alpha-hydroxy acids—designed to exfoliate the outer, loose stratum corneum, a structural effect—whereas others were closer to cosmetics, like rouge—designed to give color, a purely decorative effect.

I anticipated endorsement of a concept whose time had come. Instead, the response was immediate disapproval and even outrage. My colleagues in the industry branded me a troublemaker, unfaithful to those who had supported my research. Since then, the cosmeceutical concept has generated a huge amount of controversy. Along the way, the term has acquired political, economic, and legal connotations that are the source of controversy and argumentation to this very day (1).

I did not argue for new laws or regulations, but rather for recognition of a new reality, namely, that skin care science had made such great strides that the simplistic, legal separation of drugs and cosmetics omitted a broad domain between the two, for which a new category was needed for rational discourse (2,3). Despite continuing controversies, the term has permanently entered our vocabulary and debates about its legitimacy, while interesting, are mostly not very illuminating (4,5). The "ceutical" verbiage has unexpectedly encompassed other areas of commercial interest. Cosmeceuticals seem to have a certain semantic resonance, as witnessed by similar sounding neologisms; for example, neutraceuticals (foods with health benefits), neoceuticals (over-the-counter drugs with cosmetic effects), aquaceuticals (marine products with drug and cosmetic effects), and floraceuticals (botanicals with drug and cosmetic effects).

Skin care scientists (I decry the outmoded, misleading term of "cosmetic chemists") have not only made available a tremendous variety of products for the treatment of hair, skin, and nails but have also made impressive contributions to our basic knowledge about the structure and function of skin. Academicians are largely ignorant of the achievements of cosmetic scientists in advancing our fundamental understanding on a broad array of subjects, for example, percutaneous absorption, the anatomical and functional nature of the stratum corneum "barrier", methods for assessing the safety and efficacy of topical agents, noninvasive imaging techniques for visualizing the skin, novel drug delivery systems, many bioengineering techniques to objectively measure the effect of treatments, and other contributions which can properly be called basic science, providing multiple fundamental concepts that are pathways to the development of novel products (6).

The great interest in cosmeceuticals is reflected in the titles of scores of published reports, which now number more than 500 in the last 6 years! There have been several international seminars titled "Cosmeceuticals". These forums are well attended by specialists having widely different backgrounds and interests (regulators, basic scientists, physicians, manufacturers, publishers, merchandisers, lawyers, toxicologists, pharmacologists, and industry watchers).

Some merchandisers have realized the potential for increasing the sale of products that go well beyond the traditional view of cosmetics as being merely decorative. Consumers now want products that contain "active" ingredients and have measurable beneficial effects. Producers recognize this change in the marketplace and have generated a multitude of cosmeceuticals which are praised unashamedly for their ability to bring about beneficial effects that improve the healthiness of skin and keep it in good condition.

Prevention and treatment of some common skin disorders are frankly regarded as desirable goals, for example, dry, itchy skin, photoaged wrinkles, and blotchy skin. In recognition of this bioactive role, alternative terms for cosmeceuticals have sprung up, namely, performance cosmetics, functional cosmetics, dermoceuticals, and active cosmetics. All these imply value added benefits that move traditional cosmetics toward the realm of drugs. The market for cosmeceuticals is outpacing by at least two-fold the sale of traditional, ornamental cosmetics.

The issues regarding the necessity of new regulations for bioactive cosmeceuticals have been soundly discussed by Vermier and Gilchrest in their sensible and scholarly account (7).

Cosmeceuticals are a marketer's playground, which makes it possible to incorporate into skin care products an unlimited number of active substances, derived from a great variety of natural and synthetic sources. The variety of ingredients which have been incorporated in cosmeceuticals is staggering, including vitamins, antioxidants, minerals, herbs, hormones, anti-inflammatories, mood-influencing fragrances (aromatherapy), and even such exotica as placenta, amniotic fluid, *ad infinitum*. The claims for incorporating these "actives" range from the preposterous to the realistic and cover the spectrum from romantic fantasy to credible substantiation. Some formulations contain several dozens of actives, stretching credulity. Responsible manufacturers do not engage in such blatant hucksterism, which can occur because cosmeceuticals have no statutory status and are not regulated by the FDA. Premarketing testing for safety and efficacy are not required.

The popular "natural" and "green" movements, which have widespread political support and can have a substantial economic impact, also have to be considered in the context of marketing realities. For many credulous consumers, "natural is good and synthetic is bad". "Green" projects the image of protecting the environment, sustaining the health of the earth for future generations. The phrases, "not tested on animals" and "cruelty-free" are appealing to the activists of the animal rights movement. Manufacturers are now obliged to cater to these movements even though the underlying concepts are flawed. For example, those who applaud "natural" disregard the fact that heavy metals such as arsenic and lead are natural as are lethal poisons such as botulinus toxin and strychnine. Sunlight too, the scourge of good skin, is natural.

"Not tested on animals" is mainly a marketing ploy. Producers now have to face the prospect of educating consumers who generally have little understanding of the complexities involved in bringing to market the products which they fervently want.

THE ORIGIN OF THE COSMECEUTICAL CONCEPT

In 1938, the US Congress enacted a statute that officially defined cosmetics and drugs in specific terms, setting up formal criteria for classifying a product as either a drug or a cosmetic. No intermediate category was countenanced.

There were two poles and nothing in between. This remains the law to this very day.

The 1938 act came into being as a corrective reaction against the unregulated sale of innumerable patent medicines, some dangerous, which promised cures for all known human ailments. This was the era of the "snake oil" salesman who had a truckload of marvelous remedies bombastically and theatrically promoted. The act defined a cosmetic as an "article intended for beautifying and promoting attractiveness". In contrast, a drug was defined as a substance for use in the diagnosis, cure, treatment, or prevention of disease. However, one qualifying clause was added which is at the core of arguments concerning the legitimacy or necessitation of a third category, lying between drugs and cosmetics. The exact wording was that a "drug was intended to affect the structure and function of skin", implying that agents which had such effects would automatically require reclassification as a drug. It was this particular stricture that engendered the need to create a third category. The unassailable fact is that there are no topical substances which have no effect on the structure and function of skin. Subsequent advances in the science of skin care brought this realization to the fore, now embodied in the idea that cosmetics have genuine functions besides decoration. Many, perhaps most, skin care products contain active agents which can and do modify the anatomy and physiology of skin. However, this new awareness is in conflict with the 1938 act and is the prime source of continuing debates.

It is important also to note that it is not solely the ingredients of a product, but the claims in labeling or advertising that determine whether the substance will be classified as a cosmetic or a drug. Congress declared that the "intended" use would determine a product's classification. Thus, if the intended use relates to the diagnosis and treatment of a disease, the substance is a drug; if its intended use is limited to promoting attractiveness, the substance is a cosmetic. It has now become a high art among marketers to make functional claims which do not invite the attention of the FDA by using wording which avoids the implication that the product is a drug.

ENTER COSMECEUTICALS

When the 1938 law was written, the science of cosmetology was primitive and crude, steeped in folklore, tradition, and anecdotes. The 1938 definition of a drug is now completely archaic. With the great advances in our understanding of skin physiology, it is impossible to think of a single substance that cannot, under some circumstances, alter the structure and function of skin, especially when repeatedly applied, which daily grooming practices ensure. The most compelling example is water, the milieu in which all vital processes occur and which is intuitively deemed innocuous. However, when a water-moistened cotton patch is sealed to human skin for as little as 2 h, the intercellular lipid lamellae of the stratum corneum, which constitute the famous "barrier" are disrupted, increasing permeability (8). Dermatologists make use of this knowledge by applying drugs occlusively to promote their penetration. After 24 h of occlusive water exposure, cytotoxic injury to the viable epidermis occurs, accompanied by inflammatory changes. So water, which is an essential ingredient in formulating emulsions for the topical delivery of drugs, is certainly not inert and may be very useful for enhancing penetration of active substances into skin.

Clinicians have long appreciated that prolonged exposure to water, and not to soaps and detergents as formerly thought, is the cause of chronic hand dermatitis in many bartenders, housewives, canners, and so on. Thus, like many agents water can be beneficial under some circumstances, like in moisturizing emulsions, or harmful when superhydration disrupts the horny layer barrier (9).

Petrolatum is another substance, widely used in a great variety of creams and ointments, also as a vehicle for topical drugs, whose beneficial effects have long been appreciated in many different applications. It is generally thought to be completely inert, serving only to form an occlusive film on the surface, preventing water loss, hence, hydrating and softening the stratum corneum. We now know that petrolatum penetrates into the lipid-rich intercellular spaces of the stratum corneum, enhancing its barrier properties and making the horny layer pliable so that it does not crack when deformed. It actually becomes part of the internal structure of the horny layer, making it more resistant to external chemical, physical, and even mechanical stimuli (10). As an active moisturizer, it is still the gold standard. Studies show that petrolatum promotes healing of wounds and prevents ultraviolet-induced tumors, even though it is not a sunscreen (11). These are clearly medicinal effects that affect the structure and function of skin, yet no reasonable person would want petrolatum to be reclassified as a drug. From these and many other examples, it is apparent that nearly all cosmetic articles would have to be reclassified as drugs, if a strict interpretation of the "structure and function" proviso of the 1938 act was enforced.

The term "cosmeceuticals" recognizes the new realities of skin care products, emphasizing their functional aspects. All agree that we do not need new laws that officially define the category of cosmeceuticals in statutory terms. The FDA has always had the authority to determine from advertising claims whether a cosmetic product has crossed the line and requires reclassification as a drug. When the claims are grossly misleading, the Federal Trade Commission has the legal authority to insist on relabeling or recall.

If bioactive cosmetics were reclassified as drugs, that action would be a disaster of the highest magnitude. It would immediately stifle innovation and creativity. Drug development is slow and costly, requiring premarketing proof of safety and efficacy.

To its credit, the FDA has been flexible in the way in which it has viewed enthusiastic claims, making room for an acceptable degree of puffery. The trouble comes when some cosmetic manufacturers make frank drug claims. In this case, the FDA sends out warning letters that require rewording of the claims, sometimes without necessarily changing any of the ingredients.

Cosmeceuticals enable cosmetic scientists to communicate with each other regarding the standards that must be met to justify performance claims. At the same time, major producers of "active cosmetics" have become more scrupulous in premarketing testing for efficacy and safety.

THE INTERNATIONAL SCENE

There are three great trading blocks: the USA, Europe, and Japan. Obviously, an integrated free trade network cannot work if each block classifies and regulates skin care products differently. Unfortunately, no international consensus currently exists, inevitably sparking disputes and trade practices that may place some producers at disadvantage.

The situation is more complex and far more demanding in Europe. This is evidenced by the European Economic Cosmetic (EEC) Directive of 1993 (12). The requirements for labeling cosmetics are formidable. The information that must be made available to officials encompasses the following: qualitative and quantitative composition of the products, specifications of raw materials, methods of manufacture, safety assessments, and proof of effectiveness. Enforcement of these daunting requirements is more of a goal than a reality. On top of all this, the EEC will soon prohibit the sale of cosmetic ingredients which have been tested on animals, wrong-headedly infusing political ideology into the scientific domain. This misguided effort is based on the premise that alternative methods of assessing toxicity are already in place. Alternative tests are based on *in vitro* assays which are not even close to mimicking real-world *in vivo* situations. Only a very few *in vitro* methods have been validated as substitutes for animal testing. This overly optimistic dependence on nonanimal methods of testing has severe limitations; for example, no *in vitro* procedures are available to predict the induction of allergic contact sensitization, nonimmunologic contact urticaria, and low-level contact irritants. Creativity will fall prey to the ideology of "political correctness", if the bureaucracy seizes complete control of the industry.

Japanese authorities have been more rational in their approach to the regulation of skin care products (13). They concede that most products are neither pure drugs nor pure cosmetics but mixtures of the two. The category called cosmeceuticals is called "quasi-drugs" by the Japanese. They allow cosmetics to include pharmacologically active ingredients, provided that the therapeutic effects are modest and the products have been demonstrated to be safe. Still, the legal wording leaves a lot of room for ambiguities and ad hoc interpretations that some perceive as potential restraints of trade. For example, benzoyl peroxide, a very useful anti-acne OTC medication in the USA is unjustifiably banned in Japan.

Even a cursory look at these regulatory disparities shows the detrimental effects of not agreeing upon uniform, international standards. The following examples illustrate the quandaries which now exist.

In the USA the following agents are regulated as drugs, whereas in Europe they are sold as cosmetics:

1. antiperspirants,
2. antidandruff shampoos, and
3. sunscreens

This classification is detrimental to industry in the USA, especially in the case of the most effective broad-spectrum sunscreens which are sold in drug stores in Europe but are not available in the USA. To obtain FDA approval entails prohibitive costs to ascertain safety, an irrational demand because these superior sunscreens have been safely sold in Europe for a decade. To bring a drug to market now costs about 500 million dollars, a prohibitive sum for manufacturers of active cosmetics. Paradoxes abound in the USA. For example, retinol (vitamin A) can be sold as a cosmetic, but its oxidation product, retinoic acid, is regulated as a drug. Furthermore, claims allowed by the FDA for an approved retinoic acid product (Renova®, Ortho Pharmaceuticals) are purely cosmetic and relate only to improved appearance. However, the product is still only available by prescription!

Then too, theophyllin, a powerful drug with a narrow therapeutic index, is used in the treatment of asthma. Blood levels must be monitored to avoid life-threatening toxicity. Yet, this same agent can be sold as a cosmetic when incorporated into topical formulations for the treatment of cellulite! Manufacturers have been careful to use this ingredient in concentrations that are harmless, but which are also completely useless!

COSMECEUTICALS: A DIVERSITY OF OPINIONS

The writings on this subject cover a remarkable range of divergent and conflicting opinions from all over the globe. Recent papers reflect the beliefs of major players in the field.

Dweck's paper provides the British perspective (14). He begins as follows: "What on earth is a cosmeceutical? Is it an attempt to convince the consumer or is it a genuine category that attempts to provide a mild product that has been more stringently tested than a normal skin care product?" He recommends reading an official medicine leaflet as a guide to deciding what comprises a medicinal product. He concludes that future discussions will be marked by debate.

Wittern takes up the issue from a European perspective (15). He is decidedly not enamored by the term "cosmeceutical". He considers "that the existing legal regulations are precise and clearly distinguish between cosmetic and pharmaceutical efficacy. They do not allow for the introduction of a new class of products such as cosmeceuticals". He recounts that A.M. Kligman introduced the term but did not bother to define it. "Obviously, he didn't know what he was starting". I plead guilty to not foreseeing what controversial storms would follow the introduction of this concept.

The *piece de resistance* of the cosmeceutical imbroglio is the article by Urbach who states (16):

> At the moment, there is hardly a topic in the cosmetic industry as controversial as cosmeceuticals. Cosmeceuticals meet consumer demands for high efficacy. From a consumer and regulatory point of view, having a separate cosmeceutical class is neither helpful, scientifically suitable or juridically necessary. The cosmeceutical concept is superfluous. The most sensible and useful service we can give the consumer legislator and manufacturer is to advise against the further use of this term.

Steinberg presents the American perspective (17). He endorses the term and thinks its introduction has made it necessary to reconsider the statutory definition of a drug and a cosmetic and to seek international agreements on the kinds of regulatory actions that might be enacted.

Cosmeceuticals, regardless of casuistic controversies by over-wrought partisans, are here to stay. The reason is obvious. The term has heuristic value. It serves a useful function in recognition of the cosmetic industries' laudable achievements in bringing to the marketplace a great assay of skin, hair, and nail products which improve the quality of life!

REFERENCES

1. Hutt Deter Barton. The legal distinction in the United States between a cosmetic and a drug. In: Elsner P, Maibach H, eds. Cosmeceuticals: Drugs and Cosmetics. New York, NY: Marcel Dekker, 2000:223–227.
2. Kligman AM. Why cosmeceuticals? Cosmetics Toiletries 1993; 108:37–40.
3. Kligman AM. Cosmeceuticals as a third category. Cosmetics Toiletries 1995; 113:33–38.
4. Lavrijsen ADM, Vermier BJ. Cosmetics and drugs: Is there a need for a third group, cosmeceuticals? Br J Dermatol 1991; 124:503–504.
5. Lubell A. Cosmecuticals: A new breed of cosmetic products. Cosmetic Dermatol 1993; 6:10–11.
6. Gans EH. Cosmeceuticals. Skin Pharmacol 1990; 3:54–57.
7. Vermier BJ, Gilchrest BA. Cosmeceuticals. A proposal for rational definition, evaluation and regulation. Arch Dermatol 1996; 132:337.
8. Warner RR, Boessy YL. Effect of moisturizing products on the structure of lipids in human stratum corneum. In: Maibach H, Loden M, eds. Dry Skin and Moisturizers. Boca Raton, FL: CRC Press, 2000:351–371.
9. Kligman AM. Hydration injury to human skin. In: van der Valk PGM, Maibach H, eds. The Irritant Contact Dermatitis Syndrome, Boca Raton, FL: CRC Press, 1991:187–194.
10. Grubauer G, Feingold KR, Elias PM. Relationship of epidermal lipogenetics to cutaneous barrier function. J Lipid Res 1987; 8:746–752.
11. Kligman LH, Kligman AM. Petrolatum and other hydrophobic emollients reduce UV-induced damage. J Dermatol Treatment 1992; 3:3–9.

12. Rogiers V. Efficacy claims of cosmetics in Europe must be scientifically substantiated from 1997 on. Skin Res Technol 1995; 1:44–50.
13. Takamatsu T. How can we define cosmeceuticals? Advanced Technology Conference Proceedings. Cosmetics Toiletries 1996; 26:30–34.
14. Dwek AC. The definition of a cosmeceutical. Advanced Technology Conference Proceedings. Cosmetics Toiletries 1996; 26:21–24.
15. Wittern P. Cosmeceuticals from a European perspective. Advanced Technology Conference Proceedings. Cosmetics Toiletries 1996; 26:24–28.
16. Urbach W. Cosmeceuticals. The future of cosmetics. Cosmetics Toiletries 1995; 110:33–37.
17. Steinberg D. An American perspective. Advanced Technology Conference Proceedings. Cosmetics Toiletries 1996; 26:26–29.

2

Definition

Bert Jan Vermeer
Leiden University Medical Center, Leiden, The Netherlands

References   13

New insights about the function of the skin, as well as the development of new products for skin care, make it necessary to question or redefine the definitions of cosmetics and drugs. Moreover, in the USA, Europe, and Japan, different definitions of cosmetics are used. The definition of a drug is more or less equivocal in these countries. According to the Food, Drug, and Cosmetic (FDC) Act, a drug is defined as an article intended for use in the diagnosis, mitigation, treatment, or prevention of disease or intended to affect the structure or any function of the body.

In the USA, according to the FDC act of 1938, a cosmetic is defined as an article intended to be rubbed, poured, sprinkled, or sprayed on, introduced into, or otherwise applied to the human body or any part thereof for cleansing, beautifying, promoting attractiveness, or altering the appearance without affecting structure or function (1). It is noteworthy that in this definition the cosmetic is not allowed to have any activity (i.e., without affecting structure or function). In Europe, the definition of a cosmetic was reevaluated and described by the council directive 93/35/EEC of June 14, 1993 (2). The cosmetics directive contains 15 articles. The definition of a cosmetic is described in article 1 and is as follows:

A "cosmetic product" shall mean any substance or preparation intended to be placed in contact with the various external parts of the human body epidermis, hair system, nails, lips and external genital organs or with the teeth and the mucous membranes of the oral cavity with a view exclusively or mainly to cleaning them, perfuming them, changing their appearance and/or correcting body odours and/or protecting them or keeping them in good condition.

The other 15 articles describe the following topics: overall safety requirements, controlled substances, potential ban of animal testing, inventory of ingredients, labeling, harmonization, product information requirement, procedure for adaptation, list of permitted ingredients, safeguard clause, and implementation.

According to the pharmaceutical affairs law, the Japanese definition of a cosmetic is as follows:

The term cosmetic means any article intended to be used by means of rubbing, sprinkling or by similar application to the human body for cleansing, beautifying, promoting attractiveness and altering appearance of the human body, and for keeping the skin and hair healthy, provided that the action of the article on the human body is mild.

The Japanese definition is only slightly different from the definition of a cosmetic within Europe. Both definitions allow a cosmetic to have mild activity and possess pharmaceutical activity. This is in sharp contrast to the definition of a cosmetic in the USA.

Moreover, in Article 7a of the European cosmetics directive, which describes the product information requirement, it is stated that a proof of effect should be included (2). In the USA, however, a product would be regarded as a drug if a proof of effect was mentioned.

Extensive research on the physiological activity of the skin has provided evidence that even small changes in the environment can modify the activity of skin tissue (3,4). Application of inert creams (5), humidity, UV light (4), water (6), and so on, all influence the activity of the skin and therefore possess pharmaceutical activity that may affect structure or function of the skin. Thus even water or the humidity of the air could be defined as a drug, according to the FDC act! As mentioned by Vermeer and Gilchrest (7), the Food and Drug Administration asked them to define water as a drug, when water was applied on the skin under experimental conditions.

Registration of a product as a drug requires many elaborate and costly procedures; therefore, the manufacturer of a product with pharmaceutical activity would prefer to have the product registered as a cosmetic. This might mean that the pharmaceutical activity of the product is not mentioned and/or investigated, and, as a result of these confusing and old-fashioned regulatory rules, important information is not given to the public.

The introduction of the term "cosmeceutical" enables us to classify more precisely a product with an activity that is *intended* to treat or prevent a (mild) skin (abnormality). In order to avoid introducing new definition criteria, we

Table 1 Cosmeceuticals as a Subclass of Cosmetics (Europe and Japan) and as a Subclass of Drugs (USA)

	Cosmetic	Cosmeceutical	Drug
Pharmaceutical activity	+	+	+
Intended effect in skin disease	−	(+)	+
Intended effect in mild skin disorder	−	+	(+)
Side effects	−	(±)	+

suggest that cosmeceuticals are only regarded as a subclass within the domain of a cosmetic or drug. In Europe and Japan, cosmeceuticals can be regarded as a subclass of cosmetics; however, in the USA, cosmeceuticals can only be regarded as a subclass of drugs. Cosmeceuticals could be characterized as follows: (i) the product has pharmaceutical activity and can be used on normal or near-normal skin; (ii) the product should have a defined benefit for minor skin disorders (cosmetic indication); and (iii) as the skin disorder is mild the product should have a very low-risk profile (see Table 1). The definition of minor skin disorders or mild skin abnormalities is difficult and can be regarded as cosmetic indications. Even socioeconomic factors may have an impact on whether a skin disorder is regarded as a disease or as a cosmetic indication (8,9). Nevertheless, in most western countries there is no written consensus that skin abnormalities that are treated by over-the-counter drugs may be regarded as mild skin disorders or may be termed cosmetic indications (9,10).

The procedure for registration of a cosmeceutical should not be as cumbersome as for drugs. The intended activity of the cosmeceutical for treatment of a minor skin disorder should be demonstrated by clinical studies within the framework of good clinical practice. Moreover, it should be shown that safety requirements are optimal and that no side effects can be expected (11). The safety evaluation is mandatory for cosmetics in Europe, according to articles 2, 12, and 13.

In the USA, this would mean that a subclass of drugs (cosmeceuticals) are registered in a similar manner as over-the-counter products (12). It would be beneficial if these countries could agree on the definitions of cosmetics and drugs and, in so doing, define cosmeceuticals as a subclass of cosmetics. This would prevent the current situation in which certain products are registered as drugs in the USA (sunscreens) and as cosmetics or cosmeceuticals in Europe and Japan.

REFERENCES

1. 21 USC Sections 301–393.
2. Council directive 78/768 EEC of July 27, 1976. Official Journal of the European Communities no. L 151 dated June 23, 1993.

3. Lundström A, Egelrud T. Evidence that cell shedding from plantar stratum corneum in vitro involves endogenous proteolysis of desmosomal protein desmogein. J Invest Dermatol 1990; 94:216–220.
4. Noonan FP, De Fabo EC. Immunosuppression by ultraviolet B radiation, initiation by urocanic acid. Immunol Today 1992; 7:250–254.
5. Mertz PM, Davis SC, Ovington LG. Cosmeceuticals: predicting their influence on compromised skin. Cosmet Toilet 1992; 107:43–44.
6. Harris JR, Farrel AM, Grunfeld C, Holleram WM, Elias PM, Feingold KR. Permeability barrier disruption coordinately regulates RNA levels for key enzymes or cholesterol, fatty acid and ceramide synthesis in the epidermis. J Invest Dermatol 1997; 109:783–788.
7. Vermeer BJ, Gilchrest BA. Cosmeceuticals. Arch Dermatol 1996; 132:337–340.
8. O'Donoughue MN. Sunscreen: the ultimate cosmetic. Dermatol Clin 1991; 9:99–104.
9. Neher JO. Cosmetics by prescription. J Fam Pract 1989; 29:534–536.
10. Nightingale SL. FDA proposes new labeling for over-the-counter sunscreen products. J Am Med Assoc 1992; 270–302.
11. Stern RS. Drug promotion for an unlabeled indication: the case of topical tretinoin. N Engl J Med 1994; 331:1348–1349.
12. De Salva SJ. Safety evaluation of over-the-counter products. Regul Toxicol Pharmacol 1985; 5:101–108.

Classes

3

Amino Acids and Derivatives

Kazutami Sakamoto
Ajinomoto Co., Inc., Chuo-ku, Tokyo, Japan

Introduction	17
Amino Acids: Basic Features	18
Existence and Roles of Amino Acids in the Skin	18
Harmonized Integrity of Skin Function with Amino Acids	30
Effective Amino Acid Delivery into Skin	30
Amino Acid Derivatives for Extended Applications	31
Conclusion	34
References	34

INTRODUCTION

Amino acids are molecules with both an amino group and a carboxylic group. There are 20 kinds of naturally occurring amino acids with optically active structures at α-position (L-amino acids) except glycine (Gly). In their preface of *Chemistry of the Amino Acids* in 1961, Greenstein and Winitz said, "Few products of natural origin are versatile in their behavior and properties as are the amino acids, and few have such a variety of biological duties to perform" (1). Subsequently, significant progress has been made on the knowledge of amino acids, and technical achievements to utilize such progress are remarkable, including cosmetic and cosmeceutical applications. This is because of the market growth and cost reduction of certain amino acids for many industrial applications. For example, in food applications there is a huge and still growing consumption generated for glutamic acid (Glu) and Gly as food additives and aspartic acid (Asp) and phenylalanine (Phe) as raw materials of the artificial sweetener aspartame. Consumption of lysine (Lys), methionine (Met), and threonine (Thr) is expanding for the animal food additives market. Cysteine (CysH) and proline (Pro) are major amino acids utilized in the flavor industry to manufacture natural flavors by the Milliard reaction with sugars. Health food and pharmaceutical intermediates are other rapidly growing markets for many amino acids. In this chapter, the role of amino acids and their derivatives are reviewed as functional molecules for cosmeceutical applications.

AMINO ACIDS: BASIC FEATURES

According to Greenstein and Winitz, "Amino acids are at once water soluble and amphoteric electrolytes, with the ability to form acid salts and basic salts and thus act as buffers over at least two range of pH; dipolar ions of high electric moment with a considerable capacity to increase the dielectric constant of the medium in which they are dissolved; compounds with reactive groups capable of a wide range of chemical alterations leading readily to a great variety of degradation, synthetic, and transformation products such as esters, amides, amines, polymers and etc" (1). Such general features of amino acids are summarized in the tables as follows (2): solubility in water in Table 1, solubility in aqueous alcohol in Table 2, dissociation constants and isoelectric points in Table 3, optical rotations in Table 4, reactivity in Tables 5 and 6, and acute oral toxicity in Table 7. These properties of amino acids have become practical importance for cosmetic applications in recent decades. Other forces driving the increasing use of amino acids for cosmetic preparations are consumer's growing concerns of the environmental and health impacts of the traditional chemical substances, and in this regard amino acids are environmentally friendly and sustainable resources. Typical examples include application of arginine (Arg) as an alternative base to triethanolamine and Glu as an alternative acid to hydrochloric acid as neutralizers.

Actual results are greater than expected. For example, soap neutralized with Arg not only displayed better biodegradability and mildness as expected but also provided weakly alkalic mild soap formulations and moist after-feeling to lessen the tightness of regular soap, while preserving superior lathering properties (3). Arg is widely used to neutralize polyacryrate polymers too, which results in weakly acidic gels that adapt to skin pH. These gels further show improved treatment effect as hair conditioners to give enhanced smoothness (4).

Existence and Roles of Amino Acids in the Skin

As building blocks of proteins, amino acids are supplied mainly through blood circulation to the living cells. Skin has integrated structures consisting of stratum

Table 1 Solubility of Amino Acid in Water (g/100 g H_2O)

Amino acid	0°C	10°C	20°C	25°C	30°C	40°C	50°C	60°C	70°C	75°C	80°C	90°C	100°C
L-Alanine	12.73	14.17	15.78	16.51	17.68	19.57	21.79	24.26	27.02	28.51	30.08	33.50	37.30
DL-Alanine	12.11	13.77	16.02	16.72	17.83	20.29	23.09	26.27	29.90	31.89	34.01	38.70	44.04
L-Arginine	8.3		14.8				40.0						174.1
L-Asparagine · H_2O	0.86	1.43	2.36	3.00	3.78	5.94	9.12	13.68	20.09	24.1	28.77	40.32	55.21
L-Aspartic acid	0.21	0.30	0.42	0.50	0.60	0.85	1.20	1.70	2.41	2.88	3.43	4.88	6.89
DL-Aspartic acid	0.26	0.41	0.63	0.78	0.95	1.39	2.00	2.81	3.84	4.46	5.14	6.73	8.59
L-Cystine	0.0050	0.0069	0.0094	0.011	0.013	0.018	0.024	0.033	0.045	0.052	0.061	0.084	0.114
DL-Cystine	0.0016	0.0021	0.0030	0.0049	0.0049	0.0076	0.0104						
L-Glutamic acid	0.34	0.50	0.72	0.84	1.04	1.51	2.19	3.17	4.59	5.53	6.66	9.66	14.0
DL-Glutamic acid	0.86	1.21	1.72	2.05	2.45	3.48	4.93	7.01	9.95	11.86	14.13	20.05	28.49
L-Glutamic acid · HCl	31.5						52.0						81.0
L-Glumatic acid · Na · H_2O	64.1			74.22			91.57						172.0
L-Glutamine			3.25(18°C)	4.25	4.8								
Glycine	14.18	18.04	22.52	24.99	27.59	33.16	39.10	45.26	51.39	54.89	57.29	62.53	67.17
L-Histidine	2.3			4.29		6.4							42.8
L-Histidine · HCl · H_2O	29.1			39.0			50.1						93.5
L-Hydroxyproline	28.96	31.56	34.52	36.11	37.76	41.39	45.18	49.41	54.04		59.10	64.64	70.70
L-Isoleucine	3.79	3.88	4.03	4.12	4.22	4.48	4.82	5.24	5.77	6.08	6.40	7.21	8.22
DL-Isoleucine	1.83	1.95	2.12	2.23	2.35	2.65	3.03	3.54	4.20	4.61	5.08	6.24	7.80
L-Leucine	2.27	2.30	2.37	2.19	2.49	2.66	2.89	3.19	3.58	3.82	4.10	4.78	5.64
DL-Leucine	0.80	0.86	0.94	0.99	1.05	1.20	1.41	1.68	2.05	2.28	2.55	3.24	4.21
L-Lysine · HCl	53.6			40**			111.5		142.8				
L-Methionine	3.0				5.6		7.4						
DL-Methionine	1.82	2.34	3.00	3.35	3.81	4.82	6.07	7.55	9.45	10.52	11.72	14.39	17.60
L-Phenylalanine	1.98	2.33	2.74	2.97	3.21	3.77	4.48	5.20	6.11	6.62	7.18	8.43	9.90
DL-Phenylalanine	11.	1.13	1.31	1.41	1.53	1.82	2.19	2.67	3.31	3.71	4.17	5.32	6.88
L-Proline	127.2	140.3	154.6	162.3	170.3	187.6	206.7	227.7	250.9		276.4	304.4	335.4

(*continued*)

Table 1 Continued

Amino acid	0°C	10°C	20°C	25°C	30°C	40°C	50°C	60°C	70°C	75°C	80°C	90°C	100°C
L-Serine	2.20	3.10	38.0	5.02	5.85	60.5	10.34	83.0					
DL-Serine			4.30			7.84		13.41	17.11	19.21	21.48	26.53	32.24
L-Threonine		36 (14°C)			10.6		14.1(52°C)	19.0(61°C)					
DL-Threonine				20.5							55.0		
L-Tryptophan	0.82	0.93	1.06	1.14	1.22	1.44	1.71	2.06	2.51	2.80	3.12	3.92	4.99
DL-Tryptophan					0.25								
L-Tyrosine	0.020	0.027	0.038	0.045	0.054	0.075	0.105	0.15	0.21	0.24	0.29	0.40	0.57
DL-Tyrosine	0.015	0.021	0.029	0.035	0.042	0.064	0.084	0.13	0.17		0.24	0.34	0.48
L-Valine	8.34			8.85			9.62	10.24(65°C)					
DL-Valine	5.96	6.39	6.81	7.09	7.42	8.17	9.11	10.28	11.74	12.61	13.58	15.89	18.81

**w/v

Source: Greenstein, Winitzz. Chemistry of Amino Acids. Vol. 1. New York: John Wiley, 1961:564; Dunn, Lookland. Advances in Protein Chemistry. Vol. 1, III, New York: Academic Press, 1947:37; Akabori, Mizushima. Protein Chemistry. Vol. 1. Kyouritu: 1969:272; The Merck Index. 11th ed. New Jersey: Merck & Co., Inc., 1989.

Table 2 Solubility of Amino Acid in Aqueous Alcohol Solution (mol/L at 25°C)

Amino acid	0	5	10	15	20	40	50	60	70	80	90	95	100
DL-Alanine	1.660	1.160	1.250		0.877	0.402		0.158		0.0359	0.00794		0.00076
L-Arginine	0.350(20°C)												
L-Asparagine	0.186				0.0750	0.0306		0.0105					0.000023
L-Aspartic acid	0.0375				0.0749	0.00575	0.00441	0.00264	0.00149	0.00070	0.00021		0.0000116
L-Cystine	0.0005												
L-Glutamic acid	0.0585												0.0000185
L-Glutamine	0.291												0.0000315
Glycine	2.886	2.156	2.041	1.670	1.343	0.507		0.157		0.0218	0.00556		0.00039
L-Histidine	0.270												
L-Isoleucine	0.314									0.0305(20°C)			0.00534(20°C)
L-Leucine	0.171				0.0977	0.0320		0.0441		0.0204	0.00770		0.00123
DL-Leucine	0.0744	0.0661	0.0575	0.0494	0.0423	0.0264		0.0186		0.00848			
L-Lycine · HCl												0.00547	
DL-Methionine	0.1218												
L-Phenylalanine	0.1792												
D-Phenylalanine	0.1705(16°C)												
L-Proline	1.4071												5.78(19°C)
DL-Serine	0.4780												
DL-Threonine													0.00588
L-Tryptophan	0.0558												
DL-Tyrosine	0.0025												
L-Tyrosine	0.0025												
L-Valine	0.706	0.506	0.444	0.382	0.409	0.231		0.123		0.0373	0.00922		
DL-Valine	0.571				0.318	0.187		0.086		0.0280			0.00123

Source: Cohn EJ, McMeekin TL, Edsall JT, Weare JH. J Am Chem Soc 1934; 56:2270; McMeekin TL, Cohn EJ, Weare JH. J Am Chem Soc 1935; 57:626; McMeekin TL, Cohn EJ, Weare JH. J Am Chem Soc 1936; 58:2173; The Merck Index. 11th ed. New Jersey: Merck & Co., Inc., 1989.

Table 3 Dissociation Constant (pK) and Isoelectric Point (pI) of Amino Acid

Amino acid	pK_1	pK_2	pK_3	pK_4	pI
Ala	2.34	9.69			6.00
Arg	1.82	8.89	12.48		10.76
Asn	2.02	8.80			5.41
Asp	1.88	3.65	9.60		2.77
CysH	1.92	8.35	10.46		5.07
Cys	<1.00	2.1	8.02	8.71	4.60
Glu	2.19	4.25	9.67		3.22
Gln	2.17	9.13			5.65
Gly	2.35	9.78			5.97
His	1.78	5.97	8.97		7.59
Hyp	1.82	9.66			5.83
Ile	2.36	9.68			6.02
Leu	2.36 (DL)	9.60 (DL)			5.98
Lys	2.20	8.90	10.28		9.74
Met	2.13 (DL)	9.28 (DL)			5.74
Phe	2.16	9.18			5.48
Pro	1.95	10.64			6.30
Ser	2.19	9.21			5.68
Thr	2.15	9.12			6.16
Trp	2.38	9.39			5.89
Tyr	2.20	9.11	10.07		5.66
Val	2.32	9.62			5.96

Source: Kagaku-binran (Chemical Handbook). Basic Data by Chem Soc Jpn, Vol. 1. 4th ed, Maruzen, 1993.

corneum (SC), epidermis, and dermis, consecutively in order from outside to inside of the body. The epidermis and dermis are the organs based on the structured cells where blood capillaries exist only in the dermis. Thus amino acids as nutrients are supplied by blood flow to fibroblast cells in the dermis, then to keratinocyte, melanocyte, and other cells in the epidermis through intercellular liquid channels. SC consists of corneocyte, dead and cornified cell, and intercellular lipid bilayers between corneocytes. Every corneocyte is interconnected with cholesterol sulfate and desmosome protein (5).

In the SC there are materials called natural moisturizing factors (NMF) that control hydration, which consequently is an important function of the SC. Amino acids and pyrrolidone carboxylic acid (PCA) are the major constituents of NMF, which are the end metabolite from filaggrin digested by enzyme in the lower part of the SC (5,6). This is confirmed by the fact that amino acid compositions between NMF and filaggrin are identical (6). Note that each major amino acid in the NMF has a unique property corresponding to the elemental functions of the SC. PCA, composed of Glu, is the most abundant protein metabolite in NMF and has a high moisturizing effect (7).

Table 4 Optical Rotation

Amino acid			Optical rotation (JP[a], JPC[b], EP[c], DAB[d], USP[e])				Merck Index[f]			
			$[\alpha]_D$ (°)	c	Solvent	t (°C)	$[\alpha]_D$ (°)	c	Solvent	t (°C)
Ala	L-		+13.5 to +15.5[a,b,c,d]	10	6 NHCl	20	+2.8	6	H_2O	25
		HCl	+13.7 to +15.1[e]	10	6 NHCl	25				
Arg	L-		+25.5 to +28.5[c,d]	8	25%HCl	20	+8.5	9.3		26
			+26.3 to +27.7[e]	8	6 NHCl	25	+26.9	1.65	6 NHCl	20
		HCl	+21.0 to +23.5[c,d]	8	25%HCl	20	+12.5	3.5	H_2O	20
			+21.4 to +23.6[e]	8	6 NHCl	20	+11.8	0.87	0.5 NNaOH	20
							+12.0	4		20
Asn	L-,	H_2O	+33.7 to +36.0[d]	10	11%HCl	20	+21.9	12	dilHCl	20
							−5.42	1.3		20
							+20.	1mol	1 MHCl	20
							−9.3	1mol	1MNaOH	20
							+5.41	1.3		20
	D-									
Asp	L-		+24.0 to +26.0[b,c,d]	8	25%HCl	20	+25.0	1.97	6 NHCl	20
	D-						−23.0	2.30	6 NHCl	27
CysH	L-		+8.0 to +9.5[d]	12	7%HCl	20	+6.5		5 NHCl	25
		HCl					+13.0			25
							+10.0			25
		HClH_2O	+5.5 to +7.0[c,d]	8	25%HCl	20	+5.0		5 NHCl	25
			+5.7 to +6.8[e]	8	6 NHCl	25				

(*continued*)

Table 4 Continued

Amino acid			Optical rotation (JP[a], JPC[b], EP[c], DAB[d], USP[e])				Merck Index[f]			
			$[\alpha]_D$ (°)	c	Solvent	t (°C)	$[\alpha]_D$ (°)	c	Solvent	t (°C)
Cys	L-		+215 to −230[b]	2	1 NHCl	20	−223.4		1 NHCl	20
Glu	L-		+31.5 to +32.5[b,c,d]	10	2 NHCl	20	+31.4		6 NHCl	22.4
	L-	HCl	+25.2 to +25.8[d]	10	7%HCl	20	+22.4	6		22
	D-						−30.5	1.00	6 NHCl	20
Gln	L-		+6.8 to +7.3[b]	4	H$_2$O	20	+6.1	3.6		23
	L-		+31.5 to +33.0[d]	10	7%HCl	20				
His	L-		+11.8 to +12.8[b,c,d]	11	6 NHCl	20	−39.74	1.13		20
			+12.6 to +14.0[e]	11	6 NHCl	25				
		HCl					+8.0	2	3 MHCl	26
		2HCl	+8.5 to +10.0[b]	11	6 NHCl	20	+47.6	2		20
		HClH$_2$O	+9.2 to +10.6[c,d]	11	25%HCl	20				
Hyp	L-						−76.5	2.5	H$_2$O	–
	cis						−58.1	5.2	H$_2$O	18
Ile	L-		+39.5 to +41.5[a]	4	6 NHCl	20	+11.29	3		20
			+39.0 to +42.0[c,d]	4	25%HCl	20				
			+38.9 to +41.8[e]	4	6 NHCl	25				
Leu	L-		+14.5 to +16.0[a]	4	6 NHCl	20	+40.61	4.6	6.1 NHCl	20
			+14.5 to +16.5[c,d]	4	25%HCl	20	+11.09	3.3	0.33 NNaOH	20
			+14.9 to +17.3[e]	4	6 NHCl	25	−10.8	2.2		25
							+15.1		6 NHCl	26
							+7.6		3 NNaOH	20

Amino Acids and Derivatives

			[α] range	c	solvent	T (°C)	[α]	c	solvent	T (°C)
Lys	L-	HCl	+19.0 to +21.6	8	6 NHCl	20	+14.6	6.5	6.0 NHCl	20
			+21.0 to 22.5[c,d]	8	25%HCl	20	+25.9	2	6.0 NHCl	23
			+20.4 to +21.4[e]	8	6 NHCl	25	+14.6	2	0.6 NHCl	25
		2HCl								
Met	L-		+21.0 to +25.0[a]	2	6 NHCl	20	+15.3	2		20
			+22.5 to +24.0[d]	2	22%HCl	20	−8.2			25
			+21.9 to +24.1[e]	2	6 NHCl	25				
Phe	L-		−33.0 to −35.5[a,c,d]	2	H$_2$O	20	−35.1	1.94		20
			−32.7 to −34.7[e]	2	H$_2$O	25				
	D-						+35.0	2.04		20
Pro	L-		−84.0 to −86.0[b,c,d]	4	H$_2$O	20	+7.1	3.8	18%HCl	20
			−84.3 to −86.3[e]	4	H$_2$O	25	−85.0			23.4
Ser	L-		+13.5 to +16.0[b]	10	2 NHCl	20	−52.6	0.58	0.5 NHCl	20
			+14.0 to +16.0[c,d]	10	7%HCl	20	−93.0	2.4	0.6 NKOH	20
			+14.0 to +15.6[e]	10	2 NHCl	25	−6.83	15g in	15g aq.soln	20
Thr	L-		−26.0 to −29.0[a]	6	H$_2$O	20	+14.45	0.5g in	5.6 NHCl	25
			−27.6 to −29.0[d]	6	H$_2$O	20	−28.3	1.1		26
			−26.7 to −29.1[e]	6	H$_2$O	25				
Trp	L-		−30.0 to −33.0[a,d]	1	H$_2$O	20	−31.5	1		23
			−29.4 to −32.8[e]	1	H$_2$O	25				
							+2.4		0.5 NHCl	20

(continued)

Table 4 Continued

Amino acid		Optical rotation (JP[a], JPC[b], EP[c], DAB[d], USP[e])				Merck Index[f]			
		$[\alpha]_D$ (°)	c	Solvent	t (°C)	$[\alpha]_D$ (°)	c	Solvent	t (°C)
Tyr	L-	−10.5 to −12.5[b]	5	1 NHCl	20	+0.15	2.43	0.5 NNaOH	20
		−11.0 to −12.3[d]	5	7%HCl	20	−10.6	4	1 NHCl	22
		−9.8 to −11.2[e]	5	1 NHCl	25				
	D-					−13.2	4	3 NNaOH	18
Val	L-	+26.5 to +29.0[a,c,d]	8	6 NHCl	20	+10.3	4	1 NHCl	25
		+26.6 to +28.8[e]	8	6 NHCl	25	+13.9	0.9		26
						+22.9	0.8	20%HCl	23

[a]JP: Japanese Pharmacopoeia 12th Rev. Amend. 1&2;
[b]JPC: Japanese Pharmacopoeia(1993);
[c]EP: European Pharmacopoeia 2nd Ed.;
[d]DAB: German Pharmacopoeia 10th Ed;
[e]USP: United States Pharmacopoeia 23rd Ed;
[f]Merck Index 11th Ed. (1989).

Table 5 General Reactivity and Flavor Characteristics of Milliard Reaction Product by Heating at 150°C with Glucose

Amino acid	Reactivity	Flavor characteristics (heating at 180°C with glucose)
Ala	—	Caramel-like
Arg	Hydrolyzed by heat or alkali to convert to citroline or Orn	Burned sugar
Asn	Hydrolyzed by acid or alkali to convert to Asp	
Asp	—	Caramel-like
CysH	Chemicaly unstable, trace amount of heavy metal (Fe, Cu, etc.) accelarates oxidation; air oxidation occurs under neutral or alkalic aqueous conditions to convert to Cys	
Cys	Decomposes by heat or alkali in aqueous solution	Sulfur
Glu	Dehydrates to PCA over 160°C	Burned sugar
Gln	Hydrolyzed by acid, alkali, or hot water to convert to Glu then cyclilized to PCA	Butter
Gly	Heating with glucose produces formaldehyde	Caramel-like
His	—	Corn, bread
Ile	Heating with glucose produces 2-methyl-butanal	Burned cheese
Leu	Heating with glucose produces isovaleric acid	Burned cheese
Lys	Becomes di-hyrdate over 60%RH; heat with acid or alkali causes racemization	Bread
Met	Heat with strong acid causes demethylation; identical biological activity for L and D isomers	Potato
Phe	Decomposes under alkalic condition to produce benzaldehyde; heating with glucose produce α-toluic acid	Violet, lilac, saffron
Pro	Heating with glucose produces acetaldehyde	Bread
Ser	Racemization at pH 9, decomposes by hot alkalic condition, heating with glucose produces glycolic acid	Caramel-like
Thr	Decomposes by heat or alkali in aqueous solution; heating with glucose produces lactic acid	Burned fume
Trp	Decomposes by heating with strong alkali; long exposure to light causes colorization	
Tyr	—	Caramel-like
Val	Heating with glucose produces isolactic acid	Chocolate

Table 6 Sensitivity to Decomposition under Each Condition

Amino acid	Ala	Arg	Asn	Asp	CysH	Cys	Glu	Gln	Gly	His	Ile	Leu	Lys	Met	Phe	Pro	Ser	Thr	Trp	Tyr	Val
Sensitive to																					
Heat																					
Boil			X					X													
Broil (dry heating)		X	X	X	X	X	X	X		X			X	X			X	X	X		X
pH																					
Acidic			X		X			X					X				X	X	X		
Alkalic		X	X		X	X		X					X								
Oxidation																					
In air																					
With oxidant					X	X								X					X	X	
Photosensitive dye										X				X					X	X	
Peroxidized lipid	X				X					X			X	X					X	X	
Maillard reaction with sugar	X												X						X		

Note: X, amino acid sensitive to decomposition under each condition.

Table 7 Acute Oral Toxicity (LD_{50}) (g/kg rat body weight)

Amino acid	LD_w
L-Ala	>16
L-Arg	≃16
L-Asn	>16
L-Asp	>16
L-CySH · HCl · H$_2$O	3.0 (2.7 ~ 3.6)
L-Cys	11.2 (9.0 ~ 14.0)
L-Gln	>15
Gly	≃16
L-His	>16
L-Hyp	>16
L-Ile	>16
L-Leu	>16
L-Lys · HCl	10.9 (9.5 ~ 11.0)
L-Met	>16
L-Phe	≃16
L-Pro	>16
L-Ser	14.0 (12.5 ~ 15.3)
L-Thr	>16
L-Trp	>16
L-Tyr	>16
L-Val	>16
	2.75*
L-Glu · Na	>19.9**

Note: >16, greater than 16; =16, in the region of 16; 3.1 (2.7 ~ 3.6), 3.1 (95% confidence limit 2.7 ~ 3.6); Acute oral toxicity to rat of twenty-five amino acids/Huntingdon Research Center, 1971.
Source: *Merck Index 11th ed. (1989);
**Finchemical & Intermediates Vol. 1. CMC pub. 1990.

Arg is second to PCA when combined with its metabolite ornithine (Orn) and citroline (Cit). Arg is a water-soluble basic amino acid; its roles in the skin have been extensively investigated in the past decade (8,9). Skin suppleness depends on the hydration and elasticity of keratin fibers in the corneocyte. Arg stimulates aggregation of keratin filament to make organized and elastic structures in the SC (9).

Pro has unique characteristics: it is highly soluble in water and at the same time soluble in alcohol (2). Pro has the highest water holding capacity among other amino acids under dry conditions. Synergistic hygroscopicity was found for Pro when combined with PCA, which supports the rationale for their abundant coexistence in NMF (10). Urocanic acid (UA) is an end metabolite of histidine (His); its role has been unveiled recently as an immune regulator rather than an ultraviolet (UV) absorber, which it was long considered to be (11,12). UV exposure converts trans UA to cis isomer, which has an immune suppressing effect. All these functions are interconnected and controlled under homeostatic regulation (13).

Harmonized Integrity of Skin Function with Amino Acids

As explained earlier, NMF are a metabolite of filaggrin; their production requires an optimally moisturized enzymatic condition at the lower part of the SC (5). Similarly, enzymatic decomposition of desmosome for the exfoliation of corneocyte depends on the moisture content in the upper part of the SC (5,14). Brouwstra et al. (15) showed that water distributions in the SC layers are not a simple gradient, high at the stratum granulosum (SG) border and declining toward outside of the SC; instead, by careful examination through TEM and NIR they found the highest water content at the middle of SC layers. By advanced NIR measurement and analysis, Lucassen (16) found similar water distribution along with molecular distribution attributed to the amino acids. Ino et al. (17) also observed incremental amino acid existence for the tape-stripped SC up to mid-SC layers (17). As Rawlings et al. (5) precisely explained, structures of SC and distribution of key constituents that make SC functions are not uniform from the bottom to the top of the SC layers. At the bottom of the SC, bordering SG (living cells with full hydration), enzymes are activated by suitable water content to produce NMF and cellamide. The middle of the SC layers are fully functioning in their structure and constituents, with highest barrier capacity and flexible physical strength (5). Scott et al. (13) explained pH distribution in the SC by similar integration of functions.

These facts indicate that the existence and amount of NMF in the SC are the cause and result of skin condition. Changes in the skin amino acid contents and composition in the SC of aged dry skin (senile xerosis), disordered skin in atopic dermatitis, or chemically induced dry skin are the actual evidence of this assumption (18,19). Furthermore, we found decreased hydration and barrier function in subjects suffering seasonal respiratory allergic reactions but with no obvious signs or changes in the skin conditions. Fairly good correlations between skin hydration and level of amino acid contents in the SC were found for these patients (20). In each case, lack of sufficient NMF caused loss of skin hydration and even suggested that analysis of skin amino acids can be a useful diagnostic tool as shown in the case of respiratory allergic patients (20).

EFFECTIVE AMINO ACID DELIVERY INTO SKIN

There are several effects found for the topical application of amino acids. Application of ointment with an amino acid mixture with similar composition to infusion nutrients showed improved healing with decreased keroid formation (21). Occlusive application of a similar ointment with amino acids on the backs of rats fed protein-deficient food showed faster weight gain and even hair growth than rats treated with placebo (22). These transepidermal effects were found under abnormal conditions, which might have enhanced percutaneous penetration of amino acids. Cutaneous absorption of amino acids is low because of their hydrophilic nature (23). Intercellular lipid bilayers in the SC work as a barrier for water soluble molecules and water is held mostly in the corneocyte as the water holding capacity of bilayers are limited approximately up to <15% of total water contents in normal conditions (15,24). Therefore, it is assumed that water in the corneocyte works primarily as a reservoir for hydrophilic molecules. Interestingly, the amount of Pro in the SC increased when combined with other NMF constituents such as Na PCA, Na lactate, and glycerin, which lead to enhanced Pro penetration through skin because of the increased concentration gap between the SC and epidermis by Fick's equation (25). It is noteworthy that these combinations are exactly the same ones to show the synergistic hygroscopicity mentioned before (10).

Other enhancements of amino acid penetration can be achieved by modifying amino acids to be more hydrophobic than those regularly used for percutaneous drug delivery. For example, esters of Phe showed higher transepidermal penetration compared with Phe itself. Only Phe was detected in receiver solution, which indicates that esterase in epidermis hydrolyzed esters of Phe to Phe (26).

As mentioned before, roles of amino acids in the SC depend on their physicochemical properties such as hygroscopicity, water holding capacity, and pH buffering. On the contrary, physiological functions of amino acids are more prominent in the living skin. For example, Arg is a precursor of NO, which is an important regulator of micro blood circulation in dermis. We found stimulated NO production *in vitro* and temporal redness *in vivo* when PCA was topically administered (27). It was found in this phenomena that PCA stimulated transportation of Arg through cationic amino acid transporter CAT II channel, but not stimulation of constitutive NO synthase (cNOS) nor activation of induced NO synthase (iNOS). Thus, more Arg was available for cNOS in the endothelial cell, which resulted in increased NO production. Stimulation of Arg and Lys intake to the other skin-related cells, keratinocyte and fibroblast, was also observed (28). Tyr, cystine (Cys), and Pro are key molecules for the generation and differentiation of melanin (29). As such, amino acids play important physiological roles for the generation and integration of skin function. Therefore, the enhanced utilization of amino acids by delivery on demand is an important task for cosmeceutical advancement.

AMINO ACID DERIVATIVES FOR EXTENDED APPLICATIONS

Apart from straightforward application of amino acids to the skin, there are different aspects of utilization of amino acids for skin care products. Amino acids are reactive molecules easily converted to a variety of functional materials (1). A key factor of the practical utilization of amino acid derivatives is the development of a novel molecule superior in function and competitive in cost. Strategic molecular design should be applied to enhance physiological functions of amino acids while restoring their friendliness to humans in use and to the environment after use. Understanding both basic features of amino acids and the processing of molecular modification are the basics of such development. As details of each functional amino acid derivative have been introduced in some articles, historical trends for such development are reviewed here.

As a general statement, it can be said that history evidently shows that whenever characteristics of an amino acid derivative matched market demand there was creation of new applications. In the area of skin care, Na PCA was developed when the concept of NMF was created in the 1970s (6). Behind the scene at that time, mass production of monosodium glutamate as a food additive was established and industrial utilization of it that stimulated its modification to PCA was explored. Combination of other molecules in NMF with cosmetic formulations was not popular until the synergistic effect of PCA with Pro and lactate was found along with the establishment of production of Pro on a reasonable scale. Formulated NMF moisturizers were developed as a result (10). About the same time, the gel emulsification method by amino acids was established by Kumano et al. (30), which opened the door for the use of amino acids in their physicochemical aspects. In the 1980s, applications of UA and its ester as a natural UV absorber and amino acid fatty esters with EO moieties as super fatting agents or coemulsifiers followed (31).

In the 1990s, cholesterol esters of *N*-acylamino acid were developed as novel emollients with functions similar to celamides, which are the key components of lipid bilayers in SC as a barrier (32). Several advancements in the understanding of physiology in the SC and role of amino acids also occurred in the 1990s. As an example, Ala or Ser were found to stimulate activation of enzymes for desquamation (33). Further functional modification of these molecules would be expected for practical effectiveness.

Solar UV light contributes to skin photo damage, such as skin cancer, photo aging, photosensitization, and other light-related skin pathologies (34,35). Reactive oxygen species (ROS) are deeply involved in UV-induced photo damage. Iron is involved in the oxidative stress caused by both UVA and UVB (36). Therefore, it is important to design antioxidants with an iron sequestering capacity as Bisset et al. (37) have pioneered the development. Conjugates of amino acids with naphtylaldehyde or salicylaldehyde are designed by mimicking the active site of iron sequestering proteins, transferrine and feritine (38). These molecules suppress iron-induced hydroxyl radical generation and reduce the UV-induced oxidative stress by sequestering the catalytically active iron. To create an ideal cosmetic antioxidant that is not only functional but also provides cosmetic usefulness, a conjugate of vitamin B_6 with an amino acid, *N*-(4-pyridoxylmethylene)-L-serine (PYSer), was developed. These molecules are structurally similar to the amino acid iron chelator mentioned before and show antioxidative effect against UV radiation. PYSer suppresses iron-induced hydroxyl radical generation and UV-induced wrinkle formation. As the compound forms stable complexes with Fe^{3+} and inhibits iron-induced hydroxyl radical generation, it is expected to suppress free radical reactions by sequestering the catalytic iron in the body. PYSer has shown a protective effect on photo aging in hairless mice. The mechanism of the photo protection seems to be through the suppression of hydroxyl radical generation, as shown in an *in vitro* assay (38). UV exposure generates various cytokines, such as IL-1α and NF-κB, which lead to many physiological and cosmetic skin deteriorations, such as inflammation and hyperpigmentation. For example, Cys and cystein derivatives have shown suppression of UV-induced inflammation (39).

Besides the development of biofunctional molecules mentioned before, many amino acid-based surfactants have been produced as safe alternatives for people and the environment (40). In the 1970s, *N*-acylglutamate was launched first into the Japanese market as a new amino acid-based, mild, and functional anionic surfactant. With its weakly acidic nature, similar to skin pH, and gentleness to the skin, *N*-acylglutamate led to the creation of a mild cleanser market in Japan (41), coincidently promoted by the consumer's desire for safe products because of phenomenal hyperpigmentation troubles caused by some cosmetic products. Lys and Arg were the next amino acids commercially modified to surfactants because of their stable supply and reasonable cost to convert to functional surfactants. *N*-Lauroyl lysine has a superior surface modifying effect for various inorganic powders and a smooth touch to the skin; thus, it is used for cosmetic products, especially for powder formulations (42,43). *N*-cocoylarginine ethylester PCA (CAE) salt is a cationic surfactant with hair conditioning, antimicrobial, and many other properties, but is mild in terms of eye and skin irritation and highly biodegradable, inferiorities of common cationic surfactants (44). Hence CAE has been used in many skin preparations as an antimicrobial and for hair care as a conditioning and antistatic agent. Further additions are made for Arg as an amphoteric surfactant but with a strongly cationic character. *N*-Alkylether-hydroxypropyl arginine was developed to endow market needs for an environmentally friendly alternative to quaterammonium cationics, as it is mild in irritation, reasonably biodegradable, and a sufficient hair conditioner (45).

In the past decade, other amino acid-based anionic surfactants became common even for mass-market products. *N*-Acylmethyltaurate helped further the expansion of the amino acid surfactant share in the anionic surfactant market, especially for shampoo preparations (46). *N*-Acyl glycinate and alanate boosted this trend further with their excellent lathering properties in use and refreshed skin touch after. These are the characteristics highly rated in the consumer's subjective expectation for cleansers, which glutamate and other aforementioned *N*-acylamino acids could not fulfill as per the market needs (47,48).

These functional amino acid derivatives have many advantages compared with the traditional synthetic molecules. Principally those materials are safe and friendly to humans and the environment. Functionalities of these materials are even better than traditional synthetic materials because of the structural similarity or affinity of such amino acid derivatives to the human body.

CONCLUSION

The roles and functions of amino acids in the skin were reviewed here. Each amino acid has its own role and function in the skin, but more importantly every molecule is interrelated for harmonized integrity to maintain homeostasis of the skin. Further advancement of skin research will lead us to develop better uses for amino acids and their derivatives.

REFERENCES

1. Greenstein JP, Winitz M. Chemistry of the Amino Acids. New York: John Wiley & Sons Inc., 1961.
2. Amino Acid Data Book 1996 Edition, Japan Essential Amino Acids Association.
3. Abe H et al. J Soc Cosmet Chem Jpn 1996; 30(4):396; Okumura H, Fragrance J. 1996; 7:42; JP52-15687, 01-238521, 01-238522.
4. FRP2040954_ A; Ajinomoto Technical Data 3000-0200, Jun. 1998.
5. Rawlings AV et al. J Invest Dermatol 1994; 103:731.
6. Jacobi OT. Pro Sci Sect Good Assoc 1959; 31:22; Laden K. Am Perf Cosmet 1967; 82:77; Tatsumi S. Am Cosmet Perfum 1972; 87:61.
7. Pascher G et al. Klin Exp Dermatol 1956; 203:334; Pascher G et al. Klin Exp Dermatol 1957; 204:140.
8. Sauermann G, Hoppe U. IFSCC Venezia 1994.
9. Kawada Y et al. Annual Scientific Seminar of Society of Cosmetic Chemists Japan, June 1998, Osaka, Japan.
10. Sakamoto K. Cosmet Toileteries 1984; 99(3):109.
11. Igata S et al. J Soc Cosmet Chem Jpn 1993; 27(3):450.
12. Noonan FP, de Fabo EC. Immunol Today 1992; 13:259.
13. Scott I et al. Biochim Biophys Acta 1982; 719:110.
14. Kitamura K et al. J Soc Cosmet Chem Jpn 1995; 29:133.
15. Brouwstra JA et al. IFSCC Edinburg 2002; Brouwstra JA et al. J Invest Dermatol 1991; 97:1005; Brouwstra JA et al. J Control Release 1991; 15:209.
16. Lucassen GW. IFSCC/ISBS Workshop. Edinburg, Sept. 27, 2002.
17. Ino M et al. Conference of Society of Cosmetic Chemists Japan, October 2002, Tokyo, Japan.
18. Hara M et al. J Geriatr Dermatol 1993; 1:111.
19. Watanabe M et al. Arch Dermatol 1991; 137:1689.
20. Tanaka M et al. Br J Dermatol 1998; 139:618.
21. Fumiiri et al. Conference for Plastic Surgery Japan, 1962, Tokyo.
22. Katayama Y et al. XIII International Congress of Nutrition, Brighton, England.
23. Sznitowska M et al. Int J Pharm 1993; 99:43.
24. Imokawa G et al. Invest Dermtol 1991; 96:845.
25. Kawasaki Y et al. J Soc Cosmet Chem Jpn 1996; 30:55.

26. Kouzuki Y et al. Drug Der Syst 1995; 10:37.
27. Ogasahara K et al. J Soc Cosmet Chem Jpn 2003; 6(3):229–232.
28. Ogasahara K et al. IFSCC Conference, September 2003:Seoul.
29. Ito S et al. J Invest Dermatol 1993; 100:166; Kobayashi T et al. Pig Cell Res 1994; 7:227; Kobayashi T et al. EMBO J 1994; 13:5818.
30. Kumano Y et al. J Soc Cosmet Chem Jpn 1977; 28:285.
31. Sagawa K et al. Fragrance J 1988; 89:109.
32. Ishii H et al. J Soc Cosmet Chem 1996; 47:351.
33. Koyama J et al. 19th IFSCC Congress, Proceedings, Sidney, 1996.
34. Witt EH et al. In: Fuchs J, Packer L, eds. Oxidative Stress in Dermatology. New York: Marcel Dekker, 1993:29–47.
35. Black HS. Photochem Photobiol 1987; 46:213.
36. Pourzand C et al. Proc Natl Acad Sci USA 1999; 96:6751.
37. Bissett DL et al. Photochem Photobiol 1991; 54:215.
38. Kitazawa M, Iwasaki K. Biochem Biophys Res Commun 1996; 220:36.
39. Kitazawa M et al. FEBS Lett 2002; 526:106.
40. Sakamoto K et al. In: Xia, Nnann, eds. Surfactant Science Series Vol. 101, Protein Based Surfactants Chapter 4, New York: Marcel Dekker Inc., 2001:75; Sakamoto K, Yukagaku J Oleo Sci 1995; 44:256–265.
41. Sakamoto K. In: Xia and Nnann, eds. Surfactant Science Series Vol. 101, Protein Based Surfactants Chapter 10, New York: Marcel Dekker Inc., 2001:261; Saito T. Cosmet Toilet 1983; 98:111.
42. Yokota H et al. J Am Oil Chem Soc 1985; 62(12):1716.
43. Sagawa K et al. Fragrance J 1986; 14:71.
44. Yoshida R et al. Yukagaku J Oleo Sci 1976; 25(7):404.
45. Tabohashi T et al. Fragrance J 1998; 26:58.
46. Tabohashi T et al. Colloid Surf B: Biointerfaces 2001; 20:79–86; Kouchi J et al. J Oleo Science 2001; 50:847.
47. Miyazawa K et al. Yukagaku J Oleo Sci 1989; 38:297.
48. Shiojiri E et al. J Soc Cosmet Chem Jpn 1996; 30(4):410.

4

Antioxidant Defense Systems in Skin*

Jens J. Thiele
Department of Dermatology, Northwestern University, Chicago, Illinois, USA

Frank Dreher
Department of Dermatology, University of California, San Francisco, California, USA
TOPALIX, Topical Product Development, San Francisco, California, USA

Introduction	38
Constitutive Skin Antioxidants	39
Water-Soluble Antioxidants	39
Ascorbate	39
Glutathione	42
Urate	44
Lipid-Soluble Antioxidants	44
Vitamin E	44
Ubiquinols/Ubiquinones ("Coenzyme Q")	45
Carotenoids and Vitamin A	48
Enzymatic Antioxidant Systems	49
Enzymatic GHS System	49
Superoxide Dismutases	50
Catalase	51
Effect of Environmental Stressors on Skin Antioxidants	51
Hydrophilic Skin Antioxidants	52
Lipophilic Skin Antioxidants	53

*This chapter is dedicated to our scientific mentors, Lester Packer and Howard Maibach.

Enzymatic Skin Antioxidants	54
Role of Antioxidants in the Photoprotection of Skin	55
Topical Application of Antioxidants	55
Vitamin E	55
Vitamin C	63
Other Antioxidants	63
Antioxidant Combinations	70
Topical Application of Antioxidants after UVR Exposure	73
Topical Application of Substances Other than Conventional Antioxidants	74
Summary and Conclusion	74
Acknowledgments	75
References	75

INTRODUCTION

As the outermost organ of the body, the skin is frequently and directly exposed to a pro-oxidative environment, including ultraviolet radiation, drugs, and air pollutants (1). Besides dealing with external inducers of oxidative attack, the skin has to cope with endogenous generation of reactive oxygen species (ROS) and other free radicals, which are continuously produced during physiological cellular metabolism. To counteract the harmful effects of ROS, the skin is equipped with antioxidant systems, which maintain an equilibrium between pro- and antioxidants.

In the course of skin evolution, a variety of primary (preventive; e.g., vitamin C) and secondary (interceptive; e.g., vitamin E) antioxidant mechanisms have been developed, which form an "antioxidative network" of closely interlinked components (Fig. 2). Although some antioxidants such as glutathione (GSH) or ubiquinol-10 can be synthesized by humans, others have to be supplied by intake, for example, antioxidant vitamins C and E and trace metals. Antioxidants intervene at different levels of oxidative processes, for example, by (i) scavenging free radicals, (ii) scavenging lipid peroxyl radicals, (iii) binding metal ions, or (iv) by removing oxidatively damaged biomolecules (2).

However, the antioxidant defense in cutaneous tissues can be overwhelmed by either an increased exposure to exogenous (e.g., UV exposure) or endogenous (e.g., inflammatory disorders) sources of ROS, or a primarily depleted antioxidant defense (e.g., by malnutrition) facing a normal level of pro-oxidative challenge. Such a disturbance of the pro-oxidant/antioxidant balance may result in oxidative damage of biomolecules, such as lipids, proteins, and DNA, and has been termed "oxidative stress" (3,4). In skin, the induction of oxidative damage by environmental stimuli such as UVA, UVB, and ozone was demonstrated to occur in lipids (5–7), proteins (8), and DNA (9,10).

The objective of this review is to summarize the currently available knowledge on (i) the presence and physiological distribution of natural antioxidants in skin, (ii) their response to oxidative environmental stressors, and (iii) the photoprotective potential of topically applied antioxidants.

CONSTITUTIVE SKIN ANTIOXIDANTS

Water-Soluble Antioxidants

Ascorbate

Antioxidant Properties: Ascorbate, a ketolactone, is also known as vitamin C (Fig. 1). Although most mammals are able to synthesize ascorbate from glucose-derived glucuronic acid, guinea pigs, monkeys, and humans lack the enzyme gulonolactase, and therefore require the dietary intake of this vitamin. Dietary ascorbate is absorbed and distributed throughout the body within a few hours. The biochemical importance of vitamin C is primarily based on its reducing potential, as is required in a number of hydroxylation reactions. Several hydroxylases involved in collagen synthesis require ascorbate as a reductant (11). Owing to its high reduction potential, ascorbate is an efficient scavenger of superoxide anion radicals, hydroxyl radicals, hypochlorite, singlet oxygen, thiyl radicals, and water-soluble peroxyl radicals (2,12,13). Oxidation of ascorbate results in the formation of dehydroascorbate via the ascorbyl radical, which can be recycled back to ascorbate in the presence of thiols (Fig. 2), or irreversibly decomposed to the unstable diketogulonic acid. Although ascorbate is not able to scavenge lipophilic radicals directly, in the presence of vitamin E, it synergistically reduces lipid peroxyl radicals by reacting with tocopheroxyl radicals. This leads to regeneration of active tocopherol [Fig. 2, (14)]. Ascorbate has also been reported to show pro-oxidant properties. Mixtures of copper or iron salts with ascorbate are well known to stimulate lipid peroxidation *in vitro* (15). However, with the exception of pathological metal overload disease states, the pro-oxidative potential of ascorbate is not considered to be of relevance *in vivo* (16).

Prevalence in Skin: The data available on ascorbate concentrations in skin are limited and variable owing to differences in species, skin layer analyzed, and method of analysis (Table 2). Importantly, however, vitamin C is present at significant levels in both the dermis and epidermis of animals and humans (Table 1). In hairless mice, vitamin C levels are only slightly higher in the epidermis than in the dermis (5,17). In human skin, which is dependent on dietary vitamin C, the epidermis apparently contains approximately fivefold higher levels than the dermis (18). This difference in dermal and epidermal vitamin C levels may reflect an increased utilization in the dermis for the regulation of

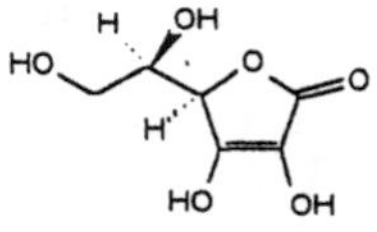

Figure 1 Chemical structures of selected antioxidants. (1) L-ascorbic acid (176.1 g/mol, pKa$_1$ = 4.2, pKa$_2$ = 11.6), (2) uric acid [168.1 g/mol, pKa$_1$ (37°C) = 5.2 (215)}, (3) D-α-lipoic acid (206.3 g/mol, pKa = 5.4), (4) tocopherols (α: R$_1$ = R$_2$ = CH$_3$, 430.7 g/mol; β: R$_1$ = CH$_3$, R$_2$ = H, 416.7 g/mol; γ: R$_1$ = H, R$_2$ = CH$_3$, 416.7 g/mol; δ: R$_1$ = R$_2$ = H, 402.7 g/mol), (5) tocotrienols (α: R$_1$ = R$_2$ = CH$_3$, 424.7 g/mol; β: R$_1$ = CH$_3$, R$_2$ = H, 410.6 g/mol; γ: R$_1$ = H, R$_2$ = CH$_3$, 410.6 g/mol; δ: R$_1$ = R$_2$ = H, 396.6 g/mol), (6) ubiquinone (n = 9: 795.3 g/mol; n = 10: 863.4 g/mol), (7) ubiquinol (n = 9: 797.3 g/mol; n = 10: 865.4 g/mol), (8) vitamin A precursors (R = H: β-carotene, 536.9 g/mol; R = OH: cryptoxanthin, 552.9 g/mol), (9) vitamin A (all-*trans*-retinol: R = CH$_2$-OH, 286.5 g/mol; all-*trans*-retinoic acid: R = COOH, 300.4 g/mol).

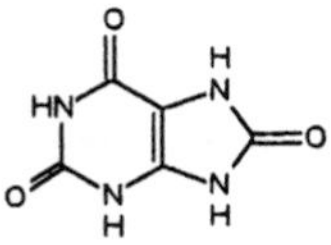

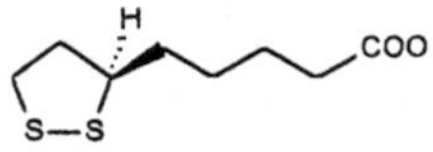

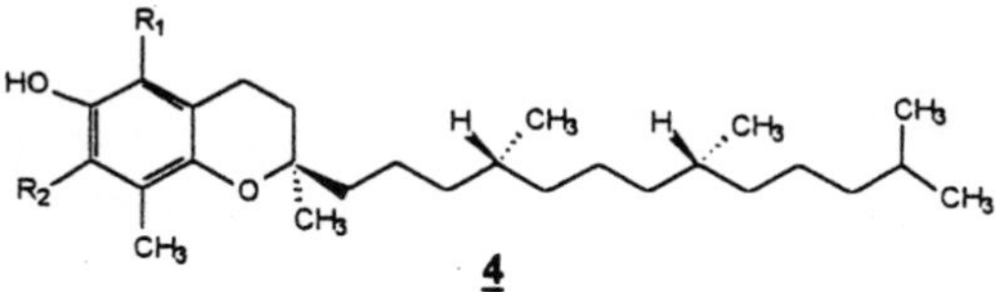

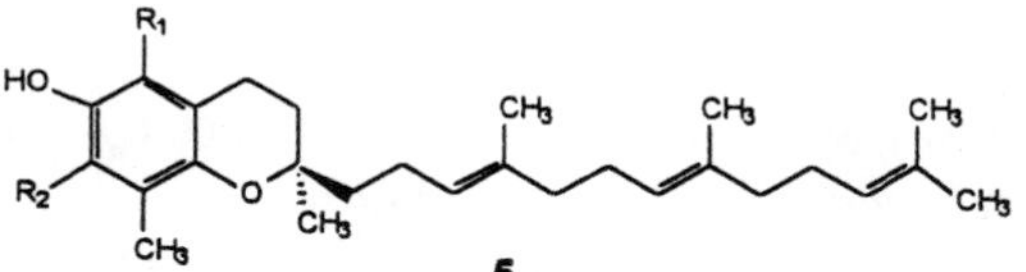

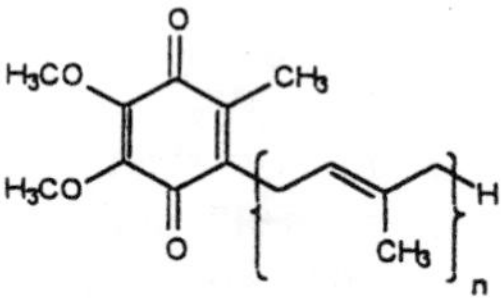

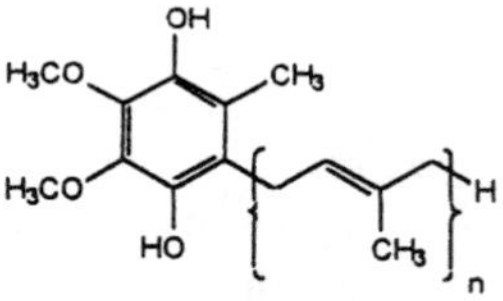

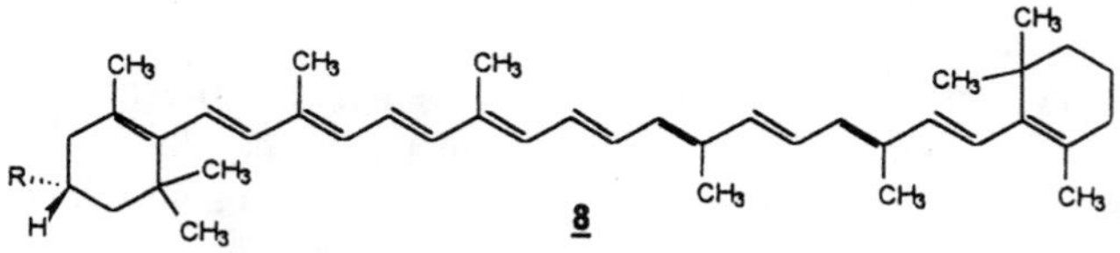

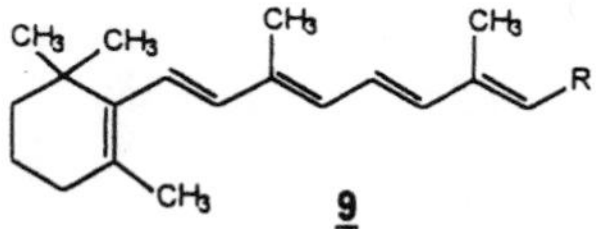

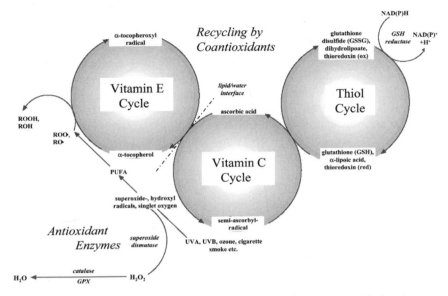

Figure 2 Activation of the antioxidant network by environmental oxidative stressors. $O_2^{-\bullet}$: Superoxide anion radical; PUFA: polyunsaturated fatty acids; $ROO^{\bullet}$, $RO^{\bullet}$: lipid (per-) oxy radicals; ROOH, ROH: Lipidhydro(per)oxides. Some of the depicted recycling mechanisms have been found in other than cutaneous systems (see section Antioxidant Properties).

Table 1 Physiological Levels of Ascorbate in Cutaneous Tissues

Skin layer	Species	Concentration	Authors	Year
Total skin	Rat	0.2 g/kg tissue	Salomon and Stubbs (216)	1961
Total skin	Human	41 µg/g dry weight	Stüttgen and Schaefer (217)	1974
Total skin	Mouse	6–7 nmol/mg protein	Fuchs et al. (103)	1989
Epidermis	Mouse	1321 ± 77 nmol/g tissue	Shindo et al. (17)	1993
Dermis	Mouse	1064 ± 54 nmol/g tissue	Shindo et al. (17)	1993
Epidermis	Human	3798 ± 1016 nmol/g tissue	Shindo et al. (18)	1994
Dermis	Human	723 ± 320 nmol/g tissue	Shindo et al. (18)	1994
Stratum corneum	Mouse	208 ± 82.5 pmol/10 tape strips	Weber et al. (106)	1999

collagen and elastin biosynthesis (19), or facilitated transport mechanisms for vitamin C from the dermal vasculature to the epidermis. The epidermis is not only more directly exposed to the environment than the underlying dermis and therefore might have a higher demand of antioxidant protection, but also requires the presence of ascorbate for efficient formation of the stratum corneum barrier (20). Isolated human stratum corneum was reported to contain only very low ascorbate levels, as compared with levels in subjacent epidermal layers (6). The latter phenomenon is most likely due to both the hydrophobicity and, due to its location, the high degree of environmental exposure of the stratum corneum.

Glutathione

Antioxidant Properties: GSH (γ-glutamyl-cysteinyl-glycine), present intracellularly at millimolar concentrations, is an important water-soluble antioxidant and reducing compound. Oral GSH is poorly absorbed and is not required to be provided by dietary intake (21). In cells, GSH is synthesized from glutamate, cysteine, and glycine (22). It acts as a substrate for numerous reducing enzymes, such as glutathione peroxidase (GSH-Px) and phospholipid hydroperoxide glutathione peroxidase. Therefore, the absence of GSH may lead to an accumulation of lipid hydroperoxides (2). Importantly, GSH also protects cells by reacting directly with ROS such as singlet oxygen ($^1O_2$), hydroxyl radicals (HO$^\bullet$), and superoxide radicals (O$^{\bullet-}_2$), resulting in the formation of thiyl radical (GS$^\bullet$), and subsequently, glutathione disulfide (GSSG). The latter can be recycled to GSH by the NADPH-dependent enzyme glutathione reductase (Fig. 2). The ratio of GSH/GSSG in tissues is normally high (i.e., >100) (23). In many biological systems, the GSH/GSSG ratio is lowered upon pro-oxidative conditions and therefore is frequently used as indicator of oxidative stress. In mice, ascorbate supplementation increases GSH levels in lung epithelial tissue (24), and GSH deficiency increases hepatic ascorbic acid synthesis (25), suggesting that the antioxidant actions of GSH and ascorbate are closely linked. In humans, who are dependent on dietary vitamin C intake, this link remains to be clarified.

Prevalence in Skin: Although a number of studies are available on GSH and GSSG, absolute values obtained for levels in total skin, epidermis, and dermis are highly variable (Table 2). However, comparing the relative levels, most studies demonstrated higher GSH levels in the epidermis than in the dermis. Furthermore, the epidermis reveals a higher ratio of GSH/GSSG than the dermis, indicating either a lower oxidative challenge or a better antioxidative protection. As the epidermis is more directly exposed to the environment, it also seems possible that the pathways leading to the endogenous formation of epidermal GSH are upregulated by chronic environmental factors, as was shown for GSH-Px in ozone-exposed lung epithelium (26). It must be considered that the cell turn-over rate in the epidermis, as well as cellular differentiation processes,

Table 2 Physiological Levels of Glutathione in Cutaneous Tissues

Skin layer	Species	Concentration	Authors	Year
Epidermis	Human	1.8 µmol/g tissue (GSH); 0.09 µmol/g tissue (GSSG)	Halprin and Ohkawara (218)	1967
Total skin	Guinea pig	0.7–1.1 µmol/g tissue (GSH); 1.4–1.5 µmol/g tissue (GSSG)	Benedetto et al. (219)	1981
Epidermis	Mouse	0.75 µmol/g tissue (GSH)	Wheeler et al. (65)	1986
Dermis	Mouse	0.32 µmol/g tissue (GSH)	Wheeler et al. (65)	1986
Epidermis	Human	1.2 µmol/g tissue (GSH)	Connor and Wheeler (66)	1987
Total skin	Mouse	3.9–6.3 µmol/g protein (GSH); 1–1.5 µmol/g protein (GSSG)	Fuchs et al. (27,103)	1989
Epidermis	Mouse	1.16 µmol/g tissue (GSH); 0.07 µmol/g tissue (GSSG)	Shindo et al. (17)	1993
Dermis	Mouse	0.59 µmol/g tissue (GSH); 0.16 µmol/g tissue (GSSG)	Shindo et al. (17)	1993
Epidermis	Human	0.46 µmol/g tissue (GSH); 0.02 µmol/g tissue (GSSG)	Shindo et al. (18)	1994
Dermis	Human	0.08 µmol/g tissue (GSH); 0.01 µmol/g tissue (GSSG)	Shindo et al. (18)	1994
Stratum corneum	Mouse	283.7 pmol/10 tape strips (GSH)	Weber et al. (106)	1999

is very high; as GSH is an important substrate for essential enzymes, and GSSG can inactivate enzymes by forming disulfides (27), a high GSH/GSSG ratio could be essential for the stratified and keratinized epidermis.

Urate

Antioxidant Properties: Uric acid (deprotonated form: urate) is a small water-soluble molecule (Fig. 1) that accumulates in human tissues as the end-product of purine metabolism. In blood plasma, urate has been shown to be a powerful scavenger of singlet oxygen, peroxyl radical, and hydroxyl radical (28). Further studies have demonstrated that urate scavenges ozone (15) and hypochlorous acid (29). In addition to its radical scavenging potential, urate was proposed to stabilize reduced vitamin C in serum. This stabilizing effect appears to be due to inhibition of iron-catalyzed oxidation of ascorbate, which largely results from the formation of a stable, noncatalytic urate–iron complex (30). Unlike radical scavenging reactions, this protective effect provided by iron chelation is not associated with depletion of urate. Direct free radical attack on urate generates allantoin, which has therefore been proposed as a marker molecule for free radical reactions *in vivo* (31).

Prevalence in Skin: Only little data are available on urate levels in cutaneous tissues. Lopez-Torres et al. reported values of 147 ± 5 nmol/g tissue in the epidermis, and 75 ± 9 nmol/g tissue in the dermis of hairless mice (32). In humans, Shindo et al. reported levels of 1071 ± 242 nmol/g tissue in the epidermis, and 182 ± 24 nmol/g tissue in the dermis (18). Thus, as found for other antioxidants, highest cutaneous urate levels are present in epidermal tissue.

Lipid-Soluble Antioxidants

Vitamin E

Antioxidant Properties: Vitamin E is the major lipophilic antioxidant in plasma, membranes, and tissues (33). The term "vitamin E" collectively refers to the eight naturally occurring molecules (four tocopherols and four tocotrienols), which exhibit vitamin E activity. Tocotrienols differ from tocopherols in that they have an isoprenoid instead of a phytyl side chain (Fig. 1); the four forms of tocopherols and tocotrienols differ in the number of methyl groups on the chromanol nucleus (α- has three, β- and γ- have two, and δ- has one). In humans, α-tocopherol is the most abundant vitamin E homolog, followed by γ-tocopherol.

Vitamin E is among the early recognized biological antioxidants, and its redox and free radical chemistry are well documented (33). Vitamin E acts as an antioxidant by scavenging free radicals, which can, either directly or indirectly, initiate ($HO^{\bullet}$ and $O_2^{\bullet -}$) or propagate (lipid peroxyl radicals) lipid chain reactions (34). Vitamin E can also react with nitric oxide (35). The major antioxidant role of vitamin E is generally considered to be the arrest of chain propagation by scavenging lipid peroxyl radicals. The initial oxidation product of tocopherol is the metastable tocopheroxyl radical (Fig. 2), which can either be reduced to tocopherol by coantioxidants, or can react with another lipid peroxyl radical, yielding tocopherol-quinone (36). Thus, one molecule of tocopherol is able to scavenge two peroxyl radical molecules. As the physiological molar ratio of tocopherols to polyunsaturated phospholipids, first-line targets of oxidative attack, is less than about 1:1000 in most biological membranes, regeneration of tocopherol is essential for its high antioxidant efficacy *in vivo*. As mentioned earlier, several hydrophilic coantioxidants, such as ascorbate and GSH, can regenerate vitamin E from the tocopheroxyl radical and thus enhance the antioxidant capacity of vitamin E (14). Furthermore, there is some *in vitro* evidence that ubiquinol-10 protects α-tocopherol from photo-oxidation by recycling mechanisms (37). *In vitro*, unphysiologically high concentrations of α-tocopherol were reported to induce pro-oxidative effects leading to acceleration of lipid peroxidation (38,39). However, in human skin *in vivo*, such adverse health effects have not been reported.

Prevalence in Skin: As demonstrated in other body tissues, α-tocopherol is the predominant vitamin E homolog in murine and human skin (5,6,18). In addition, γ-tocopherol is present in murine and human epidermis, dermis, and stratum corneum (Table 3). The α-tocopherol/γ-tocopherol molar ratio in the human dermis and epidermis is approximately 10:1. Notably, a vitamin E gradient has been recently demonstrated in human upper arm stratum corneum. The highest α-tocopherol levels were found in the lower stratum corneum, whereas the lowest levels were present in the upper layers. The α-tocopherol/γ-tocopherol ratio decreased from about 10:1 in the lower layers to about 3:1 in the upper stratum corneum. The α-tocopherol levels in human dermis and epidermis were several-fold higher than in corresponding layers of hairless mouse skin (17,18). Consistently, human stratum corneum contains almost 10-fold higher α-tocopherol levels than measured in murine stratum corneum (5,6). As observed for hydrophilic antioxidants, higher vitamin E levels were found in murine and human epidermis, as compared with dermal levels. It remains to be clarified whether the uptake and transport of α-tocopherol in the epidermis is an unspecific and passive process or, as described for human hepatocytes (33), is regulated by a mechanism involving a specific binding enzyme (α-tocopherol transfer protein).

Ubiquinols/Ubiquinones ("Coenzyme Q")

Antioxidant Properties: The terms "coenzyme Q" and "ubiquinone" are commonly used for the redox couple ubiquinol/ubiquinone (Fig. 1). Ubiquinones are lipid-soluble quinone derivatives with an isoprenoid side chain. In nature, ubiquinone homologs containing 1–12 isoprene units occur; the predominant form of ubiquinone in humans is ubiquinone-10 (contains 10 isoprene units), and in mice, ubiquinone-9. In liver cells, $\sim$40–50% of the total cellular

Table 3 Physiological Levels of α- and γ-Tocopherol in Cutaneous Tissues

Skin layer	Species	Concentration	Authors	Year
Total skin	Mouse	200 pmol α-tocopherol/mg protein	Fuchs et al. (27,103)	1989
Epidermis	Mouse	4.8 ± 0.5 nmol α-tocopherol/g tissue	Shindo et al. (17)	1993
Dermis	Mouse	3.3 ± 0.3 nmol α-tocopherol/g tissue	Shindo et al. (17)	1993
Epidermis	Human	31 ± 3.8 nmol α-tocopherol/g tissue; 3.3 ± 1 nmol γ-tocopherol/g tissue	Shindo et al. (18)	1994
Dermis	Human	16.2 ± 1.1 nmol α-tocopherol/g tissue; 1.8 ± 0.2 nmol γ-tocopherol/g tissue	Shindo et al. (18)	1994
Stratum corneum	Mouse	8.4 ± 1.3 nmol α-tocopherol/g tissue; 2.9 ± 0.9 nmol γ-tocopherol/g tissue	Thiele et al. (5)	1997
Stratum corneum	Human	33 ± 4 nmol α-tocopherol/g tissue; 4.8 ± 0.8 nmol γ-tocopherol/g tissue	Thiele et al. (6)	1998
Sebum	Human	76.5 ± 1.5 nmol α-tocopherol/g sebum; 8.7 ± 1.8 nmol γ-tocopherol/g sebum	Thiele et al. (220)	1999

ubiquinone is located in the mitochondria, 25–30% in the nucleus, 15–20% in the endoplasmatic reticulum, and only 5–10% in the cytosol (40). *In vitro*, the reduced forms of ubiquinones, the ubiquinols, are by two to three orders of magnitude more potent antioxidants (41). The role of ubiquinol/ubiquinone as a redox carrier in the respiratory chain is well established, by participating in the transfer of protons across the inner mitochondrial membrane (42). Ubiquinols can react with ROS and prevent direct damage to biomolecules and initiation of lipid peroxidation. Although ubiquinones cannot prevent autocatalytic free radical reactions by donating a phenolic hydrogen atom (unlike ubiquinols and tocopherols), they scavenge singlet oxygen and inhibit lipid peroxidation in model membranes (43). Furthermore, there is some *in vitro* evidence that ubiquinol-10 protects α-tocopherol against superoxide-driven oxidation (37). In low density lipoproteins, its protective potential against lipid peroxidation was shown to exceed that of α-tocopherol (44). However, it must be noted that the antioxidant properties reported for ubiquinones are strongly dependent on the length of the side chain and the model systems used. A growing scientific and commercial interest in ubiquinones has led to their incorporation into skin care products; however, further research is needed to better understand their protective antioxidant mechanisms in human skin.

Prevalence in Skin: In both mouse and human skin, highest ubiquinol levels were found in the epidermis. In human skin, the majority of ubiquinone is present in its oxidized form (ubiquinone-10) (Table 4). This is in accordance with the ratios determined in brain and lung tissues, but different from those in heart, kidney, liver, and blood plasma, where the majority of ubiquinone is present in the reduced form (45). Interestingly, all three organs, skin, brain, and lung, are well known to be challenged by a high load of oxidative stress. Despite its high lipid content, the stratum corneum appears to be very low in

Table 4 Physiological Levels of Ubiquinone/Ubiquinol in Skin

Skin layer	Species	Concentration	Authors	Year
Total skin	Mouse	20–48 pmol ubiquinol-9/mg protein; 98–136 pmol ubiquinone-9/mg protein	Fuchs et al. (27,103)	1989
Epidermis	Mouse	1.9 ± 0.2 nmol ubiquinol-9/g tissue; 15.2 ± 1.1 nmol ubiquinone-9/g tissue	Shindo et al. (17)	1993
Dermis	Mouse	1.2 ± 0.2 nmol ubiquinol-9/g tissue; 10.0 ± 0.7 nmol ubiquinone-9/g tissue	Shindo et al. (17)	1993
Epidermis	Human	3.5 ± 0.8 nmol ubiquinol-10/g tissue; 4.1 ± 0.6 nmol ubiquinone-10/g tissue	Shindo et al. (18)	1994
Dermis	Human	0.4 ± 0.1 nmol ubiquinol-10/g tissue; 2.9 ± 0.8 nmol ubiquinone-10/g tissue	Shindo et al. (18)	1994
Stratum corneum	Mouse	Ubiquinol-9 and ubiquinone-9: not detectable (<0.1 pmol/mg)	Thiele et al. (5)	1997
Stratum corneum	Human	Ubiquinol-10 and ubiquinone-10: not detectable (<0.1 pmol/mg)	Thiele et al. (6)	1998

ubiquinol/ubiquinone levels (5,6). Most likely, this results from the loss of nuclei and organelles, both rich in ubiquinones, during the terminal differentiation process of keratinocytes into the stratum corneum barrier.

Carotenoids and Vitamin A

Antioxidant Properties: Dietary vitamin A is available in the form of provitamin A compounds (e.g., α- and β-carotene and cryptoxanthin; Fig. 1), or directly from animal food (liver, milk, egg, and fish) (46). In comparison with α-tocopherol, β-carotene membrane levels are several-fold lower; however, β-carotene accumulates significantly in skin and may achieve levels far exceeding those of α-tocopherol in subjects on a β-carotene supplemented diet (47). There are at least three known mechanisms by which carotenoids protect cells from oxidative stress: (i) by quenching triplet-state sensitizers, (ii) by quenching singlet oxygen, and (iii) by scavenging peroxyl radicals (48,49). Triplet sensitizers, such as flavins and porphyrins, may abstract a hydrogen atom or an electron from various molecules; this can lead to further radical-mediated damage (type I) or formation of singlet oxygen (type II) by reaction with ground-state oxygen. The quenching of singlet oxygen by carotenoids is almost entirely an energy transfer process yielding ground-state oxygen and a triplet-excited carotenoid (2). The role of carotenoids within the "antioxidant-network" is not clear. It has been demonstrated in liver homogenates that dietary carotenoids increase the resistance to lipid peroxidation primarily by enhancing α-tocopherol membrane levels, whereas direct antioxidant effects provided by carotenoids were less protective (50). Several forms of vitamin A (13-*cis*-retinoic acid, all-*trans*-retinoic acid, all-*trans*-retinol; Fig. 1), however, were shown to effectively inhibit lipid peroxidation in liver microsomes (2,51). Carotenoids protect biological systems against triplet sensitizers and singlet oxygen-mediated oxidative damage largely without being sacrificed. Both carotenoids and retinoids act at physiological oxygen tension as peroxyl radical scavengers, preventing oxidative damage (49). As opposed to the reducing antioxidants, ascorbate and dihydrolipoic acid, β-carotene was not effective in recycling α-tocopherol in mouse skin homogenates irradiated with solar simulated UV irradiation (52).

Prevalence in Skin: Data available on carotenoid and vitamin A levels in skin are very limited. Vahlquist et al. revealed that the levels of β-carotene in human skin (epidermis: 2.2 μg/g protein; dermis: 0.7–0.8 μg/g protein; subcutis: 18.9 μg/g protein) is several-fold higher than that of vitamin A (retinol; epidermis: 0.3 μg/g protein; dermis: 0.2–0.4 μg/g protein; subcutis: 6.4 μg/g protein) (53). The same authors furthermore detected carotene and retinol in skin surface lipids, but no data are yet available on stratum corneum levels of these compounds (53). Recently, Stahl et al. (54) detected relatively high basal levels of carotenoids in human skin of the forehead (0.40 ± 0.09 nmol/g), back (0.22 ± 0.13 nmol/g), and palmar hand (0.32 ± 0.08 nmol/g), but significantly lower levels were present in the skin of the dorsal hand (0.03 ± 0.10 nmol/g) and the inside of the forearm (0.07 ± 0.05 nmol/g). Furthermore, skin carotenoid levels increased after oral carotenoid supplementation (with daily doses of 20–25 mg carotenoids), and correlated well with increased serum carotenoid levels. Higher levels of β-carotene (1.4 ± 0.7 nmol/g tissue) and lycopene (1.6 ± 0.6 nmol/g tissue) in human skin samples were found when the subcutaneous fat was included in the whole skin samples (55). Thus, as was reported for other skin antioxidants, β-carotene levels are higher in the epidermis than in the dermis. This difference seems to be less pronounced for vitamin A (53,56).

Enzymatic Antioxidant Systems

Enzymatic GHS System

Antioxidant Properties: The major components of the enzymatic GSH system are GSH-Px, GSSG reductase, phospholipid hydroperoxide GSH-peroxidase, and GSH-S-transferase (GST). GSH-Px is a selenoenzyme consisting of four identical subunits, each of which contains a selenocysteine residue in its active site. In eukaryotes, the majority of its enzymatic activity is localized in the cytosol, and, to a lesser extent, in mitochondria (57,58). GSH-Px reduces H_2O_2 and lipid hydroperoxides at the expense of two molecules of GSH, which are oxidized to GSSG. GSSG-reductase, a dimeric enzyme containing FAD in its active site, catalyzes the reduction of GSSG using reducing equivalents such as NADPH (59) (Fig. 2). Nonselenium-dependent GSH-Pxs (GSTs) and phospholipid hydroperoxide GSH-Px are able to catalyze the reduction of lipid hydroperoxides, but not of hydrogen peroxide (60). An increasing volume of data indicates that polymorphism at GST genes influences skin cancer susceptibility. It was proposed that GSTs influence tumorigenesis because these enzymes detoxify the products of UV-induced oxidative stress (61), and that heritable deficiency of specific GSTs may be a genetic determinant of individual skin sensitivity toward UV irradiation (62). Recently, increased tumorigenesis has been demonstrated in mice lacking π-class GSTs (63).

Prevalence in Skin: As compared with that of liver, kidney, and brain, skin GSH-Px and GSH-reductase activities are markedly lower (47). The baseline levels measured in epidermis and dermis vary considerably between different studies and therefore do not point to a clear preferential distribution of GSH-Px in skin (Table 5). GST is expressed during all stages of differentiation of cultured human keratinocytes, but was reported to lack substrate specificity and catalytic activity for reduction of lipid hydroperoxides (64). GST and GSH-reductase activities have been detected at similar levels in murine epidermis (19.6–53.3 U/mg protein and 22.5–31.6 U/mg protein, respectively) and dermis (33.8–64.8 U/mg protein and 14.3–27.6 U/mg protein, respectively) (65,66). Although little is known about absolute levels of GSTs in distinct layers of human skin, π-, μ-, and α-class GSTs have been localized

Table 5 Activities of GSH-Px in Cutaneous Tissues

Skin layer	Species	Concentration (U/mg protein)	Authors	Year
Epidermis	Mouse	80.2	Wheeler et al. (65)	1986
Dermis		37.0		
Epidermis	Mouse	80.2	Connor and Wheeler (66)	1987
Dermis		36.5		
Total skin	Mouse	35	Fuchs et al. (27,103)	1989
Epidermis	Mouse	11.7 ± 1.4	Shindo et al. (17)	1993
Dermis		27.5 ± 2.5		
Epidermis	Human	17.8 ± 1.0	Shindo et al. (18)	1994
Dermis		15.0 + 1.3		

immunohistologically in normal skin, naevi, and melanoma (67): π-GSTs were found in the stratum basalis and, to a lesser extent, in the superficial epidermal layers. Distribution of π-GST in the epidermis showed that only the stratum basale, where melanocytes are located, stained well. The α-GSTs were relatively abundant in the upper strata and, to a lesser extent, in the basal layers.

Superoxide Dismutases

Antioxidant Properties: Superoxide dismutase (SOD) catalyzes in the dismutation reaction of superoxide radicals ($O_2^{\cdot -}$) to H_2O_2. SODs are found in virtually all eukaryotic cells. Three types of human SODs have been purified: Cu/Zn-SOD (a cytosolic enzyme); Mn-SOD (a mitochondrial enzyme), and an extracellular SOD (EC-SOD; a tetrameric glycoprotein which contains Cu^{II} and Zn^{II}) (68,69). Cu/Zn-SOD consists of two protein subunits, each of which has an active site containing one Cu^{II} and one Zn^{II}. The Cu-ion serves as an active redox site, whereas the Zn-ion maintains the protein structure (68). The Mn-SOD consists of four subunits, each containing Mn^{II}, and is more labile than Cu/Zn-SOD. The presence of SOD in various compartments of the body may facilitate immediate dismutation of $O_2^{\cdot -}$ at the site where it is generated.

Prevalence in Skin: Many investigators measured SOD activities in epidermal and dermal tissues, mostly using unspecific spectrophotometric activity assays determining total SOD activity (70). The reported activity levels are highly variable and do not allow clear conclusions about the preferential distribution of SOD within layers of skin (Table 6). In both human and pig epidermis, the Cu/Zn-SOD activity seems to be 5- to 10-fold higher than that of Mn-SOD (71,72). As compared with other body tissues, SOD activity is relatively low in skin (47).

Table 6 Physiological Activities of Superoxide Dismutase in Cutaneous Tissues

Skin layer	Species	Concentration (U/mg protein)	Authors	Year
Epidermis	Human	12.0	Kim and Lee (221)	1987
Epidermis	Pig	11.4	Ohkuma et al. (72)	1987
Dermis	Human	10.5	Kim and Lee (221)	1987
Epidermis	Mouse	0.6	Carrao and Pathak (222)	1988
Epidermis	Guinea pig	0.5	Carrao and Pathak (222)	1988
Total skin	Mouse	3.0–4.3	Fuchs et al. (27,103)	1989
Epidermis	Mouse	11.7 ± 1.4	Shindo et al. (17)	1993
Dermis	Mouse	27.5 ± 2.5	Shindo et al. (17)	1993
Epidermis	Human	17.8 ± 1.0	Shindo et al. (18)	1994
Dermis	Human	15.0 + 1.3	Shindo et al. (18)	1994

Catalase

Antioxidant Properties: Catalase is a tetrameric enzyme which is expressed in all major body organs. Each of its four subunits contains a heme group in its active site and one tightly bound molecule of NADPH (73). Highest catalase activities are found in the peroxisomes, where it constitutes ∼50% of the peroxisomal protein. The main characteristic of catalase as an antioxidant is its ability to detoxify H_2O_2 by decomposing two H_2O_2 molecules to two molecules of water and one molecule of oxygen. Recently, high levels of catalase were found in the human stratum corneum, with an age- and solar exposure-dependent decline of the protein level (74). These results were confirmed on the activity level of the enzyme by Hellemans et al. (75).

Prevalence in Skin: Epidermal activities were first measured in mice by Solanki et al. (76), who reported 78–175 U/mg protein. Shindo et al. measured activities of 30.4 ± 4.3 U/mg protein in murine epidermis, and 33.3 U/mg protein in murine dermis. The same authors reported higher catalase activities in human epidermis (62 ± 6 U/mg protein), but lower activities in human dermis (14.6 ± 2.9 U/mg protein).

Effect of Environmental Stressors on Skin Antioxidants

UVB and UVA irradiations induce the formation of ROS in cell cultures (77,78), skin homogenates (52,79,80), and intact murine and human skin (81,82). Evaluation of the protective mechanisms of skin has included measurements of baseline levels of antioxidants in the dermis and epidermis (17,18) and the antioxidant response to UVB and UVA light in these layers (27,83). Terrestrial UVR consists of UVB (280–320 nm) and UVA (UVA II: 320–340 nm, UVA

I: 340–400 nm). Radiation <280 nm (UVC) does not reach the earth's surface, as they are absorbed by stratospheric ozone.

Although ozone (O_3) in the upper atmosphere (stratosphere) occurs naturally and protects skin by filtering out harmful solar ultraviolet radiation, O_3 at ground level (troposphere) is a noxious, highly reactive oxidant pollutant. The precursors of photochemical oxidants are volatile organic compounds (e.g., vapor-phase hydrocarbons and halogenated organics), oxides of nitrogen (NO_x), NO and other radicals, O_2, and sunlight (84). As a major pollutant in photochemical smog, O_3 occurs at concentrations between 0.1 and 0.8 ppm and represents a severe urban air quality problem (85). In addition to photochemical smog, O_3 is generated during operation of high voltage devices and dermatologic phototherapy equipment (85). There is ample evidence that acute (2–6 h) and chronic *in vivo* exposure to O_3 causes airway inflammation and affects pulmonary function in humans (86–88). The biological effects of O_3 are attributed to its ability to cause ozonation, oxidation, and peroxidation of biomolecules, both directly and via secondary reactive reactions. Hydrogen peroxide, hydroperoxide, hydroxyl radical, superoxide anion, and singlet oxygen have been proposed as intermediates in these secondary reactions (85,89–92). Analogous to the respiratory tract and the surface tissues of plants, a primary function of the skin is to provide a protective barrier against noxious environmental agents including oxidative air pollutants.

Numerous studies have documented the effects of O_3 on the respiratory tract in animals and humans (85,93,94) and on plants (95–98). In contrast, only little is known about the effect of O_3 on cutaneous tissues. Recently, a series of studies were published investigating the impact of O_3 on skin antioxidants (1,5,7,99). As O_3 levels are frequently highest in areas where exposure to ultraviolet radiation is also high, the concomitant exposure to O_3 and ultraviolet radiation in photochemical smog could be of relevance for skin pathologies, as has been implicated for plants (95,100).

Hydrophilic Skin Antioxidants

Ascorbate and Urate: High acute doses of solar simulated UVA/UVB (SSUV) have been demonstrated to deplete ascorbate and urate in cultured human skin equivalents. The SSUV dose needed to deplete these hydrophilic antioxidants was much higher than those necessary to deplete lipophilic antioxidants ubiquinol-10 and α-tocopherol (101). In hairless mice, however, Shindo et al. (102) observed depletion of ascorbate at lower SSUV doses than those needed to deplete lipophilic antioxidants or GSH. A single acute ozone exposure depletes ascorbate in the upper epidermis of hairless mice, but not in lower skin layers (7).

Glutathione: Fuchs et al. (27,103) reported that single exposures to UVB, but not to UVA, depleted GSH and increased GSSG in excised mouse skin, whereas ascorbate levels remained unchanged. However, UVA irradiation of human fibroblasts depleted intracellular GSH levels (104). Treatment of hairless mice with 8-methoxypsoralen plus UVA (PUVA) resulted in a significant depletion of cutaneous GSH after 24–48 h (65). Epidermal GSH levels of UVB-treated hairless mice were depleted by 40% within minutes after exposure and returned to regular levels after half an hour (66).

Lipophilic Skin Antioxidants

Vitamin E: Single, suberythemogenic doses of SSUV light (UVA and UVB; 0.75 MED) depleted human stratum corneum α-tocopherol by almost 50%, and murine stratum corneum α-tocopherol by 85% (6). These findings were in contrast to previous studies investigating the effects of SSUV light on dermal and epidermal antioxidants, in which doses equivalent to 3 MED or more were necessary to detect a significant depletion of α-tocopherol (17,83,105). Hence, it was concluded that α-tocopherol depletion in the stratum corneum is a very early and sensitive event of photo-oxidative damage in skin (6). The high susceptibility of stratum corneum vitamin E to SSUV may be due, at least in part, to lack of coantioxidants in the stratum corneum. Ubiquinol-10 was undetectable in human stratum corneum at levels found in epidermis and dermis (6). Additionally, ascorbate, the major hydrophilic coantioxidant that is capable of recycling photo-oxidized α-tocopherol (52,80), is present only at very low levels in murine and human stratum corneum, as compared with epidermal and dermal tissue (106).

Vitamin E may be depleted (i) directly, by absorption of UVB radiation, and/or (ii) indirectly, by excited-state singlet oxygen or reactive oxygen intermediates that are generated by photosensitizers upon UV absorption also in the UVA range. As both UVB and UVA have been shown to deplete murine α-tocopherol (6), both mechanisms may be relevant. The absorption maxima of α- and γ-tocopherols fall between 290 and 295 nm (107,108) and extend well into the solar UV spectrum. Interestingly, a large part of terrestrial UVB $\sim$290–300 nm is absorbed in the human stratum corneum (109). Furthermore, depletion of α-tocopherol by UVR is maximal at wavelengths in the range of its absorption maximum in skin homogenates of hairless mice (52). This congruency suggests that α-tocopherol is directly destroyed upon short wavelength UVB absorption. Indeed, tocopheroxyl radical formation occurs in UVB irradiated skin homogenates (52). Direct depletion of α-tocopherol and formation of its radical may also affect other endogenous antioxidant pools. As mentioned previously, α-tocopherol is readily regenerated from its radical at the expense of reductants like ascorbate (52,110) (Fig. 2), which itself can be regenerated by GSH (25). In addition to direct depletion by UVB, skin α-tocopherol levels may also be consumed as a consequence of its chain-breaking antioxidant action. The absorption of UVB and UVA photons by endogenous photosensitizers (e.g., porphyrins, riboflavin, quinones, and bilirubin) results in their electronically excited state (111,112). The excited sensitizer subsequently reacts with another substrate (type I reaction) to form radicals or radical ions, or with oxygen (type II reaction) to generate singlet oxygen (113). Photosensitizers, such as melanin, are present in variable amounts in the stratum corneum (114). Hence, their wavelength-dependent potential to generate or to quench free radicals, and to absorb UVR, may modulate α-tocopherol depletion during and after solar exposure.

Recently, Thiele et al. investigated the effects of the air pollutant ozone on skin antioxidants. Although no depletion of vitamin E was observed in whole skin (99), α-tocopherol depletion was detected in the outer epidermis when skin layers were analyzed separately (7). It was concluded that ozone itself is too reactive to penetrate deeply into skin and reacts rapidly with skin barrier lipids and proteins (8). Consequently, it was demonstrated that the stratum corneum is the most susceptible skin layer for ozone-induced vitamin E depletion (5). Recently, we have demonstrated that stratum corneum vitamin E is highly susceptible to topical treatment with benzoyl peroxide (115).

Ubiquinol/Ubiquinone: Ubiquinol-9 has been shown to be the most susceptible non-enzymatic antioxidant in murine skin, with respect to SSUV-induced (280–400 nm) depletion *in vivo* (17). Similar results were obtained for ubiquinol-10 in SSUV-irradiated human cell culture models (101). Exposure of purified ubiquinol-9 and α-tocopherol to SSUV *in vitro* resulted in the depletion of both compounds, which have similar absorption maxima $\sim$295 nm (83). As ubiquinol depletion precedes that of α-tocopherol in UVR-challenged skin *in vivo*, it is thought that ubiquinol protects vitamin E, as demonstrated *in vitro* (37).

Vitamin A/Carotenoids: A single exposure of human volar forearm skin to SSUV (3 MED) was found to lower the skin lycopene (ψ,ψ-carotene) level by 31–46%, whereas the same UV dose did not induce significant changes in the skin β-carotene level (55). However, repeated exposures of human volunteers to solar light (total UV dose of $\sim$10 kJ/cm) also depleted β-carotene levels in skin (116).

Enzymatic Skin Antioxidants

Catalase, SOD, GSH-Px, GSSG-Reductase: It was demonstrated by Aronoff et al. more than three decades ago that photo-oxidation of a single porphyrin ring in catalase results in complete inhibition of its activity (117). Superoxide anion radicals (118) and ozone (119) have also been shown to inactivate catalase activity. Punnonen et al. demonstrated that UVB (120), as well as UVA or PUVA therapy (121), decreases the activity of both catalase and SOD in cultured human keratinocytes. In cultured human fibroblasts, a single UVA exposure decreased catalase activities immediately, whereas GSH-Px and GSSG-reductase remained unaffected, and SOD activity decreased only 3 days after exposure (122). *In vivo* exposures of hairless mouse skin to SSUV light demonstrated that dermal and epidermal catalases are more susceptible to photoinactivation than SOD, and far more than GSH-Px and GSSG-reductase (17,83). *In vitro*, purified catalase was demonstrated to be directly inactivated by SSUV light, whereas SOD activity remained unaffected (83). Hence, although direct photodestruction appears to account for catalase inactivation, other mechanisms, possibly involving free radical-mediated oxidative protein damage, may account for the observed UV-induced loss of skin SOD activity *in vivo*. Notably, chronic UVB irradiation was recently shown to upregulate human epidermal SOD activity *in vivo*, whereas the activities of other antioxidant enzymes remained unchanged (123).

ROLE OF ANTIOXIDANTS IN THE PHOTOPROTECTION OF SKIN

Topical Application of Antioxidants

UVR-induced skin damage includes acute reactions, such as erythema, edema, and pain, followed by exfoliation, tanning, and epidermal thickening. Premature skin aging ("photoaging") and carcinogenesis are generally believed to be consequences of chronic UVR exposure (124). ROS and other free radicals, particularly the highly damaging hydroxyl radical, deplete the skin of its antioxidant defense and, when the latter is overwhelmed, can damage biomolecules such as lipids, proteins, and nucleic acids (27,83,103). Therefore, apart from using chemical and/or physical sunscreens to diminish the intensity of UVR reaching the skin, preventing ROS from reacting with these biomolecules by strengthening the skin's antioxidative capacity is an emerging approach in limiting UVR-induced skin damage (125–128). Topical application of antioxidants, such as vitamin E, provides an efficient means of increasing antioxidant tissue levels in epidermis and dermis (105,129). The stratum corneum, which was shown to be the most susceptible skin layer for UVR-induced depletion of vitamin E (6), may particularly benefit from an increased antioxidant capacity.

A selected overview of animal and human studies investigating acute and chronic photoprotection of skin by topical administration of antioxidants is given in Tables 7–10.

Vitamin E

The photoprotective effect of vitamin E (α-tocopherol) and its esters has been studied extensively (Table 7). Numerous topical studies demonstrate that when vitamin E was applied before UVR exposure there was a significant reduction in acute skin responses, such as erythema and edema (130–133), sunburn cell formation (134,135), lipid peroxidation (108,129,136), DNA adduct formation (10,137,138), immunosuppression (108,139), as well as UVA-induced binding of photosensitizers (140,141) and chemiluminescence (142). Chronic skin reactions, such as skin wrinkling (82,143–145) and skin tumor incidence (133,139, 143–145) due to prolonged UVR exposure were also diminished by topical vitamin E. Numerous studies used animal models, whereas some studies exist

Table 7 Photoprotective Effects of Topically Applied Vitamin E (α-Tocopherol) and Derivatives *In Vivo*

Compound(s)	Species	Endpoint(s)	Efficacy	Remarks	Authors	Year
Vitamin E	Rabbit	Erythema (MED)	Vitamin E protective; vitamin E acetate not protective	BHT also protective; Vitamin E also protective when applied after UVR exposure	Roshchupkin et al. (130)	1979
Vitamin E acetate						
Vitamin E	Human	Mechanoelectrical properties of skin	Protection against UVR- and PUVA-induced damage		Potapenko et al. (147)	1983
Vitamin E	Human, rabbit	PUVA-induced erythema and changes in mechanoelectrical properties of skin	Vitamin E and derivatives with shorter hydrocarbon chain protective; vitamin E acetate not protective	No protection of vitamin E and derivatives when applied after UVR exposure	Potapenko et al. (146)	1984
Vitamin E derivatives with shorter hydrocarbon chains						
Vitamin E acetate						
Vitamin E	Mouse	Lipid peroxidation	Protective	Vitamin A, BHT, and β-carotene also protective	Khettab et al. (136)	1988

Compound	Species	Endpoint	Effect	Comments	Reference	Year
Vitamin E	Mouse	Skin wrinkling, skin tumor incidence, and histology	Protective		Bissett et al. (144)	1989
Vitamin E	Human	Erythema (MED)	Protective	SPF-determination	Möller et al. (131)	1989
Vitamin E	Mouse	Skin wrinkling and sagging, skin tumor incidence, and histology	Vitamin E esters not as protective as vitamin E or vitamin E analog Trolox®; no protection against UVA-induced skin sagging	GSH, β-carotene, BHT, and mannitol not protective	Bissett et al. (145)	1990
Trolox®						
Vitamin E acetate						
Vitamin E succinate						
Vitamin E linoleate						
Vitamin E nicotinate						
Vitamin E	Mouse	Skin tumor incidence and immunosuppression	Protective	Prolonged pretreatment	Gensler et al. (139)	1991
Vitamin E	Rat	UVA-induced binding of 8-MOP and CPZ to epidermal biomacromolecules	Vitamin E protective after single application; vitamin E acetate only protective after prolonged application	Limited conversion of vitamin E acetate into vitamin E after single application	Schoonderwoerd et al. (141)	1991
Vitamin E acetate						

(continued)

Table 7 Continued

Compound(s)	Species	Endpoint(s)	Efficacy	Remarks	Authors	Year
Vitamin E acetate	Mouse	Lipid peroxidation and DNA synthesis rate	Protective		Record et al. (148)	1991
Vitamin E	Mouse	Skin wrinkling, skin tumor incidence, and histology	Protective	Additive protection in combination with anti-inflammatory agents	Bissett et al. (143)	1992
Vitamin E acetate	Mouse	Erythema, edema, and skin sensitivity	Protective	Treatment immediately after UVR exposure	Trevithick et al. (149)	1992
Vitamin E acetate	Mouse	Edema and histology	Protective	Delayed treatment after UVR exposure; increased skin vitamin E concentration	Trevithick et al. (150)	1993
Vitamin E Vitamin E acetate Vitamin E sorbate	Mouse	Skin wrinkling	Vitamin E and sorbate ester protective; vitamin E acetate ester only modestly protective	Sorbate ester more protective than free vitamin E	Jurkiewicz et al. (82)	1995

Vitamin E	Human	Erythema (skin color)	Moderate protection of vitamin E and vitamin E acetate when applied occlusively after UVR exposure	No protection when applied occlusively before UVR exposure	Montenegro et al. (204) 1995
Vitamin E acetate					
Vitamin E	Rat	UVA-induced binding of 8-MOP to epidermal biomacromolecules	Vitamin E protective; vitamin E acetate only protective after prolonged application	Conversion of vitamin E acetate into vitamin E flow	Beijersbergen van Henegouwen et al. (140) 1995
Vitamin E acetate					
Vitamin E acetate	Mouse	Skin tumor incidence and immunosuppression	No protection		Gensler et al. (151) 1996
Vitamin E succinate					
Vitamin E	Yorkshire pig	Sunburn cell formation	Protection against UVR-induced damage	Minimal protection in reducing PUVA-induced damage	Darr et al. (134) 1996
Vitamin E	Mouse	Immunosuppression and lipid peroxidation	Protective	No protection when applied after UVR exposure	Yuen et al. (108) 1997

(continued)

Table 7 Continued

Compound(s)	Species	Endpoint(s)	Efficacy	Remarks	Authors	Year
Vitamin E	Mouse	Histology (sunburn cell formation and skin thickness)	Protective		Ritter et al., 1997 (135)	
Vitamin E	Mouse	Formation of DNA photoadducts	Vitamin E derivatives less protective than vitamin E	Sunscreening properties of vitamin E	McVean et al. (10)	1997
Vitamin E acetate Vitamin E methyl ether						
Vitamin E	Mouse	Chemiluminescence after UVA exposure	Protective	β-Carotene also protective	Evelson et al. (142)	1997
Vitamin E	Mouse	Formation of DNA photoadducts in epidermal p53 gene	Protective		Chen et al. (137)	1997
Vitamin E	Mouse	Lipid peroxidation	Protective	Skin's enzymatic and non-enzymatic antioxidant capacity investigated	Lopez-Torres et al. (129)	1998
Vitamin E	Human	Erythema (skin color and skin blood flow)	Moderate protection	No protection when applied after	Dreher et al. (132,205)	1998

Vitamin E	Mouse	Formation of DNA photoadducts	Vitamin E, γ-tocopherol and δ-tocopherol protective; vitamin E acetate and vitamin E methyl ether not protective	UVR exposure; SPF (determined *in vitro*) = 1 Application as dispersion in cream	McVean et al. (138) 1999
γ-Tocopherol					
δ-Tocopherol					
Vitamin E acetate					
Vitamin E methyl ether					
Vitamin E	Mouse	Erythema, pigmentation, skin tumor incidence	Protective after prolonged application	No sign of toxicity observed for vitamin E and vitamin E succinate	Burke et al. (133) 2000
Vitamin E succinate					

Note: BHT, butylated hydroxytoluene; CPZ, chlorpromazine; MED, minimal erythema dose; 8-MOP, 8-methoxypsoralen; PUVA, 8-methoxypsoralen and UVA-treatment; SPF, sun protection factor.

demonstrating photoprotection by topical application of vitamin E in humans (131,132,146,147).

Vitamin E esters, particularly vitamin E acetate, were also shown to be promising agents in reducing UVR-induced skin damage (82,133,140,141,145, 148–150) (Table 7). However, their photoprotective effects appeared to be less pronounced as compared with vitamin E; moreover, some studies failed to detect photoprotection provided by vitamin E esters (130,138,146,151). As the free aromatic hydroxyl group is responsible for the antioxidant properties of vitamin E, vitamin E esters need to be hydrolyzed during skin absorption to show activity. Vitamin E acetate was shown to be absorbed and penetrate skin (152–154). A skin bioavailability study demonstrated that vitamin E and vitamin E acetate behave similarly with regard to penetration of rat epidermis (140). The difference between physicochemical parameters determining skin transport for vitamin E and its esters seems negligible. Notably, the bioconversion of vitamin E acetate to its active antioxidative form, α-tocopherol, was found to be slow and to occur only to a minor extent *in vivo* (140,155). As demonstrated in recent studies with viable micro-Yucatan pig skin (156,157) or viable human skin (158) *ex vivo*, vitamin E acetate was not found to be hydrolyzed in the skin penetration limiting layer, the stratum corneum. In the nucleated epidermis, however, the bioconversion of vitamin E acetate into vitamin E occurs, but seems to be dependent on formulation (156,158). Consequently, the controversial observations of photoprotective effects of topically applied vitamin E acetate may be explained by a limited bioavailability of the active, ester-cleaved form during oxidative stress at the site of action (e.g., superficial skin layers). Furthermore, photoprotection was often obtained only after several topical applications of vitamin E acetate (140,141). Some evidence exist, however, that the bioconversion of vitamin E acetate into vitamin E might be enhanced due to UVR exposure (159). UVB exposure was demonstrated to cause an increase in esterase activity in murine epidermis.

In addition to the antioxidative properties of vitamin E, further photoprotective mechanisms have been discussed. Recent studies on vitamin E, using a liposome dispersion model to estimate the photo-oxidation of biomolecules (160), or measuring DNA adduct formation *in vivo* (10), indicated that vitamin E may also have substantial sunscreening properties. On the other hand, determination of the sun protection factor (SPF) of a vitamin E lotion (2 w%) *in vitro* resulted in no significant sunscreening effect when administered at a dose of 2 mg/cm^2 (132). Different vitamin E concentrations and applied doses as well as differing experimental setups used might explain the nonconforming results regarding the determination of vitamin E's sunscreening properties. Additionally, interactions of vitamin E with the metabolism of arachidonic acid have been described. Vitamin E was shown to modulate the activity of cyclo-oxygenase and to depress the biosynthesis rate of prostaglandin E_2, possibly by inhibiting the release of arachidonic acid by phospholipase A_2 (33,161). Interactions with the eicosanoid system may result in an anti-inflammatory effect and thus complement antioxidative photoprotection in skin.

Vitamin C

Few studies have reported photoprotective effects for vitamin C (Table 8). Using a porcine skin model, Darr and associates proposed that topically applied vitamin C is effective only when formulated at high concentration in an appropriate vehicle (162). Vitamin C is unstable and is preferentially absorbed into the skin at low pH (163). Vitamin C can be protected from degradation by selecting appropriate, sophisticated vehicles such as triple emulsions (164). Hence, chemical instability and poor skin bioavailability partially explain its modest photoprotective effect when applied topically using unsuitable formulations. Furthermore, lipophilic and more stable vitamin C esters, such as its palmitatyl, succinyl, or phosphoryl ester (165–167), might be promising derivatives providing increased photoprotection, as compared with vitamin C. As described for vitamin E esters, such compounds must be hydrolyzed to vitamin C to be effective as antioxidants.

Other Antioxidants

Besides vitamin E and vitamin C, several other compounds with antioxidative potential have been suggested to lower photodamage when topically applied (Table 9). Administration of different plant, vegetable, or fruit extracts were reported to diminish acute and chronic skin damage after UVR exposure (168–175). Such extracts may contain flavonoids (e.g., apigenin, catechin, epicatechin, α-glycosylrutin, and silymarin). Flavonoids are polyphenolic compounds and exhibit antioxidative capacity because of their free phenolic groups. Green tea extracts contain such polyphenolic compounds and were shown to inhibit UVR-induced skin tumorigenesis in different animal models after topical treatment (176,177). Furthermore, topical application of ($-$)-epigallocatachin-3-gallate, the major polyphenolic green tea constituent, before UVB exposure, significantly decreased UVB-induced erythema in humans (178). Flavonoids have been shown to modulate biochemical pathways involved in inflammatory responses as well as UVR-induced inflammatory markers of skin inflammation (176,177,179). The observed photoprotective effect of topical flavonoids may thus be partially attributed to their anti-inflammatory properties.

Thiols, such as N-acetyl-cysteine and derivatives, are another important group of potent radical scavengers (180,181). It was demonstrated in several rat studies that topical administration of thiols diminishes UVA-induced binding of photosensitizers to epidermal lipids and DNA (182,183) and affords some protection against the damaging effects of UVB on epidermal DNA (184). Treatment with cysteine derivatives, like N-acetyl-cysteine, resulted in increased intracellular GSH levels in human keratinocytes (185). Thus, thiol-induced stimulation of GSH biosynthesis might be a key mechanism accounting for the observed photoprotective effects. However, this mechanism is currently debated, as it was lately shown in mice that the antioxidant effect of N-acetyl-cysteine itself seems sufficient to provide protection against UVB

Table 8 Photoprotective Effects of Topically Applied Vitamin C (Ascorbic Acid) and Derivatives *In Vivo*

Compound(s)	Species	Endpoint(s)	Efficacy	Remarks	Authors	Year
Vitamin C	Mouse	Skin wrinkling and sagging, skin tumor incidence, and histology	Vitamin C plamitate less protective than vitamin C; no protection against UVA-induced skin sagging		Bissett et al. (145)	1990
Vitamin C palmitate						
Vitamin C	Yorkshire pig	Erythema (skin blood flow) and sunburn cell formation	Protection against UVR- and PUVA-induced damage	High vitamin C concentration	Darr et al. (162)	1992
Vitamin C	Mouse	Skin wrinkling, skin tumor incidence, and histology	Protective	Additive protection in combination with anti-inflammatory agents	Bissett et al. (143)	1992
Vitamin C	Human	Erythema (skin color)	Poor protection when applied occlusively after UVR exposure	No protection when applied occlusively before UVR exposure	Montenegro et al. (204)	1995
Vitamin C palmitate	Yorkshire pig	Sunburn cell formation	No protection against UVR-induced damage, protective against PUVA-induced damage	Additive protection in combination with sunscreens	Darr et al. (134)	1996
Vitamin C	Human	Erythema (skin color and skin blood flow)	Poor protection	SPF (determined *in vitro*) = 1	Dreher et al. (132)	1998

Note: For abbreviations see Table 7.

Table 9 Photoprotective Effects of Topically Applied Plant Extracts, Flavonoids, N-Acetyl-cysteine and Derivatives, and other Antioxidants In Vivo

Compound(s)	Species	Endpoint(s)	Efficacy	Remarks	Authors	Year
Green tea extract	Mouse	Skin tumor incidence	Protective	Green tea contains catechin and epicatechin derivatives	Wang et al. (168)	1991
Polypodium leucotomos (tropical fern) extract	Guinea pigs, human	Erythema (skin color)	Protection against UVR- and PUVA-induced damage	Extract with immunomodulating properties	González et al. (169)	1996
Polypodium leucotomos (tropical fern) extract	Human	Erythema (MED), immediate pigment darkening, delayed tanning, minimal phototoxic dose and histology	Protection against UVR- and PUVA-induced damage		González et al. (170)	1997
Epigallocatechin-3-gallate	Mouse	Skin tumor incidence	Protective	Not immunosuppressive; isolated from green tea	Gensler et al. (171)	1996
Apigenin	Mouse	Skin tumor incidence	Protective		Birt et al. (172)	1997
Silymarin	Mouse	Edema, sunburn and apoptotic cell formation, and skin tumor incidence	Protective	Isolated from milk thistle plant	Katiyar et al. (173)	1997

(continued)

Table 9 Continued

Compound(s)	Species	Endpoint(s)	Efficacy	Remarks	Authors	Year
Epigallocatechin-3-gallate	Human	Erythema (skin color)	Protective	Epigallocatechin-3-gallate without UVB-sunscreening properties; reduced leukocyte infiltration and myeloperoxidase activity observed	Katiyar et al. (178)	1999
Epigallocatechin-3-gallate	Mouse	Production of H_2O_2 and NO	Protective	Reduced leukocyte infiltration, myeloperoxidase activity, and number of antigen-presenting cells observed	Katiyar et al. (177)	2001
Resveratrol	Mouse	Lipid peroxidation and edema	Protective	Resveratrol (*trans*-3,4′,5-trihydroxystilbene) is found in grapes, nuts, fruits, and red wine; with anti-inflammatory and antiproliferative properties	Afaq et al. (175)	2003

Caffeic acid	Human	Erythema (skin color)	Protective, ferulic acid more protective than caffeic acid	Caffeic and ferulic acids represent hydroxycinnamic acids; ferulic acid with UV-absorbing properties	Saija et al. (174) 2000
Ferulic acid					
N-acetyl-cysteine	Rat	UVA-induced binding of 8-MOP and CPZ to epidermal biomacromolecules	N-acetyl-cysteine and captopril most protective thiols	Vitamin E less protective	Van den Broeke et al. (183) 1993
Captopril					
Other thiols					
N-acetyl-cysteine	Rat	DNA synthesis rate	Protective		Van den Broeke et al. (184) 1994
N-acetyl-cysteine	Rat	UVA-induced binding of 8-MOP and CPZ to epidermal biomacromolecules	Protective	High epidermal bioavailability of N-acetyl-cysteine	Van den Broeke et al. (182) 1995
Several cysteine derivatives					
Melatonin	Human	Erythema (skin color)	Protective	Also protective when applied after UVR exposure	Bangha et al. (223) 1996

(continued)

Table 9 Continued

Compound(s)	Species	Endpoint(s)	Efficacy	Remarks	Authors	Year
Melatonin	Human	Erythema (skin color)	Protective	No protection when applied after UVR irradiation; melatonin without sunscreening properties	Bangha et al. (191)	1997
Melatonin	Human	Erythema (skin color and skin blood flow)	Protective	No protection when applied after UVR irradiation; melatonin with sunscreening properties	Dreher et al. (132,205)	1998
Melatonin	Human	Erythema (skin color)	Protective	No protection when applied after UVR irradiation	Fischer et al. (230)	1999

Antioxidant Defense Systems

Compound	Species	Endpoint	Result	Notes	Reference	Year
Superoxide dismutase	Guinea pig	PUVA-induced erythema and edema	Protective	β-Carotene also protective; vitamin E, vitamin E acetate, and GSH not protective	Carraro et al. (195)	1988
Superoxide dismutase	Guinea pig	Erythema	Not protective		Hamanaka et al. (198)	1990
Superoxide dismutase	Human	Erythema (skin color)	Protective when applied occlusively after UVR exposure	No protection when applied occlusively before UVR exposure	Montenegro et al. (204)	1995
Superoxide dismutase	Mice, Human	PUVA-induced erythema and edema	Protective	Prolonged pretreatment	Alaoui et al. (196)	1994
					Filipe et al. (197)	1997
2,4-Hexadienol	Mouse	Skin wrinkling and sagging, and skin tumor incidence	Protective, not protective against UVA-induced skin sagging	Also other conjugated dienes tested	Bissett et al. (224)	1990

Note: For abbreviations see Table 7.

immunosuppression, independently of GSH synthesis (186). Exogenously applied GSH penetrates the cell membrane and the skin only poorly and does not prevent photodamage in mice when applied topically (145) or injected intraperitoneally (187).

A photoprotective effect for the redox couple α-lipoate/dihydrolipoate (also referred to as "α-lipoic acid") has been proposed for skin (188). Dihydrolipoate, the reduced form of lipoic acid, is a reductant with a more negative redox potential (-0.32 V for the couple lipoate/dihydrolipoate) than ascorbate (0.08 V for the couple dehydroascorbate/ascorbate), which is able to regenerate ascorbate from its oxidation products (Fig. 2). In liposomes irradiated with solar-simulated UV light, dihydrolipoate in combination with ascorbate was shown to strongly enhance the recycling of α-tocopherol (52). It was demonstrated in hairless mice that α-lipoate readily penetrates skin and thereafter is reduced to its more potent antioxidant form, dihydrolipoate (189). In addition, α-lipoic acid was reduced to dihydrolipoate and significantly protected against UVA-induced loss of lipid-soluble antioxidant in human keratinocytes (190). Furthermore, Fuchs et al. reported anti-inflammatory properties of dihydrolipoate in dermatitis induced by reactive oxidants in hairless mice (188).

Regarding the pineal hormone melatonin (N-acetyl-5-methoxytryptamine), suppression of UVR-induced erythema by topical melatonin in humans was reported (191). Besides melatonin's antioxidant (192) and dose-dependent sunscreening properties (132,191), it might also act in an immuno-modulatory way (193,194). It remains to be elucidated to what degree antioxidant mechanisms, or rather the known UVB absorbing properties, of melatonin account for to the moderate inhibition erythema formation *in vivo*. Photoprotective effects were also reported for topical application of several other substances with antioxidant properties. Interestingly, topical administration of SOD resulted in reduction of PUVA-induced skin reactions after single application in guinea pigs (195), or after prolonged pretreatment of murine (196) and human skins (197). In contrast, Hamanaka and associates did not observe significantly lowered UVB-induced erythema reaction after topical administration of SOD in guinea pigs (198). However, they demonstrated that while cutaneous SOD activity was decreased in nontreated control animals after UVB exposure, topical SOD diminished this decrease in activity. Owing to its high molecular weight, SOD is unlikely to significantly penetrate into deeper skin layers. Yet, it was shown to be capable of inhibiting PUVA-induced erythema, which suggests that oxidative processes initiated at the skin surface may induce an inflammatory response in lower skin layers (127,196).

Antioxidant Combinations

The cutaneous antioxidant system is complex and far from completely understood. As pointed out, the system is interlinked and operates as an antioxidant network (Fig. 2). Thus, an enhanced photoprotective effect may be obtained by applying appropriate combinations of antioxidants (Table 10). As was shown

Table 10 Photoprotective Effects of Topically Applied Antioxidant Combinations *In Vivo*

Compounds	Species	Endpoint(s)	Efficacy	Remarks	Authors	Year
Vitamins E and C, BHT, and GSH	Mouse	Erythema (MED)	Protective	BHT alone also protective	De Rios et al. (225)	1978
Vitamins E and C	Yorkshire pig	Sunburn cell formation	Protective	Maximal protection in combination with sunscreens	Darr et al. (134)	1996
Vitamin E acetate and α-glycosylrutin	Human	Chemiluminescence and reflection spectrometry of experimentally provoked polymorphous light eruption	Protective	Polymorphous light eruption induced by UVA radiation	Hadshiew et al. (199)	1997
Vitamin E acetate, α-glycosylrutin, and ferulic acid						
Vitamins E and C	Human	Erythema (skin color and skin blood flow)	Protective; maximal protection when vitamins E and C are combined with melatonin	No protection when administered after UVR exposure; melatonin with sunscreening properties	Dreher et al. (132,205)	1998
Vitamins E and C and melatonin						

(continued)

Table 10 Continued

Compounds	Species	Endpoint(s)	Efficacy	Remarks	Authors	Year
Vitamin E linoleate, magnesium ascorbyl phosphate, BHT, nordihydroguaradinic acid	Mouse	Sunburn cell formation	Protective after prolonged application	Antioxidants formulated as oil-in-water emulsion possessing no detectable UVR absorbance	Muizzuddin et al. (226)	1998
Vitamin E linoleate, magnesium ascorbyl phosphate, BHT, nordihydroguaradinic acid	Human	Erythema (MED) and immediate pigment darkening	Protective after single application	Antioxidants formulated as oil-in-water emulsion possessing no detectable UVR absorbance	Muizzuddin et al. (227)	1999
Vitamin E acetate, magnesium ascorbyl phosphate, green tea extract, BHT	Human	Lipid peroxidation in extracted stratum corneum lipids	Protective after prolonged application	Antioxidants formulated in standard cosmetic vehicle	Pelle et al. (228)	1999
Vitamins E and C	Mouse	Erythema, tanning, and immunosuppression	Protective	Study duration 15 days	Quevedo et al. (229)	2000

Note: For abbreviations see Table 7.

in a human study by Dreher and coworkers, application of vitamin C or vitamin E alone resulted in modestly decreased erythema reaction (132). However, a much more pronounced effect was obtained by combining these two vitamins. Notably, the most dramatic improvement resulted from the coformulation of melatonin together with vitamin E and vitamin C. Studying the effect of distinct mixtures of topically applied antioxidants in photodermatoses, Hadshiew and associates demonstrated that the development and severity of polymorphous light eruption were significantly reduced by administration of a combination consisting of α-glycosylrutin, ferulic acid, and tocopheryl acetate (199). The authors hypothesized that a sunscreening effect of the substances employed was negligible, and that the photoprotective observed was due to reduction of UVA-induced oxidative stress. Another human study demonstrated that 5% vitamin E linoleate combined with 1% magnesium ascorbyl phosphate incorporated into an oil-in-water emulsion, containing also 0.03% butylated hydroxytoluene as well as 0.01% nordihydroguaradinic acid, significantly reduced UVR-induced erythema.

Furthermore, topically applied vitamin E and/or vitamin C efficiently protected against UVB radiation (200) as well as simulated solar radiation-induced (201) lipid peroxidation in the presence of polyunsaturated fatty acids, such as eicosapentaenoic acid (C20:5), as was shown using pig skin *ex vivo* as a skin model for assessing short-term biochemical effects related to UVR. Eicosapentaenoic acid is also known to reduce or prevent UVB radiation-induced immunosuppression when applied topically in mice (202) and to reduce sensitivity to UVB radiation-induced erythema when taken as dietary fish-oil supplementation in humans (203).

Topical Application of Antioxidants after UVR Exposure

Though the photoprotective effect of topical antioxidants applied before UVR exposure has been recognized, the effect of these compounds administered after irradiation is less obvious (Tables 7–10). Diminished erythema formation was reported when antioxidants, such as α-tocopherol or α-tocopherol acetate, were topically administered after UVR exposure (130,149,150,204). However, these findings are in contrast to other studies that found no diminished UVR-related skin damage when antioxidants were applied after the irradiation (108,146,191). As was shown in a human study, neither vitamin E, vitamin C, nor melatonin, nor combinations thereof, led to a significantly lowered erythema formation when administered after UVB exposure (205). Therefore it seems that UVR-induced ROS formation and the subsequent reaction of ROS with skin biomolecules lead to acute skin damage, which is a very rapid process. As antioxidants applied after irradiation possibly do not reach the site of action (e.g., superficial skin layers) in relevant amounts during occurrence of oxidative stress, they do not significantly reduce UVR-induced erythema formation as compared with their vehicles. Possibly, such skin damage may be more efficiently treated at an inflammatory level by classical anti-inflammatory drugs.

Topical Application of Substances Other than Conventional Antioxidants

Apart from antioxidants, which increase the skin's antioxidant capacity by topical application, other substances may serve to enhance the antioxidative capacity by preventing the formation of ROS or by increasing the formation, stability, or activity of constitutive skin antioxidants. Skin contains substantial amounts of iron, and chronic exposure to UVR was shown to increase the skin levels of nonheme iron (206). Iron participates as a catalyst in the formation of the highly damaging hydroxyl radical (15). Hence, topical application of certain iron chelators, such as 2-furildioxime, was demonstrated to be efficient in providing photoprotection alone (207) or in combination with sunscreens (208). Furthermore, a possible role of 1,25-dihydroxy-vitamin D_3-induced formation of metallothionein in cutaneous photoprotection was reported; Hanada and coworkers found a significantly lowered level of sunburn cell formation in mouse skin after UVB exposure, by topical application of the active form of vitamin D_3 (209). The authors postulated that the cysteine-rich metallothionein may act as radical scavenger. Supplementation with selenium is a further interesting approach in reducing UVR-induced skin damage. Selenium is an essential trace element in humans and animals and is the required constituent for GSH-Px. Applying topical selenium in the form of L-selenomethionine proved to reduce acute and/or chronic skin damage in mice (210), as well as in humans (211). Topical application of L-selenomethionine led to increased skin selenium levels, whereas free selenium was apparently not absorbed (212,213). In addition, zinc's supporting role as antioxidant in providing photoprotection for skin was recently reported after topical application (214).

SUMMARY AND CONCLUSION

Animal and human studies have convincingly demonstrated significant photoprotective effects of natural and synthetic antioxidants when applied topically before UVA and UVB exposure. However, particularly with respect to UVB-induced skin damage, the photoprotective effects of most antioxidants were modest, as compared with sunscreens. More successful in preventing such damage were appropriate combinations of antioxidants resulting in a sustained antioxidant capacity of the skin, possibly due to antioxidant synergisms. On the other hand, regarding photoprotective effects against UVA-induced skin alterations, which are largely determined by oxidative processes, topical administration of antioxidants might be particularly promising. In fact, topical application of antioxidants resulted in a remarkable reduction of UVA-induced ROS generation in mice, and diminished UVA-induced polymorphous light eruption in humans. Furthermore, topical application of antioxidants, particularly of vitamin C, was reported to diminish PUVA-induced erythema and sunburn cell formation.

As UVA- and UVB-induced skin damage is not solely dependent on ROS formation and their reaction with numerous skin biomolecules, topical (as well as systemic) antioxidant supplementation cannot be presumed to give complete photoprotection. Other ROS-independent processes, such as DNA dimer formation, will persist causing skin damage, regardless of the effectiveness of the antioxidants administered. Therefore, efficient sunscreens are indispensable in the effective prevention of skin photodamage. However, antioxidants, in combination with sunscreens or other photodamage-reducing agents, seem to be highly effective adjuncts increasing the safety and the efficacy of photoprotective topical products.

ACKNOWLEDGMENTS

This work was supported by a grant from the Deutsche Forschungsgemeinschaft (Th 620/2-2).

REFERENCES

1. Thiele JJ, Podda M, Packer L. Tropospheric ozone: an emerging environmental stress to skin. Biol Chem 1997; 378:1299–1305.
2. Briviba K, Sies H. Nonenzymatic antioxidant defense systems. In: Frei B, ed. Natural Antioxidants in Human Health and Disease. New York: Academic Press, 1994.
3. Sies H. Introductory remarks. In: Sies H, ed. Oxidative Stress. Orlando, FL: Academic Press, 1985:1–7.
4. Sies H. Biochemie des oxidativen Streß. Angew. Chem 1986; 98:1061–1075.
5. Thiele JJ, Traber MG, Polefka TG, Cross CE, Packer LP. Ozone exposure depletes vitamin E and induces lipid peroxidation in murine stratum corneum. J Invest Dermatol 1997; 108(5):753–757.
6. Thiele JJ, Traber MG, Packer L. Depletion of human stratum corneum vitamin E: an early and sensitive *in vivo* marker of UV-induced photooxidation. J Invest Dermatol 1998; 110(5):756–761.
7. Thiele JJ, Traber MG, Tsang KG, Cross CE, Packer L. *In vivo* exposure to ozone depletes vitamins C and E and induces lipid peroxidation in epidermal layers of murine skin. Free Radical Biol Med 1997; 23(3):385–391.
8. Thiele JJ, Traber MG, Re R et al. Macromolecular carbonyls in human stratum corneum: a biomarker for environmental oxidant exposure? FEBS Lett 1998; 422:403–406.
9. Beehler BC, Przybyszewski J, Box HB, Kulesz-Martin MF. Formation of 8-hydroxydeoxyguanosine within DNA of mouse keratinocytes exposed in culture to UV-B and hydrogen peroxide. Carcinogenesis 1992; 13(11):2003–2007.
10. McVean M, Liebler DC. Inhibition of UVB induced DNA photodamage in mouse epidermis by topically applied alpha-tocopherol. Carcinogenesis 1997; 18(8):1617–1622.
11. Englard S, Seifter S. The biochemical functions of ascorbic acid. Annu Rev Nutr 1986; 6:365–406.
12. Frei B, Stocker R, Ames BN. Antioxidant defenses and lipid peroxidation in human blood plasma. Proc Natl Acad Sci USA 1988; 85(24):9748–9752.

13. Niki E, Tsuchiya J, Tanimura R, Kamiya Y. Regeneration of vitamin E from alpha chromanoxyl radical by glutathione and vitamin C. Chem Lett 1982; 13(6):789–792.
14. Packer JE, Slater TF, Willson RL. Direct observation of a free radical interaction between vitamin E and vitamin C. Nature 1979; 278(5706):737–738.
15. Halliwell B, Gutteridge JMC. Free Radicals in Biology and Medicine. 2nd ed. Oxford: Clarendon Press, 1989.
16. Halliwell B. How to characterize a biological antioxidant. Free Radical Res Commun 1990; 9:1–32.
17. Shindo Y, Witt E, Packer L. Antioxidant defense mechanisms in murine epidermis and dermis and their responses to ultraviolet light. J Invest Dermatol 1993; 100(3):260–265.
18. Shindo Y, Witt E, Han D, Epstein W, Packer L. Enzymic and non-enzymic antioxidants in epidermis and dermis of human skin. J Invest Dermatol 1994; 102(1):122–124.
19. Davidson JM, Luvalle PA, Zoia O, Quaglino D, Jr., Giro M. Ascorbate differentially regulates elastin and collagen biosynthesis in vascular smooth muscle cells and skin fibroblasts by pretranslational mechanisms. J Biol Chem 1997; 272(1):345–352.
20. Ponec M, Weerheim A, Kempenaar J et al. The formation of competent barrier lipids in reconstructed human epidermis requires the presence of vitamin C. J Invest Dermatol 1997; 109(3):348–355.
21. Witschi A, Reddy S, Stofer B, Lautenberg BH. The systemic availabilty of oral glutathione. Eur J Clin Pharmacol 1992; 43:667–669.
22. Meister A, Anderson ME. Glutathione. Annu Rev Biochem 1983; 52:711–760.
23. Akerboom TPM, Sies H. Assay of glutathione, glutathione disulfide, and glutathione mixed disulfides in biological samples. In: Jakoby W, ed. Detoxication and Drug Metabolism: Conjugation and Related Systems. Vol. 77. New York: Academic Press, 1981:373–382.
24. Jain A, Martensson J, Mehta T, Krauss AN, Auld PA, Meister A. Ascorbic acid prevents oxidative stress in glutathione-deficient mice: effects on lung type 2 cell lamellar bodies, lung surfactant, and skeletal muscle. Proc Natl Acad Sci USA 1992; 89(11):5093–5097.
25. Martensson J, Meister A. Glutathione deficiency increases hepatic ascorbic acid synthesis in adult mice. Proc Natl Acad Sci USA 1992; 89(23):11566–11568.
26. Rahman I, Clerch LB, Massaro D. Rat lung antioxidant enzyme induction by ozone. Am J Physiol 1991; 260(6 Pt 1):L412–L418.
27. Fuchs J, Huflejt ME, Rothfuss LM, Wilson DS, Carcamo G, Packer L. Impairment of enzymic and nonenzymic antioxidants in skin by UVB irradiation. J Invest Dermatol 1989; 93(6):769–773.
28. Ames BN, Cathcart R, Schwiers E, Hochstein P. Uric acid provides an antioxidant defense in humans against oxidant- and radical-caused aging and cancer: a hypothesis. Proc Natl Acad Sci USA 1981; 78:6858–6862.
29. Wagner DK, Collins-Lech C, Sohnle P. Inhibition of neutrophile killing of *Candida albicans* pseudohyphae by substances which quench hypochlorous acid. Infect Immunol 1986; 51:731–736.
30. Sevenian A, Davies KJA, Hochstein P. Serum urate as an antioxidant for ascorbic acid. Am J Clin Nutr 1991; 54:1129–1134.
31. Grootveldt M, Halliwell B. Measurement of allantoin and uric acid in human body fluids. J Biochem 1987; 243:803–808.

32. Lopez-Torres M, Shindo Y, Packer L. Effect of age on antioxidants and molecular markers of oxidative damage in murine epidermis and dermis. J Invest Dermatol 1994; 102(4):476–480.
33. Traber MG, Sies H. Vitamin E in humans—demand and delivery. Annu Rev Nutr 1996; 16:321–347.
34. Sies H, Stahl W, Sundquist AR. Antioxidant functions of vitamins. Ann NY Acad Sci 1992; 669:7–20.
35. De Groot H, Hegi U, Sies H. Loss of alpha-tocopherol upon exposure to nitric oxide or the sydnonimine SIN-1. FEBS Lett 1993; 315:139–142.
36. Kamal-Eldin A, Appelqvist LA. The chemistry and antioxidant properties of tocopherols and tocotrienols. Lipids 1996; 31:671–701.
37. Stoyanovsky DA, Osipov AN, Quinn PJ, Kagan VE. Ubiquinone-dependent recycling of vitamin E radicals by superoxide. Arch Biochem Biophys 1995; 323(2):343–351.
38. Cillard J, Cillard P, Cormier M. Effect of experimental factors on the prooxidant behaviour of α-tocopherol. Am J Oil Chem Soc 1980; 57:255–261.
39. Husain SR, Cillard J, Cillard P. Alpha-tocopherol, prooxidant effect and malondialdehyde production. J Am Oil Chem Soc 1987; 64:109–111.
40. Sustry PC, Jayaraman J, Ramasarma T. Distribution of coenzyme Q in rat liver cell fractions. Nature 1961; 189:577–580.
41. Mellors A, Tappel AL. The inhibition of mitochondrial peroxidation by ubiquinone and ubiquinol. J Biol Chem 1966; 241:4353–4356.
42. Gutman M. Electron flux through the mitochondrial ubiquinone. Biochim Biophys Acta 1980; 594:53–84.
43. Cabrini L, Pasquali P, Tadolini B, Sechi AM, Landi L. Antioxiant behaviour of ubiquinone and beta-carotene incorporated in model membranes. Free Radical Res Commun 1986; 2:85–92.
44. Ingold KU, Bowry VW, Stocker R, Walling C. Autoxidation of lipids and antioxidants by alpha-tocopherol and ubiquinol in homogenous solution and in aqeous dispersion of lipids: unrecognized consequences of lipid particle size as exemplified by oxidation of human low density lipoprotein. Proc Natl Sci USA 1993; 90:45–49.
45. Aberg F, Appelkvist EL, Dallner G, Ernster L. Distribution and redox state of ubiquinones in rat and human tissues. Arch Biochem Biophys 1992; 295(2):230–234.
46. Romiu I, Stampfer MJ, Stryker WS, Hernandez M, Kaplan L. Food predictors of plasma beta-carotene and alpha-tocopherol: validation of a food frequency questionaire. Am J Epidemiol 1990; 131:864–876.
47. Fuchs J. Oxidative Injury in Dermatopathology. Berlin, Heidelberg, New York: Springer, 1992.
48. Sies H. Strategies of antioxidant defense. Eur J Biochem 1993; 215:213–219.
49. Krinsky NI. Antioxidant functions of carotenoids. Free Radical Biol Med 1989; 7:617–635.
50. Mayne ST, Parker RS. Antioxidant activity of dietary canthaxantine. Nutr Cancer 1989; 12:225–236.
51. Samokyszyn VM, Marnett LJ. Inhibition of liver microsomal lipid peroxidation by 13-*cis*-retinoic acid. Free Radical Biol Med 1990; 8:491–496.
52. Kagan V, Witt E, Goldman R, Scita G, Packer L. Ultraviolet light-induced generation of vitamin E radicals and their recycling. A possible photosensitizing effect of vitamin E in skin. Free Radical Res Commun 1992; 16(1):51–64.

53. Vahlquist A, Lee JB, Michaelsson G, Rollman O. Vitamin A in human skin. II: concentrations of carotene, retinol, and dehydroretinol in various components of normal skin. J Invest Dermatol 1982; 79:94–97.
54. Stahl W, Heinrich U, Jungmann H et al. Increased dermal carotenoid levels assessed by noninvasive reflection spectrophotometry correlate with serum levels in women ingesting betatene. J Nutr 1998; 28(5):903–907.
55. Ribaya-Mercado JD, Garmyn M, Gilchrest BA, Russell RM. Skin lycopene is destroyed preferentially over beta-carotene during ultraviolet irradiation in humans. J Nutr 1995; 125(7):1854–1859.
56. Törmä H, Vahlquist A. Vitamin A uptake by human skin *in vitro*. Arch Dermatol Res 1984; 276:390–395.
57. Flohe L, Schlegel W. Glutathion peroxidase IV. Intrazelluläre Verteilung des Gluthation-Peroxidase-Systems in der Rattenleber. Hoppe-Seyler's Z Physiol Chem 1971; 352:1401–1410.
58. Zakowski JJ, Forstrom JW, Condell RA, Tappel AL. Attachment of selenocysteine in the catalytic site of glutathione peroxidase. Biochem Biophys Res Commun 1978; 84:248–253.
59. Sies H, Cadenas E. Biological basis of detoxification of oxygen free radicals. In: Caldwell J, Jacoby WB, eds. Biological Basis of Detoxification. New York: Academic Press, 1983:181–211.
60. Fridovich I. The biology of oxygen radicals. Science 1978; 201:875–880.
61. Strange R, Lear J, Fryer A. Polymorphism in glutathione S-transferase loci as a risk factor for common cancers. Arch Toxicol Suppl 1998; 20:419–428.
62. Kerb R, Brockmoller J, Reum T, Roots I. Deficiency of glutathione S-transferases T1 and M1 as heritable factors of increased cutaneous UV sensitivity. J Invest Dermatol 1997; 108:229–232.
63. Henderson C, Smith A, Ure J, Brown K, Bacon E, Wolf C. Increased skin tumorigenesis in mice lacking pi class glutathione S-transferases. Proc Natl Acad Sci USA 1998; 95(9):5275–5280.
64. Blacker K, Olson E, Vessey DA. Characterization of glutathione-S-transferase in cultured human keratinocytes. J Invest Dermatol 1991; 97:442–446.
65. Wheeler LA, Aswad A, Connor MJ, Lowe M. Depletion of cutaneous glutathione and the induction of inflammation by 8-methoxypsoralen plus UVA radiation. J Invest Dermatol 1986; 87:658–662.
66. Connor MJ, Wheeler LA. Depletion of cutaneous glutathione by ultraviolet radiation. Photochem Photobiol 1987; 47:239–245.
67. Moral A, Palou J, Lafuente A et al. Immunohistochemical study of alpha, mu and pi class glutathione S-transferase expression in malignant melanoma. Br J Dermatol 1997; 136(3):345–350.
68. Fridovich I. Superoxide dismutases. Annu Rev Biochem 1975; 44:147–159.
69. Marklund SL. Properties of extracellular superoxide dismutase from human lung. J Biochem 1984; 220:269–272.
70. Thiele JJ, Lodge JK, Choi JH, Packer L. Measurements of antioxidants in cutaneous tissues. In: Sternberg H, Timiras PS, eds. Studies of Aging-Springer Lab Manual. Heidelberg: Springer-Verlag, 1999:15–33.
71. Sugiura K, Ueda H, Hirano K, Adachi T. Studies on superoxide dismutase in human skin. 2: Contents of superoxide dismutase and lipoperoxide in normal human skin. Jpn J Dermatol 1985; 95:1541–1545.

72. Ohkuma N, Izka H, Mizumoto T, Ohkawara A. Superoxide dismutase in epidermis: its relation to keratinocyte proliferation. In: Hayaishi O, Immamura S, Miyachi Y, eds. The Biological Role of Reactive Oxygen Species in Skin. New York: Elsevier, 1987:231–237.
73. Kirkman HN, Gaetani GF. Catalase: a tetrameric enzyme with four tightly bound molecules of NADPH. Proc Natl Acad Sci USA 1984; 81:4343–4347.
74. Sander CS, Chang H, Salzmann S et al. Photoaging is associated with protein oxidation in human skin *in vivo*. J Invest Dermatol 2002; 118(4):618–625.
75. Hellemans L, Corstjens H, Neven A, Declercq L, Maes D. Antioxidant enzyme activity in human stratum corneum shows seasonal variation with an age-dependent recovery. J Invest Dermatol 2003; 120(3):434–439.
76. Solanki V, Rana RS, Slaga TJ. Diminution of mouse epidermal superoxide dismutase and catalase activities by tumor promotors. Carcinogenesis 1982; 2:1141–1146.
77. Wlaschek M, Briviba K, Stricklin GP, Sies H, Scharffetter-Kochanek K. Singlet oxygen may mediate the ultraviolet A-induced synthesis of interstitial collagenase. J Invest Dermatol 1995; 104(2):194–198.
78. Grether-Beck S, Olaizola-Horn S, Schmitt H et al. Activation of transcription factor AP-2 mediates UVA radiation- and singlet oxygen-induced expression of the human intercellular adhesion molecule 1 gene. Proc Natl Acad Sci USA 1996; 93(25):14586–14591.
79. Nishi J, Ogura R, Sugiyama M, Hidaka T, Kohno M. Involvement of active oxygen in lipid peroxide radical reaction of epidermal homogenate following ultraviolet light exposure. J Invest Dermatol 1991; 97(1):115–119.
80. Kitazawa M, Podda M, Thiele JJ, et al. Interactions between vitamin E homologues and ascorbate free radicals in murine skin homogenates irradiated with ultraviolet light. Photochem Photobiol 1997; 65(2):355–365.
81. Jurkiewicz BA, Buettner GR. EPR detection of free radicals in UV-irradiated skin: mouse versus human. Photochem Photobiol 1996; 64(6):918–935.
82. Jurkiewicz BA, Bissett DL, Buettner GR. Effect of topically applied tocopherol on ultraviolet radiation-mediated free radical damage in skin. J Invest Dermatol 1995; 104(4):484–488.
83. Shindo Y, Witt E, Han D, Packer L. Dose-response effects of acute ultraviolet irradiation on antioxidants and molecular markers of oxidation in murine epidermis and dermis. J Invest Dermatol 1994; 102(4):470–475.
84. Finlayson BJ, Pitts JN. Photochemistry of the polluted troposphere. Science 1976; 192:111–119.
85. Mustafa MG. Biochemical basis of ozone toxicity. Free Radical Biol Med 1990; 9(3):245–265.
86. Koren HS, Devlin RB, Graham DE et al. Ozone-induced inflammation in the lower airways of human subjects. Am Rev Respir Dis 1989; 139:407–415.
87. Kerr HD, Kulle TJ, McIlhany ML, Swidersky P. Effects of ozone on pulmonary function in normal subjects. Am Rev Respir Dis 1975; 111:763–773.
88. Schelegle ES, Stefkin AD, McDonald RJ. Time course of ozone-induced neutrophilia in normal humans. Am Rev Respir Dis 1991; 143:1253–1358.
89. Whiteside C, Hassan HM. Role of oxy radicals in the inactivation of catalase by ozone. Free Radical Biol Med 1988; 5(5–6):305–312.
90. Hewitt CN, Kok GL, Fall R. Hydroperoxides in plants exposed to ozone mediate air pollution damage to alkene emitters. Nature 1990; 344(6261):56–58.

91. Pryor WA, Church DF. Aldehydes, hydrogen peroxide, and organic radicals as mediators of ozone toxicity. Free Radical Biol Med 1991; 11(1):41–46.
92. Kanofsky JR, Sima PD. Singlet oxygen generation from the reaction of ozone with plant leaves. J Biol Chem 1995; 270(14):7850–7852.
93. Menzel DB. Ozone: an overview of its toxicity in man and animals. J Toxicol Environ Health 1984; 13:183–204.
94. Lippmann M. Health effects of ozone. A critical review. J Air Pollut Control Assoc 1989; 39(5):672–695.
95. Runeckles VC. The impact of UV-B radiation and ozone on terrestrial vegetation. Environ Pollut 1994; 83:191–213.
96. Foyer CH, Lelendais M, Kunert KJ. Photooxidative stress in plants. Physiol Plantarum 1994; 92:696–717.
97. Polle A, Rennenberg H. Significance of antioxidants in plant adaptation to environmental stress. In: Fowden L, Mansfield T, Stoddard J, eds. Plant Adaptation to Environmental Stress. New York: Chapman & Hall, 1993:263–273.
98. Schraudner M, Langebartels C, Sandermann J. Plant defence systems and ozone. Biochem Soc Trans 1996; 24:456–461.
99. Thiele JJ, Traber MG, Podda M, Tsang K, Cross CE, Packer L. Ozone depletes tocopherols and tocotrienols topically applied to murine skin. FEBS Lett 1997; 401:167–170.
100. Rao MV, Ormrod DP. Impact of UVB and O_3 on the oxygen free radical scavenging system in *Arabidopsis thaliana* genotypes differing in flavonoid biosynthesis. Photochem Photobiol 1995; 62(4):719–726.
101. Podda M, Traber MG, Weber C, Yan LJ, Packer L. UV-irradiation depletes antioxidants and causes oxidative damage in a model of human skin. Free Radical Biol Med 1998; 24:55–65.
102. Shindo Y, Witt E, Han D et al. Recovery of antioxidants and reduction in lipid hydroperoxides in murine epidermis and dermis after acute ultraviolet radiation exposure. Photodermatol Photoimmunol Photomed 1994; 10(5):183–191.
103. Fuchs J, Huflejt ME, Rothfuss LM, Wilson DS, Carcamo G, Packer L. Acute effects of near ultraviolet and visible light on the cutaneous antioxidant defense system. Photochem Photobiol 1989; 50(6):739–744.
104. Basu-Modak S, Luescher P, Tyrrell RM. Lipid metabolite involvement in the activation of the human heme oxygenase-1 gene. Free Radical Biol Med 1996; 20(7):887–897.
105. Weber C, Podda M, Rallis M, Thiele JJ, Traber MG, Packer L. Efficacy of topically applied tocopherols and tocotrienols in protection of murine skin from oxidative damage induced by UV-irradiation. Free Radical Biol Med 1997; 22(5):761–769.
106. Weber SU, Thiele JJ, Cross CE, Packer L. Vitamin C, uric acid and glutathione gradients in murine stratum corneum and their susceptibility to ozone exposure. J Invest Dermatol 1999; 113(6):1128–1132.
107. Baxter JG, Robeson CD, Taylor JD, Lehman RW. Natural alpha, beta, and gamma-tocopherols and certain esters of physiological interest. J Am Chem Soc 1943; 65:918–924.
108. Yuen KS, Halliday GM. Alpha-tocopherol, an inhibitor of epidermal lipid peroxidation, prevents ultraviolet radiation from suppressing the skin immune system. Photochem Photobiol 1997; 65(3):587–592.

109. Anderson RR. Tissue optics and photoimmunology. In: Parrish JA, ed. Photoimmunology New York: Plenum Medical, 1983:73.
110. Kagan VE, Serbinova EA, Forte T, Scita G, Packer L. Recycling of vitamin E in human low density lipoproteins. J Lipid Res 1992; 33(3):385–397.
111. Kochevar IE, Lambert CR, Lynch MC, Tedesco AC. Comparison of photosensitized plasma membrane damage caused by singlet oxygen and free radicals. Biochim Biophys Acta 1996; 1280(2):223–230.
112. Rosenstein BS, Ducore JM, Cummings SW. The mechanism of bilirubin-photosensitized DNA strand breakage in human cells exposed to phototherapy light. Mutat Res 1983; 112(6):397–406.
113. Foote CS. Definition of type I and type II photosensitized oxidation. Photochem Photobiol 1991; 54(659).
114. Jimbow K, Fitzpatrick TB, Wick MM. Biochemistry and physiology of melanin pigmentation. In: Goldsmith LA, ed. Physiology, Biochemistry, and Molecular Biology of the Skin. New York: Oxford University Press, 1993:873–909.
115. Weber SU, Thiele JJ, Han N et al. Topical alpha-tocotrienol supplementation inhibits lipid peroxidation but fails to mitigate increased transepidermal water loss after benzoyl peroxide treatment of human skin. Free Radical Biol Med 2003; 34(2):170–176.
116. Biesalski HK, Hemmes C, Hopfenmuller W, Schmid C, Gollnick HP. Effects of controlled exposure of sunlight on plasma and skin levels of beta-carotene. Free Radical Res 1996; 24:215–224.
117. Aronoff S. Catalase: kinetics of photooxidation. Science 1965; 150:72–73.
118. Kono K, Fridovich I. Superoxide radical inhibits catalase. J Biol Chem 1982; 257:5751–5754.
119. Whiteside C, Hassan HM. Induction and inactivation of catalase and superoxide dismutase of escherichia-coli by ozone. Arch Biochem Biophys 1987; 257(2):464–471.
120. Punnonen K, Puntala A, Jansen CT, Ahotupa M. UV-B irradiation induces lipid peroxidation and reduces antioxidant enzyme activities in human keratinocytes *in vitro*. Acta Derm Venereol 1991; 71(3):239–242.
121. Punnonen K, Jansen CT, Puntala A, Ahotupa M. Effects of *in vitro* UV-A irradiation and PUVA treatment on membrane fatty acids and activities of antioxidant enzymes in human keratinocytes. J Invest Dermatol 1991; 96(2):255–259.
122. Shindo Y, Hashimoto T. Time course of changes in antioxidant enzymes in human skin fibroblasts after UVA irradiation. J Dermatol Sci 1997; 14(3):225–32.
123. Punnonen K, Lehtola K, Autio P, Kiistala U, Ahotupa M. Chronic UVB irradiation induces superoxide dismutase activity in human epidermis *in vivo*. Photochem Photobiol 1995; 30(1):43–48.
124. Gilchrest BA. Photodamage. Cambridge, Massachusetts, USA; Oxford, England, UK: Blackwell Scientific Publications, 1995.
125. Fryer MJ. Evidence for the photoprotective effects of vitamin E Photochem Photobiol 1993; 58:304–312.
126. Trevithick JR. Vitamin E prevention of ultraviolet-induced skin damage. In: Fuchs J, Packer L, eds. Oxidative Stress in Dermatology. New York: M Dekker, Inc., 1993:67–80.
127. Darr D, Pinnell SR. Reactive oxygen species and antioxidant protection in photodermatology. In: Lowe NJ, Shaath NA, Pathak MA, eds. Sunscreens—Development,

Evaluation, and Regulatory Aspects. 2nd ed. New York: M Dekker, Inc., 1997:155–173.
128. Dreher F, Maibach H. Protective effects of topical antioxidants in humans. Curr Probl Dermatol 2001; 29:157–164.
129. Lopez-Torres M, Thiele JJ, Shindo Y, Han D, Packer L. Topical application of α-tocopherol modulates the antioxidant network and diminishes ultraviolet-induced oxidative damage in murine skin. Br J Dermatol 1998; 138:207–215.
130. Roshchupkin DI, Pistsov MY, Potapenko AY. Inhibition of ultraviolet light-induced erythema by antioxidants. Arch Dermatol Res 1979; 266:91–94.
131. Möller H, Ansmann A, Wallat S. Wirkungen von Vitamin E auf die Haut bei topischer Anwendung. Fat Sci Technol 1989; 91(8):295–305.
132. Dreher F, Gabard B, Schwindt DA, Maibach HI. Topical melatonin in combination with vitamins E and C protects skin from UV-induced erythema: a human study *in vivo*. Br J Dermatol 1998; 139(2):332–339.
133. Burke KE, Clive J, Combs GF, Jr., Commisso J, Keen CL, Nakamura RM. Effects of topical and oral vitamin E on pigmentation and skin cancer induced by ultraviolet irradiation in Skin. 2: hairless mice. Nutr Cancer 2000; 38(1):87–97.
134. Darr D, Dunston S, Faust H, Pinnell S. Effectiveness of antioxidants (vitamin C and E) with and without sunscreens as topical photoprotectants. Acta Dermatol Venereol 1996; 76:264–268.
135. Ritter EF, Axelrod M, Minn KW et al. Modulation of ultraviolet light-induced epidermal damage: beneficial effects of tocopherol. Plast Reconstr Surg 1997; 100:973–980.
136. Khettab N, Amory MC, Briand G et al. Photoprotective effect of vitamins A and E on polyamine and oxygenated free radical metabolism in hairless mouse epidermis. Biochimie 1988; 70:1709–1713.
137. Chen W, Barthelman M, Martinez J, Alberts D, Gensler HL. Inhibition of cyclobutane pyrimidine dimer formation in epidermal p53 gene of UV-irradiated mice by alpha-tocopherol. Nutr Cancer 1997; 29(3):205–211.
138. McVean M, Liebler DC. Prevention of DNA photodamage by vitamin E compounds and sunscreens: roles of ultraviolet absorbance and cellular uptake. Mol Carcinog 1999; 24(3):169–176.
139. Gensler HL, Magdaleno M. Topical vitamin E inhibition of immunosuppression and tumorigenesis induced by ultraviolet radiation. Nutr Cancer 1991; 15:97–106.
140. Beijersbergen van Henegouwen GMJ, Junginger HE, de Vries H. Hydrolysis of RRR-α-tocopheryl acetate (vitamin E acetate) in the skin and its UV protecting activity (an *in vivo* study with the rat). J Photochem Photobiol B: Biol 1995; 29:45–51.
141. Schoonderwoerd SA, Beijersbergen van Henegouwen GMJ, Persons KCM. Effect of alpha-tocopherol and di-butyl-hydroxytoluene (BHT) on UV-A-induced photobinding of 8-methoxypsoralen to Wistar rat epidermal biomacromolecules *in vivo*. Arch Toxicol 1991; 65:490–494.
142. Evelson P, Ordóñez CP, Llesuy S, Boveris A. Oxidative stress and *in vivo* chemiluminescence in mouse skin exposed to UVA radiation. J Photochem Photobiol B: Biol 1997; 38(2–3):215–219.
143. Bissett DL, Chatterjee R, Hannon DP. Protective effect of a topically applied antioxidant plus an anti-inflammatory agent against ultraviolet radiation-induced chronic skin damage in the hairless mouse. J Soc Cosmet Chem 1992; 43:85–92.

144. Bissett DL, Hillebrand GG, Hannon DP. The hairless mouse as a model of skin photoaging: its use to evaluate photoprotective materials. Photodermatology 1989; 6:228–233.
145. Bissett DL, Chatterjee R, Hannon DP. Photoprotective effect of superoxide-scavenging antioxidants against ultraviolet radiation-induced chronic skin damage in the hairless mouse. Photodermatol Photoimmunol Photomed 1990; 7:56–62.
146. Potapenko AY, Abijev GA, Pistsov MY et al. PUVA-induced erythema and changes in mechanoelectrical properties of skin. Inhibition by tocopherols. Arch Dermatol Res 1984; 276:12–16.
147. Potapenko AJ, Piszov MJ, Abijev GA, Pliquett F. α-Tokopherol, ein Inhibitor von durch UV-Strahlung induzierten Veranderungen mechanoelektrischer Hauteigenschaften. Dermatologische Monatsschrift 1983; 169:300–304.
148. Record IR, Dreosti IE, Konstantinopoulos M, Buckley RA. The influence of topical and systemic vitamin E on ultraviolet light-induced skin damage in hairless mice. Nutr Cancer 1991; 16(3–4):219–226.
149. Trevithick JR, Xiong H, Lee S et al. Topical tocopherol acetate reduces post-UVB, sunburn-associated erythema, edema, and skin sensitivity in hairless mice. Arch Biochem Biophys 1992; 296(2):575–582.
150. Trevithick JR, Shum DT, Redae S et al. Reduction of sunburn damage to skin by topical application of vitamin E acetate following exposure to ultraviolet B radiation: effect of delaying application or of reducing concentration of vitamin E acetate applied. Scanning Microsc 1993; 7(4):1269–1281.
151. Gensler HL, Aickin M, Peng YM, Xu M. Importance of the form of topical vitamin E for prevention of photocarcinogenesis. Nutr Cancer 1996; 26(2):183–191.
152. Kamimura M, Matsuzawa T. Percutaneous absorption of α-tocopheryl acetate. J Vitaminol 1968; 14:151–159.
153. Norkus EP, Bryce GF, Bhagavan HN. Uptake and bioconversion of α-tocopheryl acetate to α-tocopherol in skin of hairless mice. Photochem Photobiol 1993; 57:613–615.
154. Trevithick JR, Mitton KP. Topical application and uptake of vitamin E acetate by the skin conversion to free vitamin E. Biochem Mol Biol Int 1993; 31(5):869–878.
155. Alberts DS, Goldman R, Xu MJ et al. Disposition and metabolism of topically administered α-tocopherol acetate: a common ingredient of commercially available sunscreens and cosmetics. Nutr Cancer 1996; 26(2):193–201.
156. Rangarajan M, Zatz JL. Effect of formulation on the delivery and metabolism of alpha-tocopheryl acetate. J Cosmet Sci 2001; 52(4):225–236.
157. Rangarajan M, Zatz JL. Kinetics of permeation and metabolism of alpha-tocopherol and alpha-tocopheryl acetate in micro-Yucatan pig skin. J Cosmet Sci 2001; 52(1):35–50.
158. Baschong W, Artmann C, Hueglin D, Roeding J. Direct evidence for bioconversion of vitamin E acetate into vitamin E: an *ex vivo* study in viable human skin. J Cosmet Sci 2001; 52(3):155–161.
159. Kramer-Stickland K, Liebler DC. Effect of UVB on hydrolysis of alpha-tocopherol acetate to alphatocopherol in mouse skin. J Invest Dermatol 1998; 111(2):302–307.
160. Kramer KA, Liebler DC. UVB induced photooxidation of vitamin E. Chem Res Toxicol 1997; 10(2):219–224.
161. Meydani SN, Meydani M, Blumberg JB et al. Vitamin E supplementation and *in vivo* immune response in healthy elderly subjects: a randomized controlled trial. J Am Med Assoc 1997; 277(17):1380–1386.

162. Darr D, Combs S, Dunston S, Manning T, Pinnell S. Topical vitamin C protects porcine skin from ultraviolet radiation-induced damage. Br J Dermatol 1992; 127(3):247–253.
163. Pinnell SR, Yang H, Omar M et al. Topical L-ascorbic acid: percutaneous absorption studies. Dermatol Surg 2001; 27(2):137–142.
164. Gallarate M, Carlotti ME, Trotta M, Bovo S. On the stability of ascorbic acid in emulsified systems for topical and cosmetic use. Int J Pharm 1999; 188(2):233–241.
165. Kameyama K, Sakai C, Kondoh S et al. Inhibitory effect of magnesium L-ascorbyl-2-phosphate (VC-PMG) on melanogenesis *in vitro* and *in vivo*. J Am Acad Dermatol 1996; 34:29–33.
166. Kobayashi S, Takehana M, Itoh S, Ogata E. Protective effect of magnesium-L-ascorbyl-2 phosphate against skin damage induced by UVB irradiation. Photochem Photobiol 1996; 64(1):224–228.
167. Austria R, Semenzato A, Bettero A. Stability of vitamin C derivatives in solution and topical formulations. J Pharm Biomed Anal 1997; 15:795–801.
168. Wang ZY, Agarwal R, Bickers DR, Mukhtar H. Protection against ultraviolet B radiation-induced photocarcinogenesis in hairless mice by green tea polyphenols. Carcinogenesis 1991; 12:1527–1530.
169. González S, Pathak MA. Inhibition of ultraviolet-induced formation of reactive oxygen species, lipid peroxidation, erythema and skin photosensitization by *Polypodium leucotomos*. Photodermatol Photoimmunol Photomed 1996; 12:45–56.
170. González S, Pathak MA, Cuevas J, Villarrubia VG, Fitzpatrick TB. Topical or oral administration with an extract of *Polypodium leucotomos* prevents acute sunburn and psoralen-induced phototoxic reactions as well as depletion of Langerhans cells. Photodermatol Photoimmunol Photomed 1997; 13:50–60.
171. Gensler HL, Timmermann BN, Valcic S et al. Prevention of photocarcinogenesis by topical administration of pure epigallocatechin gallate isolated from green tea. Nutr Cancer 1996; 26(3):325–335.
172. Birt DF, Mitchell D, Gold B, Pour P, Conway-Pinch H. Inhibition of ultraviolet light induced skin carcinogenesis in SKH-1 mice by apigenin, a plant flavonoid. Anticancer Res 1997; 17:85–91.
173. Katiyar SK, Korman NJ, Mukhtar H, Agarwal R. Protective effects of silymarin against photocarcinogenesis in a mouse model. J Natl Cancer Inst 1997; 89:556–566.
174. Saija A, Tomaino A, Trombetta D et al. *In vitro* and *in vivo* evaluation of caffeic and ferulic acids as topical photoprotective agents. Int J Pharm 2000; 199(1):39–47.
175. Afaq F, Adhami VM, Ahmad N. Prevention of short-term ultraviolet B radiation-mediated damages by resveratrol in SKH-1 hairless mice. Toxicol Appl Pharmacol 2003; 186(1):28–37.
176. Katiyar SK, Ahmad N, Mukhtar H. Green tea and skin. Arch Dermatol 2000; 136(8):989–994.
177. Katiyar SK, Mukhtar H. Green tea polyphenol (−)-epigallocatechin-3-gallate treatment to mouse skin prevents UVB-induced infiltration of leukocytes, depletion of antigen-presenting cells, and oxidative stress. J Leukoc Biol 2001; 69(5):719–726.
178. Katiyar SK, Matsui MS, Elmets CA, Mukhtar H. Polyphenolic antioxidant (−)-epigallocatechin-3-gallate from green tea reduces UVB-induced inflammatory responses and infiltration of leukocytes in human skin. Photochem Photobiol 1999; 69(2):148–153.

179. Katiyar SK, Elmets CA, Agarwal R, Mukhtar H. Protection against ultraviolet-B radiation-induced local and systemic suppression of contact hypersensitivity and edema responses in C3H/HeN mice by green tea polyphenols. Photochem Photobiol 1995; 62:855–861.
180. Van den Broeke LT, Beijersbergen van Henegouwen GMJ. Thiols as potential UV radiation protectors: an *in vitro* study. J Photochem Photobiol B: Biol 1993; 17:279–286.
181. Aruoma OI, Halliwell B, Hoey BM, Butler J. The antioxidant action of N-acetylcysteine: its reaction with hydrogen peroxide, hydroxyl radical, superoxide, and hypochlorous acid. Free Radical Biol Med 1989; 6:593–597.
182. Van den Broeke LT, Beijersbergen van Henegouwen GMJ. UV radiation protecting efficacy of cysteine derivatives, studies with UVA-induced binding of 8-MOP and CPZ to rat epidermal biomacromolecules *in vivo*. Int J Radiat Biol 1994; 67:411–420.
183. Van den Broeke LT, Beijersbergen van Henegouwen GMJ. UV-radiation protecting efficacy of thiols, studied with UVA-induced binding of 8-MOP and CPZ to rat epidermal biomacromolecules *in vivo*. Int J Rad Biol 1993; 63:493–500.
184. Van den Broeke LT, Beijersbergen van Henegouwen GMJ. The effect of N-acetylcysteine on the UVB-induced inhibition of epidermal DNA synthesis in rat skin. J Photochem Photobiol B: Biol 1994; 26:271–276.
185. Steenvoorden DPT, Beijersbergen van Henegouwen GMJ. Cysteine derivatives protect against UV-induced reactive intermediates in human keratinocytes: the role of glutathione synthesis. Photochem Photobiol 1997; 66:665–671.
186. Steenvoorden DP, Beijersburgen van Henegouwen GM. Glutathione synthesis is not involved in protection by N-acetylcysteine against UVB-induced systemic immunosuppression in mice. Photochem Photobiol 1998; 68(1):97–100.
187. Kobayashi S, Takehana M, Tohyama C. Glutathione isopropyl ester reduces UVB-induced skin damage in hairless mice. Photochem Photobiol 1996; 63(1):106–110.
188. Fuchs J, Milbradt R. Antioxidant inhibition of skin inflammation induced by reactive oxidants: evaluation of the redox couple dihydrolipoate/lipoate. Skin Pharmacol 1994; 7(5):278–284.
189. Podda M, Rallis M, Traber MG, Packer L, Maibach HI. Kinetic study of cutaneous and subcutaneous distribution following topical application of [7,8-^{14}C]rac-α-lipoic acid onto hairless mice. Biochem Pharmacol 1996; 52:627–633.
190. Podda M, Zollner TM, Grundmann-Kollmann M, Thiele JJ, Packer L, Kaufmann R. Activity of alpha-lipoic acid in the protection against oxidative stress in skin. Curr Probl Dermatol 2001; 29:43–51.
191. Bangha E, Elsner P, Kistler GS. Suppression of UV-induced erythema by topical treatment with melatonin (N-acetyl-5-methoxytryptamine). Influence of the application time point. Dermatology 1997; 195:248–252.
192. Reiter RJ, Melchiorri D, Sewerynek E et al. A review of the evidence supporting melatonin's role as an antioxidant. J Pineal Res 1995; 18:1–11.
193. Martinuzzo M, Del Zar MM, Cardinali DP, Carreras LO, Vacas MI. Melatonin effect on arachidonic acid metabolism to cyclooxygenase derivatives in human platelets. J Pineal Res 1991; 11:111–115.
194. Franchi AM, Gimeno MF, Cardinali DP, Vacas MI. Melatonin, 5-methoxytryptamine and some of their analogs as cyclooxygenase inhibitors in rat medial basal hypothalamus. Brain Res 1987; 405:384–388.

195. Carraro C, Pathak MA. Studies on the nature of *in vitro* and *in vivo* photosensitization reactions by psoralens and porphyrins. J Invest Dermatol 1988; 90:267–275.
196. Alaoui Youssefi A, Emerit I, Feingold J. Oxyradical involvement in PUVA-induced skin reactions. Protection by local application of SOD. Eur J Dermatol 1994; 4:389–393.
197. Filipe P, Emerit I, Vassy J et al. Epidermal localization and protective effects of topically applied superoxide dismutase. Exp Dermatol 1997; 6:116–121.
198. Hamanaka H, Miyachi Y, Imamura S. Photoprotective effect of topically applied superoxide dismutase on sunburn reaction in comparison with sunscreen. J Dermatol 1990; 17:595–598.
199. Hadshiew I, Stäb F, Untiedt S, Bohnsack K, Rippke F, Hölzle E. Effects of topically applied antioxidants in experimentally provoked polymorphous light eruption. Dermatology 1997; 195:362–368.
200. Moison RM, Beijersbergen van Henegouwen GM. Topical antioxidant vitamins C and E prevent UVB-radiation-induced peroxidation of eicosapentaenoic acid in pig skin. Radiat Res 2002; 157(4):402–409.
201. Moison RM, Doerga R, G MJBVH. Increased antioxidant potential of combined topical vitamin E and C against lipid peroxidation of eicosapentaenoic acid in pig skin induced by simulated solar radiation. Int J Radiat Biol 2002; 78(12):1185–1193.
202. Moison RM, Steenvoorden DP, Beijersbergen van Henegouwen GM. Topically applied eicosapentaenoic acid protects against local immunosuppression induced by UVB irradiation, *cis*-urocanic acid and thymidine dinucleotides. Photochem Photobiol 2001; 73(1):64–70.
203. Rhodes LE, O'Farrell S, Jackson MJ, Friedmann PS. Dietary fish-oil supplementation in humans reduces UVB-erythemal sensitivity but increases epidermal lipid peroxidation. J Invest Dermatol 1994; 103(2):151–154.
204. Montenegro L, Bonina F, Rigano L, Giogilli S, Sirigu S. Protective effect evaluation of free radical scavengers on UVB induced human cutaneous erythema by skin reflectance spectrophotometry. Int J Cosmet Sci 1995; 17:91–103.
205. Dreher F, Denig N, Gabard B, Schwindt DA, Maibach HI. Effect of topical antioxidants on UV-induced erythema formation when administered after exposure. Dermatology 1999; 198(1):52–55.
206. Bissett DL, Chatterjee R, Hannon DP. Chronic ultraviolet radiation-induced increase in skin iron and the photoprotective effect of topically applied iron chelators. Photochem Photobiol 1991; 54(2):215–223.
207. Bissett DL, Oelrich DM, Hannon DP. Evaluation of a topical iron chelator in animals and in human beings: short-term photoprotection by 2-furildioxime. J Am Acad Dermatol 1994; 31:572–578.
208. Bissett DL, McBride JF. Synergistic topical photoprotection by a combination of the iron chelator 2-furildioxime and sunscreen. J Am Acad Dermatol 1996; 35:546–549.
209. Hanada K, Sawamura D, Nakano H, Hashimoto I. Possible role of 1,25-dihydroxyvitamin D_3-induced metallothionein in photoprotection against UVB injury in mouse skin and cultured rat keratinocytes. J Dermatol Sci 1995; 9:203–208.
210. Burke KE, Combs GF, Gross EG, Bhuyan KC, Abu-Libdeh H. The effects of topical and oral L-selenomethionine on pigmentation and skin cancer induced by ultraviolet irradiation. Nutr Cancer 1992; 17:123–137.
211. Burke KE, Bedford RG, Combs GF, French IW, Skeffington DR. The effect of topical L-selenomethionine on minimal erythema dose of ultraviolet irradiation in humans. Photodermatol Photoimmunol Photomed 1992; 9:52–57.

212. Sanchez JL, Torres VM. Selenium sulfide in tinea versicolor: blood and urine levels. J Am Acad Dermatol 1984; 11:238–241.
213. Cummins LM, Kimura ET. Safety evaluation of selenium sulfide antidandruff shampoos. Toxicol Appl Pharmacol 1971; 20:89–96.
214. Rostan EF, DeBuys HV, Madey DL, Pinnell SR. Evidence supporting zinc as an important antioxidant for skin. Int J Dermatol 2002; 41(9):606–611.
215. Yoshimura H, Asada T, Iwanami M. Some measurements of dissociation constants of uric acid and creatinine. J Biochem Tokyo 1959; 46:169–176.
216. Salomon L, Stubbs DW. Some aspects of the metabolism of ascorbic acid in rats. Ann NY Acad Sci 1961; 92:128–140.
217. Stüttgen G, Schaefer E. Vitamine und Haut. In: Stüttgen G, Schaefer E, eds. Funktionelle Dermatologie. Berlin: Springer, 1974; 78–79.
218. Halprin K, Ohkawara A. The measurement of glutathione in human epidermis using glutathione reductase. J Invest Dermatol 1967; 48:149–152.
219. Benedetto JP, Ortonne JP, Voulot C, Khatchadourian C, Prota G, Thivolet J. Role of thiol compounds in mammalian melanin pigmentation. J Invest Dermatol 1981; 77:402–405.
220. Thiele JJ, Weber SU, Packer L. Sebaceous gland secretion is a major physiological route of vitamin E delivery to skin. J Invest Dermatol 1999; 113(6):1006–1010.
221. Kim YP, Lee SC. Superoxide dismutase activities in the human skin. In: Hayashi O, Imamura S, Miyachi Y, eds. The Biological Role of Reactive Oxygen Species in Skin. New York: Elsevier, 1987; 225–230.
222. Carrao C, Pathak MA. Characterization of superoxide dismutase from mammalian skin epidermis. J Invest Dermatol 1988; 90:31–36.
223. Bangha E, Elsner P, Kistler GS. Suppression of UV-induced erythema by topical treatment with melatonin (*N*-acetyl-5-methoxytryptamine). A dose response study. Arch Dermatol Res 1996; 288:522–526.
224. Bissett DL, Majeti S, Fu JJL, McBride JF, Wyder WE. Protective effect of topically applied conjugated hexadienes against ultraviolet radiation-induced chronic skin damage in the hairless mouse. Photodermatol Photoimmunol Photomed 1990; 7:63–67.
225. De Rios G, Chan JT, Black HS, Rudolph AH, Knox JM. Systemic protection by antioxidants against UVL-induced erythema. J Invest Dermatol 1978; 70:123–125.
226. Muizzuddin N, Shakoori AR, Marenus KD. Effect of topical application of antioxidants and free radical scavengers on protection of hairless mouse skin exposed to chronic doses of ultraviolet B. Skin Res Technol 1998; 4:200–204.
227. Muizzuddin N, Shakoori AR, Marenus KD. Effect of antioxidants and free radical scavengers on protection of human skin against UVB, UVA and IR irradiation. Skin Res Technol 1999; 5:260–265.
228. Pelle E, Muizzuddin N, Mammone T, Marenus K, Maes D. Protection against endogenous and UVB-induced oxidative damage in stratum corneum lipids by an antioxidant-containing cosmetic formulation. Photodermatol Photoimmunol Photomed 1999; 15(3–4):115–119.
229. Quevedo WC, Jr., Holstein TJ, Dyckman J, McDonald CJ, Isaacson EL. Inhibition of UVR-induced tanning and immunosuppression by topical applications of vitamins C and E to the skin of hairless (hr/hr) mice. Pigment Cell Res 2000; 13(2):89–98.
230. Fischer T, Bangha E, Elsner P, Kistler GS. Suppression of UV-induced erythema by topical treatment with melatonin. Influence of the application time point. Biol Signals Recept 1999; 8(1–2):132–135.

5

Botanical Extracts

Alain Khaiat
Johnson & Johnson Asia Pacific, Singapore

Origin of Botanical Extracts	90
Extraction Process	90
Total Extracts	91
Selective Extracts	91
Purification	91
Biotechnology Extracts	92
Usage	92
Activity	92
Antioxidants	92
Lipids of the Epidermis and Barrier Function	93
Fat Storage and Slimming	94
Antiage	95
Conclusion	96
Acknowledgment	97
References	97

The existence of the word "cosmeceuticals" is very much linked to the US FDA definition of drugs and cosmetics in the 1938 FD&C Act. One can only speculate as to why 60 years of scientific knowledge and research have been ignored by the FDA in not revising the definition! The European Commission has been wiser and its 1976 definition of cosmetics was modified in 1993 to acknowledge the fact that everything put on the skin or hair may have a physiological effect (1). It puts the responsibility on the industry to ascertain product safety and efficacy (claims justification) (2).

Natural extracts, whether from animal, botanical, or mineral origin, have been used as "active ingredients" of drugs or cosmetics for as long as human history can trace. Oils, butter, honey, beeswax, lead, and lemon juice were common ingredients of beauty recipes from ancient Egypt. Many botanical extracts are used today in traditional medicine and large pharmaceutical companies are rediscovering them.

The major differences between the drug and the cosmetic approach rely on intent (i.e., cure or prevention of a disease vs. beautifying) as well as how the extract is considered. In the cosmetic industry, the botanical extract is the active ingredient. It may contain hundreds of chemical structures and it has a proven activity. In the drug industry, one needs to know the chemical structure of the active ingredient within the extract, very often to synthesize it, to purify it, sometimes to discover that isolation and purification leads to a loss in the biological activity, or to realize that, despite all the skills of organic chemists, nature is not easy to reproduce.

ORIGIN OF BOTANICAL EXTRACTS

Botanical extracts have been used for centuries and are present in today's products either for their own properties or as substitutes of animal materials that may have to be removed from products because of pressure from animal rights associations or diseases like bovine spongiform encephalopathy. There are plant powders for hair coloring (Henna), scrubs (apricot kernel, corn), and masks (oat flour); plant extracts ("as is" or purified); and biotechnology extracts obtained through fermentation, cloning, soilless culture (aquaculture, artificial media, etc.), which are developed from micro-organisms, plant organs, and total plants, or through the use of specific enzymes (3).

EXTRACTION PROCESS

Active ingredients are not present in equal amounts in all parts of a plant or an organism. Most of the time, a higher concentration can be found in certain parts. Therefore, it is usually only one part of the plant that is used: fruit, bark, root, bud, flower, leaves, and so on.

Depending on the future use of the extract, various extraction processes can be performed. As mentioned, it is industry's responsibility to ensure the absence of toxic substances that could lead to unwanted side effects. The drug approval process allows side effects to be present, provided the benefits outweigh the disadvantages. The cosmetics consumer has the choice of using a product that may have side effects or using another that has none; obviously, the product with side effects would be less acceptable.

Total Extracts

Total extracts are most common in the cosmetics industry and are rarely, if ever, used in drugs. They are generally known from traditional usage. Their activity is often empirical and their active ingredients are not always identified, but their benefits are, very often, without possible doubt. Their mode of preparation can be found in traditional pharmacopeias (China, India, Africa, Europe, America) or from observing shamans or traditional practitioners. Very often, plants are blended in order to better control or synergize their effects, but sometimes also to preserve the secret of the active ingredient.

Modern techniques include (a) pressing, for plants rich in water or oil (e.g., fresh plants, fruits, vegetables); (b) percolation, with one solvent or a mixture of solvents (water, glycols, ethanol) at room temperature or at elevated temperature (this process is the same as the one used to obtain coffee); and (c) maceration, with the same type of solvents (this process is the same as the one used to obtain tea).

These processes allow for better control: stability, preservation, and manufacturing reproducibility.

The content of the extract is very much a function of the type of solvent, the temperature, the plant–solvent ratio, the time of contact, the part of the plant used, and its species. Sometimes it is also dependent on the plant culture conditions and the season of harvest.

In the drug industry, especially, the extract must be concentrated and the active material isolated by selective precipitation, chromatography, electrophoresis, and so on.

Solvents have to be carefully chosen, not only for their extraction properties, but also for their compatibility with the final formulation and their harmlessness.

Selective Extracts

Special extraction processes or the use of specific solvents will lead to the obtention of a specific class of molecules.

The fragrance industry has for centuries obtained essential oils or floral water by water vapor extraction or "enfleurage"—a process by which the plant flowers are put in contact with solid fats and terpenes and sesquiterpenes migrate into the oil phase.

The use of vegetable oils as solvents allows for the extraction of oil-soluble vitamins or lipids. More recently, the use of supercritical CO_2 has been developed to extract aroms, essential oils, and oleoresins.

Purification

Extract purification to separate specific molecules from others is done following classic physicochemical processes—cryoprecipitation, column chromatography, electrophoresis, use of selective solvents and salts, and the like.

Biotechnology Extracts

Biotechnology can be used to obtain, purify, or transform extracts. The use of enzymes as tools in this area is booming (4). One can find different enzymes to be used for very specific reactions in certain conditions. They could become alternatives to chemical reactions as they provide stereospecificity or eliminate the risk of solvent residues. Today, protein hydrolysates obtained by enzymatic reaction are free of the chlorine residues formed when acid hydrolysis is used. In addition, the use of exo-, endo-, or amino acid-specific proteases allows for a better control of the end result.

Enzymes will allow for better yields by transforming or releasing specific molecules (use of pectinases, β-glucosidase, β-glucanase, lipases, transferases, esterases, etc.).

Amino acids, polyols, esters of fatty acids, polyol organic acids, more stable lipo-soluble vitamin esters with slow release properties, and new molecules (5) can be obtained.

Usage

Extracts or purified botanical molecules can be incorporated directly into solutions, emulsions, or vectors or can be used to form a vector (liposomes, phytosomes, phytospheres) (6). They can be topically applied, ingested, or injected, depending on the intended use, provided absence of toxicity has been shown.

Activity

Are botanical extracts really active? How does their activity compare to that of synthetic materials? Are all natural ingredients safe?

Certainly one learns a lot about these questions by studying traditional uses. Centuries of human experience can prove safety. For example, lilium bulb oil extract use for sunburns has been reported since ancient Greece, whereas the water extract has been shown to be toxic. Natural ingredients have been shown to have a broad spectrum of activity, including hallucinogenic mushrooms and cardiotonic belladona. Scientific research conducted on plant extracts described in traditional pharmacopeias (7,8) has led to a broader range of potential applications.

Furthermore, research conducted on skin biology during the last 10 years allows us to better understand the biological mechanisms involved in dehydration, aging, and so on. This, in turn, leads to the search for extracts with specific activities for targeted applications.

Antioxidants

Free radicals have been shown to play a major role in sun damage as well as in aging or in pollution (tobacco, stress). They act by degrading the skin structural fibers (collagen, elastin), cell membranes, and DNA, or by creating inflammatory reactions (9). Free-radical actions can be blocked by the following:

Vegetable oils rich in tocopherols and tocotrienols. α-Tocopherol contributes directly to cell membrane structure by stabilizing it and allowing for proper functioning of membrane enzymes. Wheat germ oil and palm oil are particularly rich in tocopherols and α-, β-, and γ-tocotrienols.

Carotenoids, such as β-carotene, found in plants or in part of plants exposed to the sun. Of particular interest is a unicellular microalgae, *Dunaliella.* Under normal conditions of light, temperature, or salt, these algae are green. However, under extreme conditions (high salinity, low pH, high sunlight, lack of nitrogen or phosphorus), they protect themselves by multiplying their β-carotene concentration by 10. The ponds become red, and the β-carotene concentration can reach 14% of their dry weight.

As first shown by Kligman (10), the action of retinoids and carotenoids (11) on sun damage has led to numerous works.

SOD is an enzyme that deactivates free radicals. Its concentration decreases with age. It has been possible to obtain *Bifidus* extracts that are rich in SOD (12).

Ascorbic acid, which can be found in *Rosa canina* (dog rose) fruits, *Actinidia* (kiwi fruits), or *Malphigia punicifolia* (West Indian cherry) is an antioxidant that is also used for many of its other properties. It is active in the synthesis of carnitin, a molecule intervening in the transfer of lipids inside the mitochondria. Ascorbic acid thus plays a role in improving cell resistance owing to a better use of lipids. Ascorbic acid is an anti-inflammatory agent that degrades and eliminates histamine. It can be used in after-sun products; it protects against free-radical damage, helps maintain the elasticity and the integrity of the extracellular matrix (ECM), and has immunostimulating activity.

Flavonoids, rich extracts from *Gingko*, *Fagopyrum* (buckwheat), *Eucalyptus sambucus* (European elder), or *Sophora japonica*, are used for their antioxidant and anti-free-radical properties (13).

Rosmarinus (rosemary) extracts, rich in carnosic acid, are very potent antioxidants, used to protect food.

Syzygium aromaticum or *Germanium thumbergii* extracts can be used to protect collagenase activity and the ECM from free radicals (14).

Lipids of the Epidermis and Barrier Function

Fish oils, rich in polyunsaturated fatty acids (PUFA) of the n-3 type [e.g., EPA (eicosapentaenoic acid) or DHA (docosapentaenoic acid)], act directly on cell membranes by increasing their fluidity. They favor the exchanges between the inner and the outer compartment of the cells or between cells. In addition, they have anti-inflammatory activity (15).

Thanks to the use of microalgae cultures in photobioreactors, plant oils rich in PUFA (EPA and DHA) can be produced.

Other plant oils rich in PUFA of the n-6 type [e.g., *Oenothera biennis* (evening primrose), *Borage officinalis* (borage), and *Ribes nigrum* (black currant)] are important in bringing essential fatty acids (EFA) to the skin, contributing to the maintenance or the restoration of epidermal lipids.

Oil and plant butters (rice, wheat, coffee, mango, sorgho, baobab, soya, corn, carob) are rich in EFA (e.g., oleic and linoleic) or squalene (olive oil), which maintains skin suppleness and reduces water loss. They also contain a nonsaponifiable fraction rich in sterols. Some of these have exceptional healing properties that make them of particular value in sun or antiage products: *Camelia* (tea), *Argania*, *Medicago* (alfalfa), *Spinacia* (spinach), *Butyrospermomum* (shea butter), *Cucurbitaceae*, *Pongamia* (hongay or pongamia oil). β-Sitosterol is well known for its inflammatory properties. The nonsaponifiable fraction is also a stimulant of collagen or elastin synthesis.

Phytosterols slow down the aging process by favoring fatty acid desaturation, which in turn maintains membrane fluidity and catalytic activity. γ-Orizanol (ferulic esters of cycloartanol, cycloartenol, and β-sitosterol) extracted from rice, topically applied, stimulates sebaceous gland activity, which slows down with age.

One can also find plant waxes (sugar cane, *Camauba*, *Ceroxylon*, *Jojoba*, rose), which are used to protect lips, hands, or face from dehydration.

Certain plants (yeast, wheat, apple, potato, rice bran, *Agaricus*, *Morus alba*, or white mulberry) are rich in ceramides and glycosylceramides. These may be used for their action on skin or hair to provide hydration or reconstitute epidermal barrier function.

Other plants are rich in oils containing very long-chain fatty acids (C22, 24, 26), like *Pentaclethra* or ewala oil used in Africa as a massage oil or *Limnanthes alba* or shambrilla oil.

Fat Storage and Slimming

We are currently using botanical extracts with very specific actions that act at various levels of adipocyte metabolism.

Garcinia cambodgia decreases the transformation of sugars into fat.

Extracts of *Guarana*, tea, coffee, and cocoa, which are rich in methylxanthines (caffeine, theobromin) are cAMP-phosphodiesterase inhibitors and thus accelerate lipid degradation.

Flavonoids, like quercetin or its derivatives, are also inhibitors of this enzyme and could lead to a 40% increase in cAMP.

Methylxanthins of the same plants will act on lipoprotein lipase, reducing the passage of fatty acids into the adipocyte.

Phytosterols from plant oils are being investigated for their potential action on fat storage or degradation and on adipocyte differentation or multiplication.

Antiage

Ascorbic acid is a key element in collagen synthesis (also in "botanical collagen"). It stimulates the production of RNA coding for collagen and contributes to the synthesis of hydroxyproline and hydroxylysine (which is responsible for collagen's 3D structure).

Tests on cells have shown that procyanidol oligomers from pine barks or grape pits were active in reinforcing and protecting the structure of the ECM. They improve microcirculation, leading to a better irrigation of the tissues and thus to nutrition, hydration, hormone transport, and so forth.

Protection of elastic fibers (collagens, elastin) is promoted by extracts having free-radical scavenging properties, activating the synthesis of these proteins or inhibiting the enzymes responsible for their degradation: *Streptomyces*, black currant, *Centella asiatica* (rich in asiatic acid), *Rudbeckia purpurea*, *Coleus*, and *Areca*.

Apigenin, extracted from *Chamomile* and its derivatives, and rutin from *Fagopyrum* have anti-inflammatory properties (by inhibiting histamine release), but they are also β-glucuronidase inhibitors. They protect mucopolysaccharides from degradation. Other extracts rich in polyphenols—tanins—also have antihyaluronidase activity (16–18).

Amino acids obtained by biotechnology through the action of microorganisms or enzymes on plant extracts are used for stimulation of systems that are active in aging as well as slimming (arginin, glutamin, HGH), hair growth (glutamic acid), or immunity (arginin) (19,20). Recent studies show the importance of amino acids in protecting the skin barrier function.

Tryptophan (from *Spirulina*, soy bean, pumpkin), vitamin B3 (from *Saccharomyces*), vitamin B6 (from avocado, banana, yeast, wheat germ), calcium, and magnesium stimulate melatonin (MSH) synthesis. This hormone is very important to many biological processes and decreases rapidly with age. Melatonin is present in animals as well as plants. The highest concentration is found in *Festuca*, oats, corn, rice, and ginger (21).

α- or β-Hydroxyacids that have been in vogue in recent years, not only in cosmetics but also in OTC drugs, are common in the botanical world. Whether from fruits (e.g., bilberry, apple, lemon, orange, kalanchoe), *Tamarindus*, *Hibiscus*, *Saccharum officinalis* (sugar cane), *Acer saccharum* (sugar maple), *Salix*, *Betula* (sweet birch), or *Gaultheria* (wintergreen) (22), their efficacy has been shown in smoothing, brightening, and sloughing skin. They contribute to the elimination of dead cells from the skin surface, hydration, as well as cell renewal. These acids are broadly used in facial, body, and even scalp care.

Oligoelements and minerals like silicium can be found in *Equisetum* (horsetail), *Oryza* (rice), or *Diatoma*. They contribute directly to the synthesis of collagen or proteoglycans and to the stabilization of the ECM (23).

Selenium (*Astrogalus*) is said to play an important role in antiaging (immunity, inflammation, free-radical scavenging), zinc (*Taraxacum*) in hair growth (action on testosterone) (24), and mother of pearl from shellfish in wound healing or tissue repair.

Saponins, a huge family of compounds, whether of a steroidal or triterpenic structure, are known for their detergent activity. They probably have other activities, which are yet to be established. Constant research shows that saponins, present in botanical extracts, have tremendous pharmacological and metabolic properties.

Ginseng and *bupleurum* stimulate biosynthesis of proteins, RNA, cholesterol, and lipogenesis.

Centella asiatica (asiaticosides) stimulates synthesis of collagen and fibronectin.

Hedera ficaria (hederagenin) inhibits proteases.

Sterols from *Sabal* and *Serenoa* as well as $\Delta 7$ sterols are inhibitors of 5-α-reductase, an enzyme involved in androgenic alopecia, hyperseborrhea of the scalp or the skin, as well as acne.

Glycyrrhizin from *glycyrrhiza* and harpagosides from *harpagophytum* are broadly used for their anti-inflammatory properties.

Saponins have also been shown to increase stress resistance by increasing cortisol and prostaglandins, to protect membranes (*Eleutherococcus*), to increase metabolic efficacy (*Medicago*), and to stimulate cells (*Ginseng*, *Bupleurum*).

Extracts from *Ganoderma* are immunostimulating and immunoregulating, they prolong all life in culture, and act on endocrine functions. They have been used in traditional Chinese medicine to slow down aging. This mushroom is rich in polysaccharides, triterpenes, and steroids.

Extracts from *Arctophylos uva-ursi*, *Coactis*, and *Adenotricha* rich in arbutin and methylarbutin are used for their depigmenting effect. So are kojic acid, ascorbic acid and its derivatives, and SOD-rich bifidus extracts. Rosmarinic acid from rosemary also has a tyrosinase-inhibiting activity.

CONCLUSION

Many other activities of botanical extracts have been shown and are used in cosmetics and drugs (OTC or traditional). The main difference between cosmetics and drugs is the intention of the manufacturer (i.e., cure or disease prevention rather than improvement of overall condition of the skin or hair), by maintaining or improving the natural processes.

Most cosmetic products today address both the rational and the emotional aspects that characterize their need in society, though they are often still considered as a "dream in a bottle" (Charles Revson).

Botanicals are playing an increasingly important role in the activity and safety of cosmetics; they allow for a renewal of the source of active ingredients in drugs.

ACKNOWLEDGMENT

I would like to thank Mrs. A. M. Scott de Martinville for her help in the preparation of this manuscript.

REFERENCES

1. EU Directive 93/35.
2. Khaiat A. Cosmeceuticals or cosmetics: industry responsibility. Cosmet Toilet 1993; 108:23.
3. Bocchietto E, Allan N. Case for biotechnology. Soap Perf Cosmet 1996; 69:43–47.
4. Lalonde J. Enzyme catalysis: cleaner, safer, energy efficient. Chem Eng 1997; 108–112.
5. Yvergnaux F, Bonnefoy I, Callegari JP, Coutable J, Scott de Martinville AM, Khaiat A. French Patent 9414229.
6. Kurata Y. New raw materials and technologies in cosmetics. Properties and applications of plant extract complexes. Fragr J 1994; 22:49–53.
7. Kushibashi K, Yamaki H. New raw materials and technologies in cosmetics. Recent topics of plant extracts and their applications to cosmetics. Fragr J 1994; 22:54–61.
8. Lee OS, Kang HH, Han SH. Oriental herbs in cosmetics: plant extracts are reviewed for their potential as cosmetic ingredients. Cosmet Toilet 1997; 112:57–64.
9. Rice-Evans CA, Burdon RH. Free radical damage and its control. N Compr Biochem 1994; 28.
10. Kligman LH, Kligman AM. The effect on rhino mouse skin of agents which influence keratinization and exfoliation. J Invest Dermatol 1979; 73:354–358.
11. XI International Symposium on carotenoids, Leyde, 18–23 August 1996.
12. Katsuta K. New raw materials and technologies for cosmetics: ROD extractive Bifidus. Fragr J 1996; 24:118–123.
13. Leung AY, Foster S. Encyclopedia of Common Ingredients Used in Food, Drugs and Cosmetics, 2d ed. New York: Wiley, 1996.
14. Ito M, Tanaka H, Kojima H. New raw materials and new technologies in cosmetics: Chouji and Gennoshouko extracts as a useful scavenger of reactive oxygen species for cosmetics. Fragr J 1994; 22:38–42.
15. Muto Y, Moriwaki H, Ninomiya M, Adachi S, Takasaki KT, Tanaka T, Tsurumi K, Okuno M. Prevention of second primary tumors by an acyclic retinoid, polyprenoic acid, in patients with hepatocellular carcinoma. N Engl J Med 1996; 334:1561–1567.
16. Kakegawa H, Matsumoto H, Satoh T. Inhibitory effects of some natural products on the activation of hyaluronidase and their antiallergic actions. Chem Pharm Bull 1992; 40:1439–1442.
17. Lee J, Lee SH, Min KR, Ro JS, Ryu JC, Kim Y. Inhibitory effects of hydrolyzable tannins on calcium activated hyaluronidase. Planta Med 1993; 59:381–382.
18. Hara M, Ponda Y. Patent JP 9409391.
19. Adjei AA, Yamauchi K, Nakasone Y, Konishi M, Yamamoto S. Arginine supplemented diets inhibit endotoxin—induced bacterial translocation in mice. Nutrition 1995; 11:371–374.
20. Welhourne TC. Increased bicarbonate and growth hormone after an oral glutamine load. Am J Clin Nutr 1995; 61:1058–1061.

21. Hattori A, Migitakia H, Reiter RJ. Identification of MSH in plants and its effects on plasma melatonin levels and biding to melatonin receptors in vertebrates. Biochem Mol Biol Int 1995; 35:627–634.
22. Eppensperger H, Wilker M. Hibiscus extract: cosmetic effects. Parfumerie Kosmet 1996; 77:582–584; 622–625.
23. Lassus A. Colloidal silicic acid for oral and topical treatment of aged skin, fragile hair and brittle nails in females. J Int Med Res 1993; 21:209–215.
24. Prasad AS, Mantzoros CS, Beck FWJ, Hess JW, Brewer GJ. Zinc status and serum testosterone levels of healthy adults. Nutrition 1996; 12:344–348.

6

Cutaneous Barrier Repair

Karl Lintner, Claire Mas-Chamberlin, Philippe Mondon, François Lamy, and Olivier Peschard
Sederma, Paris, France

Introduction	99
Stratum Corneum, the Lipid Barrier and Its "Repair"	101
Short-Term "Repair"	106
Long-Term Study	107
Visualization of Barrier Disruption and Lipid Integration (="Repair")	108
Barrier Repair Leads to Improved Water Retention	110
Epidermis: How to Build the Stratum Corneum Barrier	112
Dermis: The Final Frontier	119
Conclusion	124
References	125

INTRODUCTION

Cosmeceuticals—the title of this book—and cutaneous barrier repair are two powerful concepts, words, and ideas that we all encounter frequently in our activity in cosmetic research and product development.

    The problem with both items is that there is no generally defined meaning for these terms. Coined by Prof. Kligman more than 15 years ago, the word "cosmeceuticals" has entered our language and is still being debated upon very controversially (1–3). In an article entitled "Cosmetics and Life Sciences, a Continuing Courtship", Greive, who received the Maison G. de Navarre prize for her contribution (4), defines cosmeceuticals as "... a substance that will achieve cosmetic results [...] by means of some degree of physiological action (5)". With this definition in hand, she then demonstrates that substances as widely used and universally accepted as petrolatum might (should?) be considered cosmeceuticals, or even "drugs".

As other chapters in this book address this controversial question more specifically, we shall limit our discussion to products, ideas, and concepts that participate in cutaneous barrier repair, be they called active ingredients, functional ingredients, cosmeceuticals, or anything else. Petrolatum will not be discussed in detail.

Cutaneous barrier repair is as equally ambiguous a term as cosmeceuticals, although no legal conundrums are likely to arise from differing interpretations of what is meant by it. A quick Internet search with these key words turns up thousands of sites, from purely commercial advertising of creams claiming barrier repair to extremely pinpointed research papers that address a particular aspect of skin physiology.

In the narrowest sense (and by the general jargon of the cosmetic industry), barrier repair is often understood as providing the skin, in particular the stratum corneum, with some lipids that re-establish or reinforce the "cement" between the corneocytes. Petrolatum is a good candidate for this.

A much broader view of the barrier function of the skin can also be found in the many documents that turn up in an Internet search with "barrier repair" as search items. A few examples will illustrate this:

1. "The major function of the skin is to generate a **protective barrier**..."
2. "The skin is a **physical barrier** to the environment".
3. "When the skin **barrier** is violated, bacteria, viruses, fungi are introduced into the wound".
4. "The skin **barrier** protects us from dehydration. It provides a **protective layer** from ultraviolet light by causing tanning".
5. "It is likely that transglutaminases contribute to additional components of **the cutaneous barrier** through cross-linking of proteins at the dermal–epidermal junction (DEJ) or in the dermal extracellular matrix".
6. "Integrin receptors are essential in maintaining tissue integrity, thereby providing an effective **barrier** against the outside environment".
7. "The **barrier** function of the basal cell layer of the epidermis is maintained by cadherin mediated cell–cell junctions and integrin-mediated cell–matrix adhesions".
8. "Immune responses against bacteria, protozoa, viruses and fungi are an integral part of the **barrier function** of the skin".

9. "**Cutaneous barrier** and dermal immunity to *Staphylococcus aureus* [...]"
10. "Exposure to UVA irradiation [...] challenges the **barrier** function of the skin and will increase the incidence of cancers and photoaging".

Thus we realize that cutaneous barrier means many different things to many different people in the field:

The lipid barrier of the stratum corneum
A mechanical barrier of general nature, against invasion and abrasion
A physical barrier against dehydration of the underlying organism
A sunscreen barrier against damages from UV light
An immunological barrier

Research subjects focusing on wound healing, transepidermal water loss, microbiological defense, free radical damages, melanogenesis, skin elasticity and the dermal–epidermal junction (DEJ), and cell to cell communication and attachment are therefore all within the scope of cutaneous barrier and its repair.

Between the severely limited definition where cutaneous barrier is equated with the lipid barrier of the stratum corneum and the broadest view that would require us to describe all skin related research as relevant to barrier repair, we shall compromise, navigate among the three layers of stratum corneum, epidermis, and dermis, and look at a few examples of recent work.

A note on the word "repair"—cosmetic products should generally be used on healthy skin. Does healthy skin need "repair"? Again, where is the boundary between drugs and cosmetics? Is it the type or strength of the activity of a product on the skin, or is it the type and strength of the claims associated with it that define a product as one or as the other? As no worldwide unified interpretation exists, we have to leave the readers to their own analysis.

STRATUM CORNEUM, THE LIPID BARRIER AND ITS "REPAIR"

The outermost layer of the epidermis consists of 25–30 stacked sheets of flat, dead cells filled with keratin. It is continually renewed by the desquamation process, by which the intercellular adhesion forces (covalent and noncovalent bonding) are broken such that the corneocytes can be shed. Keratinocytes from the lower layers migrate during the differentiation process to the surface, and replenish the stratum corneum by turning into cornified, anucleated cells (Fig. 1).

Since the pioneering papers by Wertz et al. (6) and Elias and Friend (7) on epidermal lipids, we know that the cement that holds the stratum corneum cells together, which constitutes the "lipid barrier", is a mixture of ceramides, cholesterol, free fatty acids, and a few minor components (triglycerides and cholesterol sulfate) that also include water ($\sim 13\%$). The "brick and mortar" model is usually evoked to explain and illustrate the structure of the stratum corneum (8). Closer

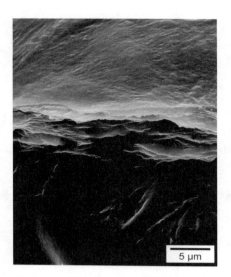

Figure 1 Scanning electron micrograph of stripped human corneocytes. The flattened sheet like structure of the stratum corneum is clearly visible.

examination reveals that the "mortar" or "cement" between the cells is of marvellous complexity (Fig. 2).

The chemistry of the seven (so far) identified ceramides is challenging to the synthetic chemist who tries to reproduce these molecules in the laboratory (Fig. 3). Also, the physical arrangement of the ceramides and other lipids in the intercellular space follows precise rules that assure the functionality of the

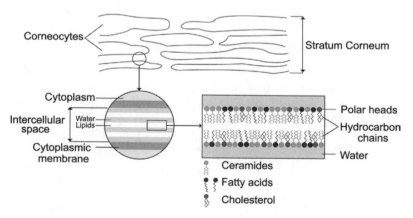

Figure 2 A schematic representation of the stratum corneum barrier and the lipid arrangement in the intercellular space.

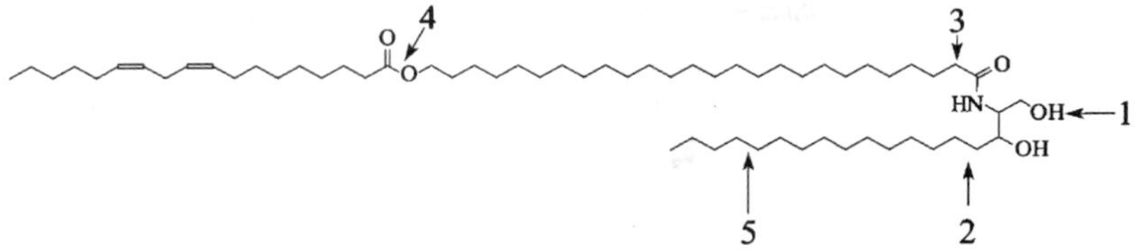

Figure 3 A general structure of ceramides: Position 1: glucocerebrosides (sphingolipids) have sugar molecules attached; Position 2: this position may contain a single bond, a double bond, or a hydroxyl group; Position 3: some ceramides contain an alpha-hydroxyl group here; Position 4: ceramide 1 and 6a contain a hydroxyl group here that often is esterified; Position 5: the chain lengths range from C_{14} to C_{30}.

structure. The lamellar bilayers visible in the electron micrograph (Fig. 4) show some resemblance to the simplified bilayer structure than can be observed in liposomes (models of cell membrane vesicles) (Fig. 5).

However, certain interactions with proteins from the corneocyte cell wall (in particular with involucrine), the extreme length of the fatty acid chains on ceramide 1 (which allows for molecular anchoring across bilayers), and the still poorly understood role of cholesterol sulfate (at the low level of $\sim 1\%$ of the

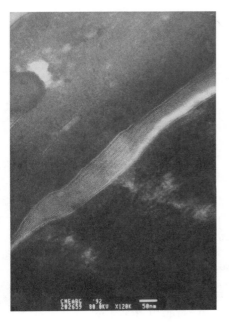

Figure 4 Transmission electron micrograph of the intercellular lipid-filled space between corneocytes from human stratum corneum. The bilayer structure is clearly visible.

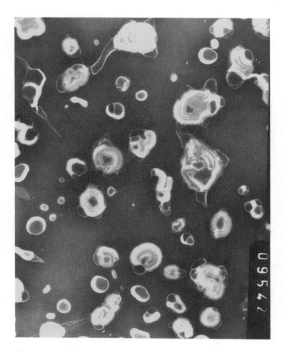

Figure 5 Transmission electron micrograph of a lecithin based liposome: the bilayers, modeling those of living cells, are well defined.

epidermal lipids) and cholersterolsulfatase in cell cohesion and desquamation demonstrate the care with which evolution has provided the skin—and thus the entire organism—with a highly efficient layer of protection against uncontrolled "traffic" of various entities (molecules, microorganisms, particles, water vapor, and radiation). A detailed description of the lipids constituting the stratum corneum barrier, their chemical structure, their analysis, and their function and role in the skin can be found in *Cosmetic Lipids and the Skin Barrier* (9). It would go far beyond the scope of this chapter to review and summarize this book and similar works.

Lipid barrier repair implies, first of all, damages that need repairing. The appearance of dry, flaky, rough skin, which can easily be irritated, is often a sign of damaged stratum corneum barrier function (10). This may arise as a consequence of aging (reduced capacity to synthesize the lipids needed for efficient barrier building) or external influences, such as the use of aggressive soaps, detergents, sanitizers (alcohol), mechanical stress, and UV irradiation, which lead to peroxidation of the lipids which then break down and lose their barrier ability. A major result of disrupted lipid barrier in the stratum corneum is a measurable increase in transepidermal water loss (TEWL), which leads to increased dryness of the skin. Although TEWL is controversially discussed as a measure of barrier integrity, it is still a useful tool that complements visual scoring of dry skin, corneometry, and many other parameters that have been proposed (11). Absolute values of TEWL are difficult to interpret, as great interindividual differences exist. Denda (12) states that aged skin does not necessarily show greater TEWL values than young skin; however, the TEWL of older skin increases more strongly and is more slowly returned to initial values after chemical (surfactant treatment) or mechanical (tape stripping) stress. Thus the inherent barrier repair function of the skin decreases with age.

UVB radiation is also known to diminish skin barrier function *in vivo* (13) and to increase TEWL. However, this appears to be true only for living human skin, and not for *ex vivo* models, where the inflammatory response is lacking (14). No changes in TEWL or tritiated water permeation through UVB (from 600 mJ/cm^2 to 10 J/cm^2) irradiated skin could be observed by these authors, thus again confirming the difficulty of extrapolating *in vitro*, *ex vivo*, or animal studies to living human skin.

The following study describes such an observation. A single dose of UVB (70 mJ) caused an increase of TEWL, which peaked at 72–96 h parallel to which a decrease in free ceramide and an increase in glucosylceramide was observed. As glucosylceramidase activity appeared reduced in a dose-dependent fashion, it might be inferred that UVB inhibits the maturation of the intercellular membrane structure (15). Cosmetic attempts to repair the barrier function of the lipids in the stratum corneum were more or less consciously initiated with the use of petrolatum. It has been shown more recently, though, that the use of physiological lipids instead of a simple occlusive film as afforded by petrolatum (16) is preferable: petrolatum acts quicker (as measured by TEWL recovery after insult) but physiological lipids (a mixture of the intercellular lipids in the "right" concentration ratios) truly repair the barrier by penetrating into the nucleated layers of the epidermis and integrating themselves into the intercellular lipid structures. A number of very carefully orchestrated studies, albeit on animals, appeared to show that barrier repair with topical application of lipids (single lipids, various mixtures thereof: ceramides, cholesterol, free fatty acids, etc.) did not occur unless the lipids were presented and used in precise molar ratios (17,18). Can these results from standardized tests (interindividual variations in mouse skin are not likely to be large) be extrapolated to the widespread of human skin conditions as found in cosmetic, consumer-oriented application? The studies did indicate that initial conditions of the skin had a profound influence on the barrier repair capacity of the lipid mixtures; and there is a sufficient number of peer reviewed work that seems to show beneficial effects of less complex lipid mixtures on impaired skin barrier function (19–21). Rieger (22) reviewed the "promise" of ceramides in skin care very critically, nevertheless admitting the potential for skin benefits that topical application of stratum corneum lipids, especially ceramides, would afford. As always, the question hinges on the term "healthy" or "normal" skin (the domain of cosmetics, see earlier discussion). A consumer perceivable benefit is always much more difficult to demonstrate on perfectly healthy skin than on age-impaired or otherwise damaged skin. The gradual progression from merely "dry" skin (a cosmetic condition) to "xerotic" skin (a medical problem) can be seen as a parallel to the difficulty of defining the borders between cosmetics (make-up?), cosmeceuticals (active skin care?), and drugs (medical treatment).

Therefore, studies on barrier repair (in the narrow sense of lipid barrier as discussed in the first section) focus on repair after artificial insult [this might simulate the aging process, as Ghadially et al. (23) suggest]. An example of vehicle-controlled barrier repair studies with or without insult to human skin on volunteer panels is given in more detail subsequently [see also Ref. (20)].

First, two studies were carried out to measure the capacity of ceramide-2 to repair the damages caused by treating healthy skin of volunteers with detergent washing [sodium lauryl sulfate (SLS)] or by repeated tape stripping.

Short-Term "Repair"

The volar forearms of 13 panelists with dry skin were treated with 10% SLS solution in a standardized washing procedure. Prior to and 15 minutes after this washing, the TEWL was measured with a TEWAMETER on the test sites. Two creams, one containing 1% ceramide-2 (N-stearoylsphinganine) and the other serving as control, were then applied to the respective test sites, and 2 h later, the TEWL values were measured again. The cream contained a sufficient amount of cosmetic unpolar lipids (5% myreth-myristate, 2.5% cetyl palmitate, and 5% jojoba oil emulsified in water) so as to make the additional lipid content (1% ceramide) negligible but for the specific chemical nature of the molecule.

The test was designed to verify the hypothesis that application of a ceramide by cosmetic treatment (cream in topical usage) would lead to rapid barrier repair after a delipidating insult with a strong, irritating detergent.

Indeed, the washing of the skin with 10% SLS leads to a strong increase (+75% on the average) of transepidermal water loss. This indicates a partial disruption of the cutaneous barrier. The topical use of a cosmetic cream is expected to reduce the irritation caused by this treatment, particularly if the cream (emulsion) contains oily, emollient substances as in the case investigated. The specific repair effect of the ceramide should then show up as a difference in the reduction of TEWL values between the treated and placebo sites.

Figure 6 illustrates the observed effects of ceramide: after 2 h, the SLS-induced TEWL has somewhat diminished (control site); the baseline cream has reduced the SLS-induced TEWL values to a small, but not insignificant degree over and beyond the natural return (control site). Statistical analysis shows, however, that the ceramide-2-treated site led to a drop in TEWL that is significant with respect to T0 and to the placebo site ($p < 0.05$).

Clearly, the ceramide in the cream had contributed to specific barrier repair that reduces the undesirable drying out of the skin, although such a rapid effect may in this case be attributed to occlusive mechanisms.

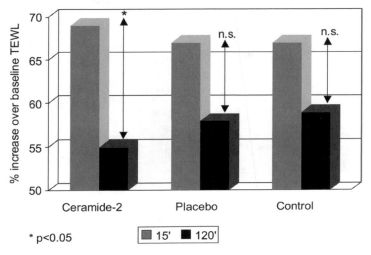

Figure 6 Changes in TEWL over baseline, 15 min after SLS washing, application of creams, and a waiting period of 120 min.

Long-Term Study

The second study was designed to evaluate the repair effect on epidermal lipids as afforded by longer treatment with the ceramide-2-containing emulsion.

For this study, we have determined the TEWL value at time $T = 0$ on the skin in its initial state, and then immediately after successive removal of several corneocyte layers (20 successive tape strippings) (Fig. 7). As expected, this led to considerable increase in TEWL.

The sites "placebo" and "treated with ceramide-2" were then treated daily with the application of an emulsion (either placebo or a cream containing 0.5% ceramide-2) over 3 weeks.

If the application of the ceramide-2-containing cream on the sites stressed at $T = 0$ led to improved rebuilding of the cutaneous barrier, one should expect a lower increase of the TEWL induced by stripping on day $T = 21$, when compared with the one observed for the placebo.

Indeed, we observed that after stripping 20 times, the TEWL increased significantly over the initial value, going from about 10 to an average of 14 g/m^2 per h. This was true for the two sites "ceramide-2" and "placebo" at $T = 0$ (beginning of the study). After 3 weeks, the protocol was repeated. After having carried out the same stripping as on T0 on the two sites, the TEWL values were different; specifically, the rate in increase in TEWL between the basic value and the TEWL after stripping showed a significant difference (Fig. 7). The increase in TEWL induced by 20 strippings on the lower arm treated with ceramide-2 was less than half of the one observed for the "placebo" site.

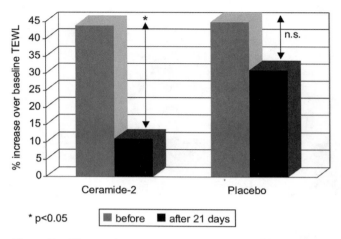

Figure 7 Changes in TEWL over baseline (in % increase) after 20 tape strippings. Results are significant ($p < 0.05$) with respect to baseline and to placebo.

Visualization of Barrier Disruption and Lipid Integration (="Repair")

The effect of impairing the lipid barrier and its "repair" by ceramide treatment can also be visualized, albeit only with electron microscopy, by investigating the events that occur at the bilayer level when the human skin is harshly treated with solvents and then repaired with a cosmetic cream containing a ceramide type ingredient.

On the arms of volunteers, four zones were predefined: one untreated site and three sites where skin lipids were removed by repeated washing with alcohol/ether/hexane mixture; one site was then retained as the control site, one treated with the placebo cream, and one with the cream containing the ceramide-2 at 1% (w/w). After 30 min, cyanoacrylate strippings were obtained from the four sites, which after inclusion in a resin were thinly sliced (60 nm thickness) for electron microscopy observation at 20,000× and 120,000× magnification. At these scales, it is possible to observe the lamellar bilayer structures of ceramides between corneocytes, their disappearance, and their repair by appropriate treatment.

Figures 8–10 show these effects. The untreated site (Fig. 8) shows well-organized layers of lipid strata as described by Landmann (24). Treatment of the skin with aggressive solvents leads to a complete disorganization and removal of these lipids (Fig. 9); *in vivo* this is accompanied by strong increase in TEWL and some irritation and redness of the skin. However, as Fig. 10 shows, treatment of the insulted skin with a ceramide-2-containing cream leads to a rapid recovery of the bilayer structure and concomitant soothing effect on the skin.

Somewhat different protocols in other studies lead to similar results. Berardesca et al. (25), for instance, investigated the prevention of SLS-induced

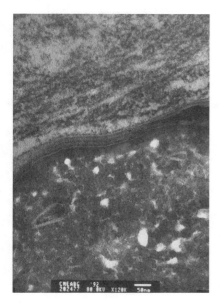

Figure 8 Transmission electron micrograph of the intercellular bilayers of the stratum corneum, obtained on healthy volunteer skin by cyanacrylate stripping.

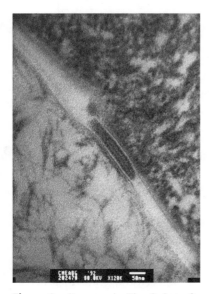

Figure 9 Same as in Fig. 8, but after washing of the skin with alcohol/ether/hexane mixture: the intercellular space is devoid of lipids and bilayer structure.

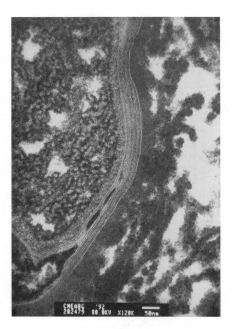

Figure 10 Same as in Figs. 7 and 8, but after treatment with ceramide-2-containing cream.

skin damage by pretreating skin with ceramides of type I for 7 days. These authors demonstrate that the increase in TEWL after SLS treatment is higher on the placebo and the untreated sites when compared with the ceramide-treated site and conclude on the fortification of the skin barrier induced by treatment with the ceramide.

The conclusion that the ceramide molecules have penetrated deeply into the stratum corneum layers and have contributed to strengthening the cutaneous barrier against water loss, as well as to reinforce intercellular cohesion, appears justified.

This is supported by the electron microscopy study conducted with ceramide-2 on the formation of lamellar bilayers in the epidermis. It showed that the typical multilayer band structure could be repaired in the upper layers of the stratum corneum by a single application of a ceramide-containing emulsion after solvent delipidation of the skin.

Barrier Repair Leads to Improved Water Retention

Further support for the beneficial effect of topically applied lipid barrier repair comes from a study on "dry" and "very dry" skin (without previous insult) (26). A study was carried out by topical magnetic resonance imaging (MRI) on the improvement of water retention in the epidermis after ceramide-2 treatment.

The method uses the capacity of hydrogen atoms in water to absorb specific radio frequencies. An increase in the quantity of free water in the sample under study, and thus an increase in the mobility of the protons, will generate an increase in magnetic signals. Thus MRI makes it possible to evaluate the variations of hydration of the epidermis (27).

The use of MRI techniques and a special surface probe with high resolution allows one to measure *in vivo*, in real time, the variation of T2, and thus the quantity of water contained in the epidermis (Fig. 11).

Contrary to the measurement of TEWL, one does not observe water fluxes, but the capacity of the epidermis to retain the water supplied by a cosmetic emulsion.

We have studied the case of five volunteers chosen for their state of dry or very dry skin. During 8 days, the volunteers applied twice daily (morning and evening) a nonhydrating cream against a cream containing 1% ceramide-2 on the designated zones on the lower arm.

Hydration of the epidermis was monitored over 6.5 h, 30 min after the last application of the creams. The curve in Fig. 12 shows the evolution of T2 over time. One remarks that the T2 values collected on the sites treated with the placebo cream for 8 days change only little with respect to the initial value throughout the day. The treatment with the placebo cream—in itself nonmoisturising—has had no hydrating effect on the dry skin.

The situation is different for the cream containing 1% ceramide-2. The MRI study *in vivo* shows that the treatment of dry skin with ceramide-2 during 8 days leads to a strong increase in the capacity of the epidermis to retain the water supplied by the cream, and this in the entire epidermis (Fig. 12)

All the above studies used a synthetic molecule representing "ceramide-2". As Rieger (22) points out, between the different chain lengths of the fatty acid and

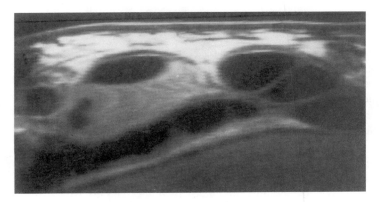

Figure 11 MRI image of the wrist of a human volunteer. The epidermis and dermis are visible, where it is possible to measure T2 relaxation times of the protons contained in epidermal water.

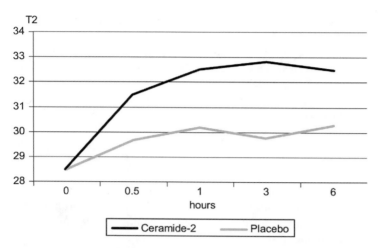

Figure 12 T2 relaxation times measured in human skin, in real time, by MRI, after treatment with either a ceramide-2-containing cream or a placebo cream. The increases follow 30 min after the last application of the creams.

the amino base, saturated or not, there are more than 200 possible structures in the skin, all lumped together under the name "ceramide-2". Nevertheless, this family of ceramides appears to be the most abundant in human skin, slowly decreasing in proportion with age (12) and thus deficient in dry skin. A stearoyl-sphinganine as tested in the earlier studies is a reasonably good representative of ceramides in general, and its cosmetic use in skin care (to reduce barrier damage in threatened skin or to repair deficient lipid barrier in older, insulted skin) is justified and compatible with the notion of "cosmeceutical".

EPIDERMIS: HOW TO BUILD THE STRATUM CORNEUM BARRIER

Technically, the stratum corneum is part of the epidermis. However, the fact that it is dead (although not totally inert, biochemically), not nucleated, and not innervated, and of quite different morphology and physical aspect, sets it apart from the living epidermis. It is undeniably an emanation of the epidermis, which renews itself every 3 weeks or so: the cells at the basal level divide, some cells stay to continue mitosis; the others (keratinocytes) start to differentiate, changing aspect and biochemical priorities a number of times until they end up as desquamating corneocytes. There can be no doubt that the epidermis also plays an important role in the barrier function of the skin as a whole. It turns out to be even more complex than the one of the stratum corneum, which is essentially based on the hydrophobicity of its components and the physical toughness of its structure.

The scientific and even the specifically cosmetic scientific literature on the epidermis is extremely voluminous. As stated before, almost all aspects (keratinocyte growth, differentiation, melanogenesis, sunlight-induced damages, enzymatic protection against free radicals, cell signaling, inflammation, nerve transmission, and immune response) of epidermal physiology have some bearing on its function as a second barrier. We must therefore be extremely selective to remain within the scope of this chapter and will thus discuss only a few items destined to the interconnectivity of all these aspects.

Möller (28) and Denda (12) reviewed the role, distribution, and appearance of ceramides in the stratum corneum. But the synthesis of all the components of the stratum corneum (proteins, lipids, and proteoglycans) occurs in the viable epidermis, which is why "barrier repair" via cosmetic means may legitimately address the question of whether it is possible to stimulate and reinforce the basic level of barrier "manufacturing" in the epidermis.

Similar to petrolatum, where the short-term effect of occlusion was seen as beneficial long before TEWL and lipid barrier function were understood, cosmetic formulators used alpha hydroxy acids (AHAs) (lactic acid and glycolic acid) with visible benefits on the skin without knowing that cell renewal, stimulation of ceramide synthesis, and barrier repair were sped up by these products. Initially, mainly the keratolytic effect was observed and sought. The abundant literature on AHAs shows, however, that more intricate mechanisms are at play. For instance, it has been demonstrated that lactic acid and its derivatives (or salts) contribute to an increase in ceramide levels in the skin, clearly a barrier repair reaction.

Rawlings et al. (29) measured the effect of different isomers of lactic acid on the synthesis of ceramide in the skin after topical application over a 4 week period. The D(−) form showed no increase, the racemic form a 25% increase, and the L(+) form a 38% increase in ceramide levels. A clinical study with a protocol similar to the one described for the topical application of ceramides to SLS-insulted skin showed that treatment of the skin with L+-lactic-acid-containing lotion led to lower TEWL values, hinting at improved barrier function, possibly due to increased ceramide synthesis.

Other active ingredients that could be called "cosmeceuticals" also have been investigated in this context. Matts et al. (30) report the effects of niacinamide (vitamin B3) on keratinocyte differentiation: incubating normal human epidermal keratinocytes with niacinamide leads first to an increase in cell proliferation and subsequently to an upregulation in involucrin and filaggrin synthesis. Furthermore, Tanno et al. (31) have shown vitamin B3 to increase ceramide and free fatty acid levels in skin by topical application and to prevent skin from losing water content, particularly after peeling sessions.

Almada (32) reports that a substance called avocadofuran displayed increased cholesterol and ceramide synthesis in human skin without altering the total lipid content of the skin (unlike that seen with lactic acid). Even more refined is the response of epidermal cells to vitamin C and its derivatives: a study carried out on a 3D model of the epidermis (SkinEthic®) showed that the profile of the ceramides synthesized is modified by ascorbic acid 2 phosphate, but not by the palmitate derivative (33). Overall ceramide content remains the same, only the relative proportions change. The physiological effect on human users cannot be predicted from this, however.

A very convoluted role in ceramide synthesis and barrier buildup, especially in embryonic skin, was discovered and described for the ubiquitous calcium ion (34). The multiple roles of extra- and intracellular calcium in the human body make it difficult to pin down meaningful cosmetic activities of topical calcium application in any form. It is, however, well known that extracellular calcium concentration in keratinocyte cell cultures modulates the rate of proliferation or differentiation. Above a level of ~ 1 mM Ca in the culture medium, the keratinocytes prefer to differentiate rather than multiply. This is visualized, using the optical microscope, in the morphological changes the cells undergo.

A recent observation was reported where a fermentation broth medium, devoid of calcium, vitamin C derivatives, lactic acid, niacinamide, or similarly known stimulants of keratinocyte metabolism, induces, nevertheless, clear signs of keratinocyte differentiation (35). It appears that extremophile bacteria, living in the depth of the ocean under conditions (-2000 m, at $80°C$ and 200 bar pressure) where surface organisms would die, have not only evolved heat stable enzymes (extremozymes) (36) to protect themselves, but also thus far unidentified metabolites that mimic extracellular calcium effects on keratinocytes.

Figure 13 shows the visually observable change in normal human skin keratinocytes when incubated with the fermentation broth (obtained from *Thermus thermophilus* culture, followed by cell breakup and extraction: TTF, *Thermus Thermophilus* Ferment); the concentration dependence clearly hints at the presence of specific molecular entities. Further confirmation of the differentiation-inducing activity comes from analysis of the involucrin synthesis, carried out by tagging the synthesized involucrin with a fluorophore-containing antibody. Again, a dose–response relationship is observed: the fluorescence increases strongly with increasing amounts of TTF in the culture medium of keratinocytes (Fig. 14).

The final observation concerns the synthesis of epidermal lipids by the keratinocytes: cultivating them for 7 days in standard culture medium, supplemented or not with TTF, and then extracting the lipids from the cells for analysis by HPTLC leads to the conclusion that TTF also stimulates the increased production of barrier lipids in the keratinocytes (data not shown).

What impact would these *in vitro* effects have on human skin in a clinical trial (Mondon P, in preparation)? Again, barrier repair needed to be investigated indirectly by normalizing the insult to the healthy skin of volunteers. A study on 15 volunteers was carried out in the following manner: TEWL was measured on the legs with a TEWAMETER (Courage & Khasaka), under strictly controlled conditions of temperature, humidity, and imposed rest period, on day 1. Insult to the skin was in the form of 10 and 20 strippings on different sites with DSQUAM® adhesive tape, leading to an increase, 20 min later, in TEWL values by 33% (10 strippings) and 210% (20 strippings) on average. This

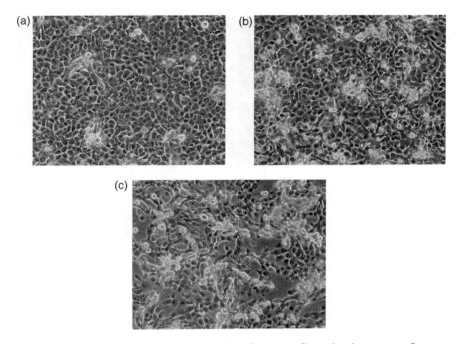

Figure 13 Normal human keratinocytes in culture. (a) Control culture at confluence; (b) culture incubated with 1% TTF medium; and (c) culture incubated with 3% TTF medium.

indicated strong disruption of the skin barrier on the second site. The panelists then used a light gel with 3% TTF on one leg and the same gel without TTF on the other leg for a period of 56 days. After 2 months, the same protocol of TEWL measurement and stripping was applied. In parallel, corneometer measurements were used to evaluate skin hydration status.

Figures 15 and 16 summarize the results. The use of TTF over this period of time led to a strong and significant strengthening of the cutaneous barrier, the stratum corneum, and the upper layers of the epidermis. This can be concluded from the fact that the insult by stripping the skin is drastically reduced on the TTF-treated side, whereas no change in response to the aggression can be observed on the placebo-treated side. Although topical application of barrier components such as ceramides lead to similar results (20), TTF stimulated barrier repair from the inside of the skin, by increasing the energy supply via ATP synthesis (Mondon P, personal communication) and by keratinocyte differentiation. It therefore constitutes a perfect complement to skin treatment with topical ceramides.

The corneometer measurements on the nonstripped sites confirmed the improvement of skin hydration status. This result is particularly interesting: it

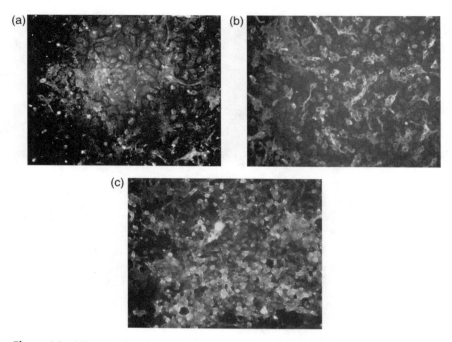

Figure 14 Micrographs of normal human keratinocytes in culture, tagged with fluorescent antibody to involucrine. (a) Control culture at confluence; (b) culture incubated with 1% TTF medium; and (c) culture incubated with 3% TTF medium.

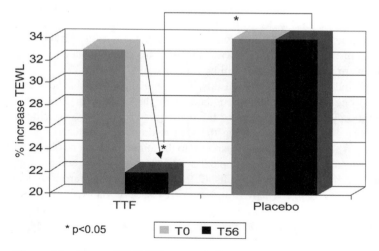

Figure 15 Changes in TEWL values after light insult (10 tape strippings), before and after treatment with TTF (3% w/w)-containing gel or vehicle for 2 months.

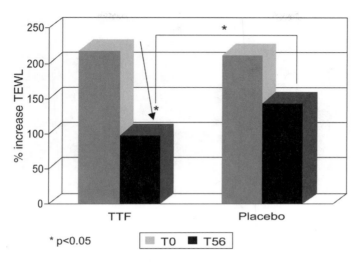

Figure 16 Changes in TEWL values after strong insult (20 tape strippings), before and after treatment with TTF (3% w/w)-containing gel or vehicle for 2 months.

shows that the increase in hydration after 2 months usage of the two gels was comparable, as both contained equal amounts of glycerine. Stopping the use of the gel for 24 h, however, led to a difference in hydration state. The TTF-treated sites retained their moisture, whereas the placebo sites lost much of this benefit (Fig. 17); the difference between the sites was significant ($p = 0.02$).

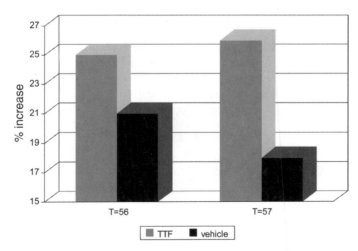

Figure 17 Changes in moisturization (corneometer values) over baseline ($T = 0$) after treatment with TTF (3%)-containing gel or vehicle after $T = 56$ days and $T = 57$ days. Last product application occurred on $T = 55$.

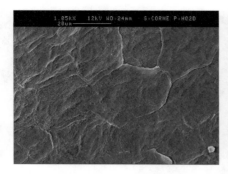 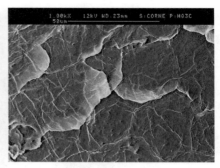

Figure 18 Scanning electron micrographs of corneocytes obtained from the skin of the volunteers having used TTF-containing gel on one leg and vehicle on the other for 2 months: (left) TTF treatment; (right) vehicle treatment.

The improvement of the stratum corneum barrier thus clearly has led to improved moisture retention capacity of the skin.

As a corollary, strippings of corneocytes were analyzed by scanning electron microscopy in order to compare the visible hydration state and morphology of treated and untreated sites. Figure 18 confirms the positive influence of TTF on this parameter.

Barrier repair at the epidermal level has another aspect that has not been fully appreciated until recently. The epidermis is relatively densely packed with keratinocytes; the connective tissue between the cells is much less evident than, say, in the dermis where the fibroblasts are sparsely distributed within the fibrous network of macromolecules. Nevertheless, hyaluronan (hyaluronic acid) is present in the epidermis, acting as a lubricant, a water-retaining entity, and a homeostasis-regulating molecule, according to Martikainen (37). This long chain polysaccharide undergoes very rapid turnover (2 days) without interference by hyaluronidase (absent in the epidermis).

Hyaluronan in the epidermis is, however, exposed to ROS inflicted damage (38), and this noxious effect is a key factor in the control of epidermal matrix cohesion (Table 1).

Table 1 Influence of UV-Induced ROS on the Catabolism of Epidermal Hyaluronan

	Decrease in hyaluronan
Control	$-37 \pm 7\%$
Control + SOD (33 U/mL)	$-19 \pm 13\%, p < 0.05$
Control + catalase (1300 U/mL)	$-23 \pm 9\%, p < 0.05$

Note: Mean results from $n = 7$ explants (38).

In an experiment on human skin biopsies, a protective effect of superoxide-dismutase (SOD) and of catalase on the catabolism of epidermal hyaluronan was shown.

Thus, the quality of the epidermis and its barrier function is also based on the maintenance of its intercellular cohesion, mediated by hyaluronan, and placed under the protection of antioxidant enzymes. Furthermore, the works by Sander (39), Sasaki (40), and recent investigations by Maes and colleagues (41) teach us the pivotal role played by SOD and catalase in maintaining a young looking epidermis. Indeed, Sasaki shows immediate stimulation of the synthesis of Cu, Zn-SOD after UVB irradiation (+145%). Maes argues, however, that SOD alone would not be good protection, as the absence of a functional catalase would lead to accumulation of deleterious H_2O_2 in the skin. Only the combined presence of SOD and catalase on or in the surface layers of the skin will contribute to the preservation of epidermal integrity—and barrier function.

Now it turns out that the TTF described earlier possesses exactly this combination of SOD, catalase, and peroxide enzymatic activity. The latter is also described as essential to skin protection (42), which the epidermis needs in time of solar irradiation. These enzymes, extracted from extremophile bacteria have the advantage of extremely high stability and lend themselves, therefore, to cosmeceutical use in barrier repair/maintenance applications extremozymes.

The combined activity of TTF consisting of thermostable antioxidant, detoxifying enzymes on the one hand, and cell differentiation stimulating activity (involucrin, ceramide production) on the other, represents a novel approach for improving the epidermal structural integrity and functionality. To protect the skin against environmental aggression and to ensure its moisture retaining capacity, it is now possible to stimulate the endogenous mechanisms that prevent and repair damages, in addition to supplying topically administered ceramides, antioxidants, biomimetic enzymes, and other active ingredients.

According to a recent publication (43), the lack of epidermal lipids in the barrier layers of the human scalp is also correlated with the appearance of dandruff. The use of barrier repair stimulating active ingredients, such as the ones described, could thus also find applications in the domain of hair care, or more precisely, in scalp care (as the term "hair care" should be reserved for treating the hair appendage itself).

DERMIS: THE FINAL FRONTIER

The dermis represents ~85–90% of the skin tissue, so if we consider the entire skin as the barrier to invasion from outside and protection for the underlying organism, then cutaneous barrier repair really means wound healing! On the other hand, wounds, even if only "skin deep", are clearly not the domain of cosmetics, or even cosmeceuticals. Band-aid® and bandages, antiseptic lotions or powders, blood clotting aids, and the like are medical devices or registered drugs, outside the cosmetic domain. So, in what way can active ingredients play a role in skin repair? If we consider wrinkles the wounds of time (Horace, Odes III), if we see stretch marks (i.e., from pregnancy) as an aesthetic problem, thin and flaccid skin as a consequence of age-related decrease in extra cellular matrix (ECM) production and of an increase in its enzymatic breakdown, then there is room for cosmetic intervention with appropriate active ingredients (cosmeceuticals).

The first visible signs of aging often occur in the face: fine lines and surface irregularities appear around the eyes (crow's feet), the mouth, and the front part of the face. Consensus about the causes of wrinkles centers on a gradual destruction of ECM, a lack of connective tissue macromolecules (collagen mostly), a deficient alignment of elastic fibers, and a relaxation of the DEJ. Cosmetic science has invested considerable efforts into understanding the appearance of wrinkles, and into subsequent attempts to prevent and/or treat them. The general approach has been, in all logic, the search for ingredients that can stimulate the synthesis of collagen and other macromolecules of the ECM. One substance that is a carryover from medical wound healing applications is the titrated *Centella asiatica* extract [for instance, sold in France under the tradename Madecassol® for speeding up the healing of small skin scratches and cuts (44)]. It contains three triterpenes (asiatic acid, madecassic acid, and asiaticoside) and possesses proven collagen synthesis stimulating activity (45). Probably because of the high price and some perceived supply problems, difficulties in formulating the actives in effective concentrations, or other such considerations, the extract did not turn into a major antiwrinkle success. Many products presently on the ingredient market claim collagen stimulation *in vitro*, many of them botanical extracts. A major step in wrinkle treatment appeared with the use of high concentrations of AHAs, mentioned before (46). The mechanism of this process is, however, complex and indirect. The peeling effect at the surface, the increased rate of cell renewal in the epidermis, and the concomitant improved moisturization may play a role as important as the reported stimulation of fibroblast proliferation. Nevertheless, the huge marketing success of the AHAs and some of the strongest claims led to scrutiny by the FDA, who established some guidelines about the boundaries that separate "cosmetic" AHA use from "drug" use. Have AHAs then become a cosmeceutical because of these overlapping applications?

This kind of question is even less rhetorical in the case of the retinoids. Retinoic acid in whatever isomer form is considered a prescription drug in most countries around the world, including for topical applications. It is prescribed by dermatologists for a variety of skin blemishes, foremost of them severe acne. Retinoic acid is an irritant, difficult to formulate and to stabilize in higher concentrations, and considered potentially teratogenic (47). It had been observed, however, that retinoic acid reduced wrinkles in subjects treated with topical RA-containing products (48). Cosmetic applications then evolved with the use of retinol, retinaldehyde, and retinol esters (acetate, palmitate, etc.), all derivatives of vitamin A. The problems of formulation, stability, and sometimes irritation remained, though (49), even if the retinoid derivatives did not require registration as a drug. Wrinkle repair with topical creams containing sufficient amounts of retinol (700–1000 ppm) could be shown in a number of clinical studies, at least if conducted over periods of ≥ 2 months (50). Again, the mechanism of action of this ubiquitous molecule is complex. A DNA array study on a 3D epidermis model reveals that retinol activates more than 40 genes of great variety (51). Collagen synthesis stimulation by retinol *in vitro* has been reported (52); a thickening of the skin of human volunteer users of topical retinol-containing creams has also been observed (50).

A concise review of the respective advantages and drawbacks of retinoids and AHAs can be found in Hermitte (53).

Parallel to vitamin A and its derivatives, vitamin C and vitamin B3 (niacinamide) were investigated and proposed as active antiwrinkle ingredients. Vitamin C is known to stimulate collagen synthesis (54) in fibroblasts *in vitro* and *ex vivo* (on biopsies). It is also needed for the hydroxylation step of the freshly synthesized collagen. Niacinamide also stimulates collagen synthesis in young and old fibroblasts, as reported by Elias et al. (34) and Oblong et al. (55). However, results of clinical, vehicle controlled *in vivo* studies using vitamin C or niacinamide for specific reduction of wrinkle parameters (depth and density) are hard to come by, even if improvements in skin texture have been described (34).

A recent approach to ECM repair involves the concept of matrikines (56). The term "matrikines" designates small peptides of defined amino acid sequence, which are set free by proteolytic processes during tissue renewal. The enzymatic breakdown of collagen and elastin during wound healing, for instance, generates small protein fragments (peptides of a few amino acids' length) that possess stimulating activity on the surrounding fibroblasts: they initiate the neosynthesis of tissue macromolecules (ECM), thus speeding the rate of renewal and healing. A number of these matrikines have been described and investigated: glycyl-histidyl-lysine is a breakdown product of serum proteins, stimulating collagen and GAG synthesis (57); valyl-glycyl-valyl-alanyl-prolyl-glycine is a fragment of elastin and has chemotactic activity [i.e., it attracts fibroblasts to the site of ECM breakdown (58)]; rigin (glycyl-glutaminyl-prolyl-arginine) and tuftsin (threonyl-lysyl-prolyl-arginine) are small fragments of immunoglobulin IgG, possessing immune modulating and tissue regulating activity (59); and lysyl-threonyl-threonyl-lysyl-serine is a fragment of pro-collagen I for which collagen I, collagen III, and fibronectin synthesis stimulation has been described (60). As an example of cosmetic use of this concept, this last matrikine peptide shall be presented in more detail in the following.

Discovered by Katayama et al. (60) during wound healing related research, the peptide KTTKS (one letter amino acid code) cannot be used as such in topical applications, as the lipid stratum corneum barrier would preclude any significant amount of penetration to the deeper layers of the skin. Palmitoylation (attaching a fatty acid to the amino end group) affords sufficient lipophilic properties to the

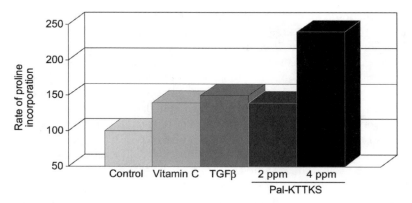

Figure 19 Stimulation of collagen synthesis in human full thickness explants in survival medium. TGFβ: 10 ng/mL; vitamin C: 1 mg/mL; Pal-KTTKS: 2 μg/mL, 4 μg/mL, resp. Expressed as % over control.

peptide (61), allowing it to penetrate into the epidermis and, to a certain extent, the dermis. *In vitro* studies on normal human fibroblasts confirm the ECM stimulation of the palmitoylated peptide: collagen I and GAG are increased over baseline by amounts varying between 50 and 250%. On full thickness skin tissue (from human biopsies), the Pal-KTTKS increases collagen I synthesis (as measured by tritiated proline incorporation) in a dose-dependent manner (Fig. 19).

It is interesting, however, to compare the amounts of active ingredient needed: 2 ppm of Pal-KTTKS achieves the same result as 1000 ppm of vitamin C; 4 ppm of the peptide doubles the effect. In contrast to the massive amounts of AHAs needed (>10% = 100,000 ppm), or even the 10,000 ppm of vitamin C, the 1000 ppm of retinol, the micromolar concentrations at which these matrikines are active, are a strong indication of their specificity. This is what nature intended them to do: initiate the repair of damaged tissue. For acting as signal molecules, no great amounts are needed.

Ongoing structure–activity relationship investigations also demonstrate that the precise sequence of these matrikines is essential: changes in the amino acid composition usually lead to loss of activity (Mondon P, unpublished).

A number of clinical, vehicle, or benchmark (retinol, moisturizer) controlled studies using the Pal-KTTKS peptide in topical antiwrinkle creams have been carried out (50,62,63).

They all demonstrate that the use of 3–5 ppm of Pal-KTTKS in a topical formula leads to significant, measurable, and consumer perceivable benefits in reducing wrinkle volume, depth, and density and to overall improvement of the facial skin when used for up to 6 months. It becomes clear from these studies that true tissue repair with matrikines needs some time, as the biological processes cannot repair damages of 30 years in 1 or 2 weeks (Fig. 20).

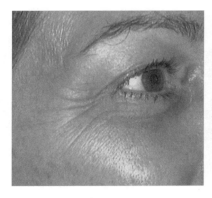 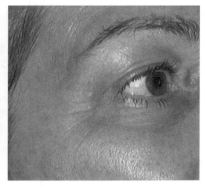

Figure 20 Two months treatment with a cream containing 5 ppm Pal-KTTKS; (left) $T = 0$; (right) $T = 56$.

This becomes apparent from skin biopsies that were taken during one of the panel studies (62) on both the Pal-KTTKS-treated group and the placebo group, at time points $T = 0$, $T = 2$ months, and $T = 4$ months. Staining of the histological slides was carried out for collagen IV (important collagen type for the maintenance of the DEJ) and for elastin. The following figures show that the treated skin has improved collagen IV and elastin fiber assemblies, whereas the control group showed no notable changes in the skin samples (Figs. 21 and 22).

In view of these results, obtained at very low concentrations of the matrikines, and considering the fact that the palmitoylated peptide does not impair the lipid epidermal barrier [as evidenced by TEWL measurements (63)] and the recognition that the peptide is a natural fragment of procollagen, it is not surprising that no adverse effects, irritation, sensitization, or mutagenicity is observed for these molecules. Matrikines such as Pal-KTTKS are thus ideal candidates for cosmetic tissue repair. The palmitoylation affords an additional advantage: the

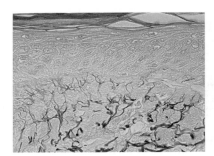 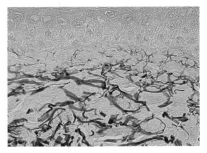

Figure 21 Skin biopsies, taken from human volunteers, at submaxillary sites; stained for elastin fibers: (left) after treatment for 4 months with 5 ppm Pal-KTTKS-containing cream; (right) after treatment for 4 months with placebo.

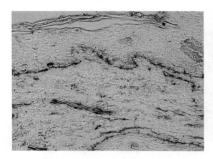 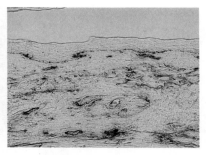

Figure 22 Skin biopsies, taken from human volunteers, at submaxillary sites; stained for collagen IV: (left) after treatment for 4 months with 5 ppm Pal-KTTKS-containing cream; (right) after treatment for 4 months with placebo.

more lipophilic nature of the peptide reduces its water solubility and thus its likelihood of being taken up into systemic fluids.

Earlier, we mentioned stretch marks and flaccid, inelastic skin as further signs of tissue damage, treatment of which could be attempted with cosmetic active ingredients. The scarcity of published data on products that could be considered cosmeceuticals (64) for these applications prevents us from delving further into this subject.

CONCLUSION

Having—arbitrarily, we admit—defined the cutaneous barrier as a three tiered structure with different functions, it became possible to select a few novel approaches for repairing some of the damages that these barrier layers can undergo during the aging process:

1. Ceramides and similar skin lipids to strengthen the intercellular cement of the stratum corneum.
2. Various active ingredients to stimulate the synthesis and renewal of the stratum corneum layer (AHAs, retinoids, vitamin B3, calcium salts, and extremozymes).
3. AHAs, vitamin A, vitamin B3, and vitamin C, but especially the matrikines to renew the dermal tissue, which after all constitutes the major part of the skin, and thus the envelope/barrier of our bodies.

At present we can only speculate on the complex interplay that is at work in living human skin among the three layers: moisture or its absence in the stratum corneum will have an influence on metabolic processes in the epidermis; free radical damages in the epidermis, leading to irritation/inflammation, will impact epidermal renewal, ceramide synthesis, and cell cohesion; and in dermal structures, the arrival of leucocytes, mastocytes, proteolytic enzymes and the like may cause destruction of the ECM.

Many of these interactions will be the subject of intense study in the coming years and will lead to novel ideas about active ingredients that can be used topically, stimulating and helping the preservation and/or repair of the cutaneous barrier. It is an exciting field to be in: at the borderline between purely decorative cosmetics and medical dermatology.

REFERENCES

1. Kligman AM. Why cosmeceuticals? Cosm Toil 1993; 108(8):37–38.
2. Umbach W. Active ingredients in cosmetic and toiletries—the current situation. Arztl Kosmetol 1985; 15:336–342.
3. Umbach W. Cosmeceuticals, the future of cosmetics? Cosm Toil 1995; 110(11):33–40.
4. Greive K. Cosmetics and life sciences: a continuing courtship. IFSCC Mag 2002; 303–305.
5. Stimson N. Cosmeceuticals: realising the reality if the 21st century. SÖFW 1994; 120(7):631–641.
6. Wertz PW, Miethke MC, Long SA, Strauss JS, Downing DT. The composition of the ceramides from human stratum corneum and from comedones. J Invest Dermatol 1985; 84:410–412.
7. Elias PM, Friend DS. The permeability barrier in mammalian epidermis. J Cell Biol 1975; 65:180–191.
8. Elias PM, Menon GK. Structural and lipid biochemical correlates of the epidermal permability barrier. In: Elias PM, ed. Advances in Lipid Research. Vol. 24. Skin Lipids, San Diego, CA: Academic Press, 1991:1–26.
9. Förster T, ed. Cosmetic Lipids and the Skin Barrier. New York: Marcel Dekker, 2002.
10. Harding CR, Watkinson A, Rawlings AV, Scott IR. Review article: dry skin, moisturisation and corneodesmolysis. Int J Cosmet Sci 2000; 22:21–52.
11. Chilcott RP, Dalton CH, Emmanuel AJ, Allen CE, Bradley ST. Transepidermal water loss does not correlate with skin barrier function *in vitro*. J Invest Dermatol 2000; 118(5):871–875.
12. Denda M. Role of lipids in skin barrier function. In: Förster T, ed. Cosmetic Lipids and the Skin Barrier. New York: Marcel Dekker, 2002:97–120.
13. Lamaud E, Schalla W. Influence of UV irradiation on penetration of hydrocortisone. *In vivo* study in hairless rat skin. Br J Dermatol 1984; 111(suppl 27):152–157.
14. Dalton CH, Chilcott RP. The effects of UVB radiation on TEWL and water barrier function *in vitro*. Proceedings of Stratum Corneum III Basel, September 12–14, 2001, Poster 32.
15. Takagi Y, Hori K, Takema Y, Imokawa G. A decrease of b-glucocerebrosidase activity induced by UVB causes a skin barrier abnormality. Proceedings of Stratum Corneum III Basel, September 12–14, 2001, Poster 14.
16. Man MQ, Brown BE, Wu-Pong S, Feingold KR, Elias PM. Exogenous nonphysiologic vs physiologic lipids. Arch Dermatol 1995; 131:809–816.
17. Man MQ, Feingold KR, Elias PM. Exogenous lipids influence permeability barrier recovery in aceton-treated murine skin. Arch Dermatol 1993; 129:728–738.
18. Yang L, Man MQ, Taljebini M, Elias PM, Feingold KR. Topical stratum corneum lipids accelerate barrier repair tape stripping, solvent treatment and some but not all types of detergent treatment. Br J Dermatol 1995; 133:679–685.

19. Imokawa G, Akasaki S, Kawamata A, Yano S, Takaishi N. Water-retaining function in the stratum corneum and its recovery properties by synthetic pseudoceramides. J Soc Cosmet 1989; 40:273–285.
20. Lintner K, Mondon P, Girard F, Gibaud C. The effect of synthetic ceramide-2 on transepidermal water loss after stripping or sodium lauryl sulfate treatment: an *in vivo* study. Int J Cosmet Sci 1997; 19:15–25.
21. Philippe M, Garson JC, Gilard P, Hocquaux M, Hussler G, Leroy F, Mahieu C, Semeria D, Vanlerberghe G. Synthesis of N-2-oleoylamino-actadecane-1,3-diol: a new ceramide highly active for the treatment of skin and hair. Int J Cosmet Sci 1995; 17:133–146.
22. Rieger M. Ceramides: Their promise in skin care. Cosm Toil 1996; 111(12):33–45.
23. Ghadially R, Brown BE, Sequeira-Martin SM, Feingold KR, Elias PM. The aged epidermal permeability barrier. J Clin Invest 1995; 95:2281–2290.
24. Landmann L. Lamellar granules in mammalian, avian and reptilian epidermis. J Ultrastruct Res 1980; 72:245–263.
25. Berardesca E, Vignoli GP, Oresajo C, Vargas A, Rabbiosi G. Prevention of barrier function damages by topically applied ceramides. Proceedings of XVIIth IFSCC Congress, Yokohama, Vol. II. 1992:881–888.
26. Lintner K, Langley N. The function and application of bioceramides in skincare. Fragrance J 1999; 10:65–70.
27. Franconi F, Akoka S, Guesnet J, Baret JM, Dersigny D, Breda B, Muller C, Beau P. Measurement of epidermal moisture content by magnetic resonance imaging: assessment of a hydration cream. Br J Dermatol 1995; 132(6):913–917.
28. Möller H. The Chemistry of natural and synthetic skin barrier lipids. In: Förster T, ed. Cosmetic Lipids and the Skin Barrier. New York: Marcel Dekker, 2002:1–35.
29. Rawlings AV, Davies A, Carlomusto M, Pillai S, Zhang K, Kosturko R, Verdejo P, Feinberg C, Nguyen L, Chandar P. Effect of lactic acid isomers on keratinocyte ceramide synthesis, stratum corneum lipid levels and stratum corneum barrier function. Arch Dermatol Res 1996; 288:383–390.
30. Matts PJ, Oblong JE, Bissett DL. A review of the range of effects of Niacinamide in human skin. IFSSC Mag 2002; 5(4):285–289.
31. Tanno O, Ota Y, Kitamura N, Katsube T, Inoue S. Nicotinamide increases biosynthesis of ceramides as well as other stratum corneum lipids to improve the epidermal permeability barrier. Br J Dermatol 2000; 143(3):524–531.
32. Almada AL. New research on vitamin E, soy and avocado. Funct Food Neutraceut Nov/Dec 2001.
33. Ramdin LSP, Richardson J, Harding CR, Rosdy M. The effect of ascorbic acid (vitamin C) on the ceramide subspecies profile in the SkinEthic epidermal model. Proceedings of Stratum Corneum III Basel, September 12–14, 2001, Poster 40.
34. Elias PM, Nau P, Hanley K, Cullander C, Crumrine D, Bench G, Sideras-Haddad E, Mauro T, Williams ML, Feingold KR. Formation of the epidermal calcium gradient coincides with key milestones of barrier ontogenesis in the rodent. J Invest Dermatol 1998; 110:399–404.
35. Lintner K, Mondon P, Mas-Chamberlin C. Stimulation of Cutaneous Barrier Repair: Involucrine, Ceramide and Stratum Corneum Structure. Proceedings of Active Ingredients, Paris 2003. Personal Care Magazine 2003; 4(3):47–49.

36. Lintner K, Lamy F, Mas-Chamberlin C, Mondon P, Scocci S, Buche P, Girard F. Heat-stable enzymes from deep sea bacteria: a key tool for skin protection against UV-A induced free radicals. IFSCC Mag 2002; 5(3):195–200.
37. Martikainen AL. Proteoglycans synthesized by adult human epidermis in whole skin organ culture. J Invest Dermatol 1992; 99:623–628.
38. Agren UM, Tammi RH, Tammi MI. Reactive oxygen species contribute to epidermal hyaluronan catabolism in human skin organ culture. Free Radic Biol Med 1997; 23:996–1001.
39. Sander CS. Photoageing is associated with protein oxidation in human skin *in vivo*. J Invest Dermatol 2002; 118:618–622.
40. Sasaki H. Effects of a single exposure to UV-B radiation on the activities and protein levels of copper-zinc and manganese superoxide dismutase in cultured keratinocytes. Photochem Photobiol 1997; 65(4):707–714.
41. Hellemans L, Corstjens H, Neven A, Declercq L, Maes D. Antioxidant enzyme activity in human stratum corneum shows seasonal variation with an age-dependent recovery. J Invest Dermatol 2003; 120(3):434–439.
42. Brooks G, Scholz DB, Parish D, Bennett S. Aging and the future of enzymes in cosmetics. Cosm Toil 1997; 112(11):79–89.
43. Harding CR, Moore AE, Rogers JS, Meldrum H, Scott AE, McGlone FP. Dandruff: a condition characterized by decreased levels of intercellular lipids in scalp stratum corneum and impaired barrier function. Arch Dermatol Res 2002; 294(5):221–230.
44. Dictionnaire des médicaments VIDAL. Paris: VIDAL, 2003.
45. Macquart FX, Bellon G, Gillery P, Wegrowski Y, Borel JP. Stimulation of collagen synthesis in fibroblast cultures y a triterpene extracted from *Centella asiatica*. Cosmet Tissue Res 1990; 24:107–120.
46. Van Scott EJ. Alpha hydroxy acids affective for acne, warts, dry skin. Skin Allergy News 1987; 18:35.
47. Nau, H. Teratogenicity of isotretinoin revisited. J Am Acad Dermatol 2001; 45:183–187.
48. Weiss JS, Ellis CN, Headington JT. Topical tretinoin improved photoaged skin. A double blind vehicle controlled study. J Am Med Assoc 1988; 259:527–532.
49. Kligman AM, Fulton JEC, Plewig G. Topical vitamin A acid in acne vulgaris. Arch Dermatol 1969; 99:469–476.
50. Lintner K. Promoting production in the extracellular matrix without compromising barrier. Cutis 2002; 70 6S(suppl):13–16.
51. Bernard FX, Pedretti N, Rosdy M, Deguercy A. Comparison of gene expression profiles in human keratinocyte mono-layer cultures, reconstituted epidermis and normal human skin; transcriptional effects of retinoid treatments in reconstituted human epidermis. Exp Dermatol 2002; 11(1):59–74.
52. Kligman LH. Preventing, delaying and repairing photoaged skin. Cutis 1988; 41:419.
53. Hermitte R. Aged skin, retinoids and alpha hydroxy acids. Cosm Toil 1992; 107(7):63–67.
54. Pinell SR, Murad S, Darr D. Induction of collagen synthesis by ascorbid acid. A possible mechanism. Arch Dermatol 1987; 123:1684–1686.
55. Oblong JE, Bissett DL, Ritter JL, Kurtz KK, Schnicker MS. Niacinamide stimulates collagen synthesis from human dermal fibroblasts and differentiation marker in normal human epidermal keratinocytes: Potential of niacinamide to normalize aged skin cells to correct homeostatic balance. Proceedings of 59th Annual Meeting American Academy of Dermatology, Washington, 2001.

56. Maquart FX, Simeon A, Pasco S, Monboisse JC. Regulation of cell activity by the extracellular matrix: the concept of matrikines. J Soc Biol 1999; 193(45):423–428.
57. Maquart FX, Pickart L, Laurent M, Gillery P, Monboisse JC, Borel JP. Stimulation of collagen synthesis in fibroblast cultures by the tripeptide-copper complex glycyl-L-histidyl-L-lysine-Cu^{2+}. FEBS Lett 1988; 238(2):343–346.
58. Senior RM, Griffin GL, Mecham RP, Wrenn DS, Prasad KU, Urry DW. Val-Gly-Val-Ala-Pro-Gly, a repeating peptide in elastin, is chemotactic for fibroblasts and monocytes. J Cell Biol 1984; 99(3):870–874.
59. Veretennikova NI, Chipens GI, Nikiforovich GV, Betinsh YR. Rigin, another phagocytosis-stimulating tetrapeptide isolated from human IgG. Confirmations of a hypothesis. Int J Pept Protein Res 1981; 17(4):430–435.
60. Katayama K, Armendariz-Borunda J, Raghow R et al. A pentapeptide from type I procollagen promotes extracellular matrix production. J Biol Chem 1993; 268(14):9941–9944.
61. Lintner K, Peschard O. Biologically Active Peptides: from a lab bench curiosity to a functional skin care product. Int J Cosm Sci 2000; 22:207–218.
62. Mas-Chamberlin C, Lintner K, Basset L, Revuz P et al. Relevance of antiwrinkle treatment of a peptide: 4 months clinical double blind study vs excipient. Ann Dermatol Vener 129 (Proceedings 20th World Congress of Dermatology, Book II, PO 438, Paris, 2002).
63. Robinson L, Fitzgerald NC, Doughty DG, Dawes NC, Berge CA, Bissett DL. Palmitoyl-pentapeptide offers improvement in human photoaged facial skin. Ann Dermatol Vener 129 (Proceedings 20th World Congress of Dermatology, Book II, PO 179, Paris).
64. Lintner K. Purified Plant Extracts Demonstrating the cosmetic activity of darutoside, esculoside and ursolic acid. Cosm Toil 1998; 113:67–72.

7

Seborrheic Dermatitis (Dandruff)

Jan Faergemann
Department of Dermatology, Sahlgrenska University Hospital, Gothenburg, Sweden

Etiology and Pathogenesis	130
Treatment	132
References	133

Dandruff and seborrheic dermatitis are often mentioned together. Dandruff is the mildest manifestation of seborrheic dermatitis and it cannot be separated from seborrheic dermatitis. Therefore, what is mentioned in the literature for seborrheic dermatitis is also true for dandruff and vice versa. It is characterized by inflammation and desquamation in areas with a rich supply of sebaceous glands, namely the scalp, face, and upper trunk (1). It is a common disease, and the prevalence ranges from 8 to 10% in different studies. It is more common in males than in females. The disease usually starts during puberty and is more common around 40 years of age. Seborrheic dermatitis is characterized by red scaly lesions predominantly located on the scalp, face, and upper trunk. The skin lesions are distributed on the scalp, eyebrows, nasolabial folds, cheeks, ears, presternal and interscapular regions, axillae, and groin. Around 90 to 95% of all patients have scalp lesions and lesions on glabrous skin are found in ~60% of the patients. The lesions are red and covered with greasy scales. Itching is common in the scalp. Complications include lichenification, secondary bacterial infection, and otitis externa. The course of seborrheic dermatitis tends to be chronic with recurrent flare-up. A seasonal variation is observed, with the majority of patients doing better during the summertime. Mental stress and dry air are factors that may aggravate the disease. A genetic predisposition is also of importance. Seborrheic dermatitis is seen more frequently than expected in patients with pityriasis versicolor, *Malassezia* (*Pityrosporum*) folliculitis, Parkinson's disease, major truncal paralysis, mood depression, and acquired immunodeficiency syndrome (1).

ETIOLOGY AND PATHOGENESIS

Molecular biology using rRNA sequence analysis and nDNA comparisons as well as GC ratios in extracted DNA has clearly divided the genus *Malassezia* into seven different species (2,3). *M. pachydermatis* is the nonlipophilic member of the genus and is isolated primarily from animals. *M. furfur*, *M. sympodialis*, *M. globosa*, *M. obtusa*, *M. restricta*, and *M. slooffiae* are the lipophilic members of the genus.

The lipophilic yeasts *Malassezia* are members of the normal human cutaneous flora in adults but are also associated with several skin diseases, such as pityriasis versicolor, *Malassezia* folliculitis, seborrheic dermatitis (dandruff), and atopic dermatitis (4,5). There are now many studies indicating that *Malassezia* (former *Pityrosporum ovale*) plays an important role in seborrheic dermatitis (4,6). Many of these are treatment studies that describe effectiveness of antimycotics, paralleled by a reduction in number of *Malassezia*, and recolonization leading to a recurrence of seborrheic dermatitis.

The various *Malassezia* yeasts have been cultured from both healthy controls as well as from patients with various *Malassezia*-related diseases (7–11). Gemmer et al. (11) have found that *M. restricta* and *M. globosa* were the dominating species in patients with dandruff and were not able to culture *M. furfur* in these patients. However, in a study from Japan, Nakabayshi et al. (7) found *M. furfur* to be the dominating species. In a study from Canada, *M. globosa* was found to be the dominating species, but other species, including *M. furfur*, were also cultured. In Sweden, *M. obtusa* and *M. globosa* were the dominating species, but other species, including *M. furfur*, were also cultured (10). Further studies are needed to clarify which species are dominant in seborrheic dermatitis.

The increased incidence of seborrheic dermatitis in patients with immunosuppressive disorders suggests that the relationship between *Malassezia* and the immune system is of importance.

Malassezia can activate complement by both the classical and alternative pathways (12). The humoral immune response to *Malassezia* in patients with seborrheic dermatitis and pityriasis versicolor has been studied using different antigen preparations and different techniques (12,13). Elevated titers in patients when compared with controls, as well as no difference in titers, have been reported

(12,13). In patients with seborrheic dermatitis, a reduced lymphocyte transformation response when compared with healthy controls has been reported in two studies (14,15). However, in another study, an enhanced lymphocyte stimulation response was found when compared with healthy controls (16). In two recently published studies, no difference in lymphocyte stimulation response was found between patients with seborrheic dermatitis and healthy controls (17,18). In an immunological screening of patients with seborrheic dermatitis, we have found low (<0.7) responses in lymphocyte transformation tests to PHA and ConA in 13 of 30 patients (19). However, in a recent study we were not able to confirm this (17). Ashbee et al. (16) found a normal PHA stimulation response in patients with seborrheic dermatitis when compared with controls. In an earlier study, we found a normal, but lower range (<1) CD4/CD8 ratio in 26 out of 30 patients with seborrheic dermatitis (19). Ashbee et al. (16) found a normal CD4/CD8 ratio in patients when compared with controls. Kieffer et al. (20) found a low CD4/CD8 ratio in 13 of 19 patients with seborrheic dermatitis.

In a study by Neuber et al. (14), IL-2 and IFN-γ production by lymphocytes from patients with seborrheic dermatitis was markedly depressed and IL-10 synthesis was increased after stimulation with *P. ovale* extract. In another paper by Kesavan et al. (21), the *Pityrosporum* yeast suppressed the production of the proinflammatory cytokines IL-1, IL-6, and TNF-α. In an immunohistochemical study in patients with seborrheic dermatitis, deposits of complement C3c and IgG were found in the stratum corneum below clusters of *Malassezia* (22).

Given the large amount of inconsistency in the data available for both generalized responses to *Malassezia* and changes in the immune response in patients with seborrheic dermatitis, we sought to take the investigation to the site of the response (i.e., the skin). We have, therefore, in a recent study compared the number and type of inflammatory cells and mediators in skin biopsies from normal and lesional skin from the trunk and scalp in patients with seborrheic dermatitis and *Malassezia* folliculitis and in normal skin from healthy controls (23). Staining was often more intense when *Malassezia* yeast cells were present. An increase in NK1- and CD16-positive cells in combination with complement activation indicates that an irritant nonimmunogenic stimulation of the immune system is important. The result with the interleukins showed an increase in both the production of inflammatory interleukins as well as in the regulatory interleukins for both T_H1 and T_H2 cells. Similarities with the immune response described for *Candida albicans* infections indicate the role of *Malassezia* in the skin response in seborrheic dermatitis (24,25).

Malassezia are members of the normal skin flora and all individuals have both a humoral and a cellular immune response to the yeasts (4,5,12,17). This is probably one of the important explanations for why the immune response in the skin is more complex with diseases where this organism is involved. A strong stimulation of cells with natural killer function and complement activity may partly be explained by various enzymes (e.g., lipases) produced by *Malassezia*, but further studies are needed to clarify this.

Lipids are essential for the growth of *Malassezia*. Diseases with increase of lipids on the skin are associated with an increase in seborrheic dermatitis (e.g., Parkinson's disease, multiple sclerosis, and stroke). Some studies have also found an increase of lipids on the skin of patients with seborrheic dermatitis (12). However, in one study, a decreased level of intercellular lipids in scalp stratum corneum was found, indicating that a barrier defect may be an important factor in seborrheic dermatitis (26).

TREATMENT

Seborrheic dermatitis is a chronic disease, and informing the patients about the risk for relapse and predisposing factors is very important. Stress and winter climate have a negative effect on the majority of patients, and summer and sunshine have a positive effect. In patients with neurological diseases and especially in patients with immunosuppressive disorders, seborrheic dermatitis is more resistant to therapy. In a young individual with resistant lesions, always think of HIV infection. Mild corticosteroids are effective in the treatment of seborrheic dermatitis. However, the disease recurs quickly, often within a few days. Antifungal therapy is effective in the treatment of seborrheic dermatitis, and because it reduces the number of *Malassezia*, the time to recurrence is increased when compared with corticosteroids. Antifungal therapy should be the primary treatment of this disease.

Antifungal therapy for *Malassezia* is effective in treating most cases of seborrheic dermatitis, and prophylactic treatment with antifungal drugs reduces the recurrence rate much more than corticosteroids (6,27–38). In one study, the combination of hydrocortisone and miconazole in an alcoholic solution was significantly more effective than hydrocortisone alone in reducing the number of *Malassezia*, and the recurrence rate was also significantly lower with the combination therapy; 16% with the combination, compared with 82% for hydrocortisone alone (6).

Ketoconazole is very effective *in vitro* against *Malassezia* with mimimum inhibitory concentrations in the range of 0.02 to 0.5 $\mu g/mL$. Oral ketoconazole has been effective in a double-blind placebo-controlled trial in patients with seborrheic dermatitis of the scalp and other areas (29). However, oral ketoconazole should be reserved for patients not responding to topical therapy. In another double-blind placebo-controlled study, ketoconazole 2% cream has been effective in the treatment of seborrheic dermatitis of the scalp and face (28), and in a comparative study between ketoconazole and hydrocortisone cream no difference was seen in effectiveness (31).

Ketoconazole shampoo used twice weekly is very effective in treating seborrheic dermatitis of the scalp (29). In a double-blind placebo-controlled study of ketoconazole shampoo used twice weekly for 4 weeks, 89% in the ketoconazole group was cured, compared with only 14% in the placebo group (29). Ketoconazole used once weekly has also been effective in preventing recurrence of dandruff in previously treated patients. Ketoconazole shampoo has been compared to ciclopirox olamine shampoo in the treatment of seborrheic dermatitis/dandruff (25). Both shampoos were equally effective and significantly more effective than placebo. However, at a follow-up visit 2 weeks after stop of treatment, the recurrence rate was significantly lower in the ketoconazole group compared with the ciclopirox olamine group.

Zinc pyrithione is also effective in the treatment of seborrheic dermatitis (32,37). In one study, zinc pyrithione has been shown to improve stratum corneum ultrastructure and return it to normal (37). Shampoos containing selenium sulfide (27), bifonazole (36), or coal tar (38) are also effective and widely used. Propylene glycol solution and shampoo has also been used successfully (33).

In severe inflammatory seborrheic dermatitis, topical treatment with antifungal therapy alone may not be so effective. Some of these patients respond well to oral ketoconazole (30) or itraconazole. Another therapy that can be effective is to combine potent topical corticosteroids with topical antifungal therapy. After clearance, many of these patients will remain free of lesions on prophylactic topical antifungal treatment. When lesions are covered with thick adherent scales, keratolytic therapy, especially in the scalp, is necessary. Seborrheic dermatitis especially in the scalp and external ear canal may be secondary infected with bacteria. In these patients, topical or many times oral antibacterial therapy in combination with regular treatment is indicated.

REFERENCES

1. Burton JL, Holden CA. Seborrhoeic dermatitis. In: Champion RH, Burton JL, Burna DA, Breatnach SM, eds. Rook A, Wilkinsson DS, Ebling FJG. Textbook of Dermatology. Oxford: Blackwell Scientific Publications, 1998:638–643.
2. Gueho E, Midgley G, Guillot J. The genus *Malassezia* with description of four new species. Antonie Leuwenhoek. 1996; 69:337–355.
3. Guillot J, Gueho E, Lesourd M, Midgley G, Chévrier G, Dupont B. Identification of *Malassezia* species—a practical approach. J Med Mycol. 1996; 26:103–110.
4. Faergemann J. *Pityrosporum* yeasts—what's new? Mycoses 1997; 40(Suppl 1):29–32.
5. Faergemann J. Atopic dermatitis and fungi. Clin Microbiol Rev. 2002; 15:545–563.
6. Faergemann J. Seborrhoeic dermatitis and Pityrosporum orbiculare: Treatment of seborrhoeic dermatitis of the scalp with miconazole—hydrocortisone (Dactacort), miconazole and hydrocrotisone. Br J Dermatol 1986; 114:695–700.
7. Nakabayshi A, Sei Y, Guillot J. Identification of *Malassezia* species isolated from patients with seborrhoeic dermatitis, atopic dermatitis, pityriasis versicolor and normal subjects. Med Mycol 2000; 38:337–341.
8. Gupta AK, Kohli Y, Summerbell RC, Faergemann J. Quantitative culture of *Malassezia* species from different body sites of individuals with or without dermatoses. Med Mycol. 2001; 39:243–251.
9. Gupta AK, Kohu J, Faergemann J, Summerbell RC. Epidemiology of *Malassezia* yeasts associated with pityriasis versicolor in Ontario, Canada. Med Mycol. 2001; 39:199–206.

10. Sandström MH, Bartosik J, Bäck O, Scheynius A, Särnhult T, Tengval Linder M, Faergemann J. The prevalence of the *Malassezia* yeasts in patients with atopic dermatitis, seborrhoeic dermatitis and healthy controls. Poster Presentation 10th EADV meeting in Munich, Germany. JEADV 2001;15(Suppl 2):112.
11. Gemmer CM, DeAngelis YM, Theelen B, Boekhout T, Dawson TL. Fast, non invasive method for molecular detection and differentiation of *Malassezia* yeast species on human skin and application of the method to dandruff microbiology. J Clin Microbiol 2002; 40:3350–3357.
12. Bergbrant I-M. Seborrhoeic dermatitis and *Pityrosporum ovale*: cultural, immunological and clinical studies. Acta Derm Venereol (Stockh) 1991;(suppl 167).
13. Midgley G, Hay RJ. Serological responses to *Pityrosporum (Malassezia)* in seborrhoeic dermatitis demonstrated by ELISA and Western blotting. Bull Soc Fr Mycol Méd 1988; 17:267–276.
14. Neuber K, Kröger S, Gruseck E, Abeck D, Ring J. Effects of *Pityrosporum ovale* on proliferation, immunoglobulin (IgA, G, M) synthesis and cytokine (IL-2, IL-10, IFN-γ) production of peripheral blood mononuclear cells from patients with seborrhoeic dermatitis. Arch Dermatol Res 1996; 288: 532–536.
15. Wikler JR, Trago E, de Haan P, Nieboer C. Cell-mediated deficiency to *Pityrosporum orbiculare* in patients with seborrhoeic dermatitis. Abstracts of the ESDR-JSID-SID Tricontinental meeting, Washington DC, April 26–30, 1989.
16. Ashbee HR, Ingham E, Holland KT, Cunlife WJ. Cell-mediated immune responses to *Malassezia furfur* serovars A, B and C in patients with pityriasis versicolor, seborrhoeic dermatitis and controls. Exp Dermatol 1994; 3:106–112.
17. Bergbrant I-M, Andersson B, Faergemann J. Cell-mediated immunity to *Pityrosporum ovale* in patients with seborrhoeic dermatitis and pityriasis versicolor. Cin Exp Dermatol. Clin Exp Dermatol 1999; 24:402–406.
18. Pearry ME, Sharpe GR. Seborrhoeic dermatitis is not caused by an altered immune response to *Malassezia* yeast. Br J Dermatol 1998; 139:254–263.
19. Bergbrant I-M, Johansson S, Robbins D, Scheynius A, Faergemann J, Söderström T. An immunological study in patients with seborrhoeic dermatitis. Clin Exp Dermat 1991; 16:331–338.
20. Kieffer M, Bergbrant I-M, Faergemann J, Jemec GB, Ottevanger V, Skov patients with atopic dermatitis and seborrhoeic dermatitis. J Am Acad Dermatol 1990; 22:739–742.
21. Kesavan S, Walters CE, Holland KT, Ingham. The effects of *Malassezia* on pro-inflammatory cytokine production by human peripheral blood mononuclear cells in vitro. Med Mycol 1998; 36:97–106.
22. Piérard-Franshimont C, Arrese JE, Piérard G. Immunohistochemical aspects of the link between *Malassezia ovalis* and seborrhoeic dermatitis. J Eur Acad Dermatol Venereol 1995; 4:14–19.
23. Faergemann J, Bergbrant I-M, Dohsé M, Scott A, Westgate G. Seborrhoeic dermatitis and *Pityrosporum (Malassezia)* folliculitis—characterisation of inflammatory cells and mediators in the skin by immunohistochemistry. Br J Dermatol 2001; 144:549–556.
24. Romani L, Bistoni F, Puccetti P. Initiation of T-helper cell immunity to *Candida albicans* by IL-12: the role of neutrophils. Chem Immunol 1997; 68:110–135.
25. Gulay Z, Imir T. Anti-candidial activity of natural killer (NK) an lymphokine activated killer (LAK) lymphocytes in vitro. Immunobiol 1996; 95:220–230.

26. Harding CR, Moore AE, Rogers JS, Meldrum H, Scott AE, McGlone FP. Dandruff: a condition characterized by decreased levels of intercellular lipids in scalp stratum corneum and impaired barrier function. Arch Dermatol Res. 2002; 294:221–230.
27. Shuster S. The aetiology of dandruff and the mode of action of therapeutic agents. Br J Dermatol 1984; 111:235–242.
28. Skinner RB, Noah PW, Taylor RM et al. Double-blind treatment of seborrheic dermatitis with 2% ketoconazole cream. J Am Acad Dermatol 1985; 2:852–857.
29. Faergemann J. Treatment of seborrhoeic dermatitis of the scalp with ketoconazole shampoo. Acta Dermato-Vener (Stockh) 1990; 70:171–172.
30. Ford GP, Farr PM, Ive FA et al. The response of seborrhoeic dermatitis to ketoconazole. Br J Dermatol 1984; 111:603–607.
31. Stratigos ID, Katamboas A, Antoniu CH et al. Ketoconazole 2% cream versus 1% hydrocortisone cream in the treatment of seborrhoeic dermatitis: a double-blind comparative study. J Am Acad Dermatol 1988; 19:850–853.
32. Marks R, Pears AD, Walker AP. The effects of a shampoo containing zinc pyrithione on the control of dandruff. Br J Dermatol 1985; 112:415–422.
33. Faergemann J. Propylene glycol in the treatment of seborrheic dermatitis of the scalp: a double-blind study. Cutis 1988; 42:69–71.
34. Faergemann J. Treatment of seborrhoeic dermatitis with bifonazole. Mycoses 1989; 32:309–311.
35. Shuttleworth D, Squire RA, Boorman GC, Goode K. Comparative clinical efficacy of shampoos containing ciclopirox olamine (1.5%) or ketoconazole (2%; Nizoral) for the control of dandruff/seborrhoeic dermatitis. J Dermatol Treat 1998; 9:157–162.
36. Zeharia A, Mimouni M, Fogel D. Treatment with bifonazole shampoo for scalp seborrhea in infants and young children. Ped Dermatol 1996; 13:151–153.
37. Warner RR, Schwartz JR, Boissy Y, Dawson TL. Dandruff has an altered stratum corneum ultrastructure that is improved with zinc pyrithione shampoo. J Am Acad Dermatol. 2001; 45:897–903.
38. Piérard-Franchimont C, Piérard G, Vroome V, Lin GC. Comparative anti-dandruff efficacy between a tar and a non-tar shampoo. Dermatol 2000; 200:181–184.

8

Decorative Products

Mitchell L. Schlossman
*Kobo Products, Inc., South Plainfield,
New Jersey, USA*

Introduction	140
Color	141
Color Additive Regulation	141
Color Additives: Definitions	141
United States Regulations	142
21 CFR Part 73: Listing of Color Additives Exempt from Certification	142
21 CFR Part 74: Listing of Color Additives Subject to Certification	142
21 CFR Part 82: Listing of Certified Provisionally Listed Colors	142
Proposed Permanent Listing of Color Additive Lakes (FR Vol. 61 #43), March 4, 1996	143
European Community	143
Annex IV: List of Coloring Agents Allowed in Cosmetic Products	143
Lakes and Salts	143
Purity Criteria	143
Japan	144
Positive List	144
Inorganic/Natural Colorants	144
US Colorants Not Permitted/Restricted in Japan	144
Color Chemistry and Manufacture	144

Organic Pigments	145
Categories of Organic Colorants	146
Stability of Organic Pigments	146
Natural Dyes	147
Inorganic Pigments	147
Titanium Dioxide	148
Zinc Oxide	148
Iron Oxides	149
Ultramarines	149
Manganese Violet	149
Iron Blue	149
Chromium Oxide (Cr_2O_3)	149
Chromium Hydroxide ($Cr_2O(OH)_4$)	150
Hydrated Alumina	150
Barium Sulfate	150
Quality Control of Colorants	150
Establishment of Standards	150
Test Methods	150
Shade Evaluation	150
Heavy Metals	151
Particle Size	151
Bulk Density	151
Pearlescent Pigments and Other Specialty Pigments	151
Pearlescent Pigments	151
Organic Pearls	151
Inorganic Pearls	151
Pigment Pearls	152
Specialty Pigments	152
Treated Pigments	152
Microfine Pigments	154
Light Diffusing Pigments	154
Makeup Technology	154
Powder	155
Face Powders	155
Talc	155
Kaolin	156
Calcium Carbonate	156
Magnesium Carbonate	156
Metallic Soap	156
Starch	156
Mica	156
Polymers	157
Colorants	157

Decorative Products

Perfumes	157
Preservatives	157
Loose Face Powders	157
Pressed Face Powders	158
Powder Blushers	158
Pressed Powder Eye Shadows	159
Quality Assurance on Powder Products	159
Foundation	160
Emulsified Foundations	160
Formulation Considerations	160
Makeup Manufacturing Equipment	160
Manufacturing Procedure	161
Anhydrous Foundations	161
Ingredients	161
Basic Formulation	162
Manufacturing Procedure	162
Eye Makeup	163
Mascara	163
Oil-in-Water	163
Solvent-Based	164
Water-in-Oil	164
Anhydrous Mascara	165
Mascara Componentry	165
Cream Eye Shadows	166
Ingredients	166
Basic Formulation	166
Manufacturing Procedure	167
Eyeliners	167
Ingredients	167
Basic Formulations	167
Manufacturing Procedure	167
Pencils	168
Raw Materials	168
Product Types	168
Manufacturing Procedure	168
Lipsticks	168
Classical Lipstick	169
Ingredients	169
Basic Formulation	170
Manufacturing Procedure	170
Volatile Lipstick	170
Ingredients	170
Basic Formulation	171

Manufacturing Procedure	171
Nail Color	171
Makeup Formulary	172
Face Products	172
Loose Face Powder	172
Pressed Powder Foundation	173
Two-Way Powder Foundation (Wet and Dry)	173
Pressed Face Powder	174
Liquid Compact Foundation	174
Blusher	175
Eye Shadow	176
Eye Shadow	176
Solvent Mascara	177
Emulsion-Resistant Mascara	177
Waterproof Eyeliner	178
Aqueous Eyeliner	179
Makeup Pencil	179
Classical Lipstick	180
Solvent Lipstick	180
Manicure Preparations	181
Cream Nail Enamel	181
Pearlescent Nail Enamel	181
Acrylic Nail Hardener	182
References	182

INTRODUCTION

Decorative cosmetics are principally concerned with beautifying and decoration, rather than functionality. No discussion of decorative products can be complete without a full understanding of the importance of color, a prime component of every decorative cosmetic. Conventional pigments create color by absorption of certain wavelengths of incident light. The color perceived corresponds to that of the wavelengths reflected. Formulation of decorative cosmetics has been an exciting challenge for cosmetic chemists. Before formulating any color cosmetic product, one must check the current regulations in the country where the proposed product will be sold, to make sure all the colors conform to those regulations. This chapter is a practical guide for the formulator and covers a maximum of technical and regulatory issues in an "easy to use" format.

    Additionally, there has been an increasing demand for color cosmetics containing treatment "actives" or cosmeceuticals. Decorative products now contain UV filters, herbs, vitamins, and moisturizers to counteract the effects of aging and to add moisture to the skin.

COLOR

Color Additive Regulation

In the past, colorants had been used in cosmetics without any consideration given to their possible toxicity. Today, all countries have regulations that control the type and purity of colors that may be used in cosmetics.

> **USA: Food and Drug Administration (FDA)**
> *21 CFR 73, 74: positive list (1).* Colors listed for general cosmetic use, including eye area only if stated specifically, or external only, meaning no contact with mucous membranes.
> Hair dyes and true soaps are exempt.
>
> **Europe (EU): European Commission (EC)**
> Directive 76/768.
> *Annex IV (2): positive list.* Coloring agents allowed for use in cosmetic products.
> *Annex II: negative list.* Substances that must not be part of cosmetic products (not specific for colorants).
>
> **Japan: Ministry of Health and Welfare (MHW)**
> *MHW ordinance No. 30 (3): positive list.* Coal-tar colors.
> Pre-market approval by MHW for all other cosmetic ingredients, including inorganic and natural colorants.

Color Additives: Definitions

> *Primary/straight color*: A color that is pure, containing no extenders or dilutents.
> *Dye*: A color that is soluble in the medium in which it is dispersed (e.g., FD&C Blue #1).
> *Pigment*: A color that is insoluble in the medium in which it is dispersed (e.g., FD&C Blue #1 A1 lake, black iron oxide).
> *Lake**: A water insoluble pigment composed of a water-soluble straight color strongly absorbed onto an insoluble substratum through the use of a precipitant (e.g., FD&C Blue #1 A1 lake). Generally, 10–40% color.

---

*FDA has considered any certified colorant mixed with a diluent to be a lake; D&C Red #30 plus talc; D&C Red #7 CA lake on calcium carbonate.

Toner: A pigment that is produced by precipitating a water-soluble dye as an insoluble metal salt. (i.e., D&C Red #6 barium salt, D&C Red #7 calcium salt).

True Pigment: A pigment that, on the basis of its chemistry, precipitates as it is formed (e.g., D&C Red #36).

Extender: A pigment, diluted on substrate (a) during manufacture by precipitation; (b) post-manufacture by intimate milling or mixing.

United States Regulations

21 CFR Part 73 (1): Listing of Color Additives Exempt from Certification

Inorganic pigments, powdered metals, and naturally derived colorants approved for food, drug, and/or cosmetic use.

Listed permitted uses:
- Food
- Ingested/externally applied drugs
- General cosmetic
- Eye area only if mentioned
- External (no mucous membrane), that is ultramarines, ferric ammonium ferrocyanide not permitted in lip or bath products

21 CFR Part 74 (1): Listing of Color Additives Subject to Certification

Synthetic organic dyes and pigments. Each batch must be submitted by the manufacturer to the FDA for certification that specifications are met.

Permitted uses as in Part 73.

Four certified organic dyes and their lakes are now permitted for eye area use:
- FD&C Blue #1
- FD&C Red #40
- FD&C Yellow #5
- D&C Green #5

21 CFR Part 82 (1): Listing of Certified Provisionally Listed Colors

Lakes

FD&C: Aluminum or calcium salt on alumina

D&C: Sodium, potassium, barium, calcium, strontium, or zirconium salt on alumina, blanc fixe, gloss white, clay, titanium dioxide, zinc oxide, talc, rosin, aluminum benzoate, calcium carbonate.

A salt prepared from straight color (i.e., D&C Red #6) by combining the color with a basic radical.

Proposed Permanent Listing of Color Additive Lakes
(FR Vol. 61 #43), March 4, 1996 (4)

List substrate (i.e., D&C Red #27 aluminum lake on alumina).

Extenders of insoluble straight colors will no longer be called lakes (i.e., D&C Red #30).

Permit blends of previously certified straight colors in a lake (i.e., FD&C Blue #1 and Yellow #5 aluminum lake).

All lakes to be prepared from previously certified batches of straight color would necessitate process changes for D&C Reds #6, #7, and #34.

Abbreviations permitted for cosmetic ingredient labeling, omitting FD&C, precipitate and substrate designation (i.e., Blue 1).

European Community

Directive 76/768, as amended (2).

Annex IV: List of Coloring Agents Allowed in Cosmetic Products

List by color index number

Part 1: Permanently listed
Part 2: Provisionally listed

Four fields of application and restriction of use

1. All cosmetic products.
2. All cosmetic products, except those intended to be applied in the vicinity of the eyes, in particular eye makeup and makeup remover.
3. Allowed exclusively in cosmetic products intended not to come into contact with mucous membranes (including the eye area).
4. Allowed exclusively in cosmetic products intended to come into contact only briefly with skin (not permitted in nail preparations).

Lakes and Salts

If a color index number is listed in Annex IV, then the pure color plus its salts and lakes are allowed, unless prohibited under Annex II (the list substances that cosmetics may not contain). *Exception*: barium, strontium, and zirconium.

Prohibited under Annex II, but where a footnote "3" appears in Annex IV, "the insoluble barium, strontium, and zirconium lakes, salts, and pigments..." shall also be permitted. They must pass the test for insolubility which will be determined by the procedure in Article 8 (insoluble in 0.1 N HCl).

Purity Criteria

Only colors designated by an "E", those also permitted for food use, must meet the general specification for food colors.

<5 ppm	As
<20 ppm	Pb
<100 ppm	Sb, Cu, Cr, Zn, BaSO$_4$ separately
<200 ppm	of those together
None detectable	Cd, Hg, Se, Te, Th, U Cr^{6+} or soluble Ba

Sixth amendment to the directive is currently adopted. Update of purity criteria is being considered, test methods may be stipulated.

Japan

MHW ordinance No. 30 (1966) as amended by MHW ordinance No. 55 (1972) (3).

Positive List

83 Coal-tar colors.

Must be declared on cosmetic product label
Fields of application: oral, lip, eye area, external, rinse-off

Inorganic/Natural Colorants

Listing, specifications, test methods.

Japan standards of cosmetic ingredients (JSCI)
Comprehensive licensing standards of cosmetics by category (CLS)
Japan cosmetic ingredient dictionary (CLS)

US Colorants Not Permitted/Restricted in Japan

Pigments
D&C RED #6	Ba Lake
D&C RED #21	Al Lake
D&C RED #27	Al Lake
D&C RED #33	Zr Lake
D&C ORANGE #5	Al Lake

Substrates
Aluminum benzoate	0.5% maximum in lipstick
Rosin	7.0% maximum in lipstick
Calcium carbonate	Not permitted

COLOR CHEMISTRY AND MANUFACTURE

The property of a colorant that makes it absorb more in one part of the visible spectrum than in another is its chemical constitution. Molecules, like atoms, exist in different electronic states. As molecules contain two or more nuclei they also possess energies of rotation and vibration. This theory applies to both organic and inorganic colorants. With the inorganic colorants, colored compounds are obtained with the ions of the transition elements that have atomic numbers 22–29.

ORGANIC PIGMENTS

Organic pigments are chiefly conjugated cyclic compounds based on a benzene ring structure, although some heterocyclic ones exist. There are three main types of organic pigments: lakes, toners, and true pigments. Organic pigments are seldom used without a diluent or substrate, in order to maintain color consistency from batch to batch. A true pigment is an insoluble compound that contains no metal ions, for example, D&C Red #30 and D&C Red #36. They are the most stable. A lake is essentially an insoluble colorant, produced by precipitating a permitted soluble dye to a permitted substrate. In cosmetics, most lakes are based on aluminum, although zinconium lakes are also found. Stability-wise, true aluminum lakes can be effected by extremes of pH, resulting in reformation of the soluble dye or "bleeding". They are fairly transparent and not particularly light fast. Toners are colorants made with other approved metals, such as barium and calcium, besides aluminum. Generally, they are more resistant to heat, light, and pH, although extremes of pH can result in shade changes. Generally, many organic colorants are unsuitable for certain cosmetics because of there chemical nature. D&C Red #36, a typical non-soluble azo color, is not recommended for lipstick; because of its very slight solubility in oils and waxes, it tends to crystallize upon continual reheating of the lipstick mass. Soluble azo dyes, such as FD&C Yellow #5 and #6 and D&C Red #33 lakes, are often used in lipstick and nail lacquer. Sparingly soluble types such as D&C Red #6 are not highly soluble, but the barium lake of Red #6 and the calcium lake of Red #7 are the most popular colors for cosmetics. Colors in this group do not need a substrate to make them insoluble. The D&C Red #6 and #7 lakes are widely used in lipstick and nail lacquer because of high strength, bright hues, good light fastness, and chemical and heat stability. Non-azo soluble dyes such as D&C Red #21, Orange #5, and Red #27 are fluoresceins and act as pH indicators and will change accordingly. They all stain the skin, and D&C Red #27 gives the strongest bluest stain.

Organic pigments are characterized by transparency, variable chemical and physical stability, and "clean", bright colors. Color is produced by chromophoric groups, generally, electron donors such as $-N{=}N-$, $-NO_2$, $-NO$, $-C{=}O$, and $-C{=}S$. Shade is modified or intensified by auxochromes, generally, electron acceptors such as $-NH_2$, $-NHR$, $-NR_2$, $-OH$, and $-OCH_3$.

Categories of Organic Colorants

AZO colorants: $-N=N-$

Insoluble (unsulfonated): D&C Red #36; light stable.
Soluble (sulfonated): D&C Red #33, FD&C Red #40, FD&C Yellow #5, FD&C Yellow #6. Stable to acid, alkali, and light; bleed in water.
Slightly soluble (sulfonated/insoluble salt): D&C Red #6, D&C Red #7, D&C Red #34. Color shift in acid and alkali; light fast; resistant to oil bleed.
Oil-soluble (unsulfonated): D&C Red #17.

On the basis of a SCCNFP opinion, certain European member states have proposed a ban of the azo dyes that could split into aromatic amines classified as CMR 1 or 2 by the Dangerous Substances Directive. The SCCNFP has asked CTFA for data to demonstrate that there would be an acceptable risk in continuing to use azo dye in cosmetics. The issue is how the dyes can break down. The future of azo dyes in Europe is thus under active discussion, and the reader is advised to get updated information on the regulatory status of azo dyes at the time of reading.

Xanthenes

D&C Orange #5, D&C Red, D&C Red #21, D&C Red #27 "staining dyes". Structure changes with pH; poor light stability; bleed in solvent.

Triarylmethane

FD&C Blue #1, FD&C Green #3. Water soluble; poor light stability.

Anthraquinone

D&C Green #5; Good light stability.

Quinoline

D&C Yellow #10, D&C Yellow #11. Oil soluble.

Indigoid

D&C Red #30. Good chemical, light, and bleed resistance. Exception: acetone soluble.

Stability of Organic Pigments

True pigments > toners > true lakes.

Light: Anthraquinone > quinone > indigoid > azo > triarylmethane > xanthene
Heat: True pigments—stable to heat. Toners—D&C Red #7 Ca lake changes reversibly. Lakes—D&C Red #27 Al lake changes irreversibly.

pH: 4–9
Metal ions: Unstable
Solubility: True lakes tend to bleed in water; fluorescein lakes bleed in solvent.

Natural Dyes (5)

Natural dyes are generally used in foods, and there is no restriction on their use in cosmetics. Mostly, the resistance of natural dyes to heat, light, and pH instability is much inferior to their synthetic counterparts. A further disadvantage is that they often tend to exhibit strong odors.

Color	Description	Source
Yellow	Curcumim	Turmeric
Yellow	Crocin	Saffron
Orange	Capsanthin	Paprika
Orange	Annato	Annatto
Orange	Carotenoids	Carrots
Red	Cochineal	*Coccus cactii*
Red	Betanine	Beetroot
Red	Anthocyanins	Red berries
Green	Chlorophylls	Lucerne grass
Brown	Caramel	Sugars

All the natural dyes mentioned in the table are of vegetable origin, except cochineal, which is extracted from the crushed insect *Coccus cactii*. Natural pigments currently under study include sweet white lupine, alfalfa, grape, and uruku from the *Bixa orellana* plant.

INORGANIC PIGMENTS

In general, inorganic colors are more opaque, more light fast, and more solvent resistant, but not as bright as organic colors. They may be affected by alkali and acid. Inorganic colorants are formed from compounds of the transition elements. Color is produced owing to the ease with which the outer "d" electrons can absorb visible light and be promoted to the next higher energy level.

Iron oxides	Red Brown	Fe_2O_3	Good stability, opacity
	Burgundy	Fe_2O_3	
	Black	Fe_3O_4	
	Yellow	FeOOH	
Chromium oxide	Green	Cr_2O_3	Good stability, opacity

Chromium hydroxide	Aqua	$Cr_2O_3 \times H_2O$	Good stability, lower tinting strength
Ultramarines	Blue		Good light stability, lower tinting strength, unstable to acid
	Violet Pink	$Na_x(AlSiO_4)_yS_z$	
Manganese violet	Violet	$NH_4MnP_2O_7$	Good light stability, lower tinting strength, unstable to water
Ferric ammonium ferrocyanide	Deep blue	$FeNH_4Fe(CN)_6$	Lower light stability, high tinting strength, unstable to alkali and salts, difficult dispersion
Ferric ferrocyanide	Deep blue	$Fe[Fe(CN)_6]_3 \times H_2O$	Lower light stability, high tinting strength, unstable to alkali and salts, difficult dispersion, precipitated on a substrate (i.e., mica)
Titanium dioxide	White	TiO_2 Anatase Rutile	Medium light stability, good chemical stability, high opacity

Titanium Dioxide

A brilliant white pigment. Two crystal types occur: anatase and rutile. Two manufacturing processes are employed:

1. Sulfate: either crystal may be produced.
2. Chloride: only rutile crystals are formed.

Properties. Crystals of both rutile and anatase are tetragonal. Rutile crystals have greater hiding power owing to the closer packing of the atoms in the crystal. Refractive indices are 2.55 for anatase and 2.71 for rutile. Opacity is the result of the light scattering ability of titanium dioxide. Light, heat, and chemical stability are excellent. In addition, in the US, titanium dioxide is a Category I sunscreen.

Zinc Oxide

Zinc ore is roasted and purified at 1000°C. Two methods of manufacture are utilized.

1. French (indirect)
2. American (direct)

Properties. Zinc oxide forms transparent hexagonal crystals. Whiteness is due to the scattering of light by extremely fine particles. Refractive index is 2.0. Hiding power is less than that of titanium dioxide. Primary use is for antibacterial and fungicidal properties. Heat and light stability are good. It is soluble in acid and alkali. In the US, zinc oxide is a Category I skin protectant and a Category III sunscreen.

Iron Oxides

Iron oxides are used in all types of cosmetic products. By blending black, red, and yellow in certain proportion, brown, tans, umbers, and sienna may be produced. Yellow iron oxide is hydrated iron II (ferrous) oxide, $Fe_2O_3 \times H_2O$. It is produced by the controlled oxidation of ferrous sulfate. Red iron oxide is chemically Fe_2O_3, and is obtained by the controlled heating (at about $1000°C$) of yellow iron oxide. Black iron oxide is Fe_2O_4 and is a mixture of ferrous and ferric oxide, and is prepared by controlled oxidation of ferrous sulfate under alkaline conditions.

Ultramarines

Theoretically, ultramarines are polysulfide sodium/aluminum sulfo-silicates. The color of ultramarines range from blue to violet, pink, and even green. A mixture is calcined at $800-900°C$ for 4–5 days. Shades are determined by reaction time, formula variations, and particle size. Ultramarine violets and pinks are obtained by treating ultramarine blue with HCl at $275°C$, removing some sodium and sulfur from the molecule.

Manganese Violet

Manganese violet is chemically $MnNH_4P_2O_7$. It is manufactured by heating manganese dioxide with ammonium dihydrogen phosphate and water. Phosphorus acid is added and the mixture is heated until the violet color develops.

Iron Blue

Iron blue is chemically ferric ammonium ferrocyanide, $Fe[Fe(CN)_6]_3$. Sodium ferrocyanide and ferrous sulfate are reacted in the presence of ammonium sulfate. Pigments prepared with sodium or potassium salts are called ferric ferrocyanide.

Chromium Oxide (Cr_2O_3)

A dull yellowish green pigment may be prepared by blending an alkali dichromate with sulfur or with a carbonaceous material. Reduction to chrome (III) oxide is achieved in a kiln at $1000°C$.

Chromium Hydroxide ($Cr_2O(OH)_4$)

Chromium hydroxide is bright bluish green pigment prepared by the calcination of a bichromate with boric acid at 500°C. The mass, during cooling, is hydrolyzed with water, yielding a hydrate.

Hydrated Alumina

Hydrated alumina is chemically $Al_2O_3 \times H_2O$. It gives little opacity and is almost transparent.

Barium Sulfate

Barium sulfate is relatively translucent and may be used as a pigment extender.

QUALITY CONTROL OF COLORANTS

Establishment of Standards

Ensure that product development is performed with material representative of supplier's production.

Prior to purchase, evaluate at least three lots; establish standard in consultation with the supplier.

Supplier and end user should agree on specifications, standard, and test methods.

Test Methods

Shade Evaluation

Methods should predict performance of the colorant under use conditions. Light source for visual evaluations to be specified.
- *Dyes*. Visual or spectrophotometric evaluation of solutions.
- *Pigments*. Cannot be evaluated as received owing to variable degree of agglomeration. Visual or instrumental evaluation is made of wet and dry dispersions prepared under defined conditions to a defined degree of dispersion.

Vehicles	Dispersion equipment
Talc	Osterizer
Nitrocellulose lacquer	Hoover muller
Acrylic lacquer	Three roll mill
Castor oil	Ball mill

Heavy Metals

Wet chemical
Atomic absorption spectroscopy (AAS)
Inductive coupled plasma (ICP)

Particle Size

Wet/dry sieve analysis
Optical microscopy
Laser diffraction
Sedimentation

Bulk Density

Fischer-Scott volumeter
pH

PEARLESCENT PIGMENTS AND OTHER SPECIALTY PIGMENTS

Pearlescent Pigments

The most important requirement for a substance to be pearlescent is that its crystals should be plate-like and should have a high refractive index. A thin, transparent, platy configuration allows light to be transmitted. A pearlescent material should have a smooth surface to allow specular reflection and should be non-toxic. Generally, when using pearlescent pigments one must use the most transparent formulation, avoiding grinding or milling the pearl pigments and blend pearls that complement each other.

Organic Pearls

These pearls produce a bright silver effect and are obtainable from fish scales as platelets or needles, which are highly reflective. The materials responsible for the pearl effect are crystals of a purine called guanine. Guanine is chiefly used in nail enamel.

Inorganic Pearls

Bismuth Oxychloride: Bismuth oxychloride produces a silvery grey pearlescent effect and is synthesized as tetragonal crystals. Crystal sizes vary from ~8 μm, which gives a soft, opaque, and smooth luster, to 20 μm, which gives a more brilliant sparkling effect. Its major disadvantage is poor light stability, which may cause darkening after prolonged exposure. UV absorbers in the finished products are used to overcome this defect. BiOCl is chiefly used to pearl nail enamels, lipsticks, blushers, and eye shadows. BiOCl may be modified by deposition on mica, titanium dioxide and mica, or talc. Inorganic pigments may be bonded to BioCl and then deposited on mica. All these alter the final effect on the finished product.

Titanium Dioxide Coated Micas: Titanium dioxide coated micas are extensively used in decorative cosmetics. They exist in several different forms. (1) Silver-titanium dioxide uniformly coats platelets of mica. Rutile crystals give a brilliant pearl effect because of a higher refractive index than the anatase grade. (2) Interference pearlescent products can be made by altering the thickness of the film. At a certain thickness, interference of light can take place so that some wavelengths of the incident light are reflected and others transmitted. The colors created are complementary to each other. As the layers become thicker, the reflection goes from silvery white, to yellow-gold, then red, blue, and green. In addition, colorants such as iron oxides can be laminated with this interference film, providing a two-color effect.

Pigment Pearls

Colored pearls are produced by laminating a layer of iron oxides on titanium dioxide coated mica, producing a color and luster effect.

Specialty Pigments

In addition to BioCl and the titanium dioxide coated mica systems, polyester foil cut into regular shapes, which have been epoxy coated with light fast pigments, have been used for nail enamels and body makeup. Finally, aluminum powder and copper/bronze powder have been used as reflective pigments, especially in eye shadows. For cosmetic use, 100% of aluminum powder particles must pass through a 200 mesh screen; 95% must pass through a 325 mesh (44 μm) screen.

Treated Pigments

Surface treated colors and substrates allow chemists to enhance the esthetic and functional qualities of their formulations. The benefits of using these treatments may be divided into two categories: those evident in the finished cosmetic product and the benefits derived from process improvements. Consumer benefits include hydrophobicity, yielding greater wear; improved skin adhesion; smoother product feel; improved optical appearance; moisturization; and ease of application. Processing benefits include ease of dispersion, pressability, less oil absorption, uniformity, and less moisture absorbtion.

The following surface treatments are commercially available.

Amino acids: *N*-Lauroyl lysine, acyl amino acid (6)
- Natural
- Good skin adhesion

- pH balanced
- Heat sensitive

Fluorochemical: Perfluoropolymethylisopropyl ether perfluoroalkyl phosphate
- Hydrophobic and lipophobic greatly enhance wear
- Heat and shear resistance

Lecithin (7)
- Natural
- Exceptionally smooth, silky skin feel, particularly in pressed products
- Heat sensitive, slightly soluble in water

Metal soaps (Zn Mg Stearate)
- Good skin adhesion
- Enhanced compressibility

Natural wax
- Natural
- Moisturizing skin feel
- Good skin adhesion
- Heat sensitive (low m.p.)

Nylon: Pure mechanically coated
- Smooth skin feel

Polyacrylate
- Enhanced wetting in aqueous systems; feel is not very good, but is usually used in dispersion

Polyethylene
- Hydrophobic
- Waxy, smooth skin feel
- Enhanced compressibility
- Heat sensitive

Silicone (Polymethylhydrogensiloxane); methicone will be chemically bonded and cannot be removed later
- Hydrophobic
- Achieves full color development
- Main use is to improve wetting

Other silicones: No potential for hydrogen evolution
- Dimethiconol
- Absorbed dimethicone
- Silicone/lecithin

Silane
- Extremely hydrophobic, lipophilic
- No hydrogen potential

Titanate ester: Isopropyl triisostearyl titanate (8)
- Enhances wetting in oil
- Smooth skin feel

- High pigment loading
- Lowers oil absorption of pigments

Microfine Pigments

Microfine/ultrafine/nanosized pigments have a primary particle size <100 nm; larger agglomerates/aggregates can be present. Properties such as surface area, bulk density, vehicle absorption, and UV absorption differ significantly from those of conventional pigment. Microfine titanium dioxide, zinc oxide, and iron oxides can be utilized in a range of color cosmetics to provide unique visual effects as well as UV protection. In pressed powders and anhydrous and emulsified formulations, significant SPF values can be achieved in formulations having a translucent, natural looking finish. With microfine pigments, formulations for darker skin tones can be formulated, which avoid the "ashy" or "made-up" appearance caused by conventional opaque pigments.

Light Diffusing Pigments

Some of the requirements for light diffusing pigments include a high refractive index, reflection to be diffused, and translucency, and its transmission must be primarily diffuse. Skin has a refractive index of 1.60. Examples of light diffusers include $BaSO_4$, silica, silica spheres coated on mica, $TiO_2/BaSO_4$ coated mica, Al_2OH_3/mica, ultrafine TiO_2/mica, ultrafine TiO_2/polyethylene, ethylene acrylates copolymer, and polymethyl methacrylate. These products are chiefly used in powders to create illusions and to hide wrinkles.

MAKEUP TECHNOLOGY

Types of color cosmetics

Foundation
Blushers
Mascara
Eyeliner
Eye shadow
Lip color
Nail color

Purpose

Improve appearance
Impart color
Even out skin tones
Hide imperfections
Protection

Decorative Products

Types of formulations

Suspensions
Aqueous
Anhydrous

Emulsions

Oil-in-water
Water-in-oil

Powder

Pressed
Loose

Anhydrous (wax, solvent)

Stick
Pan
Tube

POWDER

Powdered cosmetics are generally used to describe face powders, eye shadows, and blushers. When the product is applied to the skin, the shade must not significantly change as is worn, feel smooth in use making it easy to apply, and lastly adhere well for a reasonable time, without need for reapplication.

Face Powders

Some attributes of a satisfactory face powder are the following: (1) gives smoothness to overall texture, (2) gives added skin translucency when excess is buffed, (3) makes the skin appear more refined and finer textured, (4) helps set the make-up base, and adds longevity to the make-up overall, and (5) suppresses surface oil and shine. Generally, there is a wide range of raw materials used in powdered cosmetics and many of these carry over into the formulation of other decorative cosmetics.

Talc

Talc is the major component of most face powders, eye shadows, and blushers. Chemically it is a hydrated magnesium silicate. Cosmetic talcs are mined in Italy, France, Norway, India, Spain, China, Egypt, Japan, and the USA. Typically, talcs are sterilized by gamma irradiation. Particle size should pass through a 200 mesh sieve. Cosmetic talc should be white, free of asbestos, should have high spreadability or slip, with low covering power. Micronized talc is generally lighter and fluffier but less smooth on the skin than regular grades. Although talc is fairly hydrophobic, treated talcs have been used to enhance its texture. In some products, talc is present up to 70% of the formulation.

Kaolin

Kaolin or china clay is a naturally occurring, almost white, hydrated aluminum silicate. It does not exhibit a high degree of slip. Kaolin has good absorbency, is dense, and is sometimes used to reduce bulk densities in loose powder products. It provides a matte surface effect, which can reduce slight sheen left by some talc products.

Calcium Carbonate

Calcium carbonate or precipitated chalk has excellent absorption properties. It provides a matte finish and has moderate covering power. High levels should be avoided otherwise an undesirable, dry, powdery feel can result.

Magnesium Carbonate

Magnesium carbonate is available in a very light, fluffy grade, which absorbs well and is often used to absorb perfume before mixing it into face powders.

Metallic Soap

Zinc and magnesium stearate are important materials for imparting adhesion to face powders. They are usually incorporated at 3–10% of the formulation. Stearates add some water repellency to formulas, but too high levels give a blotchy effect on the skin. Zinc stearate, besides imparting adhesions, gives a smoothing quality to face powders. Aluminum stearate and lithium stearates have also been used. High levels can make pressed formulations too hard.

Starch

Starch is used in face powders to give a "peach-like" bloom. It provides a smooth surface on the skin. One problem attributed to rice starch is that when moistened it tends to cake. Also, the wet product may provide an environment for bacterial growth.

Mica

Mica is chemically potassium aluminum silicate dihydrate. Cosmetic mica is refined and ground to particles of ≤ 150 μm. It imparts a natural translucence when used up to 20% in formulations of face powder blushes. Mica is available as wet ground, which is creamy, or as dry ground, which is matte. Sericite is a mineral, similar to white mica in shape and composition. It has a very fine grain size and a silky shine. It is soft and smooth and has a slippery feel on the

Decorative Products

skin. Sericite may be coated with silicone and other treatments for better water repellency and skin adhesion.

Polymers

Polymers are chiefly texture enhancers used at levels of 3–40% depending on whether they are to be included in loose or pressed powder. Among these polymers, we find nylon-12 and nylon-6, lauroyl lysine, boron nitride (makes active ingredients spread more uniformly on inactive bases), polyethylene, polypropylene, ethylene acrylates copolymer (very sheer, will not affect binder in pressed powders, processing temperature $<85-90°C$), polymethyl methacrylate (PMMA) and silica beads (can carry oily ingredients into a system; increase wear on oily skin), polyurethane powders, silicone powders, borosilicate, microcrystalline cellulose, acrylate copolymers, Teflon® and Teflon composites (effective at low concentrations, 1–5%), polyvinylidene copolymers (very light ultra low density), and composite powders, which are coated on inexpensive beads to reduce costs and to increase effectiveness, like nylon/mica, silica/mica, lauryl lysine/mica, and boron nitride/mica. Many of these polymers are treated with silicones, titanates, lecithin, etc. for increased effectiveness.

Colorants

Titanium dioxide and zinc oxide, both pigmentary and ultrafine; organics; inorganics; carmine; and pearlescent pigments, either pre-dispersed or treated, are found in all face powders because the textures of these colorants are not satisfactory. Titanium dioxide and zinc oxide have anti-inflammatory properties, and zinc is an antimicrobial.

Perfumes

The use of perfumes is important for face powder, because most of the raw materials used in face powder are earthy smelling and should be masked. Perfumes should show stability and low volatility.

Preservatives

Preservation of face powders is usually not a problem as they are used dry, but small amounts of antibacterials are recommended. Powdered eye shadows should always contain antibacterials such as parabens, imidazolidinyl urea, and others.

Loose Face Powders

This type has declined in popularity in favor of pressed face powder products. The smoothness of loose face powder can be enhanced by using the aforementioned texture enhancers. In the manufacturing process, all ingredients except the pearls, if required, are combined in a stainless steel ribbon blender. Mixing time can be as long as 1 or 2 h, depending on the size of the batch and evenness of the color. The perfume, if required, is slowly sprayed into the batch and blended until homogeneous. The batch is then pulverized through a hammer mill and the color is checked. Color adjustments are made, if necessary, in the ribbon blender and the batch is re-pulverized. Any pearl or mica is then added for a final mix. The batch is then stored and made ready for filling into appropriate containers.

Pressed Face Powders

Pressed face powders are more popular than loose powders because of their ease of application and portability. The basic raw materials are the same as loose powder except that one must use a binder to press the cake into a tin-plate godet. If water based binders are used, aluminum godets should be considered to prevent corrosion. The properties of a binder is as follows: provides creaminess to the powder, aids in compression and adhesion, develops colorants, and enhances water resistance, pick-up, and deposit. If the binder level is too high, it may be difficult to remove the powder with a puff. In addition, high levels of binder may lead to glazing of the powder surface making it waxy looking, with little or no pay-off. Fatty soaps, kaolin, polyethylene, Teflon synthetic wax, and calcium silicate are some of the binder systems used. Usage levels of binder are between 3 and 10% depending on the formulation variables. Silicone treated pigments have given rise to pressed face powders, which may by used wet or dry. When used dry, they are usually smoother than regular pressed powders. When a wet sponge is applied to the cake, no water penetrates the cake; the water is repelled. These "two way" cakes can be used either as a foundation or face powder. When formulating pressed powders, one must be careful that the raw materials used do not corrode the godets or attack the plastic packaging materials. The manufacture of pressed powders, including the mixing and color matching process, is similar to loose powders. Sometimes, the powder mix is pulverized without binder and then again after its addition. Pearls are usually added during the blending process and preferably without the milling operation, which can damage the pearl. If milling a batch containing pearl becomes necessary, it should be done with the mill screen removed. Powder pressing is often more successful if the powder is kept for a few days, to allow the binder system to fully spread, especially when pearls are present. The most commonly used presses for face powder are the ALITE-high speed hydraulic press and the KEM WALL, CAVALLA OR VE. TRA. CO. The pressure used and the speed of pressing depends on the characteristics of the individual formulation and the size of the godet.

Powder Blushers

The attributes of blushers are as follows: (1) adds color to the face; (2) can give more dimension to the cheekbones; (3) harmonizes the face-balance between eye makeup and lipstick; and (4) creates subtle changes in the foundation look when lightly dusted over the face. Pressed powder blushers are similar to face powder formulations, except that a greater range of color pigments are used. The three basic iron oxides and one or more of the lakes are used to achieve various blusher shades. Blushers are usually applied with a brush. Manufacture and pressing is similar to face powders. Care should be taken that only non-bleeding pigments are used, to avoid skin staining. Total pigment concentration ranges from 2 to 10%, excluding pearls. Pressed powder rouges were once popular and contained high levels of colorants (10–30%). Usually, they are applied from the godet with the finger so that glazing may frequently occur if the rouge is improperly formulated.

Pressed Powder Eye Shadows

Eye shadows in general have the following functions: (1) adds color and personality to the face; (2) sharpens or softens the eye ball itself; (3) creates the illusion of depth or brings out deep set eyes; (4) creates light and dark illusions for subtle character changes; and (5) can be used wet or dry for different illusions. The technology is similar to other pressed powder products, but the permitted color range is limited. In the USA, the only synthetic organic pigments that may be used in eye products are FD&C Red #40, FD&C Blue #1, FD&C Yellow #5, and Green #5. Carmine, N.F. is the only natural organic pigment allowed, and all of the inorganic pigments and a wide range of pearls may be used. Preservation is very important in eye makeup products. Problems of poor adherence to the skin, color matching, and creasing in the eyelid are common when the binder formulation is ineffective with the type and level of pearls used. High binder levels may result in uneven pressing of the godets. During manufacture, formulas with high pearl content should be allowed to settle so as to remove entrapped air, before pressing.

Quality Assurance on Powder Products

Color: Production batch and standard are placed side by side on a white paper and pressed flat with a palette-knife. Shades are compared with one another. Shades of eye shadows and blushers are checked on the skin using a brush or wand.

Bulk density: Carried out on loose powder to ensure that no entrapped air is present so that incorrect filling weights are minimized.

Penetration and drop tests: Carried out on pressed godets. A penetrometer is used to determine the accuracy of the pressure used during filling. A drop test is designed to test the physical strength of the cake. Normally, the godet is dropped onto a wooden floor or rubber matte (1–3 times) at a height of 2–3 ft to note damage to the cake.

Glazing and pay-off: The pressed cake is rubbed through to the base of the godet with a puff and any signs of glazing are noted. Pay-off must be sufficient and the powder should spread evenly without losing adhesion to the skin.

FOUNDATION

In general, foundation makeup's chief functions are to hide skin flaws, even out various color tones in the skin, act as a protectant from the environment, and make the skin surface appear smoother. Requirements for an ideal foundation makeup's application are as follows: (1) should be moderately fast drying to allow for an even application, (2) should be non-settling, pour easily, and be stable in storage, (3) should not feel tacky, greasy, or too dry, (4) should improve appearance, not artificially, and (5) should have proper "play time" and slip. Depending on the formulations, several contain treated pigments and volatile silicones to add water resistance properties. There should be shade consistency between the bottle and skin tone. Products should be uniform. Coverage or capacity will vary with skin types; finish on the skin may by matte, shiny, or "dewy". Wear is extremely important—product should not peel-off, go orangey on the skin, or rub off on clothes.

Foundation makeup is available in the following forms:

Emulsions: Oil-in-water—anionic, non-ionic, and cationic. Water-in-oil—became more popular for water proofness and contains volatile silicone, hydrocarbons, mineral oil, and light esters.
Anhydrous: Cream powder and stick
Suspensions: Oil and aqueous

Emulsified Foundations

Composition can vary widely depending on the degree of coverage and emolliency desired. Although non-ionic (usually not stable), cationic (difficult to make, not on market), and water-in-oil systems have been marketed, most emulsified foundations are anionic oil-in-water emulsions, owing to ease of formulation. Anionics possess the following properties:

1. Emulsion stability
2. Pigment wetting and dispersion
3. Easy spreading and blending
4. Good skin feel
5. Slippery (soap-like) feeling

Formulation Considerations

Prolonged skin contact—minimize emulsifier levels to avoid irritation.
Choose oils on the basis of low comedogenicity.
Preservation—foundations may be difficult to preserve if containing water, gums, etc.

Makeup Manufacturing Equipment

Emulsion makeup

Pigment extenders: Hammer mill and jet mill

Internal phase: Propeller mixer/SS steam jacketed kettle
External phase: Colloid mill, homogenizer/sidesweep and SS steam jacketed finishing kettle
Emulsification: Sidesweep, homogenizer and recirculating mill (i.e., colloid mill)
With high viscosity systems, planetary mixer is needed.

Manufacturing Procedure

The coloration of the emulsion base may be handled in different ways: direct pigment, pigment dispersions, mixed pigment blender, and monochromatic color solutions (9). Each has its own advantages and disadvantages. In the direct pigment method, the pigments are weighed directly into the aqueous phase and dispersed or colloid milled; then the emulsion is formed in the usual manner. The major problem is that there are too many color adjustments needed and accurate color matching is difficult. In the pigment dispersion method, the pigment is mixed with talc as a 50:50 dispersion and pulverized to match a standard. This reduces the number of color corrections needed, but storage as well as the time taken to make these dispersions may be a problem. In the mixed pigment blender method, the pigments and extenders are premixed, pulverized, and matched to a standard. They are then dispersed in the aqueous phase of the emulsion and the emulsion is formed in the normal way. The finished shade is color matched at the powder blender stage. Chances of error are reduced. In the last method, the monochromatic color solutions required one to make color concentrates of each pigment in a finished formula. It is easy to color match by blending finished base, but much storage space is needed and the possibility for contamination is increased.

Anhydrous Foundations

Generally are powdery, not fluid, and easy to travel with.

Ingredients

Emollients: Often texturally light and have low viscosity; include oils, esters, and silicones.

Waxes:
- *Natural*: Beeswax, jojoba, orange, carnauba, candelilla, and castor.
- *Beeswax derivatives*: Dimethicone copolyol beeswax, polyglyceryl-3 beeswax, butyloctanol, and hexanediol beeswax (nice texture, compatibility with silicone material).
- *Synthetic*: Paraffins, microcrystalline, polyethylene, and "synthetic wax" (highly branched olefin polymers).
- *Fatty alcohols and fatty alcohol ethoxylates*: Unithox and Unilin.
- *Fatty esters*: Croda (Syncrowaxes), Koster Keunen (Kester waxes), Pheonix Chemical, Scher, Flora Tech, and RTD.

Pigments: Often surface treated.
- TiO_2: Pigmentary and ultrafine.
- ZnO: Pigmentary and ultrafine.
- *Iron oxides*: Pigmentary and ultrafine (enhances SPF value).

Texturizing agents: Often surface treated; include nylon, PMMA, sericite, talc, mica, boron, nitride, Teflon, borosilicates copolymer, polyvinylidene copolymer, spherical silica, starches (oats, rice, wheat, corn, and dry flo-starch), BiOCl, microcrystalline cellulose, polyurethane powder, and silicone powder.

Wetting agents: Small amount to be used; include low HLB emulsifiers, polyglyceryl esters, for example, polyglyceryl-3 diisostearate, hydrogenated lecithin, lanolin alcohols, polyhydroxy stearic acid, and soya sterols.

Bioactives: The "actives" that have been included in foundations and liquid makeups include: algae extract (anti-inflammatory), hydrolyzed wheat protein (moisturizer and skin protectant), ginseng extract, green tea, linden extract, calcium pantothenate (antioxidants), bisabolol (antiphlogistic), liposomes containing ceramide-2 cholesterol, linoleic acid, and tocopheryl acetate. Titanium dioxide is used as a physical UV sunscreen and hydrolyzed soy protein and yeast for all respiration. Vitamins C and E are antioxidants that help protect the skin from environmental damage. Urea and panthenol have been used for moisturizing and as anti-inflammatories. Allantoin is used as an anti-irritant. Copper tripeptide-1 in concealers promises to firm and diminish dark circles under the eyes. There are many others such as AHAs, salicylic acid, and hyaluronic acid used as moisturizers.

Basic Formulation

Emollients (fluids, low melting point waxes, gel-like raws)	30–60%
Waxes	5–10%
Wetting agents	0.50–1.00%
Texturizing agents	30–60%

Surface treated raw materials are frequently utilized in these types of formulations for the following reasons:

Improves dispersibility
Enhances solids loading
- Provides drier texture
- Creates matte appearance
- Improves wear
- Overall improved aesthetics

Manufacturing Procedure

1. Emollients, waxes, and wetting agent(s) are introduced into a jacketed kettle and heated until the phase is clear and uniform.

Decorative Products

2. Pigments and texturizing agents are slowly introduced into the oil phase with higher shear mixing. Continue high shear mixing until dispersion is uniform and colorants are completely "extended".

Note: If surface treatments are temperature sensitive, care must be taken to prevent the displacement of that treatment from the surface of the powder into the oil phase itself.

EYE MAKEUP

Mascara

(1) Brings out the contrast between the iris and the white of the eye and sharpens white of the eye, (2) thickens the appearance of the lashes, (3) lengthens the appearance of the eye, (4) adds depth and character to the overall look, and (5) sharpens the color of the eye shadow, when worn. Mascara's performance is usually judged by application, appearance, wear, and ease of removal. It is critical that proper brush is supplied for the chosen formulation. Generally, mascara and eyeliners consist of one or more film formers, pigment and the vehicle that mostly evaporates to allow the film to set.

Three types of formulations are currently in use. (In the past, cake or block mascara was popular. This was basically a wax base with a soap or non-ionic emulsifier present so that color could be applied with a wetted brush.) Mascara and eyeliners consist of one or more film formers, pigment, and the vehicle which mostly evaporates to allow the film to set.

Anhydrous solvent based suspension: Waterproof but not smudge-proof and difficult to remove.

Water-in-oil emulsion: Also waterproof but not smudge-proof and can be removed with soap and water.

Oil-in-water emulsion: "Water-based"; if the film is sufficiently flexible, can be flake-proof and smudge-proof. Water resistance can be achieved with the addition of emulsion polymers, such as acrylics, polyvinyl acetates, or polyurethanes.

Oil-in-Water

Water Phase
Water
Suspending agent: Hydroxyethylcellulose
Film former/dispersing agent: Polyvinylpyrrolidone
Pigment
Hydrophilic emulsifier: Alkali, high HLB non-ionic

Wax Phase
High melting point waxes
Lipophilic emulsifier: Fatty acid, low HLB non-ionic, co-emulsifier
Plasticizer: Lanolin or derivatives, liquid fatty alcohol

Petroleum solvent (optional) as extender for water phase
Preservative: propylparaben

Additional Film Formers and Actives
Solution polyacrylate (improves flake resistance)
Emulsion polyacrylate
Polyurethane
Polyvinyl acetate
Rosin derivatives
Dimethiconol
Proteins: wheat, soy, corn, keratin, oat, silk
Melanin and tocopherol—antioxidant/anti-free radicals
Panthenol

Preservative
Formaldehyde donor (not for use in Japan)

Manufacturing Procedure: Manufacturing procedure is general oil-in-water emulsification procedure except that iron oxides are first wet and milled in the water phase prior to emulsification and final product goes through a colloid mill, roller mill, or homogenizer.

Solvent-Based

Hard, high melting point waxes
Rosin derivative (optional)
Wetting agent
Pigment
Suspending agent: organoclay
Volatile solvent: To achieve wax solubility
- Petroleum distillate
- Cyclomethicone

Preservatives: parabens
Plasticizer: lanolin or derivative, liquid fatty alcohol

Water-in-Oil

Wax Phase
High melting point waxes: Carnauba, candellila, polyethylene
Rosin derivative (optional)
Lipophilic emulsifier: Lanolin acids, low HLB non-ionic
Pigment
Preservative: Propylparaben
Petroleum solvent: some cyclomethicone

Water Phase
Hydrophilic emulsifier: Alkali, medium HLB non-ionic
Preservative: Methylparaben

Additives
Emulsion polymer (optional)
Preservative: Formaldehyde donor (not for use in Japan)

Anhydrous Mascara

Ingredients
Solvents: Branched chain hydrocarbons and petroleum distillates, iso-paraffinic hydrocarbons, and volatile silicones
Waxes: Beeswax and its derivatives, candelilla, carnauba, paraffin, polyethylene, microcrystalline, castor, synthetic, ceresin, and ozokerite
Resins: (Could be introduced, but do not have to be); include aromatic/aliphatic, hydrogenated aromatics, polyterpene, synthetic, rosin, acrylics, and silicones
Gellants: Clays (stearalkonium hectorite, quaternium-18 bentonite, quaternium-18 hectorite), metal soaps (Al, Zn stearates)
Colorants: Most often utilize a classic iron oxide without any surface treatment
Functional fillers: Spherical particles (PMMA, silica, nylon), boron nitride, starches, Teflon

Purpose
Provides body to film to enhance thickening properties
Improves transfer resistance
Improves deposit on lashes

Basic Formulation

Solvents	40–60%
Waxes	10–20%
Resins	3–10%
Gellant	3–7%
Colorants	5–15%
Fillers	2–10%

Manufacturing Procedure
1. Heat waxes, solvents, and resins in a jacketed kettle until uniform and clear. Slowly add pigments under high shear and mill until dispersion is uniform.
2. Under high shear, add gellant and mill until uniform. Activate gellant with polar additive like propylene carbonate. Under high shear, add fillers and mill until uniform. Cool to desired temperature.

Mascara Componentry

Bottle: Polyvinyl chloride (PVC) for solvent-based and H.D. polyethylene/polypropylene for water-based types.

Brush/Rod/Wiper: Works complementary with each other to deliver required product attributes

For a thickening mascara the following are required:

Larger diameter rod
Larger diameter wiper
Larger brush with significant spacing between the bristles

For a defining mascara the following are required:
Smaller diameter rod
Smaller diameter wiper
Brush with minimal spacing between the bristles

Brush materials, fiber diameter, brush shape, fiber shape, fiber length, wire diameter, and the number of turns in the wire all affect performance.

Cream Eye Shadows

Generally, cream eye shadows are another form of eye shadow not as popular as the pressed form. Care must be taken in formulation to avoid creasing and other wear problems. In the past, stick eye shadows were popular. They are similar to cream eye shadows but contain high melting point waxes to make them moldable.

Ingredients

Volatile solvents: Cyclomethicone, hydrocarbons, isoparaffins
Waxes: Similar to those utilized in the anhydrous waterproof mascaras although at lower concentrations
Emollients: Esters, oils, silicones
Gellants: Bentonite derivatives, hectorite derivatives
Colorants and pearls: Classical
Fillers: Mica, talc, sericite
Functional fillers: Boron nitride, PMMA, nylon, starches, silica, Teflon, lauroyl lysine

For enhanced textural properties, higher solids loading, and improved application and coverage, use surface treated raw materials whose coatings are neither temperature nor solvent sensitive. Balance the absorption of fillers to maintain similar textures throughout the shade range.

Basic Formulation

Solvents	35–55%
Gellants	1.50–3.50%
Waxes	7–12%
Emollients	3–8%

Colorants/pearls	5–20%
Fillers	10–20%
Functional fillers	5–15%

Manufacturing Procedure

Identical to anhydrous mascaras.

Eyeliners

Eyeliners frame the eye while adding shape or changes the shape of the eye. They give the illusion of a larger or smaller eye, bringing out the color contrast between the iris and white of the eye. Lastly, eyeliners assist in making the lashes appear thicker. Generally, liquid eyeliners are the most popular and will be chiefly outlined. Cake eyeliner was popular in the past and was a wettable pressed cake applied with a wet brush. It contained powder fillers, waxes, resins, and a soap or non-ionic.

Ingredients

Solvent: Water
Gellant: Gums (magnesium aluminum silicate and bentonite)
Wetting agents: Water-soluble esters and high HLB emulsifiers
Polyols: Propylene glycol, butylene glycol, and 2-methyl-1,3-propanediol
Colorants: Surface treatment is not essential but will enhance ease of dispersibility, maintain fluidity, improve adhesion, and may enhance water resistance. Chiefly, iron oxides and other inorganic are utilized.
Alcohol: Can solubilize resins and improve dry time
Film formers: PVP, PVA, acrylics, PVP/VA, PVP/urethanes

Basic Formulations

Water	50–70%
Gellants	0.50–1.50%
Wetting agents	1–3%
Polyol	4–8%
Colorants	10–20%
Alcohol	5–10%
Film former	3–8%

Manufacturing Procedure

1. Gellants are pre-mixed with the polyol and added to a heated water phase, which also contains the wetting agent.
2. Disperse with high shear until uniform.

3. Add colorants and disperse until uniform.
4. Cool and add alcohol and film-former with low shear.

PENCILS

In general, pencils are used for coloring the eyebrows and eyelids, although they are now popular as lipsticks, lipliner, and blushers depending on the hardness of the pencil and the color composition. Products are nearly always manufactured by a handful of contract manufacturers. Chemists' responsibility is to evaluate the finished product, rather than to create one. Evaluation includes shade, texture, sharpenability, wear, application, stability (freeze–thaw and at 40–45°C), and penetration. Generally, extruded pencils are less stable than the molded ones.

Raw Materials

Oils, esters, silicones
High melting point triglycerides
Stearic acid—helps the extrusion
Synthetic waxes
Japan wax
Bright colorants and pearls in leads increase the variety available in cosmetic pencils
Fillers: mica, talc, sericite
Functional fillers: boron nitride, Teflon, PMMA, silica

Product Types

Eyeliner, lipliner, eye shadow, lipstick, brow, blush, and concealer.

Manufacturing Procedure

Molded and extruded; significant differences exist in how these products are evaluated initially after manufacturing. Molded pencils set up within a few days. Extruded pencils set up slowly over a few weeks. The molded or extruded lead is placed in a slat of wood, grooved lengthwise. A second grooved slat is glued onto the first slat and pressed together.

LIPSTICKS

Lipsticks add color to the face for a healthier look, shape the lips, and sometimes condition. They harmonize the face between the eyes, hair, and clothes and create the illusion of smaller or larger lips depending on the color. Certain pigments act to give the illusion of thicker lips. A list of lipstick actives may include herbal products and cholesterol derivatives as moisturizers. Pigments themselves tend to filter the sun, especially titanium dioxide and zinc oxide. Several lipsticks contain organic sunscreens. There are two types of lipsticks: classical and volatile (or solvent) based.

Classical Lipstick

Ingredients

Emollients: Castor oil, esters, lanolin/lanolin oil, oily alcohols (octyl dodecanol), organically modified silicones (phenyltrimethicone and alkyl dimethicones), meadowfoam seed oil, jojoba oil, esters, and triglycerides

Waxes: Candelilla, carnauba, beeswax and derivatives, microcrystalline, ozokerite/ceresein, alkyl silicone, castor, polyethylene, lanolin, paraffin, synthetic, and ester

Wax modifiers (plasticizers): Work in conjunction with the waxes to improve texture, application, and stability. Include cetyl acetate and acetylated lanolin, oleyl alcohol, synthetic lanolin, acetylated lanolin alcohol, and petroleum (white and yellow)

Colorants widely used:
- D&Cs
  - Red #6 and Ba lake
  - Red #7 and Ca lake
  - Red #21 and Al lake (stains)
  - Red #27 and Al lake (stains)
  - Red #33 and Al lake
  - Red #30
  - Red #36
  - Yellow #10
- FD&Cs
  - Yellow #5, #6 Al lake
  - Blue #1 Al lake
- Iron oxides
- TiO_2
- ZnO
- Pearls
- No Fe blue, ultramarines, Mn violet

Actives: Raw materials are added for claims and moisturization; tocopheryl acetate, sodium hyaluronate, aloe extract, ascorbyl palmitate, silanols, ceramides, panthenol, amino acids, and beta carotene

Fillers (matting and texturizing agents): Mica, silicas (classical and spherical), nylon, PMMA, Teflon, boron nitride, BioCl, starches, lauroyl lysine, composite powders, and acrylate copolymers

Antioxidants/preservatives: BHA, BHT, rosemary extract, citric acid, propylparaben, methylparaben, and tocopherol

Basic Formulation

Formula	Gloss	Matte
Emollients	50–70%	40–55%
Waxes	10–15%	8–13%
Plasticizers	2–5%	2–4%
Colorants	0.5–3.0%	3.0–8.0%
Pearls	1–4%	3–6%
Actives	0–2%	0–2%
Fillers	1–3%	4–15%
Fragrance	0.05–0.10%	0.05–0.10%
Preservatives/antioxidants	0.50%	0.50%

Manufacturing Procedure

1. Pigments are pre-milled in either one of the emollients (e.g., castor oil) or the complete emollent phase either by a 3-roller mill, stone mill, or a type of ball mill.
2. Grind phase is added to complete emollent phase and waxes, heated, and mixed until uniform (~90–105°C).
3. Pearls and fillers are added to earlier mentioned phases and mixed with shear (if necessary) until homogeneous.
4. Add actives, preservatives, fragrance, and antioxidants and mix until uniform.
5. Maintain a temperature just above the initial set point of the waxes and fill as appropriate.

Volatile Lipstick

Ingredients

Non-transfer—the proper balance of solvents and emollients prevent transfer and allow lipstick to become too dry on the lips (10).

Solvents: Isododecane, alkyl silicones, cyclomethicone
Emollients: Phenyl trimethicone, esters, alkyl silicones (fluids and pastes), vegetable/plant oils
Waxes: Polyethylene, synthetic, ceresin, ozokerite, paraffin (not compatible with some silicones), beeswax, alkyl silicones
Fixatives: Silicone resins (MQ type from G.E.), silicone plus polymers (SA 70-5, VS 70-5)
Colorants/pearls: Identical to classical lipstick
Fillers: Identical to classical lipstick
Actives: Identical to classical lipstick
Preservatives/antioxidants: Identical to classical lipstick

Basic Formulation

Solvents	25–60%
Emollients	1–30%
Waxes	10–25%
Fixatives	1–10%
Fillers	1–15%
Colorants/pearls	1–15%
Fragrance	0.05–0.10%

Manufacturing Procedure

The procedure is identical to that of classical lipstick except the product should be prepared in a closed vessel to prevent loss of volatile components.

Two new lipsticks have recently appeared. A semi-permanent color, which is marketed as two sticks: the first one is the color and the second is a moisturizing top coat (11). The wear is exceptional compared to previous developments. A different development uses interference pearlescent pigments to optically plump the lips (12).

NAIL COLOR

Nail lacquers form the largest group of manicure preparations. They should be waterproof, glossy, and adherent, dry quickly, and be resistant to chipping and abrasion. The main constituents include a film former, modifying resin, plasticizer, and solvents. Additionally, pigments, suspending agents, and ultra-violet absorbers are usually included. Nitrocellulose is the chief film forming ingredient. Nitrocellulose is derived from cellulose, a polymer made of several anhydroglucose units connected by ether linkages. Nitrocellulose by itself will produce a hard brittle film, so it is necessary to modify it with resins and plasticizers to provide flexibility and gloss. The most commonly used modifying resin is *para*-toluene sulfonamide formaldehyde resin, which is contained at 5–10% levels. This resin provides gloss and adhesion and increases the hardness of the nitrocellulose film. The formaldehyde resin has caused allergies in a small number of consumers, so other modifiers such as sucrose benzoate, polyester resin, and toluene sulfonamide epoxy resin have been used in its place with varying results. Plasticizers used include camphor, glyceryl diesters (13), dibutyl phthalate, citrate esters, and castor oil. Other resins such as polyurethanes and acrylics have been used as auxiliary resins. Variations of plasticizers and resins will change the viscosity, dry time, and gloss of the lacquer. Colorants include titanium dioxide, iron oxides, most organics, and pearlescent pigments. Soluble dyes are never used because of their staining effects on skin and nails. In order to reduce settling of the heavier pigments, treatment such as silicone (14) and oxidized polyethylene (15) have been utilized. Modified clays derived from bentonite and/or hectorite are used to suspend the pigments and make the nail enamel thixotropic and brushable. Solvents that constitute ~70% of nail lacquers include *n*-butyl acetate, ethyl acetate, and toluene. Generally, those are cream and pearl nail lacquers. Cream shades may be sheer or full coverage with titanium dioxide as the chief pigment. Pearlescent nail polish usually contains bismuth oxychloride and/or titanium dioxide coated micas and may even contain guanine-natural fish scales. The manufacturing of nail lacquer is usually carried out by specialty manufacturing firms that are familiar with the hazards of working with nitrocellulose and solvents. The manufacture consists of two separate operations: (1) manufacture and compounding of the lacquer base and (2) the coloring and color matching of shades. Top coats that are used to enhance gloss, extend wear, and reduce dry time are usually made with high solids and low boiling point solvents. Cellulose acetate butyrate (CAB) has been used as a substitute for nitrocellulose in non-yellowing top coats but does not adhere as well to the nail (16). Most top coats are nitrocellulose based. Base coats function to create a nail surface to which nail lacquer will have better adhesion. Different auxiliary resins, such as polyvinyl butyral, have been used in nitrocellulose systems. Fibers, polyamide resins, and other treatment items have been added in order to provide advertising claims, and some may actually alter the effectiveness of the film. In the evaluation of nail enamels the following criteria are considered: color, application, wear, dry time, gloss, and hardness.

Most bioactives are found in nail care products such as cuticle massage creams and oils, cuticle removers and softeners, and nail hardeners. Vitamins, herbs such as aloe and seaweed extract, myrrh, milk and other proteins, keratin amino acids, and other botanical extracts may be present for moisturizing claims. Many new shades have been developed with higher levels of mica and aluminum flakes to give a bright mirror-like appearance on the nail. Besides new and different color effects, a two-step acrylic color and sealer (17) has been developed, which provides longer wear than most conventional nail enamels. The first component is the color and the second one provides the sealer.

MAKEUP FORMULARY

Face Products

Loose Face Powder (18)

Ingredients	w/w (%)
1. Zinc stearate	8.00
2. Magnesium carbonate	1.00
3. Iron oxides	q.s.
4. Bismuth oxychloride and mica	25.00
5. Fragrance	q.s.
6. Talc	to 100.00
7. Preservative	q.s.

Manufacturing Procedure
1. Mix ingredient 3 with a portion of ingredient 6; pulverize.
2. Add the other ingredients; mix in a ribbon or double-cone blender until uniform.

Pressed Powder Foundation (19)

Ingredients	w/w (%)
Part A	
1. Talc	6.60
2. Titanium dioxide	19.20
3. Mica and titanium dioxide	4.80
4. Iron oxides	11.20
5. Zinc oxides	6.20
6. Barium sulfate	13.70
Part B	
7. Dimethicone	5.50
8. Lanolin	8.20
9. Petrolatum	1.40
10. Mineral oil	1.40
11. Isopropyl myristate	1.40
Part C	
12. Fragrance	q.s.
13. Preservative	q.s

Manufacturing Procedure
1. Mix all of the pigments in Part A together.
2. Add Part B, Part C, and Part D with high shear mixing.
3. Press into suitable container.

Two-Way Powder Foundation (Wet and Dry)

Ingredients	w/w (%)
1. Sericite	35.0
2. Talc	24.0
3. Mica	10.0
4. Nylon-12	10.0
5. Titanium dioxide	8.0
6. Zinc stearate	3.0
7. Iron oxide pigments, silicone treated	2.0
8. Cetyl octanoate	q.s.
9. Squalane	2.0
10. Octyldodecyl myristate	2.0
11. Mineral oil	2.0

Ingredients	w/w (%)
12. Dimethicone	2.0
13. Propylparaben	0.05
14. Butylparaben	0.05
15. Perfume	q.s.

Manufacturing Procedure
1. Mix all ingredients except liquid oils and perfume in a blender.
2. Spray or add liquid oils and perfume.
3. Mix and pulverize.
4. Press into pans.

Pressed Face Powder

Ingredients	w/w (%)
Part A	
1. Polymethyl methacrylate	12.00
2. Talc and polyethylene	q.s. to 100.0
3. Sericite	10.00
4. Mica and polyethylene	5.00
5. Magnesium stearate	3.00
6. Mica and titanium dioxide	5.00
7. Kaolin	8.00
8. Color	q.s.
Part B	
9. Dimethicone	6.00
10. Glyceryl diisostearate	2.00
11. Tocopherol	0.10
12. Butylparaben	0.05
13. Propylparaben	0.05

Manufacturing Procedure
1. Mix all ingredients in Part A well.
2. Heat Part B to 80°C.
3. Mix until uniform.
4. Add Part B to Part A.
5. Mix well until uniform.
6. Pulverize and sieve.
7. Press into pans.

Liquid Compact Foundation

A hot-pour solid crème foundation that seems to "liquefy" when touched. Easy to blend to a sheer finish.

Ingredients	w/w (%)
Part A	
1. Titanium dioxide and isopropyl titanium triisostearate	12.99
2. Yellow iron oxide and isopropyl titanium triisostearate	0.33
3. Red iron oxide and isopropyl titanium triisostearate	0.33
4. Black iron oxide and isopropyl titanium triisostearate	0.10
5. Aluminum starch octenyl succinate and isopropyl titanium triisostearate	15.00
6. Sericite	6.25
7. Silica	2.00
Part B	
8. Squalene	6.50
9. Dimethicone (5 Centistoke)	11.00
10. Octyl palmitate	18.00
11. Polyglycerol-3 diisostearate	5.50
12. Mineral oil	3.00
13. Hydrogenated coco glycerines	2.00
14. Microcrystalline wax	4.00
15. Carnauba	1.00
Part C	
16. Nylon-12	12.00
	100.00

Manufacturing Procedure

1. Micronize Part A until the color is fully developed.
2. Heat Part B with stirring to 195–200°F.
3. Continue to stir for 30 min.
4. Add Part A to Part B and mix until homogeneous.
5. Cool to 180°F.
6. Add Part C and mix until homogeneous.
7. Pour into pans at 165–170°F.

Blusher (Pressed) (20)

Ingredients	w/w (%)
1. Talc	65.70
2. Zinc stearate	8.00
3. Titanium dioxide	3.50
4. Iron oxides (russet)	12.00
5. Iron oxides (black)	0.20
6. D&C Red #6 barium lake	0.30
7. Titanium dioxide and mica	6.00
8. Methylparaben	0.10
9. Imidazolidinyl urea	0.10

Ingredients	w/w (%)
10. Fragrance	0.10
11. Pentaerythritol tetraisostearate	4.00
	100.00

Manufacturing Procedure
1. Mix ingredients 1–9 well.
2. Pulverize.
3. Place into ribbon blender spray into batch number 10 then 11.
4. Repulverize.
5. Sieve.
6. Press into pans.

Eye Shadow (Pressed) (21)

Ingredients	w/w (%)
1. Mica and iron oxides and titanium dioxide	40.5
2. Talc	32.4
3. Cyclomethicone and dimethicone	13.6
4. Oleyl erucate	13.5
	100.00

Manufacturing Procedure
1. Mix and mill all ingredients through a 0.027" herring bone screen.
2. Press into a suitable container.

Eye Shadow (Pressed) (22)

Ingredients	w/w (%)
1. Talc	4.20
2. Bismuth oxychloride	10.00
3. Fumed silica	0.50
4. Zinc stearate	5.00
5. Titanium dioxide and mica	65.00
6. Methylparaben	0.10
7. Propylparaben	0.10
8. Imidazolidinyl urea	0.10
9. Lanolin alcohol	3.75
10. Mineral oil	9.75
11. Isostearyl neopentanoate	1.50
	100.00

Manufacturing Procedure
1. Mix ingredients 1–8 in a ribbon blender.
2. Mix binder 9–11 in a separate container.
3. Spray binder into 1–8.
4. Mix until uniform.
5. Pulverize, if necessary without a screen.
6. Press into pans.

Solvent Mascara (23)

Ingredients	w/w (%)
Part A	
1. Petroleum distillate	q.s. to 100.00
2. Beeswax	18.00
3. PEG-6 sorbitan beeswax	6.00
4. Ozokerite 170-D	4.00
5. Carnauba wax	6.00
6. Propylparaben	0.10
7. Glyceryl oleate and propylene glycol	1.50
Part B	
8. Iron oxides	15.00
Part C	
9. Petroleum distillate and quaternum-18 hectorite and propylene carbonate	12.50
Part D	
10. Deionized water	15.00
11. Methylparaben	0.30
12. Sodium borate	0.60
13. Quaternium-15	0.10

Manufacturing Procedure
1. Mill pigments of Part B into Part A which has been heated to 90°C.
2. After Part C has been added slowly and heated with Part A, emulsify by adding Part D at 90°C to A, B, and C mixture.
3. Continue mixing until cool.

Emulsion-Resistant Mascara (23)

Ingredients	w/w (%)
Part A	
1. Deionized water	41.00
2. Hydroxyethyl cellulose	1.00
3. Methylparaben	0.30

Ingredients	w/w (%)
4. Aqueous 0.10% phenyl mercuric acetate	4.00
5. Triethanolamine	1.00
6. Ammonium hydroxide, 28%	0.50
Part B	
7. Iron oxides	10.00
8. Ultramarine blue	2.00
Part C	
9. Isostearic acid	2.00
10. Stearic acid	2.00
11. Glyceryl monostearate	1.00
12. Beeswax	9.00
13. Carnauba wax	6.00
14. Propylparaben	0.10
Part D	
15. Quaternium-15	0.10
Part E	
16. 30% Acrylic/acrylate copolymer solution in ammonium hydroxide	20.00
	100.00

Manufacturing Procedure
1. Mill the pigments of Part B in the water phase Part B.
2. Heat to 80°C. Heat the oil phase Part C to 82°C.
3. Emulsify.
4. Cool to 50°C.
5. Add Part D and then Part E.
6. Cool to 30°C.

Waterproof Eyeliner (24)

Ingredients	w/w (%)
1. Beeswax	16.50
2. PVP/eicosene copolymer	5.00
3. Petroleum distillate	35.00
4. Petroleum distillate and quaternium-18 hectorite and propylene carbonate	33.50
5. Preservative	0.20
6. Titanium dioxide and mica and ferric ferrocyanide	9.80
	100.00

Manufacturing Procedure
1. Heat ingredient 1 at 70°C and blend in 3 (n.b. flammable).
2. Blend in 4 with low shear mixing.
3. Cool to 50°C while continuing to mix.
4. Blend in ingredients 2, 5, and 6 and mix until uniform.

Aqueous Eyeliner (25)

Ingredients	w/w (%)
Part A	
1. Ammonium vinyl acetate/actylates copolymer	55.00
2. Polysorbate 80	1.00
3. Isopropyl myristate	4.00
Part B	
4. Propylene glycol USP	2.50
5. Methylparaben USP	0.25
6. Water, deionized	29.50
7. Hectorite and hydroxyethylcellulose	0.25
8. Iron oxides	7.50
	100.00

Makeup Pencil (26)

Ingredients	w/w (%)
Part A	
1a. Cyclomethicone	40.0
1b. Bis phenylhexamethicone	40.0
1c. Diphenyl dimethicone	40.0
Part B	
2. Beeswax	15.0
3. Carnauba	7.0
4. Ozokerite	7.0
5. Paraffin	20.0
6. Mineral oil	q.s. to 100.0
7. Cetyl alcohol	1.0
Part C	
8. Pigments	q.s.
9. Titanium dioxide	q.s.

Manufacturing Procedure
1. The ingredients of Part B are melted and homogenized at 78–82°C, and then maintained by a thermostatic bath regulated at 58–62°C.
2. The ingredients of Part C are dispersed in Part A; the mixture is placed in a thermostatic bath at 58–62°C.
3. Part C is then added.
4. After homogenization, the whole is cooled in a silicone treated mold (with dimethicone).

Classical Lipstick (27)

Ingredients	w/w (%)
1. Carnauba wax	2.50
2. Beeswax, white	20.00
3. Ozokerite	10.00
4. Lanolin, anhydrous	5.00
5. Cetyl alcohol	2.00
6. Liquid paraffin	3.00
7. Isopropyl myristate	3.00
8. Propylene glycolricinoleate	4.00
9. Pigments	10.00
10. Bromo acids	2.50
11. Castor oil	q.s. to 100.00

Solvent Lipstick (28)

Ingredients	w/w (%)
1. Synthetic wax	6.00
2. Ceresin	4.00
3. Isododecane	10.00
4. Paraffin	3.00
5. Cetyl acetate/acetylated lanolin alcohol	5.00
6. Methylparaben	0.30
7. Propylparaben	0.10
8. BHA	0.10
9. D&C Red #7 calcium lake	4.00
10. FD&C Yellow #5 aluminum lake	3.00
11. Titanium dioxide/mica	5.00
12. Titanium dioxide/mica/iron oxides	3.00
13. Bismuth oxychloride	10.00
14. Cyclomethicone	41.50
15. Isostearyl trimetholpropane siloxy silicate	5.00
	100.00

Manufacturing Procedure
1. Mix the dry ingredients with the volatiles and silicone ester wax.
2. The waxes and oils are added while heating.
3. Next, the powders are added.
4. The mixture is then stirred before pouring into molds and allowed to cool.

Manicure Preparations

Cream Nail Enamel (29)

Ingredients	w/w (%)
1. n-Butyl acetate (solvent)	28.23
2. Toluene (diluent)	24.54
3. Nitrocellulose 0.5 s wet (film former)	12.00
4. Ethyl acetate (solvent)	11.00
5. Toluene sulfonamide/formaldehyde resin (secondary resin)	10.00
6. Acrylates copolymer (resin)	0.50
7. Dibutyl phthalate (plasticizer)	5.00
8. Isopropyl alcohol, 99% (diluent)	4.25
9. Stearalkonium hectorite (suspending agent)	1.00
10. Camphor (plasticizer)	1.50
11. D&C Red #6 barium lake (color)	0.08
12. Titanium dioxide	0.75
13. Iron oxides	0.15
	100.00

Pearlescent Nail Enamel (29)

Ingredients	w/w (%)
1. n-Butyl acetate	34.04
2. Toluene	30.00
3. Nitrocellulose 0.5 s wet	14.90
4. Toluene sulfonamide/formaldehyde resin	7.10
5. Dibutyl phthalate	4.80
6. Camphor	2.40
7. Stearalkonium hectorite	1.20
8. Benzophenone-1	0.20
9. D&C Red #7 calcium lake	0.08
10. D&C Red #34 calcium lake	0.05
11. FD&C Yellow #5 aluminum lake	0.08
12. Iron oxides	0.15
13. Bismuth oxychloride (25%)	5.00
	100.00

Acrylic Nail Hardener (30)

Ingredients	w/w (%)
1. Ethyl acetate	41.20
2. Butyl acetate	30.00
3. Nitrocellulose 0.5 s wet	14.00
4. Toluene sulfonamide/formaldehyde resin	10.00
5. Dibutyl phthalate	4.00
6. Camphor	0.50
7. Acrylates copolymer	0.20
8. Benzophenone-1	0.10
	100.00

REFERENCES

1. 21 CFR Parts 1–99, April 1, 1998.
2. EC Cosmetics Directive 76/768/EEC, Annex IV, Part 1, September 3, 1998.
3. MHW Ordinance No. 30, August 31, 1966.
4. 61 Federal Register 8372, March 6, 1996.
5. Knowlton JL, Pearce SEM. Decorative Cosmetics. In: Handbook of Cosmetic Science and Technology. Oxford, U.K.: Elsevier Advanced Technology, 1993; 128.
6. Miyoshi R. U.S. Patent No. 4,606,914 (1986).
7. Miyoshi R. Isao Imai, U.S. Patent No. 4,622,074 (1986).
8. Schlossman ML. U.S. Patent No. 4,877,604 (1989).
9. Dweck AC. Foundations—a guide to formulation and manufacture. Cosmetic & Toiletries 1986; 101, 4:41–44.
10. Castrogiavanni A, Barone SJ, Krog A, McCulley ML, Callelo JF. U.S. Patent No. 5,505,937 (1996).
11. Drechsler LE, Rabe TE, Smith ED. US 6,340,466 (2000).
12. Cohen ID, Oko J. US 6,428,773 (2002).
13. Castrogiavanni A, Sandewicz RW, Amato SW. U.S. Patent No. 5,066,484 (1991).
14. Socci RL, Ismailer AA, Castrogiavanni A. U.S. Patent No. 4, 832,944 (1989).
15. Weber RA, Frankfurt CC, Penicnak AJ. U.S. Patent No. 5, 174, 996 (1992).
16. Martin FL, Onofrio MV. U.S. Patent No. 5,130,125 (1992).
17. Armstrong G, Callelo J, Pabil A, Pagamo F, Sandewicz R. US Patent Application Published US 2002 20018759 (April 26, 2001).
18. Hunting ALL. Face cosmetics. In: Decorative Cosmetics. Weymouth, Dorset, England: Micelle Press, 1991:3.
19. Personal Care Formulary, Waterford, NY, GE Silicones (1996), p.151.
20. Knowlton JL, Pearce SEM. Decorative products. In: Handbook of Cosmetic Science and Technology. Oxford, U.K.: Elsevier Advanced Technology, 1993:143.
21. Personal Care Formulary, Waterford, NY., GE Silicones (1996), p. 149.
22. Knowlton JL, Pearce SEM. Decorative cosmetics. In: Handbook of Cosmetic Science and Technology. Oxford, U.K.: Elsevier Advanced Technology, 1993:145.
23. Schlossman ML. Application of color cosmetics. Cosmetics & Toiletries, 1985; 100(5):36–40.

24. Hunting ALL. Eye cosmetics. In: Decorative Cosmetics. Weymouth, Dorset, England: Micelle Press, 1991:173.
25. Hunting ALL. Eye cosmetics. In: Decorative Cosmetics. Weymouth, Dorset, England: Micelle Press, 1991:170.
26. Hunting ALL. Eye cosmetics. In: Decorative Cosmetics. Weymouth, Dorset, England: Micelle Press, 1991:174.
27. Bryce DM. Lipstick. In: Poucher's Perfumes, Cosmetics and Soaps. London, U.K.: Chapman & Hall, 1992:234.
28. Castrogiavanni A, Barone SJ, Krog A, McCulley ML, Callelo JF. U.S. Patent No. 5, 505, 937 (1996).
29. Schlossman ML. Manicure preparations. In: Poucher's Perfumes, Cosmetics and Soaps. London: Chapman & Hall, 1992:253, 254.
30. Schlossman ML. Make-up formulary. Cosmetics & Toiletries, 1994; 109(4):104.

9
Depigmentation Agents

Hideo Nakayama
Nakayama Dermatology Clinic, Tokyo, Japan

Tamotsu Ebihara
Saiseikai Central Hospital, Tokyo, Japan

Noriko Satoh
Yanagihara Hospital, Tokyo, Japan

Tsuneo Jinnai
Sansho Pharmaceutical Company, Fukuoka, Japan

Introduction	185
Screening Tests for Depigmentation Agents	190
Clinical Evaluation	194
The Case of Kojic Acid	200
References	204

INTRODUCTION

There are a variety of facial pigmentary disorders (Table 1). Among such diseases, malignant tumors should be diagnosed and treated properly because some of them are quick to develop, destructive, or fatal. Hyperpigmentation of

Table 1 Pigmentary Skin Disorders of the Face

I. Acquired
  1. Melasma (chloasma)
  2. Solar lentigo
  3. Pigmented cosmetic dermatitis
  4. Sun tanning
  5. Tattoo
  6. Ochronosis
  7. Pigmentation due to atopic dermatitis
  8. Phototoxic hyperpigmentation (Berloque dermatitis)
  9. Posttraumatic hyperpigmentation
  10. Others (lichen planus cum pigmentatione, pigmentsyphilis, etc.)
II. Hereditary
  1. Nevus pigmentosus
  2. Nevus spilus
  3. Nevus of Ota
  4. Ephelid
III. Skin tumors
  1. Melanoma
  2. Basal cell carcinoma/epithelioma
  3. Spitz nevus
  4. Solar keratosis
  5. Bowen's disease
  6. Blue nevus
  7. Others

the face of middle-aged women is most common; however, it is benign, and, if diagnosed and treated properly, it can be cured or greatly improved.

Melasma is commonly observed among middle-aged women (average age of 43) (1), and is rare in men. It is a diffuse or well-circumscribed noninflammatory brown hyperpigmentation that frequently occurs around the eyes, mouth, cheeks, and forehead.

Subjective symptoms such as itching or irritation are lacking (2). Melasma is present in middle age, but is rare in women over the age of 70. An experienced old Japanese dermatologist in Kyoto City often told melasma patients, "You need not treat melasma. Just live until the age of 70 and then the melasma you suffer from will disappear".

The main cause of melasma is considered to be an increase in progesterone (P4) in the serum at luteal phases. Sato (1) measured various hormones by tritium (3H) radioimmunoassay in two groups of age-matched middle-aged women (average age 43) with and without melasma on the seventh day of the ovarial and luteal phases. Significant differences were present only in the increased levels of progesterone (P4) and 17OH progesterone in the plasma in the luteal phases of melasma patients as compared with the age-matched female controls without melasma (Fig. 1). Other hormones, such as estradiol, follicle stimulating hormone, luteinizing hormone, prolactin, androstenedione, and cortisol (Fig. 2), showed no differences between the groups during the ovarial and luteal phases. The increase in plasma progesterone may be attributed to the fact that melasma is exacerbated by pregnancy where plasma progesterone is increased or by contraceptive pills that occasionally contained progesterone; there is gradual decline of melasma after climacterium by 70 years of age.

Histopathology of melasma shows an increase in melanin pigments in the epidermal cells, especially in the supranuclear region in the basal cells (Fig. 3). The number of epidermal melanocytes has not increased and, therefore, the hyperpigmentation of melasma is considered to be functional and reversible. Two links, however, are still missing: the connection to the increase in serum progesterone as the intracellular receptor in the melanocytes is not known, and the photosensitivity of melasma patients has not been clarified.

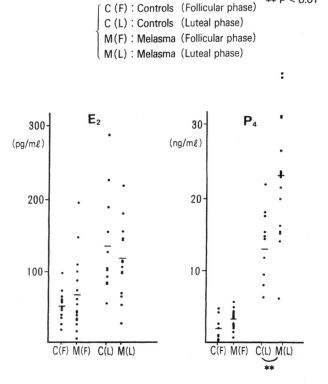

Figure 1 Progesterone levels in the plasma in the luteal phases of melasma patients as compared with age-matched female controls without melasma.

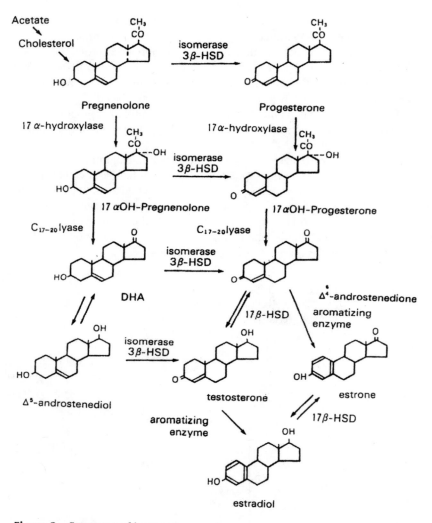

Figure 2 Structures of hormones.

When minimum erythema dosis (MED) was measured in melasma patients, 18 (24.7%) of the 73 melasma patients showed clear photohypersensitivity by lowered MED and minimum pigmentation dosis (MPD) to a mixture of UVA and UVB. Further study showed that reactivity to UVA was normal but hypersensitivity to UVB was remarkable in all 15 patients. With such photohypersensitive melasma patients, MED was lowered to approximately one-third of normal persons in summer, and a palpable erythema was observed above 2 MEDs of UVB, which produced long-lasting hyperpigmentation for weeks. Therefore, 2

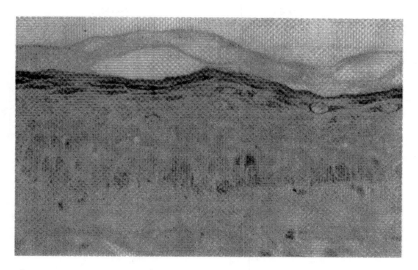

Figure 3 Increase in melanin pigments in the supranuclear region in basal cells.

MEDs were almost equal to 1 minimum quaddel dosis (MQD) and 1 MPD (Table 2; Fig. 4). All these patients did not have any medication when MED was measured, uroporphyrin and coproporphyrin levels were normal in urine, and the effect of common photoallergens such as musk ambrette or thiazides was denied. Plasma 17OH progesterone levels were elevated only in one case, but nine other cases showed normal results when these photohypersensitive cases were again examined. Therefore, the mechanism of UVB photohypersensitivity in melasma should be investigated in the future.

Melasma has been regarded as an excellent target for newly developed depigmentation agents because many middle-aged melasma patients want their skin color return to normal. Long-term therapy is necessary so that depigmentation occurs slowly, without provoking severe depigmentation (as with hydroquinone monobenzyl ether) or severe hyperpigmentation of ochronosis (as with hydroquinone at 2–4% concentrations under a tropical climate) (3). Historically, both disorders had been reported (4) and, therefore, both are disastrous pitfalls for those developing depigmentation agents.

First, unlike hydroquinone monobenzyl ether, the depigmentation agents under development should not kill melanocytes. Second, hydroquinone itself is not cytotoxic to melanocytes; however, it degenerates dermal elastic fibers under strong sunlight at high concentrations of 2–4%, which results in another disastrous strong brown hyperpigmentation called ochronosis (5). Therefore, the best depigmentation agent inhibits tyrosinase in melanocytes, and toxicity to epidermal cells, melanocytes, dermis, and other systemic organs is negligible. Also, depigmentation agents should not be strong sensitizers, oncogenic, or teratogenic. They should be stable chemically at least for more than 1 year.

Table 2 MED and MPD with Melasma Patients (1983–1987)

Apparatus: NS-9[a]
Results: 1 MPD = 1 MQD = 2 MED (general rule)

	Shortened	Normal	Total
1. MED			
Spring	9	13	22
Summer	18	55	73
Autumn	0	3	3
Winter	1	10	11
2. MPD			
Spring	10	12	22
Summer	23	49	72
Autumn	0	3	3
Winter	4	7	11

Note: NS-9 is a modified version of the previous type NCA-6, added with an inverter to shorten the irradiation time for MED.
[a]Light sources:
  FL-20 BA-37, 20W × 2 (UV-A)
  FL-20 E, 20W × 2 (UV-B)
Tube–skin distance: 10 cm
Automatic irradiation time: 10–90 s, at 10 s intervals
Performance:
  1. Normal individuals—
     MED: 70–90 s (Spring–Summer)
     MQD, MPD: more than 90 s
  2. Photodermatitis patients—
     MED: shortened to 10–60 s
     MQD, MPD: delayed erythema, and so on are detectable.

Hydroquinone cream changes color from white to brown after 3–4 months; therefore, it can be produced at pharmacies and hospitals on the condition that it is disposed of after the color changes. Therefore, it cannot be used in cosmetics or cosmeceuticals. Hydroquinone cream is an excellent preparation for the treatment of melasma with or without mild chemical peeling (6,7). However, the color change and the development of ochronosis have inhibited its usage in cosmetics and comeseuticals.

SCREENING TESTS FOR DEPIGMENTATION AGENTS

A standard method for screening depigmentation agents is the isolated tyrosinase inhibition test. Mushroom tyrosinase has been commonly used, and the suppression of tyrosinase could be demonstrated when dose-dependent inhibition was demonstrated with hydroquinone as an effective control. Another kind of tyrosinase assay is noninhibitory- or nonsuppressive-type reactions of melanogenesis. According to Mishima (8), melanogenesis can also be hindered by

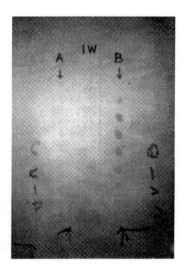

Figure 4 Measurement of MEDs.

tyrosinase production inhibition, inhibition of tyrosinase transfer, and cytotoxic inhibition (Table 3). Cultured B-16 melanoma cells have been used in this field and are useful in demonstrating several new mechanisms of melanogenesis inhibition: glycosylation turned out to be another process of the production, along with maturation of melanogenesis. Its inhibition also decreased the amount of melanin, and depigmentation agents were also found. Tyrosinase activities in ribosomes and the production of premelanosomes can also be targets for

Table 3 Mechanism of Melanogenesis Inhibition

Mechanism	Example
1. Suppression of tyrosinase	Kojic acid
	Hydroquinone
	Ascorbic acid
	Arbutin
	Ellagic acid
2. Other mechanisms	
a. Decrease in tyrosinase synthesis	Biomein®
b. Decrease in tyrosinase transfer	Glucosamine
	Tunicamycin
c. Cytotoxicity to melanocytes	Hydroquinone monobenzylether
	APTA[a]

[a] n-2,4-Acetoxyphenyl thioethyl acetamide.

melanin production inhibition (8). There are two melanins, eumelanin (black–brown) and pheomelanin (yellow or red), and eumelanin production inhibition is usually considered with depigmentation agents.

Dose-dependent reactions are requested for depigmenting agents *in vitro* tests, like tyrosinase inhibition or B-16 melanoma cell assay. This is needed because melanogenesis inhibition increases in parallel with the concentration of the depigmentation agents in the medium. When some chemical is added to the medium and the inhibition of melanogenesis disappears, it means that the added substance (Fig. 5) could successfully block the active site of metabolism, and thus the mechanism of this depigmentation agent becomes quite clear.

An example is shown in Fig. 6, where we can see that a dose-dependent melanogenesis inhibition of kojic acid was completely blocked when cupric acetate was added to the medium. These results showed that the main mechanism of kojic acid was to chelate copper ions that were indispensable for tyrosinase so that a remarkable decrease of its activity was seen by the addition of cupric acetate.

Streptomyces fervents produces melanin when it is cultured in liquid medium, and the melanin synthesis can be inhibited by the presence of depigmentation agents. An example that also shows the dose-dependent effect of kojic acid can be seen in Fig. 7. The important fact is that streptomyces was alive in all the culture medium, even though black eumelanin was not produced or decreased in

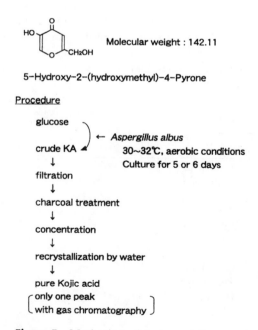

Figure 5 Mechanism of depigmentation agent.

Depigmentation Agents

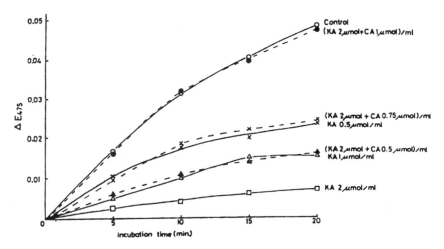

Figure 6 Blocking the dose-dependent melanogenesis inhibition of kojic acid by adding cupric acetals.

production after kojic acid was added in various concentrations: when streptomyces was transferred to another culture medium without kojic acid, it produced melanin, turning the color of the medium to black again. Various assays to detect depigmentation agents (9–12) are listed in Table 4, and the chemical structures of main depigmentation agents are shown in Table 5.

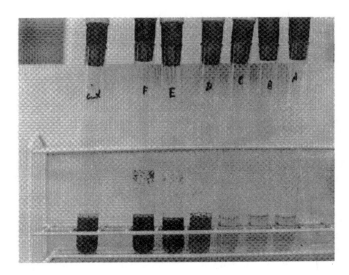

Figure 7 Dose-dependent effect of kojic acid.

Table 4 *In Vitro* and Animal Assays for Depigmentation Agents

Assays with which melanogenesis inhibition was confirmed	Depigmentation agents
1. Tyrosinase inhibition test	Kojic acid
	Hydroquinone
	Arbutin
	Ellagic acid
	4-n-butylresorcinol
2. Melanin reduction of B-16 melanoma cells	Ascorbic acid
	Liquiritin
3. Reduction of melanin pigments of *Streptomyces ferbens*	Kojic acid
	Hydroquinone
4. Reduction of melanin pigments of black goldfish	Ascorbic acid
	Kojic acid (Fig. 3)
5. Reduction of melanin pigments of pigmented mammals (C57 black mouse, Yucatan pig, etc.)	APTA[a] (topical application or intraperitoneal injection)

[a]*n*-2,4-Acetoxyphenyl thioethyl acetamide.

Cultured B-16 melanoma cells are also excellent materials for visually confirming the melanogenesis inhibition *in vitro*. A recommended method is to culture B-16 cells in Eagle's MEM with 10% fetal bovine serum, and depigmentation agents are added in the culture medium at different concentrations. After 5 days of the culture, the cells are fixed by formalin and stained by ammonical silver nitrate, then premelanosome can be visually stained in black. When the cells are alive, and such premelanosome stain is negative with the presence of depigmentation agents, melanogenesis is recognized as having been successfully inhibited (Fig. 8).

More dramatic effects of melanogenesis inhibition can be recognized when a depigmentation agent is added to the water in which black goldfish are kept. The addition of kojic acid required a month or two for the black goldfish to turn to yellowish brown; as they were alive and vivid, this demonstrated that only melanogenesis was inhibited, not systemic metabolism (Fig. 9).

CLINICAL EVALUATION

Depigmentation agents can be screened *in vivo* by tyrosinase inhibition tests or various other methods that clearly demonstrate the inhibition of melanogenesis; however, what is most important is that not only do they show definite melanogenesis inhibition *in vitro*, but also they improve the hyperpigmentation of melasma in clinical evaluation. When there is no clinical effect of depigmentation, they are of course useless, even though they showed excellent results

Table 5 Chemical Structures of Main Depigmentation Agents

1. Hydroquinone — HO—⟨benzene⟩—OH

2. Kojic acid — (pyranone ring with CH₂OH and OH substituents)

3. Arbutin — HO—⟨benzene⟩—O—(sugar ring with CH₂OH, OH, OH)

4. Ellagic acid — (fused ring structure with HO, HO, OH, OH substituents)

5. Rucinol (4-n-Butylresorcinol) — HO—⟨benzene with OH⟩—CH₂CH₂CH₂CH₃

6. N-Ac-4-S CAP (N-2,4-acetoxyphenyl thioethyl acetamid) — HO—⟨benzene⟩—SCH₂CH₂NHCOCH₃

---

in vivo trials. Laser is not effective to melasma, but is very effective to solar lentigo and nevus of Ota to which depigmentation agents are less effective or ineffective. Therefore, the best target for depigmentation agents is apparently melasma.

First, for that purpose, depigmentation agents should be mixed in vehicles, normally creams or lotions, without any alteration of the color or the effectiveness. They should be put into production without producing impurities. They should pass acute, subacute, and chronic toxicity tests, skin and eye irritation tests, skin sensitization tests (maximization and similar tests), oncogenicity tests (Ames test, micronuclei tests, carcinogenicity tests), teratogenicity tests, and stability tests. All these tests are required to develop new drugs and depigmentation agents. It is because depigmentation agents require several months to exhibit their effects and consumers may use them for several months or even several years.

Double-blind clinical tests for melasma usually are not appropriate because it takes >3 months for the effect to be recognized. Actually, depigmentation agents like kojic acid, hydroquinone, and arbutin can improve the brown hyperpigmentation of melasma by continual usage for 3–12 months. Theoretically, it is

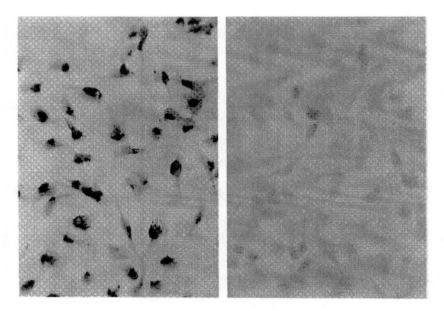

Figure 8 Melanogenesis inhibition *in vitro* using cultured B-16 melanoma cells.

possible to give active depigmentation agents to one group, whereas a second group is given a placebo cream for 3–12 months (13,14); there should be no significant differences between the backgrounds of the melasma patients as to age, severity, and exposure to sun. It is ethically acceptable to use a placebo when

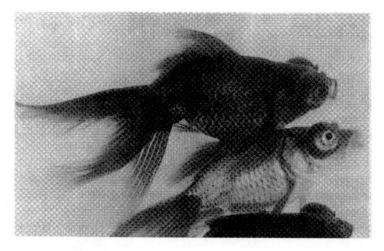

Figure 9 Effects of melanogenesis inhibition after the addition of depigmentation agent.

another effective treatment is given. However, when melasma patients are involved in the clinical trial, they have the right to see improvement in a short period of time. Therefore, the long-term use of placebo cream was abandoned because it apparently deceived patients who anticipated the effect. Double-blind tests can be used when the test ends in a week or so (as with corticosteroid ointments or antibiotics), especially when some other reliable basic treatment is given or the placebo is a competing drug having a definite effect.

Hydroquinone cream is not suitable as an active placebo because the brown color change after a few months indicates that it is hydroquinone: this is an open test (6), not a blind test.

With cosmeceuticals, double-blind tests have not always been demanded, presumably because they were not as strong as drugs and had mild effects not detectable in a short period. When some medical effects are exhibited after long-time usage, double-blind tests are difficult and, in some instances, not ethical, when the patients are to be given a placebo with no effect for months. Therefore, double-blind tests should be introduced with care with cosmeceuticals with mild and slow effects.

The evaluation of the treatment of pigmentary disorders of the face is not easy. With melasma, the brown pigmentation fades so slowly that patients often do not recognize the effects of depigmentation agents after 6 months of continual, twice-a-day application. The best way to evaluate is to take color photographs of the faces of melasma patients from three angles—front, 45° right, and 45° left. When the same camera, flashlight, and color film are used, the effect of depigmentation agents can surely be recognized (7,13,14). First, the color of melasma turns from brown to yellowish brown or normal skin color, and second, the contrast at the border of melasma becomes obscure. When colorimetry is used, it is possible to recognize the change of tint, but when the place of measurement differs at the time of measurement, the correct change of color is difficult to obtain. Mapping the human cheeks and forehead to determine the same spots at each time of measurement is usually difficult.

On the other hand, pattern recognition using color photographs from the same three angles of the face is much easier (13,14). When past color photographs from the same three angles of the patient's face are shown at the time of revisit of the patient for evaluation, the effect of whitening is easily recognized. At the very least, classification (cured, almost cured, remarkably effective, effective, slightly effective, no effect, and exacerbation) is possible. Tables 6 and 7 and Figs. 10 and 11 illustrate such evaluations.

Similar evaluation is possible with solar lentigo, ephelid, and pigmented cosmetic dermatitis; however, at the beginning of 21st century, the best treatment for solar lentigo is laser. Solar lentigo is due to the local proliferation of melanocytes; therefore, the destruction of melanocytes without serious damage to epidermal cells is ideal. Fortunately, laser can do this, and iatrogenic vitiligo is rarely formed by this treatment.

Table 6 Effect of 1% Kojic Acid Cream I on Melasma Patients (1982)

Effect	Cases treated	Duration of treatment (months, mean ± SD)	Percentage
Complete cure	0	—	0.0
Remarkably improved	37	13.9 ± 4.3	95.5
Improved	26	9.5 ± 5.5	95.5
No effect	0	—	0.0
Worsened	3	5.3 ± 4.9	4.5
Total	66	11.8 ± 5.4	100.0

Source: Ref. 13.

Pigmented cosmetic dermatitis is sometimes similar to melasma, when reticular hyperpigmentation is lacking and moderate diffuse brown hyperpigmentation is the main symptom. Biopsy shows basal liquefaction of the epidermis along with incontinentia pimenti histologica and small amount of cellular infiltration composed of lymphocytes and histiocytes in the upper dermis, unlike the basal hyperpigmentation of the basal layer cells of melasma. The most important and essential treatment for pigmented cosmetic dermatitis is not the use of depigmentation agents, but of patch testing of cosmetic series allergens including phenyl-azo-naphtol, D&C Red 31, D&C Yellow No. 11, benzyl salicylate, jasmin absolute, ylangylang oil, geraniol, sandalwood oil, artificial sandalwood, cinnamic alcohol, fragrance mix 1 and 2, and so on (15). The reading should be performed on the second, third, and seventh day so as not to overlook slow, but strong, allergic reactions. The exclusive use of allergen-free soaps and cosmetics for a year or more restores the normal skin color of the patient (15,16). It is impossible to treat the

Table 7 Effect of 1% Kojic Acid Cream II with an Improved Base Cream on Melasma Patients (1994)

Effect	Cases treated	Duration of treatment (months, mean)	Percentage
Complete cure	0	—	0.0
Remarkably improved	48	11.5	80.9
Improved	58	11.1	80.9
No effect	25	12.1	19.1
Worsened	0	—	0.0
Total	131	11.4	100.0

Note: The following side effects were noted. Those who were contact sensitized by having previously used kojic acid cream containing betacyclodextrin also developed erythema and itching by the usage of 1% kojic acid cream II. The rate of the dermatitis was 2 out of 131 patients in the table (1.5%). Those who had not used betacyclodextrin-containing kojic acid cream had not produced contact dermititis.

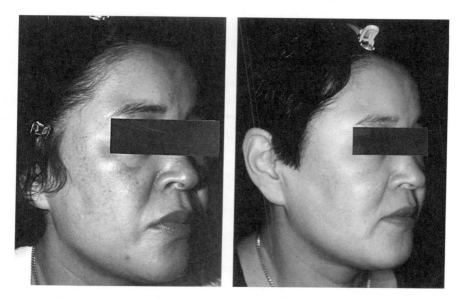

Figure 10 Effect of 1% kojic acid cream I on melamsa patients.

disease with corticosteroid ointments, even though it is a kind of allergic contact dermatitis, because only a small amount of cosmetic allergens invade the skin everyday, and these are enough to provoke the disease and maintain the hyperpigmentation. With this disease, allergen control (15) is the treatment of choice;

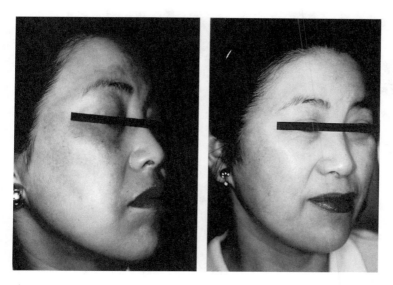

Figure 11 Effect of 1% kojic acid cream II with an improved base cream on melasma patients.

however, the additional use of a depigmentation agent accerelates the cure, presumably because the long-term inflammation at the basal layer of the epidermis enhances the melanin production and increases brown hyperpigmentation. An important fact is that sometimes melasma is complicated by pigmented cosmetic dermatitis (which is shown by biopsy with the presence of incontinentia pigmenti histologica and the inflammatory infiltrates in the upper dermis, by occasional slight erythema with itching on the face, and by positive patch test results of common cosmetic allergens). It is understandable that when melasma patients try to conceal the pigmentation by frequent use of various cosmetics, some of them become sensitized to cosmetic components, which results in the complication of pigmented cosmetic dermatitis. Such a case is shown in Fig. 12.

THE CASE OF KOJIC ACID

In 1977, a project was started to find out the cause of melasma and its reliable treatment. From 1970 to 1974, most of the causative contact cosmetic allergens that produce pigmented cosmetic dermatitis had been discovered; by 1977, the disease, which had been incurable prior to 1971, was cured, not by medication but by the exclusive use of allergen-free cosmetics and soaps. This usage of allergen-free cosmetics and soaps was designated as the allergen control system (ACS) (15). The effect of ACS had been so dramatic that a number of melasma patients whose appearance was somewhat similar to pigmented cosmetic dermatitis visited Saiseikai Central Hospital in Tokyo every day, where ACS was invented and reported by the mass media.

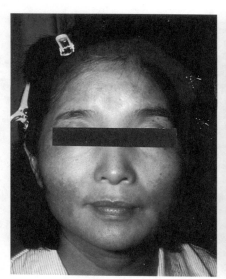 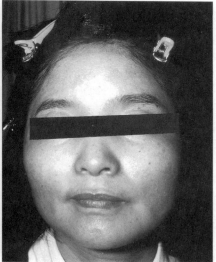

Figure 12 Complication of pigmented cosmetic dermatitis.

Depigmentation Agents

The introduction of system engineering to develop a subsystem to find the causes and how to eliminate them was key to solving the problem of pigmented cosmetic dermatitis. A new team was formed to solve the problem of melasma, adopting a similar system engineering prototype; a team investigated the role of female hormones analyzing the plasma in both the melasma patients and age-matched melasma-free women, on the seventh day of both the ovarial and luteal phases (1). The second team investigated photohypersensitivity by an automatic UVA and UVB irradiator with melasma patients. The third group started to develop a cream containing a melanogenesis inhibitor, a depigmentation agent. A plan to develop 1% hydroquinone cream was rejected by the Ministry of Health and Welfare of Japan because of the erroneous idea, at that time, that the serious and persistent leukomelanoderma caused by a depigmentation agent (hydroquinone monobenzyl ether cream banned in 1957) was an effect of hydroquinone released from hydroquinone monobenzylether. Therefore, among the known chemicals that were tyrosinase inhibitors, kojic acid was selected as the new depigmentation agent, because of its extremely long history of safe ingestion. In Japanese, kojic means ferment and had been used to brew Japanese liquor (Sake) from rice. Pure kojic acid could be produced from glucose by fermentation, and various assays to determine the mechanisms of depigmentation along with the necessary safety evaluation tests were performed. The results (Fig. 13 and Table 8) show its confirmed mechanism of action and its safety.

The initial clinical evaluation of kojic acid cream showed that 1% cream was better than 2.3% (saturated) cream, because with the latter, crystallized

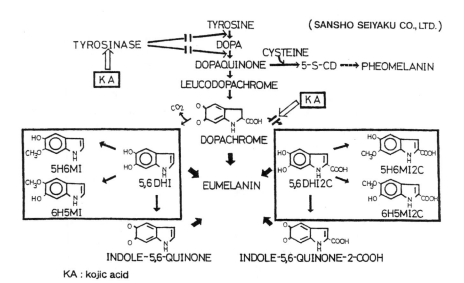

Figure 13 Kojic acid mechanism.

Table 8 Toxicity of Kojic Acid (KA) (Purity: 100%)

LD_{50}	
Subcutaneous	2050–2080 mg/kg (mice); 3010–3080 mg/kg (rats)
Oral	2650–2920 mg/kg (mice); 2260–3040 mg/kg (rats)
Chronic toxicity (rats)	
Oral 125, 250, 500, 1000 mg/kg for 26 weeks	(0/18) deaths
Teratogenicity	None (mice) None (rabbits)
Mutagenicity	
Ames test	(Negative) up to 1000 μg/plate
Mouse lymphoma assay	Negative
UDS assay	Negative
Micronucleus assay	Negative
Muta Mouse test	Negative
Dominant lethal assay	Negative
Carcinogenicity test (mouse)	Negative
Skin irritation test	
Draize method (rabbits) 50% KA aq., patch test for 24 h.	Negative (0/6)
Chronic irritation test (rabbits) Patch test for 6 h × 30 days	Negative (0/9)
Phototoxicity test (guinea pigs): 5.0% KA ethanol + UVA×5 days	(Negative)
Maximization test (guinea pigs):	(0/10)
Human skin closed patch test for 48 h.	
3% KA aq.	(1/30) ?(Positive); (29/30) Negative
1% KA aq.	(2/30) ?(Positive); (28/30) Negative

kojic acid gradually appeared and the effect of the improvement was inferior to 1% cream, with which kojic acid melted very well to the vehicle. At this time, the first and the second trials had almost ended, having shown that the cause of melasma was most likely the increase in plasma P4 levels at luteal phase, and also that 20% of melasma patients were strongly hypersensitive to UVB rays.

Sun protection was introduced to those patients who showed such photohypersensitivity. Some melasma patients were remarkably improved by the continual daily application of 1% kojic acid cream for 6 months; however, after a day of exposure to sunlight (through activities such as golf, fishing, mountaineering, etc.), melasma reappeared.

The effect of whitening was steady but too slow with this initial 1% preparation of kojic acid; 14C-labeled kojic acid cream was observed to be quickly absorbed from the skin to the liver, intestines, and kidneys in mice. When the absorption was thus quick, the depigmentation agent did not stay at the epidermis

Table 9 Safety Test Results of Kojic Acid

Experiment no.	Test	Mice Liver	Mice Hematopoietic	Rat Liver	Rat Tissue	Authors & years
1.	*In vivo/in vitro* unscheduled DNA synthesis in rat hepatocytes			Negative		RCC/CCR (1997)
2.	Comet assay	Negative				Mochizuki (2002)
3.	Comet assay	Positive		Positive	Positive	Sasaki (2002)
4.	Micronucleus assay		Negative			Nonaka et al. (1996)
5.	Micronucleus assay		Negative			Kurita (1996)
6.	Micronucleus assay		Negative			RCC/CCR (2001)
7.	Micronucleus assay			Negative	Positive	Hayashi (2002)
8.	Micronucleus assay	Positive				Sasaki (2002)
9.	Muta Mouse assay	Negative				Covance

Note: For experiments 1, 6, 8, 9, kojic acid with purity 100% was used with negative results. For experiments 2, 3, 4, 5, 7, kojic acid with unknown purities was used. RCC, Registration and Consulting Company Ltd.; CCR, Cytotest Cell Research GmbH & Co.

Source: Japanese National Institute of Health Science, December 6, 2002, from a report "On a food additive Kojic acid", chairman: Masuo Tobe.

where it had its target organ, melanocytes, for a long enough time to inhibit melanogenesis. Therefore, the second preparation conceived was 1% kojic acid cream wherein kojic acid was mixed with betacyclodextrin to slow the absorption into the dermis. This successfully sped up the whitening effect; however, contact sensitization to kojic acid occurred (17). Betacyclodextrin turned out to be a new adjuvant and, consequently, it was removed; the base cream was improved to delay the absorption without using betacyclodextrin. Owing to this improvement, contact hypersensitivity to kojic acid is rare today. Effects, as in Table 7, have been followed up every year; in 1995, 30 cases and in 2003, additional 20 cases of melasma who had used 1% kojic acid cream for >2 years were examined with CBC, liver function tests, and other tests for systemic abnormalities including carcinogenesis. No abnormal results were demonstrated, except in one person with meningioma, which was considered as coincidental. Such follow-up is always necessary whenever a new drug or cosmeceutical is introduced. Thus, depigmentation agents, kojic acid, arbutin, and rucinol, had been commercially distributed as cosmeceuticals (the Japanese term is quasi-drug) by 2003. Several others may be introduced in the future (18,19).

Kojic acid, unfortunately, had also been used as a food additive of a lower grade with unknown impurities to prevent darkening of shrimp and spicy cod ovaries; therefore, various kinds of mutagenicity tests and carcinogenicity tests were performed from 1995 to 2002 by the Japan National Institute of Health Sciences. The results are summarized in Table 9, which show that most results were negative, except for those tests performed at such high doses as $2-3$ mg/kg in mice or rats that showed some weak positive adenoma productions in the liver. There was no clear production of cancer cells. However, the quantity production of kojic acid, which lasted for almost 20 years as a whitening agent cosmeceutical in Japan, had to be suspended officially in early 2003. Therefore, hereafter, the role of the whitening agents is expected to be transferred to other chemicals in Table 5, or some newer chemical such as onion flavonoid. Though the risk amount for 1% kojic acid cream to be applied for melasma patients (Table 9) was above twice as much as the actual usage, no patient has ever produced liver function abnormalities including hepatoma or skin cancers. It follows that the risk of carcinogenicity of 1% kojic acid ointment is considered to be subclinical; for example, hydroquinone or vitamin A acid showed mild carcinogenicity experimentally, but did not produce cancer upon clinical usage.

REFERENCES

1. Sato N. Endocrine environment in adult females with chloasma. Jpn J Dermatol 1987; 97(8):937–943.
2. Sanchez NP, Pathak MA, Sato S et al. Melasma. A clinical, light microscopic, ultrastructural, and immunofluorescence study. J Am Acad Dermatol 1981; 4:698–710.
3. Findlay GH. Ochronosis following skin bleaching with hydroquinone. J Am Acad Dermatol 1982; 6:1092–1093.

4. Nakayama H. Pigmented contact dermatitis and chemical depigmentation. In Textbook of Contact Dermatitis, 2d ed. Berlin: Springer–Verlag, 1995; 637–656.
5. Hoshaw RA, Zimmerman KG, Menter A. Ochronosis-like pigmentation from hydroquinone bleaching creams in American Blacks. Arch Dermatol 1985; 121:105–108.
6. Gracia A, Fulton Jr. JE. The combination of glycolic acid and hydroquinone or kojic acid for the treatment of melasma and related conditions. Dermatol Surg 1996; 22:443–447.
7. Kang WH, Chun SC, Lee S. Intermittent therapy for melasma in Asian patients with combined topical agents (retinoic acid, hydroquinone and hydrocortisone): clinical and histological studies. J Dermatol 1998; 25:587–596.
8. Mishima Y, Hata S, Ohyama Y, Inazu M. Induction of melanogenesis suppression: cellular pharmacology and mode of differential action. Pigm Cell Res 1988; 1:367–374.
9. Kameyama K, Sakai C, Kondoh S et al. Inhibitory effect of magnesium L-ascorbyl-2-phosphate (VC-PMG) on melanogenesis *in vitro* and *in vivo*. J Am Acad Dermatol 1996; 34:29–33.
10. Akiu S, Suzuki Y, Fujinuma Y et al. Inhibitory effect arbutin on melanogenesis. Biochemical study in cultured B16 melanoma cells and effect on the UV-induced pigmentation in human skin. Proc Jpn Invest Dermatol 1988; 12:138–139.
11. Maeda K, Fukuda M. *In vitro* effectiveness of several whitening cosmetic components in human melanocytes. J Soc Cosmet Chem 1991; 42:361–368.
12. Jimbow M, Marusyk H, Jimbow K. The *in vivo* melanocytotoxicity and depigmenting potency of N-2,4-acetoxyphenyl thioethyl acetamide in the skin and hair. Br J Dermatol 1995; 133:526–536.
13. Nakayama H, Watanabe H, Nishioka K, Hayakawa R, Higa Y. Treatment of chlosama with kojic acid cream. Rinsho Hifuka 1982; 36:715–722.
14. Nakayama H, Sakurai M, Kumei A, Hanada S, Iwamoto A. The effect of kojic acid application on various facial pigmentary disorders. Nishinihon Hifuka 1994; 56:1172–1181.
15. Nakayama H, Matsuo S, Hayakawa K, Takahashi K et al. Pigmented cosmetic dermatitis. Int J Dermat 1984; 23:299–305.
16. Ebihara T, Nakayama H. Unusual and uncommon contact reactions: pigmented contact dermatitis. Clin Dermatol 1997; 15:593–599.
17. Nakagawa M, Kawai K, Kawai K. Contact allergy to kojic acid in skin care products. Contact Dermatitis 1995; 32:9–13.
18. Breathnach AS. Melanin hyperpigmentation of skin: melasma, topical treatment with azelaic acid, and other therapies. Cutis 1996; 57(suppl 1):36–45.
19. Jimbow K. N-acetyl-4-w-cyteaminylphenol as a new type of depigmenting agent for the melanoderma of patients with melasma. Arch Dermatol 1991; 127:1528–1534.

10

Hydroxyacids

E. Uhoda, C. Piérard-Franchimont, L. Petit, and G. E. Piérard
Department of Dermatopathology, University Hospital
Sart Tilman, Liège, Belgium

Introduction	207
Chemical Structure and Natural Sources of AHAs	208
Biological Activities of Hydroxyacids	209
Effects on Corneocyte Cohesion and Stratum Corneum Functions	210
Peeling and Caustic Effects	211
Hypopigmenting Effect	212
Acne and Pseudofolliculitis Treatment	212
Boosting Physiological Aspects of Skin	213
Safety	214
Conclusions	214
References	214

INTRODUCTION

Hydroxyacids are organic carboxylic acids classified into α- and β-types (AHA and BHA) according to their molecular structure. Both AHAs and BHAs exhibit almost similar effects. They are used worldwide, most probably for centuries as dermatological drugs and cosmetic ingredients. Their acceptance by physicians, cosmetologists, and consumers contrasts with the few independent, well-controlled studies demonstrating their mechanisms of action and their long-term effects.

Health care and cosmetic regulations differ among countries, although skin biology is the same throughout the world. In general, physicians consider that the current legal definitions of drugs and cosmetics are archaic and unworkable in some countries. It is evident that any environmental threat and topical product may exhibit some biological effect on the skin. Hence, some cosmetics should be viewed as skin physiology modulators. Should they all be classified as real bioactive agents? This is a matter of definition because bioactivity differs by several degrees of magnitude among product categories. There is a huge difference between decorative, suppletive compounds, and active physiology modulators in cosmetology (1).

There is vivid controversy about the concept of cosmeceuticals which aims at designating compounds that fall between cosmetics and pharmaceuticals. This concept received immediate acceptance by some people. However, many corporate leaders contend that cosmeceuticals are neither scientifically sensible nor juridically necessary. In fact, with the exception of the "quasi-drugs" in Japan, national regulatory agencies have not formally recognized the class of cosmeceuticals. The lack of clear-cut clarification might in time have negative effects. Some products are at risk to be forbidden, although they could be valuable in cosmetology. The opposite might also be true, some products being used in cosmetology without adequate evaluation of their potential biological effects. One example is provided by the widespread use of AHAs and BHAs. Despite their obvious antixerotic and peeling effects at given concentrations, there is little information available about their general toxicity and secondary biological effects. However, one should bear in mind the potential toxic effects of hydroxyacids. One example is given by the use of O-hydroxybenzoic acid (salicylic acid) when percutaneous absorption is high.

CHEMICAL STRUCTURE AND NATURAL SOURCES OF AHAs

AHAs range from simple aliphatic compounds to complex molecules. Many of these substances can be derived from natural sources and thus are commonly referred to as fruit acids. However, a number of synthetic sources provide access to structural analogs. The AHAs used in dermatology and cosmetology are usually produced by chemical synthesis. They are characterized into chemical groups based on the number of incorporated carboxylic groups (Table 1). According to their configuration, AHAs may be present under different stereoisomeric structures called enantiomers "L" and "D" or "R" and "S". Some of the common AHAs occur naturally in an enantiomerically enriched form and both enantiomers may be available.

Glycolic acid (2-hyroxyethanoic acid) is a constituent of sugarcane juice. Lactic acid (2-hydroxypropanoic acid) was first isolated in 1780. The L-lactic

Table 1 Hydroxyacid Classification

α-Hydroxyacids
  Monocarboxylic acids: Glycolic acid, lactic acid, and mandelic acid
  Dicarboxylic acids: Malic acid and tartaric acid
  Tricarboxylic acid: Citric acid
β-Hydroxyacids
  Salicylic acid (*ortho*-hydroxybenzoic acid)
  LHA (2-hydroxy-5-octanoyl benzoic acid)
  Tropic acid

acid produced by the microorganism *Lactobacillus* is responsible for the taste and odor of sour milk. The other enantiomer D-lactic acid, also called sarcolactic acid, is formed during anaerobic muscular contraction, and is found in apples, ergot, foxglove, opium, and tomatoes. Mandelic acid (2-hydroxy-2-phenylethanoic acid) can be obtained from hydrolysis of bitter almond extracts. Malic acid (2-hydroxy-1,4-butanedioic acid) was first isolated from unripened apples in 1785. Tartaric acid (2,3-hydroxy-1,4-butanedioic acid) was first isolated in 1769. It is widely distributed in plants, particularly in grapes and lees of wine. Citric acid (2-hydroxy-1,2,3-propanetricarboxylic acid) was first isolated from lemon juice in 1784. It is also found in pineapples and other citrus fruits.

BIOLOGICAL ACTIVITIES OF HYDROXYACIDS

Many biological aspects of the action of hydroxyacids still remain unknown. Numerous hydroxyacid-enriched cosmetics are present in the market with unfounded claims or little evidence of performance. Hasty conclusions have been offered from uncontrolled studies. In some instances, erroneous information and incorrect statements flourished behind promotional objectives.

At least one facet of the hydroxyacid biological activities may be ascribed to the native acid strength of the compounds. This physico-chemical characteristic is measured by the proton dissociation in solution and is expressed as the pK_a. An hydroxyacid has a stronger acid strength when its pK_a value is lower. Indeed, a decrease of 1 U in pK_a represents a 10-fold increase in the strength. If the acid strength influences some of the biological effects of hydroxyacids, it does not, however, correlate with the overall potency of the final topical formulation.

The pH of the formulations varies with both the nature of the hydroxyacid and its concentration. In order to avoid irritation as much as possible, it is desirable to formulate a cosmetic preparation with a pH close to the physiological pH range of the skin (2,3). This may be achieved by the partial neutralization and by the addition of an effective buffer. However, neutral pH AHA products seem to exert little effect on skin.

In order to prevail misunderstandings and misstatements, the biological activities of hydroxyacids should be evaluated with regard to their chemical structure irrespective of their acidity. This information is not yet rooted by scientific data. The exquisite enantio-selectivity exhibited by many biological systems suggests that enantiopurity is an important parameter in any pharmacological effect including pharmacokinetics, metabolic rate, and toxicity. Thus, the components of a racemate can differentially interact with biomolecules of the skin. Whether such a concern is of importance for some effects elicited by hydroxyacids is not settled.

The clinical indications of hydroxyacids are multiple (4). Both AHAs and BHAs exert undisputable direct effects on the stratum corneum, at least when it is affected by xerosis, ichthyosis, and analogous conditions. Some hyperpigmentation disorders may benefit from the same compounds. Comedonal hyperkeratosis in acne-prone subjects may also be improved. In the field of tumors, benign keratoses and viral warts may also be treated by high concentration formulations. The efficacy is largely related to the pH-related chemical burn. Such a caustic effect is also induced in order to realize skin peeling. The effect of hydroxyacids on heliodermatosis appears more complex, involving multifaceted mechanisms boosting some of the physiological aspects that become deficient in aging skin. Some hydroxyacids have been reported to provide protective anti-inflammatory action as an anti-oxidant in photodamaged skin (5).

Most of the aforementioned effects are in part hydroxyacid dose-dependent. In the present review, we arbitrarily define the category low concentration when there is less than 4% of active compound in the formulation. Medium concentration is applied in the range of 4–12% and high concentration for upper dosages.

EFFECTS ON CORNEOCYTE COHESION AND STRATUM CORNEUM FUNCTIONS

During the formation and maturation of the stratum corneum, the intercellular linkages by desmosomes become modified into so-called corneodesmosomes. Their numbers normally decrease toward the surface of the skin, most notably during the stratum compactum to stratum disjunctum transition (6). In xerotic, scaly, and ichthyotic conditions, ordered desquamation is impaired because desmosomes persist up to the outer stratum corneum leading to unruly accumulation of corneocytes and to skin scaling and flacking (7,8). Environmental conditions often influence these skin conditions (9).

Salicylic acid is the reference BHA used since the early days of dermatology to improve xerotic and scaly conditions. Although this compound at low and medium concentrations seems to have little or no effect on the normal stratum corneum, there is growing evidence that complete corneodesmosome degradation is helped in various xerotic and ichthyotic disorders (10,11). Therefore, it appears that the term keratolytic applied to such compound is a misnomer, whereas desmolytic agent would be more appropriate and explicit (8). The clinical effects of hydroxyacids on these hyperkeratotic conditions can be assessed using a series of biometrological methods (9,12–14).

A lipophilic derivative of salicylic acid was tested on normal human skin. It corresponds to the 2-hydroxy-5-octanoyl benzoic acid, also called lipohydroxyacid (LHA). One of the main targets is clearly the corneodesmosomes, which appear to be weakened following altered chemical bonds in the junctional complexes (15–17). Subtle differences in desmolytic activity of salicylic acid and LHA were ascribed to the respective hydrophilic and lipophilic nature of these compounds (15). LHA is likely to have a potential clinical advantage as it only interact with the more superficial layers of the stratum corneum. In addition, its activity was shown to be more highly targeted than that of salicylic acid as it looked to be channeled into the junction between the corneodesmosome and the corneocyte envelope (17). In contrast, salicylic acid destroyed the corneosome rather indiscriminately (17).

Various AHAs, particularly lactic acid and glycolic acid in the medium range of concentrations, have profound inhibitory effects on corneocyte cohesion (18,19). The usefulness of such formulations in xerotic and allied conditions is beyond doubt (20–23). The precise mechanisms of action of AHAs at that level are poorly documented. A desirable pH for inducing desquamation with AHA application lies between 2.8 and 4.8. The cutaneous surface pH changes cannot be taken lightly because they can persist several hours following applications and can affect a number of stratum corneum layers, depending on the product concentration (3). A discrete superficial lytic effect in corneodesmosomes occurs in response to low dosages. In other circumstances, when an appropriate amount of a given AHA is topically applied, the stratum corneum abruptly becomes detached at its lowermost levels within a couple of days and desquamation occurs as large flakes or sheets (23). In such instances, no disaggregation of corneocytes is apparent at upper levels of the stratum corneum (23). These changes result in skin peeling (24). To explain this situation, speculations have been made on the interaction between AHAs and various enzymatic processes involved in the maturation and disaggregation of the stratum corneum.

In addition to the therapeutic effect of the various hydroxyacids improving hyperkeratotic disorders, the same products yield cosmetic benefits by increasing plasticization and flexibility of the stratum corneum (25) without impairing the barrier function (15,19,26). This barrier function was even reported to be improved by some AHAs leading to increased resistance to SLS-induced skin irritation (27). The latter beneficial effect was not equal for all hydroxyacids, being more marked for AHAs characterized by antioxidant properties (27,28). A similar protection was not provided by applications of salicylic acid (29).

PEELING AND CAUSTIC EFFECTS

When applied to the skin at high concentration, AHAs may cause necrosis and detachment of keratinocytes leading to exogenous epidermolysis (30). Such an injury results in a chemical peel (24) depending primarily upon the disruption of the skin pH. The farther away from the physiological pH, the greater the caustic effect, the greater the risk of side effects, but the more likely the patient is to receive the resurfacing benefits of the peeling agents. A tolerable sense of burning itch is often experienced by the patients.

The indications of such treatment modality also encompass the destruction of slightly elevated seborrheic and actinic keratoses (31,32). The full-strength preparation must be applied carefully and exactly to the targeted lesion in an office procedure. After a few minutes, the entire lesion can be curetted-off. Viral warts can also be eradicated by hydroxyacids in a home-administered treatment with applications made daily for several days. To shorten the treatment period, the outer portion of the hyperkeratosis can be removed with a scalpel in an office setting.

HYPOPIGMENTING EFFECT

Glycolic acid peels can serve as a useful adjunctive treatment of epidermal hypermelanosis such as present in melasma (24). The association of 10% glycolic acid and 2% hydroquinone also improves this disorder (33–35). Still another combination therapy combines 5% glycolic acid and 2% kojic acid (34,35). It is thought that the AHA acts as a penetration enhancer and accelerates the epidermal turnover.

ACNE AND PSEUDOFOLLICULITIS TREATMENT

Salicylic acid is listed among active products to treat acne (36,37). However, clear-cut evidence for a significant benefit at low concentration in well-controlled experimental and clinical trials is scanty. Similarly, medium concentrations of AHAs such as glycolic acid, lactic acid, and mandelic acid are employed twice daily to improve mild acne (38,39). It has been postulated that hydroxyacids promote dislodgement of comedones and prevent their formation as well. Many of these treatments await for validation by independent controlled studies. In our experience, the lower AHAs concentrations as present in some cosmetic products exhibit no effect whatsoever on acne and comedones.

Another modality of acne treatment consists of using high concentrations of glycolic acid in an office setting (4). The procedure has to be repeated weekly or so. In addition to the comedolytic effect, the higher hydroxyacid concentrations help to unroof pustules and affect the follicular epithelium to the level of the sebaceous glands (38). The skin condition improvement was reported to be precipitous, while patients were also taking oral tetracyclines. Discomfort, mild diffuse erythema, and fine scaling are often experienced by patients. In addition, there is a risk for stronger irritation leading to a papular and perifollicular erythema that can persist for a few weeks.

Quite recently, a 2% LHA formulation was shown to exert a potent comedolytic effect in acne-prone subjects (40–42). The lipophilic properties of LHA allow maximum concentration inside the stratum corneum, particularly in the sebum-enriched infundibulum of pilosebaceous units. Thus, the compound is likely to be trapped in lesional sebaceous follicles which represent a critical therapeutic target in comedonal acne. The product has shown efficacy in preventing comedonal acne and treating mild acne (40,41). LHA has the capacity to decrease both the number and the size of the cornified follicular plugs induced by intense ultraviolet light exposure (41). The combination of the LHA formulation with a retinoic acid cream every other evening results in the overall decrease in the functional and physical intolerance reactions (42).

Pseudofolliculitis is another related disorder that can be improved by topical AHA treatment (43). Rosacea might also benefit from the combination of an evening AHA cream and a sun-protective daytime preparation (4).

BOOSTING PHYSIOLOGICAL ASPECTS OF SKIN

One fascinating aspect in the effects of hydroxyacids is the boosted physiology that has been claimed to occur in the epidermis and dermis (44–54). Accordingly, some of these compounds are used to correct skin atrophy (55) and to induce a gradual reduction in the aging signs including pigmentary changes (56) and wrinkles of fine and moderate depth (48,57–64). However, only a few controlled clinical trials and experimental studies have been conducted so far to validate these observations.

After a few days of application of 12% glycolic acid at low pH, fine wrinkles of the face may vanish as a result of the irritation and dermal edema (60). Besides the untoward immediate effect of stinging, such smoothing effect is rapidly alleviated upon arrest of the topical treatment. Furthermore, in long-term applications, there is some concern regarding the occurrence of chronic low-grade inflammation producing reactive oxygen species damaging collagen and elastic fibers. However, signs of repair and reverse changes of aging and photoaging have been reported on long-term therapy (48,57–59). Such findings were not confirmed in other studies which rather indicated an almost absence of AHA effects on major skin aging parameters (62,63,65). In fact, new deposits of glycosaminoglycans in the dermis represent a result of inflammation which has been mistakenly interpreted as a correction of aging. A comparative controlled study showed that tretinoin was more active than medium concentrations of glycolic acid in the improvement of the facial skin tensile properties (62). It should be noted that the combination of tretinoin and AHAs may be beneficial in improving the aspect of photoaged skin (58,66).

In contrast to salicylic acid, low concentrations of LHA elicit a dermo-epidermal stimulation (15,65,67–70) which leads to increased keratinocyte proliferation and epidermal thickness. Such an effect is more evident in older skin and remains within the physiological range of normal skin. In contrast to other AHAs and BHAs, angiogenesis is moderately increased by LHA. An increased number of Factor-XIIIa-positive dermal dendrocytes occurs after topical applications of AHAs and LHA (56,66,70). These cells may influence the metabolism of fibroblasts and endothelial cells. The increase in Factor-XIIIa expression may somehow relate increased vascularity and dermal improvements following LHA and tretinoin treatments in photoaged patients (70).

SAFETY

Adverse reactions following LHA applications are mostly represented by stinging sensations without any other clinical and histological signs of irritation. However, the higher concentrations may be responsible for severe redness, swelling (especially in the area of the eyes), burning, blistering, bleeding, rash, itching, and skin discoloration. Their long-term effects are unknown. It has been claimed that BHAs are effective as exfoliants without the occasional irritation associated with the use of AHAs.

Some people who use AHA products have greater sensitivity to sun. Indeed, it has been reported that the subjects who receive AHA products in the presence of UV radiation experience twice the cell damage than the controls in areas where the AHA is applied.

The Food and Drug Administration (FDA) stated that AHAs are readily absorbed into the skin at varying rates. The most rapid absorption occurred with AHAs having lower pHs (71). The safety of salicylic acid used as a cosmetic ingredient has been evaluated by FDA and the Cosmetic Ingredient Review. They concluded that products containing salicylic acid should contain a sunscreen or display directions advising consumers to use other sun protection (72).

CONCLUSIONS

AHAs and BHAs enjoy tremendous interest in dermatology and cosmetology. These compounds under the presentation of peels and home regimens are recognized as important preventive means and adjunctive therapy in a variety of skin conditions. Thus, they attract media attention and consumer curiosity. Claims and proven effects are contradictory in some aspects. LHA has appeared effective in the treatment of signs of skin aging and in acne treatment without the occasional irritation associated with the use of AHAs.

Much remains to be learned and speculations must be turned to facts. Improved regimens capitalizing on the various beneficial effects of hydroxyacids should be explored. Synergistic effects can be expected with some other compounds. Considering the safety status, consumers who use AHA and BHA products should follow some precautions about the ultraviolet radiation exposure.

REFERENCES

1. Piérard GE, Piérard-Franchimont C. A plea for active dermocosmetology free of unnecessary animal experimentation. Rev Med Liège 1998; 53:350–352.

2. Rippke F, Schreiner V, Schwanitz HJ. The acidic milieu of the horny layer. New findings on the physiology and pathophysiology of skin pH. Am J Clin Dermatol 2002; 3:261–272.
3. Parra JL, Paye M, the EEMCO Group. EEMCO guidance for the in vivo assessment of skin surface pH. Skin Pharmacol Appl Skin Physiol 2003; 16:188–202.
4. Tung RC, Bergfeld WF, Vidinos AT, Renzi BK. α-Hydroxy acid-based cosmetic procedures. Guidelines for patient management. Am J Clin Dermatol 2000; 1:81–88.
5. Perricone NV, Dinardo JC. Photoprotective and anti-inflammatory effects of topical glycolic acid. Dermatol Surg 1996; 22:435–437.
6. Chapman SJ, Walsh A. Desmosomes, corneosomes and desquamation. An ultrastructural study. Arch Dermatol Res 1990; 282:304–310.
7. Piérard GE. What do you mean by dry skin? Dermatologica 1989; 179:1–2.
8. Piérard GE, Goffin V, Hermanns-Lê T, Piérard-Franchimont C. Corneocyte desquamation. Int J Mol Med 2000; 6:217–221.
9. Piérard-Franchimont C, Piérard GE. Beyond a glimpse at seasonal dry skin. A review. Exog Dermatol 2002; 1:3–6.
10. Huber C, Christophers E. "Keratolytic" effect of salicylic acid. Arch Dermatol Res 1977; 257:293–298.
11. Roberts DL, Marshall R, Marks R. Detection of the action of salicylic acid on the normal stratum corneum. Br J Dermatol 1980; 103:191–196.
12. Piérard GE, Masson P, Rodrigues L, Berardesca E, Lévêque JL, Loden M, Rogiers V, Sauermann G, erup J. EEMCO guidance for the assessment of dry skin (xerosis) and ichthyosis: evaluation by stratum corneum strippings. Skin Res Technol 1996; 2:3–11.
13. Piérard-Franchimont C, Henry F, Piérard GE. The SACD method and the XLRS squamometry tests revisited. Int J Cosmet Sci 2000; 22:437–446.
14. Piérard-Franchimont C, Petit L, Piérard GE. Skin surface patterns of xerotic legs: the flexural and accretive types. Int J Cosmet Sci 2001; 23:121–126.
15. Lévêque JL, Corcuff P, Gonnord G, Montastier C, Renault B, Bazin R, Piérard GE, Poelman MC. Mechanism of action of a lipophilic derivative of salicylic acid on normal skin. Skin Res Technol 1995; 1:115–122.
16. Lévêque JL, Corcuff P, Rougier A, Piérard GE. Mechanism of action of lipophilic acid derivative on normal skin. Eur J Dermatol 2002; 12:S35–S38.
17. Corcuff P, Fiat F, Minondo AM, Lévêque JL, Rougier A. A comparative ultrastructural study of hydroxyacids induced desquamation. Eur J Dermatol 2002; 12:S39–S43.
18. Berardesca E, Maibach H. AHA mechanisms of action. Cosmet Toilet 1995; 110:30–31.
19. Fartasch M, Teal J, Menon GK. Mode of action of glycolic acid on human stratum corneum: ultrastructural and functional evaluation of the epidermal barrier. Arch Dermatol Res 1997; 289:404–409.
20. Wehr RF, Kantor I, Jones EL, McPhee ME, Krochmal L. A controlled comparative efficacy study of 5% ammonium lactate lotion versus an emollient control lotion in the treatment of moderate xerosis. J Am Acad Dermatol 1991; 25:849–851.
21. Vilaplana J, Coll J, Trullas C, Azan A, Pelejero C. Clinical and non-invasive evaluation of 12% ammonium lactate emulsion for the treatment of dry skin in atopic and non-atopic subjects. Acta Derm Venereol 1992; 72:28–33.
22. Dinardo JC, Grove GL, Moy LS. 12% Ammonium lactate versus 8% glycolic acid. J Geriatr Dermatol 1995; 3:144–147.
23. Van Scott EJ, Yu RJ. Actions of alpha hydroxy acids on skin components. J Geriatr Dermatol 1995; 3:19A–25A.

24. Murad H, Shamban AT, Premo PS. The use of glycolic acid as a peeling agent. Dermatol Clin 1995; 13:285–307.
25. Takahashi M, Machida Y. The influence of hydroxy-acids on the rheological properties of the stratum corneum. J Soc Cosmet Chem 1985; 36:177–187.
26. Effendy I, Kawangsukstith C, Lee JY, Maibach HI. Functional changes in human stratum corneum induced by topical glycolic acid: comparison with all-*trans* retinoic acid. Acta Dermatol Venereol 1995; 75:455–458.
27. Berardesca E, Distante F, Vignoli GP, Oresajo C, Green B. Alpha hydroxyacids modulate stratum corneum barrier function. Br J Dermatol 1997; 137:934–938.
28. Perricone NV. An alpha-hydroxy acid acts as an antioxidant. J Geriatr Dermatol 1993; 1:101–104.
29. Piérard-Franchimont C, Goffin V, Piérard GE. Modulation of stratum corneum properties by salicylic acid and all-*trans*-retinoic acid. Skin Pharmacol Appl Physiol 1998; 11:266–272.
30. Rubin MG. Therapeutics: personal practice. The clinical use of alpha hydroxy acids. Aust J Dermatol 1994; 35:29–33.
31. Griffin TD, Van Scott EJ. Use of pyruvic acid in the treatment of actinic keratoses: a clinical and histopathologic study. Cutis 1991; 47:325–329.
32. Marrero GM, Katz BE. The new fluor-hydroxy pulse peel. Dermatol Surg 1998; 24:973–978.
33. Lim JTE, Tham SN. Glycolic acid peels in the treatment of melasma among Asian women. Dermatol Surg 1997; 23:177–179.
34. Garcia A, Fulton JE. The combination of glycolic acid and hydroquinone or kojic acid for the treatment of melasma and related conditions. Dermatol Surg 1996; 22:443–447.
35. Petit L, Piérard GE. Skin-lightening products: revisited. Int J Cosmet Sci 2003; 25:169–181.
36. Leyden JJ, Shalita AR. Rational therapy for acne vulgaris: an update on topical treatment. J Am Acad Dermatol 1986; 15:907–914.
37. Eady EA, Burke BM, Pulling K, Cunliffe WJ. The benefit of 2% salicylic acid lotion in acne—a placebo-controlled study. J Dermatol Treat 1996; 7:93–96.
38. Van Scott EJ, Yu RJ. Alpha hydroxyacids: therapeutic potentials. Can J Dermatol 1989; 1:108–112.
39. Wang CM, Huang CL, Hu CTS et al. The effect of glycolic acid on the treatment of acne in asian skin. Dermatol Surg 1997; 23:23–29.
40. Piérard GE, Rougier A. Nudging acne by topical beta-lipohydroxy acid (LHA), a new comedolytic agent. Eur J Dermatol 2002; 12:S47–S48.
41. Uhoda E, Piérard-Franchimont C, Piérard GE. Comedolysis by a lipohydroxyacid formulation in acne-prone subjects. Eur J Dermatol 2003; 13:65–68.
42. Rougier A, Richard A. Efficacy and safety of a new salicylic acid derivative as a complement of vitamin A acid in acne treatment. Eur J Dermatol 2002; 12:S49–S50.
43. Perricone NV. Treatment of pseudofolliculitis barbae with topical glycolic acid: a report of two studies. Cutis 1993; 52:232–235.
44. Smith WP. Hydroxy acids and skin aging. Cosmet Toilet 1994; 109:41–44.
45. Bernstein EF, Uitto J. Connective tissue alterations in photoaged skin and the effects of alpha-hydroxy acids. J Geriatr Dermatol 1995; 3:7A–18A.
46. Leyden JJ, Lavker RM, Grove G, Kaidbey K. Alpha hydroxy acids are more than moisturizers. J Geriatr Dermatol 1995; 3:33A–37A.

47. Dinardo JC, Grove GL, Moy LS. Clinical and histological effects of glycolic acid at different concentrations and pH levels. Dermatol Surg 1996; 22:421–424.
48. Ditre CM, Griffin TD, Murphy GF, Sueki H, Telegan B, Johnson WC, Yu RJ, Van Scott EJ. Effect of α-hydroxy acids on photoaged skin: a pilot clinical, histologic, and ultrastructural study. J Am Acad Dermatol 1996; 34:187–195.
49. Griffin TD, Murphy GF, Sueki H, Telegan B, Johnson WC, Ditre CM, Yu RJ, Van Scott EJ. Increased factor XIIIa transglutaminase expression in dermal dendrocytes after treatment with α-hydroxyacids: potential physiologic significance. J Am Acad Dermatol 1996; 34:196–203.
50. Moy LS, Howe K, Moy RL. Glycolic acid modulation of collagen production in human skin fibroblast cultures *in vitro*. Dermatol Surg 1996; 22:439–441.
51. Smith WP. Epidermal and dermal effects of topical lactic acid. J Am Acad Dermatol 1996; 35:388–391.
52. Stiller NJ, Bartolone J, Stern R et al. Topical 8% glycolic acid and 8% L-lactic acid creams for the treatment of photoaged skin. Arch Dermatol 1996; 132:631–635.
53. Bergfeld W, Tung R, Vidimos A et al. Improving the appearance of phtoaged skin with glycolic acid. J Am Acad Dermatol 1997; 36:1011–1013.
54. Kim SJ, Park JH, Kim DH et al. Increased *in vivo* collagen synthesis and *in vitro* cell collagen synthesis and *in vitro* cell proliferative effect of glycolic acid. Dermatol Surg 1998; 24:1054–1058.
55. Lavker RM, Kaidbey K, Leyden JJ. Effects of topical ammonium lactate on cutaneous atrophy from a potent topical corticosteroid. J Am Acad Dermatol 1992; 26:535–544.
56. Burns RL, Prevost-Blank PL, Lawry MA, Lawry TB, Faria DT, Fivenson DP. Glycolic acid peels for postinflammatory hyperpigmentation in Black patients. Dermatol Surg 1997; 23:171–175.
57. Elson ML. The utilization of glycolic acid in photoaging. Cosmet Dermatol 1992; 5:12–15.
58. Hermitte R. Aged skin, retinoids, and alpha-hydroxy acids. Cosmet Toilet 1992; 107:63–67.
59. Moy LS, Murad H, Moy RL. Glycolic acid therapy: evaluation of efficacy and techniques in treatment of photodamage lesions. Am J Cosmet Surg 1993; 10:9–13.
60. Piérard-Franchimont C, Deleixhe-Mauhin F, Dubois A, Goffin V, Viatour M, Piérard GE. Rides et microrelief cutané. Modifications par un alpha-hydroxyacide. Rev Med Liège 1994; 49:268–273.
61. Newman N, Newman A, Moy LS et al. Clinical improvement of photoaged skin with 50% glycolic acid. Dermatol Surg 1996; 22:455–460.
62. Piérard GE, Henry F, Piérard-Franchimont C. Comparative effect of short-term topical tretinoin and glycolic acid on mechanical properties of photodamaged facial skin in HRT-treated menopausal women. Maturitas 1996; 23:273–277.
63. Stiller MJ, Bartolone J, Stern R, Smith S, Kollias N, Gillies R, Drake LA. Topical 8% glycolic acid and 8% L-lactic acid creams for the treatment of photodamaged skin. Arch Dermatol 1996; 132:631–636.
64. Matarasso SL, Hanke CW, Alster TS. Cutaneous resurfacing. Dermatol Clin 1997; 135:867–875.
65. Piérard GE, Kligman AM, Stoudemayer T, Lévêque JL. Comparative effects of retinoic acid, glycolic acid and a lipophilic derivative of salicylic acid on photodamaged epidermis. Dermatology 1999; 199:50–53.

66. Kligman AM. The compatibility of combinations of glycolic acid and tretinoin in acne and in photodamaged facial skin. J Geriatr Dermatol 1995; 3:25A–28A.
67. Arrese, JE, Piérard GE. El lipohidroxiacido y el envejecimiento cutaneo. Arch Argent Dermatol 1995; 45:147–150.
68. Piérard GE, Nikkels-Tassoudji N, Arrese JE, Piérard-Franchimont C, Lévêque JL. Dermo-epidermal stimulation elicited by a β-lipohydroxyacid: a comparison with salicylic acid and all-*trans*-retinoic acid. Dermatology 1997; 194:398–401.
69. Avila Camacho M, Montastier C, Piérard GE. Histometric assessment of the age-related skin response to 2-hydroxy-5-octanoyl benzoic acid. Skin Pharmacol Appl Skin Physiol 1998; 11:52–56.
70. Piérard GE, Lévêque JL, Rougier A, Kligman AM. Dermo-epidermal stimulation elicited by a salicylic acid derivative. Eur J Dermatol 2002; 12:S44–S46.
71. US Food and Drug Administration. Center for Food Safety and Applied Nutrition Office of Cosmetics and Colors Fact Sheet. Beta Hydroxy Acid in Cosmetics. March 7, 2000.
72. US Food and Drug Administration. Center for Food Safety and Applied Nutrition Office of Cosmetics and Colors Fact Sheet. Alpha Hydroxy Acid in Cosmetics. July 3, 1997.

11

Moisturizers

Marie Lodén
ACO Hud AB, Upplands Väsby, Sweden

Introduction	219
The Chemistry of "Dry" SC	221
Water	221
Humectants	222
Lipids	222
Chemistry and Use of Moisturizers	224
Fats, Oils, and Emulsifiers	224
Humectants	226
Protection of Moisturizers	227
Influence of Moisturizers on Skin Chemistry	227
Skin Structure and Desquamation	228
Influence of Moisturizers on Skin Structure and Desquamation	228
The Barrier Function of SC	232
Influence of Moisturizers on Skin Barrier Function	233
Concluding Remarks	235
References	236

INTRODUCTION

Dry and chapped skin is a common problem both in healthy individuals and in patients with skin diseases. Dry skin might be connected to some inherited disorders relating to the structure and function of the epidermis, for example, ichthyosis, atopic dermatitis, and may also be secondary to other diseases, for example, diabetes or renal failure. Moreover, the condition can occur in response to the environment with low humidity and/or low temperature. The behavior also contributes to dry skin, and exposure to solvents, cutting fluids, surfactants, acids, and alkalis may produce dryness. There are several features that give an impression of dry skin, Table 1 (1–4). The dermatologist and the affected person can judge visible and tactile characteristics of the skin surface. The affected person can also perceive sensory feelings of dryness, and instruments can be used to analyse changes in the chemical and functional characteristics, Table 1.

The term "dry skin" is not generally accepted. Some relate it to the lack of water in the stratum corneum (SC), whereas others consider the condition to belong to a group of disorders with a rough skin surface (5,6). It has not been conclusively shown that the water content of SC is reduced in all dry skin conditions. For example, reduced water content has not been detected in the pruritic and dry-looking skin in patients with chronic renal failure (7) and in the clinically dry-appearing old skin (8). There is also a discrepancy between the subjective self-assessment and the clinical assessment of the presence of dry skin (3,4). However, a decreased water content of SC has been found in elderly patients with xerosis (9,10), and the water content of SC in winter xerotic skin correlated inversely with clinical scores of dryness (1,2). Furthermore, the dry-looking skin of patients with atopic dermatitis and psoriasis is less hydrated and less capable of binding water than normal skin (8,11–15). *In-vitro* studies have also confirmed that pathological SC from atopic and psoriatic patients is less capable of binding water than normal SC (14,16).

Products used for treatment or prevention of dry skin are called emollients or moisturizers. They are able to break the dry skin cycle and maintain the smoothness of the skin. The term "emollient" implies (from the Latin derivation) a material designed to soften the skin, that is, a material that "smooths" the surface to the touch and makes it look smoother to the eye. The term

Table 1 Characteristics of "Dry" Skin

Evaluation	Common findings
Visual	Redness, a lackluster surface, dry white patches, flaky appearance, cracks, and even fissures
Tactile	Rough and uneven surface
Sensory	Feels dry, uncomfortable, painful, itchy, stinging and tingling sensation
Chemical	Reduced water content, reduced NMF content, changed lipid composition
Functional	Impaired barrier function

"moisturizer" is often used synonymously with emollient, but moisturizers usually contain humectants, aimed at potentiating the hydration of SC. In the present chapter, the term moisturizer will be used, with a possible meaning also of creams without humectants.

Large differences exist regarding the composition and function of moisturizing creams. Creams contain substances considered as actives (e.g., humectants) and substances conventionally considered as excipients (e.g., emulsifiers, antioxidants, preservatives). Recent findings indicate that actives and excipients may have other types of effects in the skin than previously considered.

The structure and barrier functions in diseased skin and in skin with normal-looking appearance are affected by moisturizers. Biophysical and biochemical techniques allow a closer examination of the functional impact of moisturizing creams. The research is focused on identifying agents that are specifically delivered into the epidermis to assist the cellular differentiation process or act as precursors to vital SC components.

New methods are supposed to facilitate tailoring of moisturizers, which will be of benefit in the treatment and prevention of skin barrier disorders. The present chapter will give an overview of the structure and function of dry skin relating to the use of moisturizers.

THE CHEMISTRY OF "DRY" SC

Water

Water is the plasticizer of keratin, allowing the SC layer to bend and stretch, avoiding cracking and fissuring. Furthermore, water increases the activity of enzymes involved in the desquamation process (17). Water in SC is associated with the hydrophilic parts of the intercellular lipids and with the keratin fibers in the corneocytes (14,18). The fibrous elements in the corneocytes have hydrophilic properties and also contain a water-soluble fraction that enhances their water-holding capacity (19–21).

In the hydrated SC, three types of water with different molecular mobilities can be found. At a water content <10%, the primary water is tightly bound, presumably to the polar sites of the proteins (14,22,23). When the degree of hydration exceeds 10%, the secondary water is hydrogen-bonded around the protein-bound water; and at >40–50%, the water resembles the bulk liquid (14,22,23). It is the secondary water that contributes to the plasticity of SC (14,21). The amount of tightly bound water is almost the same in different types of pathological skin, whereas the amount of secondary water is much smaller in SC from psoriatic patients and from elderly persons with xerosis than in normal SC (14). For example, in normal SC from glabrous skin the content is 38.2 mg/100 mg dry tissue, when compared with 31.7 mg in senile xerosis and 27.2 mg in psoriatic scales per 100 mg dry tissue (14).

Humectants

A special blend of osmotically active humectants can be found in SC, which is called natural moisturizing factor (NMF) (24), Table 2. NMF can make up $\sim 15-20\%$ of the total weight of the corneum (20,24). Substances belonging to NMF are amino acids, pyrollidone carboxylic acid (PCA), lactate, and urea, Table 2 (20,24). PCA occurs primarily in SC in the form of its sodium salt at levels reaching $\sim 2-4\%$ (20,25).

The production of NMF from profilaggrin and hydrolysis of filaggrin is critical to skin condition and for water binding in the outer layers of SC (26). A deficiency of NMF is linked to dry skin conditions, and extraction of NMF molecules from SC reduces its ability to bind water (20,21,25,27). In skin diseases such as ichthyosis vulgaris (10,28) and psoriasis (29), there is a virtual absence of NMF. In ichthyosis vulgaris, the stratum granulosum is thin or missing due to a defect in the processing of profilaggrin, which also is noticed as tiny and crumbly keratohyalin granules (30).

The moisture-binding ability of samples of SC is correlated with its PCA content (25). In xerotic skin, the amino acid compositions of the SC samples from old people are altered (10,31) and there is a decrease in the amount of water-soluble amino acids in relation to the severity of xerosis, a finding suggested to reflect decreased profilaggrin production (10). A reduced content of amino acids has also been observed in experimentally induced scaly skin (32) and in patients with ichthyosis vulgaris (10). The content of urea in the normal and affected SC of patients with atopic dermatitis is also substantially reduced (33).

Lipids

The corneocytes in SC is embedded in lipid bilayers consisting primarily of three classes of lipids: free sterols, free fatty acids, and ceramides, Table 3. The lipid composition of the epidermis changes dramatically during epidermal differentiation. There is a marked decrease in phospholipids and an increase in fatty acids and ceramides. In the final stages of this differentiation, keratinocytes discharge lipid-containing granules—lamellar bodies—into the extracellular spaces in the upper granular layer, where they form intercellular membrane

Table 2 Composition of NMF (24)

Amino acids	40.0%
Pyrrolidone carboxylic acid (PCA)	12.0%
Lactate	12.0%
Urea	7.0%
Na, Ca, K, Mg, phosphate, chloride	18.5%
NH_3, uric acid, glucosamine, creatinine 1.5	
Rest unidentified	

Table 3 Composition of Human SC Lipids

Lipid	Data from Lampe et al. (34) (facial skin)	Data from Wertz and Downing (35)
Ceramides	19.9	39.1
Fatty acids	19.7	9.1
Triglycerides	13.5	0.0
Free sterols	17.3	26.9
Cholesteryl esters		10.0
Cholesteryl sulfate		1.9
Sterol/wax esters	6.2	
Squalene, n-alkanes	9.7	
Others	6.7	11.1

bilayers (18,36). This lamellar material greatly expands the intercellular compartment and constitutes ∼5–10% of the total weight of human SC (37).

An abnormal lipid composition has been found in surfactant-irritated skin (38), in experimentally induced scaly skin (32), in normal winter dry skin (39), in dry atopic skin (40–42), in psoriatic plaques (43), and in hereditary ichthyosis (44). In particular, the content and distribution of the ceramides are changed (32,38,40,41,43–45). However, the most well-described condition might be the X-linked ichthyosis, in which there is a specific abnormality in sterol metabolism producing high levels of cholesterol sulfate in SC (44,46). Furthermore, female hormones, age, and season appear to influence the lipid composition (45,47). Changes in lipid composition may affect the normal bilayer structure, as in skin dryness (48) and in skin exposed to organic solvents (49).

Cholesterol sulfate is involved in the epidermal differentiation, and the observed drop in its concentration towards the outer layer of SC is believed to promote desquamation. Cholesterol sulfate inhibits proteases involved in the desquamation process (50) and has also been suggested to stabilize the lipid layer in the deeper layer of SC, keeping the corneocytes together (51). Cholesterol sulfate also reduces the amount of cholesterol that is present in lipid crystalline domains (51), which might induce crystallization of cholesterol and decrease the cohesion between lipid lamellae (51).

Ca^{2+} counteracts the effects of cholesterol sulfate, indicating a proper balance of SC components for appropriate SC lipid organization (51,52). Higher levels of calcium is found throughout the dry atopic skin, with a tendency to a steeper gradient than in normal skin (53). The normal calcium gradient is also lost in psoriatic plaques and substantial amounts of Ca^{2+} are present in superficial layers of SC (54).

High values of zinc have also been found in atopic skin (55). Zn has been suggested to bind to defensins and thus acts on the conformational status of the natural defensins harbored by SC allowing for free action of bacteria (55).

CHEMISTRY AND USE OF MOISTURIZERS

Creams are the most common types of delivery system used for emollients and moisturizers. They contain two phases; usually oil and water producing either an oil-in-water or a water-in-oil emulsion. The droplet size is often between 1 and 100 µm. Emulsifiers are added to the formulation to provide stability and desired reological properties. Emulsifiers have one nonpolar hydrocarbon end and one polar end, that is, they combine both hydrophilic and lipophilic components in one molecule. Thereby, they collect at the interface of the two phases and promote emulsification.

Knowledge about the interplay between ingredients in moisturizers is essential to get a stable and cosmetically attractive product with desired impact on the skin. Dermatologists propose a daily moisturizing routine as a vital part of the management of patients with eczema and other dry skin conditions even when the skin is under control (56), but greasy and sticky properties can be a nuisance and the smell of some products can be difficult to accept. Therefore, low compliance can be a problem with topical treatments and the process of treating the skin can often itself add to the burden of having the disease. The patients can also receive conflicting treatment advice, leading to frustration, noncompliance, and difficulty in following an effective regimen (56). It may also be expected that moisturizer treatment requires the same application rate on different sites due to the various severities of the dryness in the treated areas.

Differences in dosing have been noted among self-application vs. operator-assisted application of creams, where self-application resulted in larger amount applied per unit area (57,58). Moreover, jars promoted use of larger quantities than the same cream in a tube (1.7 vs. 0.7 mg/cm^2, respectively) (58). The type of vehicle may also influence the distribution within the treated area (59). A thick ointment with only a few percent of water has been found to be equally distributed in the center and periphery of the treated area, whereas formulations with lower viscosity and more volatile ingredients (e.g., creams) were less evenly spread on the skin (59).

Once applied to the skin, ingredients can stay on the surface, be absorbed into the skin, be metabolized, or disappear from the surface by evaporation, by sloughing off, or by contact with other materials. Only 50% of applied cream might remain on the surface after 8 h (60). Cream and ointments seem to allow higher transfer of the actives to surrounding surfaces than lotions and tinctures (61).

Fats, Oils, and Emulsifiers

Fats and oils may be classified into animal, vegetable, and mineral types. Common fats in moisturizers are mineral oils, waxes, long-chain esters, fatty acids, lanolin, and mono-, di-, and triglycerides. Mineral oils are derived from petroleum, and the two most important materials are liquid paraffin and petrolatum. Petrolatum and mineral oil are purified materials consisting of complex combinations of oxidation-resistant hydrocarbons. Depending on the distribution of the molecular weight, materials with different viscosity are obtained. Petrolatum has been used in skin care products since its discovery by Robert A. Chesebrough in 1872 and was included already in the 1880 edition of the U.S. Pharmacopoeia (62).

Lanolin is an animal type of wax (from the Latin *lana* for wool and *oleum* for oil) secreted by the sebaceous glands of the sheep. Lanolin is a complex mixture of esters, disesters, and hydroxy esters of high molecular weight lanolin alcohols and lanolin acids. Unlike human sebum, lanolin contains no triglycerides. Beeswax is a complicated mixture of hydrocarbons, esters, and fatty acids. A typical example of a vegetable-derived wax is carnauba, which is obtained from the leaves of the carnauba palm tree.

Triglycerides can be divided into fats and oils depending on their physical state; solids and liquids, respectively. They can have animal or vegetable origin. Nowadays, vegetable-derived materials are more widely used compared with animal sources. Refining of vegetable oils, such as peanut oil, removes proteins which can elicit sensitization reactions in allergic individuals (63).

The chemical structure of triglycerides consists of a glycerol fragment, esterified with fatty acids. There is a large variety in fatty acids, with the saturated fatty stearic acid, the monounsaturated oleic acid, and the polyunsaturated linoleic acid being the most abundant fatty acids. The fatty acid profile, which is typical for certain oil, determines to a great extent the characteristics of an oil with respect to stability, skin feel, and effects on the skin. The most important feature of a fatty acid is the number of double bonds and their distribution over the carbon chain. The degree of unsaturation has a large effect on the ease of handling. Fatty acids with a higher degree of unsaturation are oxidized more easily. Oxidation is increased by the presence of metals, heat, light, and oxygen.

Oils from vegetables and fish also contain essential fatty acids (EFA). EFA influence skin physiology via their effects on skin barrier function, eicosanoid production, membrane fluidity, and cell signaling (64). EFA are found predominantly within the epidermal phospholipids, but are also incorporated in ceramides where they play a critical role in barrier function. Fatty acids with the first double bond at the sixth C atom counting from the end of the carbon tail is called omega-6, whereas those with the first double bond at the third C atom are called omega-3 fatty acids. Omega-6 and omega-3 fatty acids are derived from linoleic and α-linoleic acid, respectively. The most abundant EFA in the skin is linoleic acid and its metabolite arachidonic acid. Evening primrose oil and borage oil have gamma-linoleic acid (GLA) levels over 9% and 20%, respectively. Seafood is known to contain omega-3 fatty acids, like eicosapentaenoic (EPA), docosahexaenoic, and stearidonic acids.

Emulsifiers can be classified as ionics (anionic or cationic) or nonionics. Long-chain fatty acids are one group of commonly used anionic emulsifiers, for example, stearic acid and palmitic acid. Fatty acids with a chain length of

14–22 carbons are found in the epidermal tissue. Cholesterol is another component of the lipid bilayer, which also is used as an nonionic emulsifier in moisturizers. Nonionic emulsifiers depend cheifly upon hydroxyl groups and ether linkages to create the hydrophilic action.

Humectants

Moisturizers often contain humectants. The majority of humectants are low molecular weight substances with water attracting properties. Some are also high molecular weight substances. Humectants differ in water-binding capacity (Table 4) as well as in ability to penetrate and influence the degree of skin hydration.

One important group of humectants is the α-hydroxy acids (AHA), for example, lactic acid, glycolic acid, and tartaric acid. AHA is an organic carboxylic acid in which there is a hydroxy group at the two, or alpha (α), position of the carbon chain. Formulations containing an AHA have an acidic pH in the absence of any inorganic alkali or organic base. Lactic acid has been used in topical preparations for several decades because of its buffering properties and water-binding capacity (68).

Urea and PCA are other physiological substances used in moisturizers. Urea occurs in human tissues, blood, and urine. Urea in solution hydrolyses slowly to ammonia and carbon dioxide (62). Urea is used as a 10% cream for the treatment of ichtyosis and hyperkeratotic skin disorders (62,69), and in lower concentrations for the treatment of less severe dryness.

Glycerin is an important ingredient in skin care products, primarily due to its humectant and smoothening properties. Glycerin can be made from a hydrolysate of olive oil, as discovered in 1779 by the Swedish scientist C.W. Scheele.

Another commonly used alcohol is propylene glycol. The substance attracts water and is widely used in cosmetics and pharmaceuticals as a solvent

Table 4 Moisture-Binding Ability of Humectants at Various Humidities

Humectant	31%	50%	52%	58%–60%	76%
Glycerin	13 (25) 11 (66)	25 (65)	26 (66)	35–38 (25,67)	67 (66)
Na-PCA	20 (25) 17 (66)	44 (65)	45 (66)	61–63 (25,67)	210 (66)
Na-lactate	19 (66)	56 (65)	40 (66)	66 (67)	104 (66)
PCA	<1 (25)			<1 (25)	
Propylene glycol				32 (67)	
Sorbitol		1 (65)		10 (67)	

Note: Description of test conditions can be found in the original articles. PCA, pyrrolidone carboxylic acid. The numbers in parentheses indicates reference numbers.

and vehicle especially for substances unstable or insoluble in water. Propylene glycol is also regarded as a penetration enhancer.

Protection of Moisturizers

Preservatives are included in formulations to kill or inhibit the growth of microorganisms inadvertently introduced during use or manufacturing. The ideal preservative has a broad spectrum of activity; it must be safe to use; it should be stable in the product and it should not affect the physical properties of the product. No single preservative meets all these requirements and usually a combination of substances is used.

The efficacy of the preservative system is influenced by pH and ingredients in the formulation. Certain substances, such as ethanol and propylene glycol, may enhance the effect of the preservatives. In addition, alcohols may on their own prevent contamination of the product when they are used at high concentrations. Propylene glycol is used as inhibitor of fermentation and mold growth (62).

Tocopherols, butylated hydroxytoluene, and alkyl gallates are included in moisturizers to inhibit oxidation by reacting with free radicals blocking the chain reaction (62). Reducing agents, such as ascorbic acid, may also act by reacting with free radicals, as well as oxidize more readily than the ingredients they are intended to protect. Citric acid, tartaric acid, and EDTA and its salts have minor antioxidant activity, but enhance the antioxidant activity by "removing" heavy-metal ions. Such substances are called chelating agents (62). The stability of the metal–edetate complex depends on the metal ion involved and on the pH. The calcium chelate is relatively weak and EDTA will preferentially chelate heavy metals, such as iron, copper, and lead (62).

Influence of Moisturizers on Skin Chemistry

Water in the applied products have an immediate hydrating effect, due to absorption into the skin from their water phase (70). Humectants in moisturizers are supposed to penetrate into the skin and exert a longer impact on the degree of hydration of SC than water. Studies on dry skin also show amplification of the clinical improvements by the content of humectants in the moisturizer (19,71–74). Absorption of urea (33) and glycerin (75) into normal SC can be followed using a simple tape-stripping technique. Furthermore, treatment of solvent-damaged guinea pig footpad corneum with humectant solutions shows that the amount of water held by the corneum increases in the following order: sorbitol < glycerin < sodium lactate < sodium PCA (68). Moreover, the water-holding capacity of normal SC and of scales from psoriatic and ichthyotic patients is substantially increased after treatment with urea and glycerin (13,71,76,77). AHA may also stimulate the keratinocyte ceramide synthesis (78).

Application of lipids to the skin surface may increase skin hydration by several mechanisms. The most conventional one is occlusion, which implies a simple reduction of the loss of water from the outside of the skin. Common occlusive substances in moisturizers are lipids, for instance, petrolatum, beeswax, lanolin, and various oils (70). These lipids have long been considered to exert their effects on the skin solely by forming an inert, epicutaneous, occlusive membrane. However, topically applied lipids also penetrate the skin (26,79–83). Furthermore, application of structural lipids from SC increases skin hydration and reduce scaling (49,84).

SKIN STRUCTURE AND DESQUAMATION

The mechanical strength of the corneocytes derives from the tightly packed keratin bundles and the cross-linked proteins of the cornified envelopes. The corneocyte envelope constitutes a backbone for the intercellular barrier lipids (85). The content and organization of these lipids have broad implications for water retention, permeability barrier function, and desquamation. The desmosomes keeping the corneocytes together is degraded by enzymes, which are dependent upon water and pH for their activity (17,86–88). In excised skin, the rate of spontaneous cell dissociation is highest at neutral to weakly alkaline pH and decreases at lower pH values (88).

Dryness disorders, such as atopic eczema (3,8, 89,90), psoriasis (91), and ichthyosis, are characterized by hyperkeratosis and scaliness. Closer examination of clinically dry skin in patients with atopic dermatitis by scanning electron microscopy shows that the surface morphology is changed from a regular pattern to a coarser one with broad, irregularly running furrows and loss of minor furrows (3). The number of peaks is less and the distance between the peaks and the valleys is increased compared with normal skin (92,93). A more coarse and irregular skin surface pattern with larger squares is also found in recessive X-linked ichthyosis (94).

In dry atopic skin, the elasticity of SC is often reduced and the cohesive forces between the cells are increased (89). These changes may explain why cracking and fissuring may be found in such conditions. Furthermore, the projected size of the corneocytes is smaller and the turnover time is shorter than in controls (89,95).

Influence of Moisturizers on Skin Structure and Desquamation

Application of moisturizers to the skin induces tactile and visual changes of the surface. The ratio between oil and water is important, as well as the type of oil and the amount and type of other ingredients (emulsifiers, humectants, etc.). The combination of substances influences the initial feel of the product, its spreading behavior on the skin, whether and how fast it is absorbed, and how the skin feels after its use. The surface friction is changed after application of moisturizers (96).

Smoothing of the surface can be observed immediately after application as a result of the filling of spaces between partially desquamated skin flakes (97,98). The influence of moisturizers on the skin structure has been evaluated using instrumental evaluation of the skin topography (75,76,93,99,100). A single application of moisturizers decreases the roughness parameters and reduces the distance between the furrows during the first hours after application (100). No change in the roughness but a decrease in the distance between the peaks was found after 21 day treatment (93).

Prolonged exposure to water induces swelling of SC in the thickness dimension with swollen corneocytes (101). Rough structures, water pools, and occasionally vesicle-like structures can be seen in the intercellular lamellar regions by means of freeze-fracture electron microscope (102). Although water is known to play an important role in maintaining skin suppleness and plasticity, the humectants in themselves may also affect its physical properties. For example, AHA and NMF increase the skin elasticity (68,103–106). Studies also indicate that if NMF is removed, water alone cannot restore elasticity (106).

Humectants might also influence the crystalline arrangement of the bilayer lipids (107). In dry skin, the proportion of lipids in the solid state may be increased, and ingredients in moisturizers may then help to maintain the lipids in a liquid crystalline state at low relative humidity (107,108). Glycerin has been found to modulate the phase behavior of SC lipids *in vitro* and prevent crystallization of their lamellar structures at low relative humidity (108). Glycerin has also been suggested to ameliorate dry flaky skin by facilitating the digestion of the superficial desmosomes in subjects with dry skin (17). In addition, divalent ions such as calcium regulate the dissociation, and chelating agents such as edetic acid (EDTA) appears to increase the rate of cell dissociation *ex vivo* (88).

AHA, especially glycolic and lactic acids, have been found beneficial for topical treatment of ichthyosis (109). Histology reveals distinct changes in the epidermis, which might mediate a prompt influence on the keratinization process. There is an abrupt loss of the entire abnormal SC, probably due to a diminished cellular cohesion between the corneocytes at the lowermost, newly forming levels of SC, at its junction with the stratum granulosum (110,111). A reduced number of SC layers is also found in ichthyotic patients after treatment with 10% urea in combination with 5% lactic acid (112). Furthermore, a soft and pliable skin was obtained in seven patients with severe ichthyosis after treatment with a 10% urea formulation (77).

Randomized and controlled studies have been performed on patients with either ichthyosis vulgaris or X-linked ichthyosis (73). The preparations (two creams without any humectants, one cream with 10% urea, 5% lactic acid, and 2% salicylic acid ointment) were applied twice daily for 2 weeks. The urea-cream was found to be better in controlling the ichthyosis than the other three preparations. X-linked ichthyosis has also been treated topically with cholesterol, and some improvement in the functional and the structural abnormalities was found (113,114).

Two preparations containing 10% urea in different vehicles were also compared in 30 patients with ichthyosis associated with atopic dermatitis (115). After 4 weeks, both investigators and patients expressed preference for a urea-cream containing multisterols, phospholipids, and fatty diols with a pH of about 6. The other urea-cream contained lactic acid and had a pH of about 3. In another study on ichthyotic patients, 10% urea in combination with lactic acid and betaine was superior to its vehicle (71). In a recent double-blind study on 60 children, it was also shown that 10% urea was superior to its placebo in reducing the severity of generalized ichthyosis (116).

Improvement in lamellar ichthyosis was recently reported after treatment of one patient with 10% N-acetylcysteine in a moisturizing cream (117). N-Acetylcysteine was found to have antiproliferative effect on a culture of human keratinocytes (117). Promising effects in reducing the signs of scaling, hyperkeratosis, and xerosis were also reported after treatment of patients with lamellar ichthyosis with 5% lactic acid combined with 20% propylene glycol (118). The authors suggested that the ingredients acted synergistically in reverting hyperkeratosis. Environmentally induced dry skin also benefits from treatment with moisturizers, where those containing humectants often are inferior to those without, Table 5.

Excipients, such as lipids and emulsifiers, have also been suggested to be able to influence the cutaneous inflammation due to a possible anti-inflammatory action. Polyunsaturated fatty acids in oils have been suggested to be transformed enzymatically by the epidermis into "putative" anti-inflammatory products (125). It has also been shown that small hydrophobic compounds, such as free fatty acids and certain oxysterols, are recognized by nuclear hormone receptors, the largest family of transcription factors. Activation of certain receptors regulates keratinocyte proliferation and differentiation. For example, peroxisome proliferating activated receptor (PPARα) has been found involved in the oxidation of long-chain fatty acids (126). Cutaneous inflammation was reduced by the PPARα-agonist linoleic acid in mice (127). Moreover, activators of liver X receptors display anti-inflammatory activity in both irritant and allergic models of dermatitis (128). Studies have also demonstrated that such activators stimulate epidermal differentiation and improve permeability homeostasis (129).

Linoleic acid is an abundant fatty acid in vegetable oils, and fatty acids are also commonly used as emulsifiers in topical drugs. Clinical studies suggest that oral or topical supplements of EPA and/or omega-3 derivatives can decrease the severity of psoriasis (81,130). However, oral treatment and topical treatment in randomized and double-blind studies could not support the effect on moderate psoriasis (131,132). Topical treatment with sunflower seed oil (rich in linoleic acid) increased the level of linoleic acid of the epidermal phospholipids, but did not improve the disease or change transepidermal water loss (TEWL) (133).

Table 5 Effect of Moisturizers on Dry Skin Conditions Not Linked to Skin Diseases

Condition	Active substance	Control	Effect on dryness	References
Dry skin	3% and 10% Urea	Untreated	Improved	(119)
Xerosis	12% Ammonium lactate	Petrolatum-based cream	Improved, active better	(120)
Xerosis on legs	12% Ammonium lactate	5% Lactic acid + 2.5% CPA	Improved, active better	(121)
Dry heels	12% Ammonium lactate	No therapy	Active improved	(122)
Xerosis on legs	12% Lactate	5% Lactic acid/emollient lotion	All improved, equally effective, but 12% lasted longer	(74)
Xerosis	5% Lactic acid	Eucerin lotion	Improved, active better	(123)
Xerosis	5% PCA	Placebo and 10% urea	Active better than placebo, and equal as urea	(19)
Senescent dryness on forearm	10% Urea	Placebo	Improved	(124)
Asteatosis, senescent dryness on leg	4% Urea + 4% sodium chloride	Placebo	Improved, active better	(72)

A range of dietary oil supplements has also been suggested effective for treatment of atopic dermatitis. Some studies have also shown promising effects of evening primrose oil, a vegetable oil rich in GLA, when administered orally to atopic patients (134). However, this has not been confirmed in more recent double-blind and placebo controlled studies, neither on children (135) nor on adult patients (136,137).

THE BARRIER FUNCTION OF SC

The rate of penetration of substances through normal skin is inversely related to the thickness of SC (138). The major route of penetration of substances through SC is considered to be the intercellular pathway. This highly convoluted and tortuous lipid pathway around the corneocytes will give a longer distance for penetration than the actual thickness of SC (139,140). Dry and scaly skin is usually associated with impaired barrier function (8,15,90,91,141–143), although normal TEWL is observed in some dry skin conditions (1). The dryness may well be confined to the outermost layer of SC, where a competent permeability barrier still resides in the lower part of SC (144).

Impairment in the barrier function might be due to cracks in the skin, resulting from a decreased softness and flexibility of SC (21,145). Moreover, in dry scaly skin the projected size of the corneocytes is decreased, which reduces the tortuous pathway and thereby allowing a greater permeability (140,146). Hyperkeratosis may therefore be one way for SC to compensate for a defect SC barrier function, indicating a failure of epidermis to produce a competent barrier with normal thickness. Hyperkeratosis may also reflect an undesired inhibition of the desquamation process.

The most important factor for restricting water loss is the lipid content and organization of the intercellular barrier lipids (18,35,85,147). The lipid membranes contain primarily cholesterol, free fatty acids, and ceramides organized in two crystalline lamellar phases with periodicities of ~ 6 and 13 nm (148,149). The structural arrangement of the lipid molecules in the transverse plane is not clearly elucidated, but recent studies suggest that the different lipids may segregate in the membrane and form separate fluid and solid phases within SC (148,150). The bulk of the lipids has been suggested to be in crystalline/gel domain bordered by lipids in a fluid crystalline state; a "domain mosaic model" (151). This model is considered an effective water barrier which allows a controlled loss of water to keep the corneocytes moistened (151).

The lipid composition of SC is highly variable among individuals, depending on a number of factors, Table 6. Changes in the lipid composition may change the normal bilayer structure and barrier function (32,40–44,49,84,152,153).

Disturbance of the epidermal barrier function induces a rapid response of the keratinocytes to restore cutaneous homeostasis. The mRNA coding for proinflammatory cytokines, adhesion molecules, and growth factors is up-regulated (154). Likewise, there is an increase in DNA synthesis, leading to epidermal

Table 6 Factors Influencing the Lipid Composition of the Skin

Anatomical region (34)
Sex (45)
Age (45)
Season (47)
Exposure to surfactants (38,144)
Exposure to solvents (49,84,152,153)
Tape-induced scaly skin (32)
Atopic dermatitis (40–42)
Psoriasis (43,143)
Ichthyosis (44)

hyperplasia, and in lipid synthesis (153,155–158). The synthetic activity includes unsaponifiable lipids (153,155,158), fatty acids (155), and sphingolipids (159). Sterols and fatty acids are synthesized immediately after barrier disruption, whereas the increase in sphingolipid synthesis is somewhat delayed (159). Over time, the content of lipids in the SC is restored to the normal level in parallel with the return of barrier function (155,156,158,159).

Influence of Moisturizers on Skin Barrier Function

It has been hypothesized that permeability barrier abnormalities drive disease activity in inflammatory dermatoses, such as atopic dermatitis (160). Therefore, improvement of the SC barrier function is central to the improvement of all dry skin conditions. However, the composition of the moisturizer determines whether the treatment strengthens or deteriorates the skin barrier function (49,118,161–165). In addition, normal skin may react differently to environmental stimuli depending on previous treatment (162,163,166,167).

A number of factors need to be considered when the effects of moisturizers on skin barrier function are to be evaluated, Table 7. Studies evaluating the effects on diseased skin have to be distinguished from those on normal skin

Table 7 Factors to Consider in Evaluating the Effects on Skin Barrier Function by Creams

Composition of the cream
Cream thickness, drying time
Test skin, animals or humans, Normal or diseased
Single application vs. repeated applications
Expected time-course for effect
Biologic endpoint
Challenging substance, application method, dosage

(i.e., treatment or prevention). Experimental models of dryness can also be used, including barrier damage by successive tape strippings, or by exposure to acetone or SLS. One way of monitoring changes in the barrier function is to measure TEWL. The level of TEWL has been suggested to serve as an indicator of the permeability of the skin to topically applied substances, and high basal values has also been found to predict increased skin susceptibility to chemical irritation stimuli (168). The TEWL measurements can be combined with challenge of the skin with exposure of the living skin to substances with biological activity and measurement of the response, Table 8 (169).

In experimental models of dryness, moisturizers usually promote normalization of the skin (49,161,170–172). Petrolatum is absorbed into delipidized skin and accelerates barrier recovery to water (173). In SLS-irritated and tape-stripped human skin, a commercially available physiological lipid mixture (containing ceramide 3) was found to promote barrier recovery compared with the untreated control area (172). However, the barrier recovery was not superior to its placebo (petrolatum) (172,174). Commercially available moisturizers have also been found to reduce elevated TEWL in acetone-treated mice skin compared with untreated areas during a 24 h test period (175). Other studies suggest that the ratios of physiological lipids are important (176), since physiological lipids have been shown to penetrate deeper into the skin. Complete mixtures of ceramide, fatty acid, and cholesterol, or pure cholesterol, were shown to allow normal barrier recovery in acetone-treated murine skin, whereas two-component mixtures of fatty acid plus ceramide, cholesterol plus fatty acid, or cholesterol plus ceramide delayed barrier recovery (49). The humectant glycerin has also been found to stimulate barrier repair in SLS-damaged human skin (170).

The percentage of lipids in the cream has also been hypothesized to be crucial for the effect, since a relationship between the rate of recovery of experimentally damaged skin and the level of lipids has been observed (161). Furthermore, not only lipids but also nonionic emulsifiers have been found to influence TEWL in irritated skin (177).

Hence, suggestions how to tailor moisturizers for various skin abnormalities have been proposed (49,161,176,178,179). It is important to support the

Table 8 Examples of Substances That Have Been Used to Test the Skin Barrier Function (169)

Substance	Biologic response
Surfactants	Irritation
Alkali resistance	Burning, itching, erythema
DMSO	Urticaria
Nicotinates	Vasodilatation
Toluene	Irritation

results from experimental studies by data from the target patient group, where the time-course for the effect ideally also should be considered.

In studies on patients, one might expect an improvement in the impaired skin barrier function in association with improvement of the clinical signs of dryness. One physiological lipid mixture has also been found to decrease TEWL and improve atopic dermatitis in an open study in children (180). One moisturizer with 5% urea also reduced TEWL in atopic patients (181) and made skin less susceptible against irritation to SLS (182). Another urea-moisturizer was also superior to a glycerin-moisturizer in lowering TEWL in a double-blind study on atopic patients (183). TEWL has also been reduced in dry skin by treatment with moisturizers containing urea (119). Reduced TEWL was found in another study of ichthyotic patients treated with 10% urea (71). However, the elevated TEWL was not normalized in cleaners and kitchen workers (165) by a lipid-rich cream and in atopics treated with ammonium lactate (184), despite clinical improvement. In addition, treatment of xerotic legs in elderly with a lotion with 15% glycolic acid increased TEWL and also the susceptibility to topically applied irritants (164). Also in patients with lamellar ichthyosis treatment with 5% lactic acid combined with 20% propylene glycol increased TEWL (118).

Despite the widespread use of moisturizers on normal skin, scant attention has been paid to their influence on the permeability barrier. Treatment with moisturizers may well influence the barrier properties of normal skin. Studies in healthy volunteers show no increase in TEWL by repeated application of moisturizers, although the treatment appeared to increase the skin hydration significantly (163). However, repeated applications of urea-containing moisturizers have been found to reduce TEWL and make skin less susceptible to SLS-induced irritation (119,163,185). A lipid-rich cream without any humectant had no significant influence on TEWL, but increased skin susceptibility to SLS-irritation compared with untreated skin (162). Increased skin reactivity was also found in a long-term study using benzyl nicotinate as a marker for permeability, where the time to maximum response was shorter for the cream-treated area compared with the untreated (167). In addition, the time to induce vasodilatation was shorter for the lipid-rich cream than for a moisturizer containing 5% urea (167). Increased sensitivity to nickel was also found when nickel-sensitive humans treated their skin with a moisturizers without humectant compared with treatment with moisturizer with humectant (166). Areas treated with the glycerol-containing cream showed less reactivity to nickel than those treated with a cream without any humectant (166).

CONCLUDING REMARKS

The structure, composition, formation, and function of SC have been the subject of intense research over the last decades. The types of problems covered by the term dry skin may not always be diminished by an increase in skin hydration.

It seems essential to identify the underlying pathogenesis and to detect agents that assist the cellular differentiation process or act as precursors to vital SC components.

Moisturizers affect the SC architecture and barrier homeostasis, that is, topically applied ingredients are not as inert to the skin as have been considered traditionally. A number of different mechanisms behind the barrier improving effects from moisturizers have been suggested. It is obvious that a reduction in TEWL may be due to a simple deposition of lipid material to the surface, and not to any deeper effects in the skin. Another explanation is increased skin hydration, which increases SC elasticity and decreases the risks of cracks and fissures. Interference with the lipid layer around the corneocytes may also help to retain the moisture content in the corneocytes and prevent cracking of SC. Moreover, it is possible that the applied moisturizer decreases the proliferative activity of epidermis, which increases the size of the corneocytes. With a larger corneocyte area, the tortuous lipid pathway gives a longer distance for penetration, which reduces the permeability.

Topically applied lipids may also penetrate deeper into the skin and interfere with the endogenous lipid synthesis, which may promote, delay, or have no obvious influence on the normal barrier recovery in damaged skin. Furthermore, other substances in the creams may influence the composition of the SC lipids, for example, lactic acid has been found to stimulate the production of ceramides by keratinocytes. Other mechanisms, such as anti-inflammatory actions, are also conceivable explanations to the beneficial actions of moisturizers on the skin.

Whether changes in TEWL are predictive also for the permeability to substances other than water is likely to be dependent on the mechanism for the change in TEWL. For example, TEWL may be reduced by absorption of certain substances from the moisturizer, but this may facilitate absorption of other exogenous substances into the skin.

In conclusion, we can foresee that the increased understanding of the interactions between topically applied substances and the epidermal biochemistry will enhance the possibilities to tailor skin care products for various SC abnormalities. Furthermore, the non-invasive bioengineering techniques will allow us to monitor treatment effects more closely and we can also expect new instruments which can diagnose specific skin abnormalities.

REFERENCES

1. Leveque JL, Grove GL, de Rigal J, Corcuff P, Kligman AM. Biophysical characterization of dry facial skin. J Soc Cosmet Chem 1987; 82:171–177.
2. de Rigal J, Losch MJ, Bazin R, Camus C, Sturelle C, Descamps V et al. Near-infrared spectroscopy: a new approach to the characterization of dry skin. J Soc Cosmet Chem 1993; 44:197–209.
3. Linde YW. "Dry" skin in atopic dermatitis. A clinical study. Acta Derm Venereol (Stockh) 1989; 69:311–314.

4. Jemec GBE, Serup J. Scaling, dry skin and gender. Acta Derm Venereol 1992; (suppl 177):26–28.
5. Rurangirwa A, Pierard-Franchimont C, Le T, Ghazi A, Pierard GE. Corroborative evidence that "dry" skin is a misnomer. Bioeng Skin 1987; 3:35–42.
6. Piérard GE. What does "dry skin" mean? Int J Dermatol 1987; 26(3):167–168.
7. Ståhle-Bäckdahl M. Stratum corneum hydration in patients undergoing maintenance hemodialysis. Acta Derm Venereol 1988; 68:53–54.
8. Thune P. Evaluation of the hydration and the water-holding capacity in atopic skin and so-called dry skin. 1989; 144:133–135.
9. Long CC, Marks R. Stratum corneum changes in patients with senile pruritus. J Am Acad Dermatol 1992; 27:560–564.
10. Horii I, Nakayama Y, Obata M, Tagami H. Stratum corneum hydration and amino acid content in xerotic skin. Br J Dermatol 1989; 121:587–592.
11. Werner Y. The water content of the stratum corneum in patients with atopic dermatitis. Measurement with the Corneometer CM 420. Acta Derm Venereol (Stockh) 1986; 66:281–284.
12. Berardesca E, Fideli D, Borroni G, Rabbiosi G, Maibach HI. In vivo hydration and water-retention capacity of stratum corneum in clinically uninvolved skin in atopic and psoriatic patients. Acta Derm Venereol 1990; 70:400–404.
13. Tagami H. Electrical measurement of the water content of the skin surface. Functional analysis of the hygroskopic property and water-holding capacity of the stratum corneum *in vivo* and technique for assessing moisturizing efficacy. Cosmet Toilet 1982; 97:39–47.
14. Takenouchi M, Suzuki H, Tagami H. Hydration characteristics of pathologic stratum corneum—evaluation of bound water. J Invest Dermatol 1986; 87:574–576.
15. Serup J, Blichmann CW. Epidermal hydration of psoriasis plaques and the relation to scaling. Measurement of electrical conductance and transepidermal water loss. Acta Derm Venereol (Stockh) 1987; 67:357–359.
16. Werner Y, Lindberg M, Forslind B. The water-binding capacity of stratum corneum in dry non-eczematous skin of atopic eczema. Acta Derm Venereol 1982; 62:334–337.
17. Rawlings AV, Harding C, Watkinson A, Banks J, Ackerman C, Sabin R. The effect of glycerol and humidity on desmosome degradation in stratum corneum. Arch Dermatol Res 1995; 287:457–464.
18. Elias PM. Lipids and the epidermal permeability barrier. Arch Dermatol Res 1981; 270(1):95–117.
19. Middleton JD, Roberts ME. Effect of a skin cream containing the sodium salt of pyrrolidone carboxylic acid on dry and flaky skin. J Soc Cosmet Chem 1978; 29:201–205.
20. Laden K. Natural moisturization factors in skin. Am Perfum Cosmet 1967; 82:77–79.
21. Blank IH. Further observations on factors which influence the water content of the stratum corneum. J Invest Dermatol 1953; 21:259–271.
22. Anderson RL, Cassidy JM, Hansen JR, Yellin W. Hydration of stratum corneum. Biopolymers 1973; 12:2789–2802.
23. Hansen JR, Yellin W. NMR and infrared spectroscopic studies of stratum corneum hydration. In: Jellinek HHG, ed. New York-London: Plenum Press, 1972:19–28.
24. Jacobi OK. Moisture regulation in the skin. Drug Cosmet Ind 1959; 84:732–812.

25. Laden K, Spitzer R. Identification of a natural moisturizing agent in skin. J Soc Cosmet Chem 1967; 18:351–360.
26. Rawlings AV, Scott IR, Harding CR, Bowser PA. Stratum corneum moisturization at the molecular level. J Invest Dermatol 1995; 103:731–740.
27. Imokawa G, Kuno H, Kawai M. Stratum corneum lipids serve as a bound-water modulator. J Invest Dermatol 1991; 96(6):845–51.
28. Sybert VP, Dale BA, Holbrook KA. Ichthyosis vulgaris: identification of a defect in filaggrin synthesis correlated with an absence of keratohyaline granules. J Invest Dermatol 1985; 84:191–194.
29. Marstein S, Jellum E, Eldjarn L. The concentration of pyroglutamic acid (2-pyrrolidone-5-carboxylic acid) in normal and psoriatic epidermis, determined on a microgram scale by gas chromatography. Clin Chim Acta 1973; 43:389–395.
30. Vahlquist A. Ichthyosis—an inborn dryness of the skin. In: Lodén M, Maibach HI, eds. Dry Skin and Moisturizers: Chemistry and Function. Boca Raton: CRC Press, 2000:121–133.
31. Jacobson TM, Yukse IU, Greesin JC, Gordon JS, Lane AT, Gracy RW. Effects of aging and xerosis on the amino acid composition of human skin. J Invest Dermatol 1990; 95:296–300.
32. Denda M, Hori J, Koyama J, Yoshida S, Nanba R, Takahashi M et al. Stratum corneum sphingolipids and free amino acids in experimentally-induced scaly skin. Arch Dermatol Res 1992; 284(6):363–367.
33. Wellner K, Wohlrab W. Quantitative evaluation of urea in stratum corneum of human skin. Arch Dermatol Res 1993; 285:239–240.
34. Lampe MA, Burlingame AL, Whitney J, Williams ML, Brown BE, Roitman E, et al. Human stratum corneum lipids: characterization and regional variations. J Lipid Res 1983; 24(2):120–130.
35. Wertz PW, Downing DT. Stratum corneum: biological and biochemical considerations. In: Hadgraft J, Guy RH, eds. Transdermal Drug Delivery. Developmental Issues and Research Initiatives. New York, Basel: Marcel Dekker, Inc.; 1989.
36. Elias PM. Epidermal lipids, barrier function, and desquamation. J Invest Dermatol 1983; 80(Suppl):44s–49s.
37. Elias PM, Cooper ER, Korc A, Brown BE. Percutaneous transport in relation to stratum corneum structure and lipid composition. J Invest Dermatol 1981; 76(4):297–301.
38. Fulmer AW, Kramer GJ. Stratum corneum lipid abnormalities in surfactant-induced dry scaly skin. J Invest Dermatol 1986; 86(5):598–602.
39. Saint-Leger D, Francois AM, Leveque JL, Stoudemayer TJ, Kligman AM, Grove G. Stratum corneum lipids in skin xerosis. Dermatologica 1989; 178(3):151–155.
40. Melnik B, Hollmann J, Hofmann U, Yuh MS, Plewig G. Lipid composition of outer stratum corneum and nails in atopic and control subjects. Arch Dermatol Res 1990; 282:549–551.
41. Imokawa G, Abe A, Jin K, Higaki Y, Kawashima M, Hidano A. Decreased level of ceramides in stratum corneum of atopic dermatitis: an etiologic factor in atopic dry skin? J Invest Dermatol 1991; 96(4):523–526.
42. Yamamoto A, Serizawa S, Ito M, Sato Y. Stratum corneum lipid abnormalities in atopic dermatitis. Arch Dermatol Res 1991; 283:219–223.
43. Motta S, Sesana S, Ghidoni R, Monti M. Content of the different lipid classes in psoriatic scale. Arch Dermatol Res 1995; 287:691–694.

44. Paige DG, Morse-Fisher N, Harper JI. Quantification of stratum corneum ceramides and lipid envelope ceramides in the hereditary ichthyosis. Br J Dermatol 1994; 131:23–27.
45. Denda M, Koyama J, Hori J, Horii I, Takahashi M, Hara M et al. Age- and sex-dependent change in stratum corneum sphingolipids. Arch Dermatol Res 1993; 285(7):415–417.
46. Williams ML, Elias PM. Stratum corneum lipids in disorders of cornification: increased cholesterol sulfate content of stratum corneum in recessive x-linked ichthyosis. J Clin Invest 1981; 68(6):1404–1410.
47. Rawlings AV, Conti A, Rogers J, Verdejo P, Harding CR. Seasonal influences on stratum corneum ceramide 1 linoleate content and the influence of topical essential fatty acids. In: 18th Int IFSCC Congr, October 3–6, 1994; 1994 October 3–6; Venice; 1994. p. 127–137.
48. Rawlings A, Hope J, Rogers J, Mayo A, Watkinson A, Scott I. Skin dryness—what is it? J Invest Dermatol 1993; 100:510.
49. Man MQ, Feingold KR, Elias PM. Exogenous lipids influence permeability barrier recovery in acetone-treated murine skin. Arch Dermatol 1993; 129(6):728–738.
50. Sato J, Denda M, Nakanishi J, Nomura J, Koyama J. Cholesterol sulfate inhibits proteases that are involved in desquamation of stratum corneum. J Invest Dermatol 1998; 111(2):189–193.
51. Bouwstra JA, Gooris GS, Dubbelaar FE, Ponec M. Cholesterol sulfate and calcium affect stratum corneum lipid organization over a wide temperature range. J Lipid Res 1999; 40:2303–2312.
52. Bouwstra JA, Dubbelaar FE, Gooris GS, Weerheim AM, Ponec M. The role of ceramide composition in the lipid organisation of the skin barrier. Biochim Biophys Acta 1999; 1419(2):127–136.
53. Forslind B, Werner-Linde Y, Lindberg M, Pallon J. Elemental analysis mirrors epidermal differentiation. Acta Derm Venereol 1999; 79:12–17.
54. Menon GK, Elias PM. Ultrastructural localization of calcium in psoriatic and normal human epidermis. Arch Dermatol 1991; 127:57–63.
55. Forslind B. The skin barrier: analysis of physiologically important elements and trace elements. Acta Derm Venereol 2000; 208:46–52.
56. Holden C, English J, Hoare C, Jordan A, Kownacki S, Turnbull R et al. Advised best practice for the use of emollients in eczema and other dry skin conditions. J Dermatolog Treat 2002; 13:103–106.
57. Schlagel CA, Sanborn EC. The weights of topical preparations required for total and partial body inunction. J Invest Dermatol 1964; 42:253–256.
58. Lynfield YL, Schechter BA. Choosing and using a vehicle. J Am Acad Dermatol 1984; 10:56–59.
59. Ivens UI, Steinkjer B, Serup J, Tetens V. Ointment is evenly spread on the skin, in contrast to creams and solutions. Br J Dermatol 2001; 145:264–267.
60. Rhodes LE, Diffey BL. Fluorescence spectroscopy: a rapid, noninvasive method for measurement of skin surface thickness of topical agents. Br J Dermatol 1997; 136(1):12–17.
61. Johnson R, Nusbaum BP, Horwitz SN, Frost P. Transfer of topically applied tetracycline in various vehicles. Arch Dermatol 1983; 119(8):660–663.
62. Kibbe AW. Handbook of Pharmaceutical Excipients. 3d ed. Washington: American Pharmaceutical Association, Pharmaceutical Press, 2000.

63. Yunginger JW, Calobrisi SD. Investigation of the allergenicity of a refined peanut oil-containing topical dermatologic agent in persons who are sensitive to peanuts. Cutis 2001; 68:153–155.
64. Rhodes LE. Essential fatty acids. In: Lodén M, Maibach HI, eds. Dry Skin and Moisturizers: Chemistry and Function. Boca Raton: CRC Press, 2000:311–325.
65. Takahashi M, Yamada M, Machida Y. A new method to evaluate the softening effect of cosmetic ingredients on the skin. J Soc Cosmet Chem 1984; 35:171–181.
66. Rieger MM, Deem DE. Skin moisturizers II. The effects of cosmetic ingredients on human stratum corneum. J Soc Cosmet Chem 1974; 25:253–262.
67. Huttinger R. Restoring hydrophilic properties to the stratum corneum—a new humectant. Cosmet Toilet 1978; 93:61–62.
68. Middleton J. Development of a skin cream designed to reduce dry and flaky skin. J Soc Cosmet Chem 1974; 25:519–534.
69. Rosten M. The treatment of ichthyosis and hyperkeratotic conditions with urea. Australas J Dermatol 1970; 11:142–144.
70. Lodén M, Lindberg M. The influence of a single application of different moisturizers on the skin capacitance. Acta Derm Venereol 1991; 71(1):79–82.
71. Grice K, Sattar H, Baker H. Urea and retinoic acid in ichthyosis and their effect on transepidermal water loss and water holding capacity of stratum corneum. Acta Derm Venereol (Stockh) 1973; 54:114–118.
72. Frithz A. Investigation of Cortesal®, a hydrocortisone cream and its water-retaining cream base in the treatment of xerotic skin and dry eczemas. Curr Ther Res 1983; 33:930–935.
73. Pope FM, Rees JK, Wells RS, Lewis KGS. Out-patient treatment of ichthyosis: a double-blind trial of ointments. Br J Dermatol 1972; 86:291–296.
74. Dahl MV, Dahl AC. 12% Lactate lotion for the treatment of xerosis. Arch Dermatol 1983; 119:27–30.
75. Batt MD, Fairhurst E. Hydration of the stratum corneum. Int J Cosmet Sci 1986; 8:253–264.
76. Batt MD, Davis WB, Fairhurst E, Gerreard WA, Ridge BD. Changes in the physical properties of the stratum corneum following treatment with glycerol. J Soc Cosmet Chem 1988; 39:367.
77. Swanbeck G. A new treatment of ichthyosis and other hyperkeratotic conditions. Acta Derm Venereol (Stockh) 1968; 48:123–127.
78. Rawlings AV, Davies A, Carlomusto M, Pillai S, Zhang AR, Kosturko R, et al. Effect of lactic acid isomers on keratinocyte ceramide synthesis, stratum corneum lipid levels and stratum corneum barrier function. Arch Dermatol Res 1996; 288:383–390.
79. Wertz PW, Downing DT. Metabolism of topically applied fatty acid methyl esters in BALB/C mouse epidermis. J Derm Sci 1990; 1:33–38.
80. Moloney SJ. The in-vitro percutaneous absorption of glycerol trioleate through hairless mouse skin. J Pharm Pharmacol 1988; 40:819–821.
81. Escobar SO, Achenbach R, Innantuono R, Torem V. Topical fish oil in psoriasis—a controlled and blind study. Clin Exp Dermatol 1992; 17:159–162.
82. Tollesson A, Frithz A. Borage oil, an effective new treatment for infantile seborrhoeic dermatitis. Br J Dermatol 1993; 129:95.
83. Feingold KR, Brown BE, Lear SR, Moser AH, Elias PM. Effect of essential fatty acid deficiency on cutaneous sterol synthesis. J Invest Dermatol 1986; 87(5):588–591.

84. Imokawa G, Akasaki S, Hattori M, Yoshizuka N. Selective recovery of deranged water-holding properties by stratum corneum lipids. J Invest Dermatol 1986; 87(6):758–761.
85. Downing DT. Lipid and protein structures in the permeability barrier. In: Lodén M, Maibach HI, eds. Dry Skin and Moisturizers; Chemistry and Function. Boca Raton: CRC Press, 2000:59–70.
86. Suzuki Y, Nomura J, Koyama J, Horii I. The role of proteases in stratum corneum: involvement in stratum corneum desquamation. Arch Dermatol Res 1994; 286: 249–253.
87. Öhman H, Vahlquist A. The pH gradient over the stratum corneum differs in X-linked recessive and autosomal dominant ichthyosis: a clue to the molecular origin of the "acid skin mantle"? J Invest Dermatol 1998; 111:674–677.
88. Lundstrom A, Egelrud T. Cell shedding from human plantar skin in vitro: evidence of its dependence on endogenous proteolysis. J Invest Dermatol 1988; 91:340–343.
89. Finlay AY, Nicholls S, King CS, Marks R. The 'dry' non-eczematous skin associated with atopic eczema. Br J Dermatol 1980; 103(3):249–256.
90. Lodén M, Olsson H, Axell T, Linde YW. Friction, capacitance and transepidermal water loss (TEWL) in dry atopic and normal skin. Br J Dermatol 1992; 126(2):137–141.
91. Ghadially R, Reed JT, Elias PM. Stratum corneum structure and function correlates with phenotype in psoriasis. J Invest Dermatol 1996; 107(4):558–564.
92. Linde YW, Bengtsson A, Lodén M. 'Dry' skin in atopic dermatitis II. A surface profilometry study. Acta Derm Venereol 1989; 69:315–319.
93. Cook TH, Craft TJ. Topographics of dry skin, non-dry skin, and cosmetically treated dry skin as quantified by skin profilometry. J Soc Cosmet Chem 1985; 36:143–152.
94. Kuokakanen K. Replica reflection of normal skin and of skin with disturbed keratinization. Acta Dermatol Venereol (Stockh) 1972; 52:205–210.
95. Watanabe M, Tagami H, Horii I, Takahashi M, Kligman AM. Functional analyses of the superficial stratum corneum in atopic dermtitis. Arch Dermatol 1991; 127:1689–1692.
96. Lodén M, Olsson H, Skare L, Axéll T. Instrumental and sensory evaluation of the frictional response of the skin following a single application of five moisturizing creams. J Soc Cosmet Chem 1992; 43:13–20.
97. Nicholls S, King CS, Marks R. Short term effects of emollients and a bath oil on the stratum corneum. J Soc Cosmet Chem 1978; 29:617–624.
98. Garber CA, Nightingale CT. Characterizing cosmetic effects and skin morphology by scanning electron microscopy. J Soc Cosmet Chem 1976; 27:509–531.
99. Murahata RI, Crowe DM, Roheim JR. Evaluation of hydration state and surface defects in the stratum corneum: comparison of computer analysis and visual appraisal of positive replicas of human skin. J Soc Cosmet Chem 1984; 35:327–338.
100. Mignot J, Zahouani H, Rondot D, Nardin P. Morphological study of human skin relief. Bioeng Skin 1987; 3:177–196.
101. Norlén L, Emilson A, Forslind B. Stratum corneum swelling. Biophysical and computer assisted quantitative assessments. Arch Dermatol Res 1997; 289:506–513.
102. Van Hal DA, Jeremiasse E, Junginger HE, Spies F, Bouwstra JA. Structure of fully hydrated human stratum corneum: a freeze-fracture electron microscopy study. J Invest Dermatol 1996; 106(1):89–95.

103. Alderson SG, Barratt MG, Black JG. Effect of 2-hydroxyacids on guinea-pig footpad stratum corneum: mechanical properties and binding studies. Int J Cosmet Sci 1984; 6:91.
104. Takahashi M, Machida Y, Tsuda Y. The influence of hydroxy acids on the rheological properties of stratum corneum. J Soc Cosmet Chem 1985; 36:177–187.
105. Hall KJ, Hill JC. The skin plasticisation effect of 2-hydroxyoctanoic acid. 1: The use of potentiators. J Soc Cosmet Chem 1986; 37:397–407.
106. Jokura Y, Ishikawa S, Tokuda H, Imokawa G. Molecular analysis of elastic properties of the stratum corneum by solid-state 13C-nuclear magnetic resonance spectroscopy. J Invest Dermatol 1995; 104:806–812.
107. Mattai J, Froebe CL, Rhein LD, Simion FA, Ohlmeyer H, Su DT et al. Prevention of model stratum corneum lipid phase transitions in vitro by cosmetic additives—differential scanning calometry, optical microscopy, and water evaporation studies. J Soc Cosmet Chem 1993; 44:89–100.
108. Froebe CL, Simion FA, Ohlmeyer H, Rhein LD, Mattai J, Cagan RH et al. Prevention of stratum corneum lipid phase transitions in vitro by glycerol—an alternative mechanism for skin moisturization. J Soc Cosmet Chem 1990; 41:51–65.
109. Van Scott EJ, Yu RJ. Control of keratinization with alpha-hydroxy acids and related compounds I. Topical treatment of ichthyotic disorders. Arch Dermatol 1974; 110:586–590.
110. Van Scott EJ, Yu RJ. Hyperkeratinization, corneocyte cohesion, and alpha hydroxy acids. J Am Acad Dermatol 1984; 11:867–879.
111. Yu RJ, Van Scott EJ. Alpha-hydroxy acids: science and therapeutic use. Cosmet Dermatol 1994(suppl):1–6.
112. Blair C. The action of a urea-lactic acid ointment in ichthyosis. With particular reference to the thickness of the horny layer. Br J Dermatol 1976; 94:145–153.
113. Zettersten E, Man MQ, Sato J, Denda M, Farrell A, Ghadially R et al. Recessive x-linked ichthyosis: role of cholesterol-sulfate accumulation in the barrier abnormality. J Invest Dermatol 1998; 111(5):784–790.
114. Lykkesfeldt G, Hoyer H. Topical cholesterol treatment of recessive X-linked ichthyosis. Lancet 1983; 2(8363):1337–1338.
115. Fredriksson T, Gip L. Urea creams in the treatment of dry skin and hand dermatitis. Int J Dermatol 1975; 32:442–444.
116. Kuster W, Bohnsack K, Rippke F, Upmeyer HJ, Groll S, Traupe H. Efficacy of urea therapy in children with ichthyosis. A multicenter randomized, placebo-controlled, double-blind, semilateral study. Dermatology 1998; 196:217–222.
117. Redondo P, Bauza A. Topical N-acetylcysteine for lamellar ichthyosis. Lancet 1999; 354:1880.
118. Gånemo A, Virtanen M, Vahlquist A. Improved topical treatment of lamellar ichthyosis: a double blind study of four different cream formulations. Br J Dermatol 1999; 141:1027–1032.
119. Serup J. A double-blind comparison of two creams containing urea as the active ingredient. Assessment of efficacy and side-effects by non-invasive techniques and a clinical scoring scheme. 1992; 177:34–43.
120. Wehr R, Krochmal L, Bagatell F, W. R. A controlled two-center study of lactate 12% lotion and a petrolatum-based cream in patients with xerosis. Cutis 1986; 37:205–209.

121. Rogers RS, Callen J, Wehr R, Krochmal L. Comparative efficacy of 12% ammonium lactate lotion and 5% lactic acid lotion in the treatment of moderate to severe xerosis. J Am Acad Dermatol 1989; 21:714–716.
122. Siskin SB, Quinlan PJ, Finkelstein MS, Marlucci M, Maglietta TG, Gibson JR. The effect of ammonium lactate 12% lotion versus no therapy in the treatment of dry skin of the heels. Int J Dermatol 1983; 32:905–907.
123. Wehr RF, Kantor I, Jones EL, McPhee ME. A controlled comparative efficacy study of 5% ammonium lactate lotion versus an emollient control lotion in the treatment of moderate xerosis. J Am Acad Dermatol 1991; 25:849–851.
124. Schölermann A, Banké-Bochita J, Bohnsack K, Rippke F, Herrmann WM. Efficacy and safety of Eucerin 10% urea lotion in the treatment of symptoms of aged skin. J Dermatol Treat 1998; 9:175–179.
125. Miller CC, Tang W, Ziboh VA, Fletcher MP. Dietary supplementation with ethyl ester concentrates of fish oil (n-3) and borage oil (n-6) polyunsaturated fatty acids induces epidermal generation of local putative anti-inflammatory metabolites. J Invest Dermatol 1991; 96:98–103.
126. Schurer NY. Implementation of fatty acid carriers to skin irritation and the epidermal barrier. Contact Dermat 2002; 47:199–205.
127. Sheu MY, Fowler AJ, Kao J, Schmuth M, Schoonjans K, Auwerx J et al. Topical peroxisome proliferator activated receptor-alpha activators reduce inflammation in irritant and allergic contact dermatitis models. J Invest Dermatol 2002; 118(1):94–101.
128. Fowler AJ, Sheu MY, Schmuth M, Kao J, Fluhr JW, Rhein L et al. Liver X receptor activators display anti-inflammatory activity in irritant and allergic contact dermatitis models: liver-X-receptor-specific inhibition of inflammation and primary cytokine production. J Invest Dermatol 2003; 120(2):246–255.
129. Komuves LG, Hanley K, Jiang Y, Elias PM, Williams ML, Feingold KR. Ligands and activators of nuclear hormone receptors regulate epidermal differentiation during fetal rat skin development. J Invest Dermatol 1998; 111(3):429–433.
130. Dewsbury CE, Graham P, Darley CR. Topical eicosapentaenoic acid (EPA) in the treatment of psoriasis. Br J Dermatol 1989; 120:581.
131. Gupta AK, Ellis CN, Goldfarb MT, Hamilton TA, Voorhees JJ. The role of fish oil in psoriasis. A randomized, double blind, placebo-controlled study to evaluate the effect of fish oil and topical corticosteroid therapy in psoriasis. Int J Dermatol 1990; 29:591–595.
132. Zepelin HHH-V, Mrowietz U, Färber L, Bruck-Borchers K, Schober C, Huber J et al. Highly purified omega-3-polyunsaturated fatty acids for topical treatment of psoriasis. Results of a double-blind, placebo-controlled multicentre study. Br J Dermatol 1993; 129:713–717.
133. Hartop PJ, Allenby CF, Prottey C. Comparison of barrier function and lipids in psoriasis and essential fatty acid-deficient rats. Clin Exp Dermatol 1978; 3:259–267.
134. Wright S, Burton JL. Oral evening-primrose-seed oil improves atopic eczema. Lancet 1982; 2:1120–1122.
135. Hederos CA, Berg A. Epogam evening primrose oil treatment in atopic dermatitis and asthma. Arch Dis Child 1996; 75:494–497.
136. Bamford JTM, Gibson RW, Renier CM. Atopic eczema unresponsive to evening primrose oil (linoleic and *-linolenic acids). J Am Acad Dermatol 1985; 13: 959–965.

137. Henz BM, Jablonska S, van de Kerkhof PCM, Stingl G, Blaszczyk M, vandervalk PGM et al. Double-blind, multicentre analysis of the efficacy of borage oil in patients with atopic dermatitis. Br J Dermatol 1999; 140:685–688.
138. Scheuplein RJ, Blank IH. Permeability of the skin. Phys Rev 1971; 51:702–747.
139. Potts RO, Francoeur ML. The influence of stratum corneum morphology on water permeability. J Invest Dermatol 1991; 96:495–499.
140. Rougier A, Lotte C, Corcuff P, Maibach HI. Relationship between skin permeability and corneocyte size according to anatomic site, age, and sex in man. J Soc Cosmet Chem 1988; 39:15–26.
141. Denda M, Koyama J, Namba R, Horii I. Stratum corneum lipid morphology and transepidermal water loss in normal skin and surfactant-induced scaly skin. Arch Dermatol Res 1994; 286:41–46.
142. Werner Y, Lindberg M. Transepidermal water loss in dry and clinically normal skin in patients with atopic dermatitis. Acta Derm Venereologica 1985; 65:102–105.
143. Motta S, Monti M, Sesana S, Mellesi L, Ghidoni R, Caputo R. Abnormality of water barrier function in psoriasis. Arch Dermatol 1994; 130:452–456.
144. Imokawa G, Akasaki S, Minematsu Y, Kawai M. Importance of intercellular lipids in water-retention properties of the stratum corneum: induction and recovery study of surfactant dry skin. Arch Dermatol Res 1989; 281(1):45–51.
145. Blank IH. Factors which influence the water content of the stratum corneum. J Invest Dermatol 1952; 18:433–440.
146. Grove GL, Kligman AM. Corneocytes size as an indirect measure of epidermal proliferative activity. In: Marks R, Plewig G, eds. Stratum Corneum. New York: Springer-Verlag, 1983:191–194.
147. Elias PM, Menon GK. Structural and lipid biochemical correlates of the epidermal permeability barrier. Adv Lipid Res 1991; 24:1–26.
148. White SH, Mirejovsky D, King GI. Structure of lamellar lipid domains and corneocyte envelopes of murine stratum corneum. An X-ray diffraction study. Biochemistry 1988; 27:3725–3732.
149. Bouwstra JA, Gooris GS, van der Spek JA, Bras W. The structure of human stratum corneum as determined by small angle X-ray scattering. J Invest Dermatol 1991; 96:1006–1014.
150. Knutson K, Krill SL, Lambert WJ, Higuchi WI. Physiochemical aspects of transdermal permeation. J Control Release 1987; 6:59–74.
151. Forslind B. A domain mosaic model of the skin barrier. Acta Derm Venereol (Stockh) 1994; 74:1–6.
152. Imokawa G, Hattori M. A possible function of structural lipids in the water-holding properties of the stratum corneum. J Invest Dermatol 1985; 84(4):282–284.
153. Feingold KR, Man MQ, Menon GK, Cho SS, Brown BE, Elias PM. Cholesterol synthesis is required for cutaneous barrier function in mice. J Clin Invest 1990; 86(5):1738–1745.
154. Nickoloff BJ, Naidu Y. Perturbation of epidermal barrier function correlates with initiation of cytokine cascade in human skin. J Am Acad Dermatol 1994; 30:535–546.
155. Grubauer G, Feingold KR, Elias PM. Relationship of epidermal lipogenesis to cutaneous barrier function. J Lipid Res 1987; 28(6):746–752.
156. Grubauer G, Elias PM, Feingold KR. Transepidermal water loss: the signal for recovery of barrier structure and function. J Lipid Res 1989; 30(3):323–333.

157. Proksch E, Feingold KR, Man MQ, Elias PM. Barrier function regulates epidermal DNA synthesis. J Clin Invest 1991; 87:1668–1673.
158. Menon GK, Feingold KR, Moser AH, Brown BE, Elias PM. De novo sterologenesis in the skin II. Regulation by cutaneous barrier requirements. J Lipid Res 1985; 26:418–427.
159. Holleran WM, Feingold KR, Man MQ, Gao WN, Lee JM, Elias PM. Regulation of epidermal sphingolipid synthesis by permeability barrier function. J Lipid Res 1991; 32:1151–1158.
160. Elias PM, Wood LC, Feingold KR. Epidermal pathogenesis of inflammatory dermatoses. Am J Contact Dermat 1999; 10:119–126.
161. Held E, Lund H, Agner T. Effect of different moisturizers on SLS-irritated human skin. Contact Dermat 2001; 44:229–234.
162. Held E, Sveinsdottir S, Agner T. Effect of long-term use of moisturizers on skin hydration, barrier function and susceptibility to irritants. Acta DermVenereol (Stockh) 1999; 79:49–51.
163. Lodén M. Urea-containing moisturizers influence barrier properties of normal skin. Arch Dermatol Res 1996; 288:103–107.
164. Kolbe L, Kligman AM, Stoudemayer T. Objective bioengineering methods to assess the effects of moisturizers on xerotic leg of elderly people. J Dermatol Treat 2000; 11:241–245.
165. Halkier-Sorensen L, Thestrup-Pedersen K. The efficacy of a moisturizer (Locobase) among cleaners and kitchen assistants during everyday exposure to water and detergents. Contact Dermat 1993; 29:266–271.
166. Hachem JP, De Paepe K, Vanpée E, Kaufman L, Rogiers V, Roseeuw D. The effect of two of moisturisers on skin barrier damage in allergic contact dermatitis. Eur J Dermatol 2002; 12:136–138.
167. Duval D, Lindberg M, Boman A, Johansson S, Edlund F, Lodén M. Differences among moisturizers in affecting skin susceptibility to hexyl nicotinate, measured as time to increase skin blood flow. Skin Res Technol 2002; 8:1–5.
168. Dupuis D, Rougier A, Lotte C, Wilson DR, Maibach HI. *In vivo* relationship between percutaneous absorption and transepidermal water loss according to anatomic site in man. J Soc Cosmet Chem 1986; 37:351–357.
169. Kolbe L. Non-invasive methods for testing of the stratum corneum barrier function. In: Lodén M, Maibach HI, eds. Dry Skin and Moisturizers: Chemistry and Function. Boca Raton: CRC Press, 2000:393–401.
170. Fluhr JW, Gloor M, Lehmann L, Lazzerini S, Distante F, Berardesca E. Glycerol accelerates recovery of barrier function in vivo. Acta Derm Venereol 1999; 79(6):418–421.
171. Loden M. Barrier recovery and influence of irritant stimuli in skin treated with a moisturizing cream. Contact Dermat 1997; 36:256–260.
172. Kucharekova M, Schalkwijk J, Van de Kerkhof PCM, Van de Valk PG. Effect of a lipid-rich emollient containing ceramide 3 in experimentally induced skin barrier dysfunction. Contact Dermat 2002; 46:331–338.
173. Ghadially R, Halkier_Sorensen L, Elias PM. Effects of petrolatum on stratum corneum structure and function. J Am Acad Dermatol 1992; 26:387–396.
174. Lodén M, Barany E. Skin-identical lipids versus petrolatum in the treatment of tape-stripped and detergent-perturbed human skin. Acta Derm Venereol 2000; 80:412–415.

175. Mortz CG, Andersen KE, Halkier-Sørensen L. The efficacy of different moisturizers on barrier recovery in hairless mice evaluated by non-invasive bioengineering methods. A model to select the potentially most effective product. Contact Dermat 1997; 36:297–310.
176. Thornfeldt C. Critical and optimal molar ratios of key lipids. In: Lodén M, Maibach HI, eds. Dry Skin and Moisturizers: Chemistry and Function. Boca Raton: CRC Press, 2000:337–347.
177. Barany E, Lindberg M, Lodén M. Unexpected skin barrier influence from nonionic emulsifiers. Int J Pharm 2000; 195(1–2):189–195.
178. Mao-Qiang M, Brown BE, Wu-Pong S, Feingold KR, Elias PM. Exogenous nonphysiologic vs physiologic lipids. Divergent mechanisms for correction of permeability barrier dysfunction. Arch Dermatol 1995; 131:809–816.
179. Zettersten EM, Ghadially R, Feingold KR, Crumrine D, Elias PM. Optimal ratios of topical stratum corneum lipids improve barrier recovery in chronologically aged skin. J Am Acad Dermatol 1997; 37:403–408.
180. Chamlin SL, Kao J, Frieden IJ, Sheu MY, Fowler AJ, Fluhr JW et al. Ceramide-dominant barrier repair lipids alleviate childhood atopic dermatitis: changes in barrier function provide a sensitive indicator of disease activity. J Am Acad Dermatol 2002; 47(2):198–208.
181. Andersson A-C, Lindberg M, Lodén M. The effect of two urea-containing creams on dry, eczematous skin in atopic patients I. Expert, patient and instrumental evaluation. J Dermatol Treat 1999; 10:165–169.
182. Lodén M, Andersson A-C, Lindberg M. Improvement in skin barrier function in patients with atopic dermatitis after treatment with a moisturizing cream (Canoderm®). Br J Dermatol 1999; 140:264–267.
183. Lodén M, Andersson AC, Andersson C, Frodin T, Oman H, Lindberg M. Instrumental and dermatologist evaluation of the effect of glycerine and urea on dry skin in atopic dermatitis. Skin Res Technol 2001; 7:209–213.
184. Vilaplana J, Coll J, Trullás C, Axón A, Pelejero C. Clinical and non-invasive evaluation of 12% ammonium lactate emulsion for the treatment of dry skin in atopic and non-atopic subjects. Acta Derm Venereol (Stockh) 1992; 72:28–33.
185. Lodén M. Barrier recovery and influence of irritant stimuli in skin treated with a moisturizing cream. Contact Dermat 1997; 36(5):256–260.

12

Alternative Drugs in Dermatology: An Overview

Cheryl Levin and Howard I. Maibach
Department of Dermatology, University of California—San Francisco Medical Center, San Francisco, CA, USA

Tea Extracts	248
Other Extracts	249
Hydroxyacids	250
Essential Fatty Acids	250
Essential Oils	253
Vitamins C and E	254
Miscellaneous	257
Conclusion	257
References	258

Recently, alternative remedies have been investigated to supplement traditional drugs in the treatment of dermatological disorders including psoriasis, phototoxicity, allergic reactions, and atopic dermatitis (AD). The following highlights recently reported medicaments. Emphasis is placed on those *in vitro* and *in vivo* controlled studies that follow the evidence-based dermatology guidelines (1) and whose results encourage further clinical research. The utilized controls, statistical approach to analysis, and validity of the experimental methodology including the possibility for extrapolation to the clinical realm were given particular importance in analyzing study results.

TEA EXTRACTS

Ultraviolet (UV) solar radiation may induce a variety of adverse effects in humans, including melanoma (2), photoaging of the skin (3,4), sunburn (5), and immune suppression (6,7). Protection against the UV-induced skin damage includes avoidance of sun exposure, application of sunscreens, low-fat diets (8,9), and pharmacologic intervention with retinoids (10). More recently, green tea extracts have been reported to be beneficial in treating UV-induced photodamage.

In a study by Elmets et al. (11) 1–10% green tea polyphenolic (GTP) fractions in ethanol/water vehicle were applied onto the backs of six volunteers. After 30 min following GTP application, patients were exposed to a 2-minimal erythema dose (MED) of UV radiation from a solar simulator. The MED was determined for each patient by exposing skin to graded doses of UV radiation from the solar simulator. Green tea extracts resulted in a dose-dependent reduction of UV-induced erythema as measured by chromametry and visual evaluation. The (−)-epigallocatechin-3-gallate (EGCG) and (−)-epicatechin-3-gallate polyphenolic fractions were most effective, whereas the (−)-epigallocatechin and (−)-epicatechin fractions had little effect. Histological examination revealed a decrease in sunburn cells in GTP-treated skin. Epidermal Langerhans cells, the antigen presenting cells involved in the skin immune response, were significantly protected against UV damage. Finally, GTP fractions reduced UV-induced mutations in DNA, as detected utilizing a phosphorus 32-postlabeling technique. Spectrophotometric analysis indicated that GTP fractions did not absorb UVB light, implying a mechanism of action different from that of sunscreens. This study demonstrates the potential benefit of GTP extracts in preventing UV-induced immunosuppression and erythema.

GTP extracts were also found to be beneficial in treating UV-induced immunosuppression in mice. GTP extracts, fruits and vegetables, and quercetin and chrysin significantly prevented the UV-induced suppression of contact hypersensitivity to picryl chloride when compared with irradiated, untreated control ($p < 0.05$). Increased ear thickness measurements were used to evaluate the response. GTP was administered in concentrations of 0.1% and 0.01% (12). Green tea extracts have been beneficial in preventing early signs of photochemical damage to mouse and human skin treated with psoralen plus UVA therapy. Psoralen plus UVA, a treatment for psoriasis, increases the patient's risk of developing melanoma and squamous cell carcinoma (SCC). Pre- and post-treatment with the green tea extracts in mouse and human skin significantly decreased markers of this photochemical damage, namely, hyperplasia and hyperkeratosis, c-fos and p53, and erythema ($p < 0.05$) when compared with vehicle controls (water given pre- and post-treatment). Further discussion of the effects of green tea on skin is discussed by Katiyar et al. (13).

Oral and topical standardized black tea extracts (SBTE) also decreased photochemical damage to the skin. In one study, SBTE significantly reduced erythema and skinfold thickness associated with UVB-induced carcinogenesis in cultured keratinocytes, mouse, and human skin ($p < 0.05$). In topically treated mice, a 64% reduction in severity of erythema and a 50% decrease in skinfold thickness were observed when compared with vehicle control. A decrease in the expression of c-fos, c-jun, and p53 in mouse skin and keratinocytes pretreated with SBTE was also noted. This study indicates that when green tea is oxidized to black tea, the extracts remain beneficial in preventing the early signs of UVB-induced phototoxicity, namely, sunburn and skin thickness (14).

A component of black tea (viz. theaflavin) was found to be a key active component in preventing UVB-induced radiation to the skin. Pretreatment with theaflavin inhibited UVB-induced activator protein-1 (AP-1) activity in a concentration-dependent manner ($p < 0.01$) through the inhibition of Erk- and JNK-dependent pathways in a mouse cell line. This is in contrast to the effects of EGCG, a major component of green tea, which inhibits AP-1 through inhibition of only the Erk-dependent pathway (15).

OTHER EXTRACTS

Persimmon leaf extract was associated with reduced scratching behavior, IgE levels, transepidermal water loss (TEWL), and clinical severity score in AD model mice ($p < 0.05$). A component of persimmon leaf extract (viz. astragalin) also induced a modest decrease in the clinical skin severity score at one time point in the study but had no statistically significant effect on scratching behavior or IgE levels. In the study, the AD model mice were fed either a control diet, a persimmon leaf extract diet, or an astragalin diet. Two studies were performed—a 4 week study assessing the therapeutic benefit of treatment and a 12 week study evaluating the preventative effects of treatment (16).

Benzoyl peroxide (BPO) is a free radical generating compound and strong oxidizer. It is commonly used in industry as a polymerization initiator (17), an additive in cosmetics (18), and a bleaching agent for flour and cheese (19). Spearmint may abrogate the effects of BPO-induced tumor promotion.

In a recent study, pretreatment with spearmint (*Mentha spicata*) induced a statistically significant decrease in the BPO oxidative damage, toxicity, and cellular hyperproliferation in adult female albino mice when compared with the BPO-treated control group. Topical spearmint extracts salvaged the levels of antioxidant enzymes glutathione peroxidase, glutathione reductase, glutathione S-transferase, and catalase that are reduced by BPO treatment alone. The BPO-elevated microsomal lipid peroxidation and hydrogen peroxide generation were significantly reduced with spearmint pretreatment. Furthermore, spearmint significantly decreased markers for cellular DNA synthesis, namely, ornithine decarboxylase activity and thymidine uptake, when compared with BPO treatment alone. Analysis was performed on excised mouse skin (20).

The anti-inflammatory efficacy of hamamelis (also known as witch hazel) has recently been tested. In one clinical study, 48 h occlusive application of one hamamelis lotion distillate significantly reduced UV-induced erythema (at 1.4 MED) when compared with vehicle. However, two other hamamelis lotion distillates were not effective in reducing UV-induced erythema when compared with placebo. Additionally, both hydrocortisone 1% cream and 0.25% lotion were more effective than hamamelis in suppressing UV-induced erythema, whereas the antihistamine dimethindene maleate did not have a greater effect (21).

The clinical benefit of oatmeal extracts in reducing inflammation was also assessed. Occlusive pretreatment for 2 h with two topically applied oatmeal extracts (viz., *Avena sativa* and *A. rhealba*) significantly reduced irritation in human volunteers when compared with placebo. Irritation was induced utilizing a 24 h sodium lauryl sulfate irritation model. Chromametry and laser-Doppler were utilized to assess irritation. There was no statistically significant difference between the two oatmeal extracts (22).

Soymilk and soybean extracts were found to have skin depigmenting capability both *in vitro* and *in vivo*. In the *in vitro* experimentation, soybean extracts reduced pigmentation in both keratinocyte–melanocyte cocultures and epidermal equivalents following daily treatment for 3 days. In addition, one of the extracts reduced pigment deposition in human skin grafted onto SCID mice following 9 week treatment. The extracts also produced visible skin depigmentation in Yukaton swine treated daily for 8–9 weeks and prevented UVB-induced skin pigmentation in Yukaton swine treated 10 times in a 2 week period. The pathogenesis is thought to be through the inhibition of protease-activated receptor 2 pathway (23).

HYDROXYACIDS

Topical β-lipohydroxyacid (β-LHA), a derivative of salicylic acid, improved some of the manifestations of aging in women by inducing a statistically significant epidermal thickening and dendrocytic hyperplasia. Both the younger and the elder populations exhibited improvement, but the changes were more diverse in the older women. When compared with placebo, 6% of the young and 16% of the elderly population experienced increased filaggrin layer thickness. Further studies are needed to understand the mechanism of hydroxyacid action and thereby their full effect on aging skin (24) Table 1.

ESSENTIAL FATTY ACIDS

A case–control study was performed to determine the association between n-3 and n-6 fatty acid intake and the development of a squamous cell carcinoma of

Table 1 Summary of Alternative Medications and Their Potential Clinical Uses in Human Studies

Therapy	Potential benefit	Experimental results	Reference
Vitamin C	Prevent nitrate tolerance	Potentiated the vasodilatory/conductivity responses provoked by GTN	(34)[a]
Vitamins C and E	Reduce sunburn reaction	Increased median MED in treated patients	(32)[b]
	Decrease UV-induced erythema	Decreased dermal blood flow, chromametry, and visual grade	(33)[b]
Green tea extract	Prevent UVII and erythema	Reduced chromametry visually and improved histologically	(11)[b]
Hamamelis (witch hazel)	Anti-inflammatory	Significantly reduced UV-induced erythema (at 1.4 MED)	(21)[b]
Oatmeal extracts		Occlusive pretreatment significantly reduced irritation as measured by chromametry and laser-Doppler flowmetry	(22)[b]
B-LHA	Improve signs of aging	Induced epidermal thickening and dendrocytic hyperplasia	(24)[b]
Ocimum oil	Treatment of acne vulgaris	Reduced the number of days taken to achieve a 50% reduction in papule and pustule count	(31)[b]
Borage oil (with GLA)	Treat AD	Improved pruritus, erythema, vesiculation, oozing in AD patients	(27)[b]

(continued)

Table 1 Continued

Therapy	Potential benefit	Experimental results	Reference
Primrose oil (with GLA)		Stabilized epidermal barrier—increased TEWL and stratum corneum hydration in AD patients	(26) (39)
GLA		No significant effect on AD patients Meta-analysis—GLA significantly improves AD pts	(28)[b] (29) (30)
n-3 Fatty acids	Association with SCC	Case–control study—tendency for a lower risk of SCC with higher intakes of n-3 fatty acids	(8)
Ocimum oil	Treatment of acne vulgaris	Reduced the number of days taken to achieve a 50% reduction in papule and pustule count	(31) (8)[b]
Quaternium-18 bentonite	Prevent poison ivy or poison oak	Reduced or prevented reaction to urushiol as evaluated visually	(35)[a]
Homeopathic gels	Reduce inflammation	Decreased LDF to methyl nicotinate	(25)[b]

Note: UVII = UV-induced immunosuppression.
[a] Compared with untreated control.
[b] Compared with placebo.

the skin. Subjects had a history of one confirmed nonmetastatic SCC of the skin and no prior history of skin cancer. Four 24 h dietary recalls were completed by each patient. The results of this study suggest a tendency for a lower risk of SCC with higher intakes of n-3 fatty acids. The association was particularly strong for intake of EPA, DHA and diet with a high n-3–n-6 ratio. The lower risk associated with n-3 fatty acids was statistically significant for men but not for women (8).

AD patients are thought to have a reduced rate of conversion from linoleic acid to γ-linolenic acid (GLA), dihomo-γ-linolenic acid, or arachidonic acid as compared with healthy subjects (26–29). Replacement of GLA, in the form of primrose oil or borage oil, may therefore benefit in the treatment of these patients.

In fact, more than 20 randomized controlled studies assessing the effects of GLA have been performed, with most studies indicating an improved epidermal barrier upon GLA application (27,30–38). In one recent study, topical application of 20% evening primrose oil caused a statistically significant stabilizing effect on the epidermal barrier in AD patients, as evaluated by TEWL and stratum corneum hydration. When compared with placebo, the water-in-oil emulsion of primrose oil proved effective whereas the amphiphilic emulsion did not, emphasizing the importance of the vehicle (37). In addition, borage oil, which contains a large quantity of GLA improved the pruritus, erythema, vesiculation, and oozing of atopic patients when compared with placebo-treated patients ($p < 0.05$). Patients were given 40 drops of borage oil twice a day for 12 weeks; dermatologists and patients visually assessed the signs (38).

In contrast, two significant studies have not observed a significant clinical effect of GLA on AD when compared with placebo. In studies by Bamford et al. (39) and Berth-Jones et al. (40), evening primrose oil capsules did not improve erythema, excoriation, and lichenification clinical scores, as evaluated by dermatologists and patients.

Meta-analysis of all previous randomized, placebo-controlled studies indicates a significant difference between treatment and placebo groups (41,42). Critics of the meta-analysis claim that it included unpublished trials and inadequate baseline data in terms of disease severity (40). Apparent differences in response between placebo and treatment groups may result from a greater severity at baseline in subjects receiving active treatment (40,43). Treatment of AD with GLA remains controversial.

ESSENTIAL OILS

Other essential oils have been investigated in treating IgE-mediated allergic reactions as well as for the treatment of acne vulgaris. Mice and rats pretreated with lavender oil inhibited mast cell degranulation indicating that the oil could inhibit immediate-type allergic reactions. Topical and intradermal lavender oil inhibited the ear swelling response in mice, and passive cutaneous anaphylaxis in rats when compared with saline control ($p < 0.05$). Peritoneal mast cells were also inhibited from releasing histamine or TNF-α *in vitro* when lavender oil was applied (44).

The essential oil from *Ocimum gratissimum* was tested for the treatment of acne vulgaris. One hundred and twenty-six subjects with acne vulgaris were treated with either placebo, 10% BPO lotion, or 2% *Ocimum* oil in either a petrolatum base or an alcohol and cetomacrogol blend for a 4 week period. A significant reduction in the number of days taken to achieve a 50% reduction in papule and pustule count was observed with both the BPO and the *Ocimum* oil alcohol and cetomacrogol lotions, when compared with placebo. *Ocimum* oil in petrolatum was less effective than the cetomacrogol blend vehicle (45). See Table 2.

VITAMINS C AND E

The hydrophobic vitamin C and lipophilic vitamin E have found an increasing use in dermatological treatment. Several studies investigated the effects of both vitamins C and E against oxidative stress. In mice, acute and chronic UVB-induced photodamage was significantly decreased with intraperitoneal postadministration of magnesium-L-ascorbyl-phosphate (MAP), a precursor to vitamin C ($p < 0.05$). Compared with irradiated, untreated mice, MAP-treated mice had a 60% decrease in UVB-induced tumor formation, a 50% decrease in skin thickness, and a 55% decrease in ODC, a marker for DNA synthesis. Additionally, upon acute exposure to UVB irradiation, MAP prevented increases of lipid peroxidation in skin and sialic acid in serum. MAP produced an immediate and transient increase in ascorbic acid in the serum, skin, and liver indicating its conversion in those tissues (46). The effect of MAP topical application in reducing UVB photodamage is unknown. The clinical significance of this study remains uncertain.

Oral ingestion of vitamin C (2000 mg/day) and vitamin E (1000 IU/day) reduced the sunburn reaction in human subjects. The volunteers' threshold dose for eliciting sunburn and their cutaneous blood flow of skin irradiated with incremental UV doses were determined before the trial and following 8 days of treatment. A statistically significant difference was observed in the median MED of vitamin-treated patients as compared with placebo-treated patients; the former MED increased 17%, whereas the latter declined 14% (47).

Topical pretreatment in man of a combination of vitamins C, E and melatonin provided a statistically significant enhanced photoprotection against UV-induced erythema. Dermal blood flow, visual grade, and chromametry parameters decreased with the combinatory treatment, as well as with each treatment alone, when compared with placebo-treated skin. The combinatory treatment was more pronounced (48).

Vitamins C and E have also proved beneficial in treating other conditions. Nitrate tolerance describes a developed tolerance to the vasodilatory effects of nitrate, because of both neurohormonal counter-regulation and enhanced response to vasoconstrictor agonists (49). Oral administration of two 500 mg vitamin C capsules daily along with the GTN for 3 days prevented nitrate tolerance in

Table 2 Summary of Alternative Medications and Their Potential Clinical Uses in Animal/*In Vitro* Studies

Therapy	Potential benefit	Experimental results	Reference
Soybean extract	Depigmentation	Reduced pigmentation in both keratinocyte–melanocyte cocultures and epidermal equivalents Reduced pigment deposition in human skin grafted onto SCID mice Produced visible skin depigmentation in Yukaton swine Prevented UVB-induced skin pigmentation in Yukaton swine	(23)[a]
Persimmon leaf extract	Improve symptoms of AD	Reduced scratching behavior, IgE levels TEWL, and clinical severity score in AD model mice when compared with mice fed a control diet	(16)
Flavonoids/Green tea extracts	Counteract UVII	Prevented UVII of contact hypersensitivity to picryl chloride	(12)[a]
Black tea extract	Decrease early symptoms of UVB-induced phototoxicity	Decreased erythema, skinfold thickness, expression of c-jun, c-fos, and p53 in mice, human skin, and keratinocytes Pretreatment with theaflavin, a component of black tea, inhibited UVB-induced AP-1 activity in a concentration-dependent manner	(14)[b] (15)[a]

(*continued*)

Table 2 *Continued*

Therapy	Potential benefit	Experimental results	Reference
Vitamin C		Decreased UVB-induced tumor formation, skin thickness, and ODC in mice	(46)[a]
Mentha spicata (Spearmint)	Prevent oxidative stress	Pretreatment decreased BPO oxidative damage, toxicity, and hyperproliferation in adult female albino mice	(20)[a]
Citrus nobiletin	Reduce skin inflammation and tumor promotion	Reduced NO-induced skin inflammation by preventing initial leukocyte infiltration and subsequent oxidative insult by leukocytes. Suppressed COX-2 expression and inducible NO synthase proteins and prostaglandin E_2 release. Reduced the number of dimethylbenz[a]anthracene/TPA-induced skin tumors in mice.	(56)[b]
Vitamin E combination[c]	Treat genital herpes simplex virus	Reduced lesion development, duration, and severity in guinea pigs and mice	(51)[a]
Lavender oil	Inhibit immediate-type allergic reactions	Inhibited mast cell degranulation in mice and rats. Prevented histamine and TNF-α release from peritoneal mast cells	(44)[b]

[a]Compared with untreated control.
[b]Compared with placebo.
[c]Vitamin E, sodium pyruvate, and membrane stabilizing fatty acid.

healthy volunteers taking transdermal glyceroltrinitrate (GTN). With those taking vitamin C, the vasodilatory/conductivity responses evoked by GTN were potentiated throughout the 3 day period (24.5% increase vs. control), whereas with those taking GTN alone, the responses slowly declined (8.2% increase vs. control) (50). This observed effect was statistically significant.

A combination of vitamin E, sodium pyruvate, and membrane stabilizing fatty acids induced a statistically significant decrease in the lesion development, duration, and severity of genital herpes simplex virus when applied postinfection to guinea pigs and mice. The combinatory treatment yielded a 36% decrease in lesion severity score in guinea pigs and 33% decrease in lesion size in hairless mice when compared with no treatment (51).

MISCELLANEOUS

Quaternium-18 bentonite, an organoclay used in cosmetics to thicken or stabilize the products, has been investigated for its ability to prevent poison ivy or poison oak contact dermatitis reactions in man. Pretreatment with 5% quaternium-18 bentonite lotion on the forearm of patients with ACD to poison oak or poison ivy significantly reduced or prevented a severe reaction to urushiol, the allergenic resin of both plants. Trained technicians blinded to the treated area visually evaluated the reactions. Statistical significance was found when comparing treated test sites with untreated controls (52).

The intrinsic vasodilator nitrous oxide (NO) may cause mutagenesis and deamination of DNA and form carcinogenic N-nitrosamines, potentially playing a role in cancer formation (53–55). In addition, NO is involved in edema formation and hyperplasia in mouse skin. Products that inhibit NO formation may help to prevent cancer formation. One such product, a component of the citrus fruit *Citrus unshiu* (satsuma mandarin), was found to have some tumor-inhibiting effects in mice. The polymethoxyflavonoid, nobiletin, inhibited NO and O_2- generation and reduced NO-induced skin inflammation [produced by 12-O-tetradecanolyphorbol-13-acetate (TPA)] by preventing initial leukocyte infiltration and subsequent oxidative insult by leukocytes. Additionally, nobiletin suppressed COX-2 expression and inducible NO synthase proteins and prostaglandin E_2 release. Finally, nobelitin reduced the number of dimethylbenz[a]anthracene/ TPA-induced skin tumors in mice (56).

CONCLUSION

The sampling of investigative medications presented by this review seems promising, though their true effects are unknown. Caution must be exhibited when interpreting animal studies. Additionally, experimental designs such as sample size, drug concentration, method of exposure to the medicine, and analytical techniques may greatly influence a study's outcome. Further exploration of these medications under different experimental conditions would better estimate their true clinical benefit. Certainly, the lower cost, wide accessibility, and possible clinical improvement with many of these newer unconventional remedies should encourage their continued research.

REFERENCES

1. Bashir S, Maibach H. Evidence Based Dermatology. Toronto: BC Dekker (in press).
2. Koh H, Kligler B, Lew P. Sunlight and cutaneous malignant melanoma: evidence for and against causation. Photochem Photobiol 1990; 51:765–779.
3. Krutmann J. Ultraviolet A radiation-induced biological effects in human skin: relevance for photoaging and photodermatosis. J Dermatol Sci 2000;23(suppl 1): S22–S26.
4. Wenk J, Brenneisen P, Meewes C et al. UV-induced oxidative stress and photoaging. Curr Probl Dermatol 2001; 29:83–94.
5. Biesalski H, Obermueller-Jevic U. UV light, beta-carotene and human skin—beneficial and potentially harmful effects. Arch Biochem Biophys 2001; 389:1–6.
6. Hart P, Grimbaldeston M, Finlay-Jones J. Sunlight, immunosuppression and skin cancer: role of histamine and mast cells. Clin Exp Pharmacol Physiol 2001; 28:1–8.
7. Gil E, Kim T. UV-induced immune suppression and sunscreen. Photodermatol Photoimmunol Photomed 2000; 16:101–110.
8. Hakim I, Harris R, Ritenbaugh C. Fat intake and risk of squamous cell carcinoma of the skin. Nutr Cancer 2000; 36:155–162.
9. Black H. Influence of dietary factors on actinically-induced skin cancer. Mutat Res 1998; 422:185–190.
10. DiGiovanna J. Retinoid chemoprevention in patients at high risk for skin cancer. Med Pediatr Oncol 2001; 36:564–567.
11. Elmets C, Singh D, Tubesing K, Matsui M, Katiyar S, Mukhtar H. Cutaneous photoprotection from ultraviolet injury by green tea polyphenols. J Am Acad Dermatol 2001; 44:425–432.
12. Steerenberg P, Garseen J, Dortant P et al. Protection of UV-induced suppression of skin contact hypersensitivity: a common feature of flavonoids after oral administration? Photochem and Photobiol 1998; 67:456–461.
13. Katiyar S, Ahmad N, Muhktar H. Green tea and skin. Arch Dermatol 2000; 136:989–994.
14. Zhao J, Jin X, E Y, Zheng ZS, Zhang YJ, Athar M. Photoprotective effect of black tea extracts against UVB-induced phototoxicity in skin. Photochem Photobiol 1999; 70:637–644.
15. Nomura M, Ma W-Y, Huang C et al. Inhibition of ultraviolet B-induced AP-1 activation by theaflavins from black tea. Mol Carcinogen 2000; 28:148–155.
16. Matsumoto M, Kotani M, Fujita A et al. Oral administration of persimmon leaf extract alemiorates skin symptoms and transepidermal water loss in atopic dermatitis model mice, NC/Nga. Br J Dermatol 2002; 146:221–227.
17. Kadoma Y, Fujisawa S. Kinetic evaluation of reactivity of bisphenol A derivatives as radical scavengers for methacrylate polymerization. Biomaterials 2000; 21:2125–2130.
18. Piérard G, Piérard-Franchimont C, Goffin V. Digital image analysis of microcomedones. Dermatology 1995; 190:99–103.
19. Karasz A, Dececco F, Maxstadt J. Gas chromatographic measurements of benzoyl peroxide in (as benzoic acid) cheese. J Assoc Anal Chem 1974; 57:706–709.

20. Saleem M, Alam A, Sultana S. Attenuation of benzoyl peroxide-mediated cutaneous oxidative stress and hyperproliferative response by the prophylactic treatment of mice with spearmint (*Mentha spicata*). Food Chem Toxicol 2000; 38:939–948.
21. Hughes-Formella B, Filbry A, Gassmueller J et al. Anti-inflammatory efficacy of topical preparations with 10% hamamelis distillate in a UV erythema test. Skin Pharmacol Appl Skin Physiol 2001; 15:125–132.
22. Via K, Cours-Darne S, Vienne M et al. Modulating effects of oatmeal extracts in the sodium lauryl sulfate skin irritancy model. Skin Pharmacol Appl Skin Physiol 2000; 15:120–124.
23. Paine C, Sharlow E, Liebel F et al. An alternative approach to depigmentation by soybean extracts via inhibition of the PAR-2 pathway. J Invest Dermatol 2001; 116:587–595.
24. Avila-Camacho M, Montastier C, Perard GE. Histometric assessment of the age-related skin response to 2-hydroxy-5-octanoyl benzoic acid. Skin Pharmacol Appl Skin Physiol 1998; 11:52–56.
25. Handschuh J, Debray M. Modification of cutaneous blood flow by skin application of homeopathic anti-inflammatory gels. STP Pharma Sci 1999; 9:219–222.
26. Biagi P, Hrelia S, Celadon M et al. Erythrocyte membrane fatty acid composition in children with atopic dermatitis compared to age-matched controls. Acta Paediatr 1993; 82:789–790.
27. Schalin-Karrila M, Mattila L, Jansen C, Uotila P. Evening primrose oil in the treatment of atopic eczema: effect of clinical status, plasma phospholipid fatty acids and circulating blood prostaglandins. Br J Dermatol 1987; 117:11–19.
28. Oliwiecki S, Burton J, Elles K, Horrobin D. Levels of essential and other fatty acids in plasma and red cell phospholipids from normal controls and patients with atopic eczema. Acta Derm Venereol 1991; 71:224–228.
29. Wright S, Sanders T. Adipose tissue essential fatty acids in the plasma phospholipids of patients with atopic eczema. Br J Dermatol 1991; 110:643–648.
30. Lovell C, Burton J, Horrobin D. Treatment of atopic eczema with evening primrose oil. Lancet 1981; 1:278 (letter).
31. Wright S, Burton J. Oral evening-primrose-seed oil improves atopic eczema. Lancet 1982; 2:1120–1122.
32. Bordoni A, Biagi P, Masi M et al. Evening primrose oil (Efamol) in the treatment of children with atopic eczema. Drugs Exp Clin Res 1988; 14:291–297.
33. Biagi P, Bordoni A, Hrelia S et al. The effect of γ-linolenic acid on clinical status, red cell fatty acid composition and membrane microviscosity in infants with atopic dermatitis. Drugs Exp Clin Res 1994; 20:77–84.
34. Biagi PBA, Masi M, Ricci G, Fanelli C, Patrizi A, Ceccolini E. A long-term study on the use of evening primrose oil (Efamol) in atopic children. Drugs Exp Clin Res 1988; 14:285–290.
35. Guenther L, Wexler D. Efamol in the treatment of atopic dermatitis. J Am Acad Dematol 1987; 17:860 (letter).
36. Humphreys F, Symons H, Brown H, Duff G, Hunter J. The effects of γ-linolenic acid on adult atopic eczema and premenstrual exacerbation of eczema. Eur J Dermatol 1994; 4:598–603.
37. Gehring W, Bopp R, Rippke F, Gloor M. Effect of topically applied evening primrose oil on epidermal barrier function in atopic dermatitis as a function of vehicle. Drug Res 1999; 49:635–642.

38. Andreassi M, Forleo P, Lorio AD, Masci S, Abate G, Amerio P. Efficacy of g-linolenic acid in the treatment of patients with atopic dermatitis. J Int Med Res 1997; 25:266–274.
39. Bamford J, Gibson R, Reiner C. Atopic eczema unresponsive to evening primrose oil (linoleic and g-linolenic acids). J Am Acad Dermatol 1985; 13:959–965.
40. Berth-Jones J, Graham-Brown R. Placebo-controlled trial of essential fatty acid supplementation in atopic dermatitis. *Lancet* 1993; 341:1557–1560.
41. Morse PH, DF, Manku MS, Stewart JC, Allen R, Littlewood S, Wright S, Burton J, Gould DJ, Holt PJ et al. Meta-analysis of placebo-controlled studies of the efficacy of Epogram in the treatment of atopic eczema. Relationship between plasma essential fatty acid changes and clinical response. Br J Dermatol 1989; 121:75–90.
42. Stewart J, Morse P, Moss M, et al. Treatment of severe and moderately severe atopic dermatitis with evening primrose oil (Epogram): a multi-centre study. J Nutr Med 1991; 2:9–15.
43. Horrobin D, Stewart C. Evening primrose oil and eczema. Lancet 1990; 335:864–865.
44. Kim H-M, Cho S-H. Lavender oil inhibits immediate-type allergic reaction in mice and rats. J Pharm Pharmacol 1999; 51:221–226.
45. Orafidiya LO, Agbani E. Oyedele A et al. Preliminary clinical tests on topical preparations of *Ocimim gratissimum* Linn leaf essential oil for the treatment of acne vulgaris. Clin Drug Invest 2002; 22:313–319.
46. Kobayashi S, Takehana M, Kanke M, Itoh S, Ogata E. Postadministration protective effect of magnesium-L-ascorbyl-phosphate on the development of UVB-induced cutaneous damage in mice. Photochem Photobiol 1998; 67:669–675.
47. Eberlein-Konig B, Placzek M, Przybilla B. Protective effect against sunburn of combined systemic ascorbic acid (vitamin C) and *d-a*-tocopherol (vitamin E). J Am Acad Dermatol 1998; 38:45–48.
48. Dreher F, Gabard B, Schwindt D, Maibach H. Topical melatonin in combination with vitamins E and C protects skin from ultraviolet-induced erythema: a human study *in vivo*. Br J Dermatol 1998; 139:332–339.
49. Munzel T, Giaid A, Kurz S, Stweart D, Harrison D. Evidence for a role of endothelin 1 and protein kinase C in nitroglycerin tolerance. Proc Natl Acad Sci 1995; 92:5244–5248.
50. Bassange E, Fink N, Skatchkov M et al. Dietary supplement with vitamin C prevents nitrate toleratnce. J Clin Invest 1998; 102:67–71.
51. Sheridan J, Kern E, Martin A, Booth A. Evaluation of antioxidant healing formulations in topical therapy of experimental cutaneous and genital herpes simplex virus infections. Antiviral Res 1997; 36:157–166.
52. Marks J, Fowler J, Sherertz E, Rietschel R. Prevention of poison ivy and poison oak allergic contact dermatitis by quaternium-18 bentonite. J Am Acad Dermatol 1995; 33:212–216.
53. Arroyo P, Hatch-Pigott V, Mower H et al. Mutagenecity of nitric oxide and its inhibition by antioxidants. Mutat Res 1992; 639.
54. Wink D, Kazprazak K, Maragos C et al. DNA deaminating ability and genotoxicity of nitric oxide and its progenitors. Science 1991; 254:1001–1003.
55. Miwa M, Stuehr D, Marletta M et al. Nitrosation of amines by stimulated macrophages. Carcinogenesis 1987; 8: 955–958.
56. Murakami A, Nakamura Y, Torikai K et al. Inhibitory effect of citrus nobiletin on phorbol ester-induced skin inflammation, oxidative stress, and tumor promotion in mice. Cancer Res 2000; 60:5059–5066.

13

Cosmeceuticals in Photoaging

William J. Cunningham
Cu-Tech, LLC, Mountain Lakes, New Jersey, USA

Background	262
Pathogenesis	263
Clinical and Histological Presentations	263
Methods of Study	265
Instrumentation	265
Clinical Methods	266
Prevention of Photoaging	267
Products for Photoaging	268
Prevention Products	268
Treatment Products	270
Moisturizers	270
Retinoids	271
Alpha Hydroxy Acids	272
Beta Hydroxy Acids	272
Vitamins	273
Hormones	273
Depigmenting Agents	274
Miscellaneous Agents	274
Future Trends	274
References	275

The popular will has spoken. Having no patience with the polemics of scientists, governmental regulatory agencies, and the like, the consumer has accepted the concept and reality of the positive effects of the cosmeceutical and has purchased or used them by the tons in all countries of the earth. Looking better and feeling better are intuitively and emotionally affirmed and embraced, no matter how elusive the logical definition of the cosmeceutical remains to the pedant. Whether it is purchased at hundreds of Euros a milliliter on the Champs Elysees or concocted from the most exotic natural source deep in the Congo, everyone understands that to look and feel your best, a little help from the cosmeceutical is most welcome.

Photoaging provides the nearly optimum paradigm for discussion of this often vigorously argued concept as it is a very cosmetically visible process yet requires significant pharmaceutical or surgical intervention for optimum treatment. We will thus approach the topic from its scientific perspectives of pathogenesis, prevention, and treatment, although we note that always significantly in the background are the primary driving force of the cosmetic concerns of the consumer and the commercial opportunities which that force creates.

BACKGROUND

Photoaging is a life-long process in most individuals, beginning even in infancy and progressing steadily until prevention, treatment, or death intervenes. The rate of change in the skin due to photoaging is dependant upon many intrinsic and extrinsic or environmental factors such as genetic background of the individual, environmental latitude at which sun exposure takes place, intensity and duration of sun exposure in outdoor activities of sport, employment, or leisure, and to some extent, vigor of prevention or treatment. The clinical, histological, and functional damage to the skin, that is, photodamage, can be quantitated in several ways at any point of a wide, life-long spectrum of effects; and the type and degree of change are specific manifestations of this nearly universal process.

In the background, and additionally contributing to the totality of change in sun-exposed skin, is the seemingly inevitable aging process itself. Much has been made of the clinical or histological differences between photoaging and aging, but in reality so much of the skin surface has been sun exposed in most individuals that differentiation of causation is frequently extremely difficult. Still, as more is learned about the basic process of aging, there are several fundamental differences in the two processes even if clinically they both produce old looking skin. Most notably in chronological aging, telomere shortening and subcellular damage by reactive oxygen species (ROS) due to intrinsic metabolic processes are prominent and difficult or perhaps impossible to prevent or reverse (1). Photoaging, also partly related to damage by ROS generated by exposure to ultraviolet radiation (UVR) and also involves direct sun-related DNA changes but may be entirely prevented and somewhat effectively treated by a number of cosmeceutical and surgical modalities.

PATHOGENESIS

However, for the protective effects of the atmosphere, the full spectrum of solar irradiation would eliminate much of the earth's flora and fauna. As it is, even the select transmission of UVR at wavelengths >290 nm, while allowing the benefits of photosynthesis, permits devastating skin effects when exposure is intense or prolonged. Although some argue that even infrared or visible light may play some role in photoaging, it is those UVR wavelengths of ~290–400 nm which are most incriminated in DNA damage and generation of ROS in human skin (2,3). UVR absorption by DNA results in damage by generation of photoadducts including pyrimidine dimers. The damaged DNA, if incompletely repaired, results in mutations that result in incorrect cellular function or in the extreme, of cellular (especially epidermal) dysplasia or neoplasia. Many cellular chromophores such as DNA, lipids, and proteins absorb UVR. The complex protein melanin may, by its absorption, mitigate against other chromophore absorption and damage. However, UVR absorption by DNA, membrane lipids, cellular enzymes, and so on produces, through multiple and complex mechanisms, ROS including superoxide anion, peroxide, and singlet oxygen, all of which may be damaging to multiple cellular structures and mechanisms (4).

Much elegant research has resulted in a more complete understanding of how these subcellular events result in the structural and functional abnormalities observed during photoaging (5). ROS cause cell surface receptor activation for a number of cytokines including epidermal growth factor and tumor necrosis factor alpha (TNF alpha). When these receptors are activated by their ligand, signal transduction is initiated, followed by activation of nuclear transcription factor AP-1. AP-1 in turn initiates transcription of genes responsible for translation of enzymes such as metaloproteinase (MMP) 1 (collagenase), MMP-3 (stromeolysin 1), and MMP-9 (gelatinase) which can degrade collagen.

Many, although not all, of the dermal effects of photoaging appear related to this profound damaging effect on the principal structural protein of the dermis. Other effects upon the elastin fiber network, anchoring fibrils, proteoglycans, and glycosaminoglycans have been repeatedly observed but are not as completely understood. Epidermal effects of photoaging play a significant role in the clinical presentation, and the pathogenesis of these changes initiated by DNA and ROS damage are being elucidated.

CLINICAL AND HISTOLOGICAL PRESENTATIONS

Again, the consumer speaks the loudest and most succinctly "I don't want to look old". All of the clinical and functional defects that are a consequence of photoaging make the subject and the observer believe that they look older than their chronological age (6). As only some of the clinical appearances of photoaging overlap with those of strictly chronological aging, this is primarily a perceptual issue. No one complains about "old skin" but about "looking old" and this complaint is primarily related to skin which is sun damaged.

Photoaging is already underway in many children with significant sun exposure (7). The appearance of freckles in the preschool child reflects both the genetic propensity to sun-induced damage and the fact of life that excessive sun exposure is occurring. This is a common pattern in countries like Australia with both a celtic genetic heritage and extremes of latitude. At the other end of the spectrum may be found the most darkly pigmented African farmer with leathery, furrowed skin after decades of all day exposure to equatorial sun. In between is seen every combination and permutation of epidermal changes, dermal damage, and cutaneous carcinogenesis, which are determined by the various combinations of genes, sex, skin type, age of induction, latitude of habitation, intensity of UVR, chronicity of exposure, degree of prevention, and type of treatment. It is in fact a constellation rather than a spectrum and reflects the diversity of skin cell types which have been damaged.

Thus, irregular hyperpigmentation and hypopigmentation, both discrete and limited or diffuse and irregular may be noted and clinically represented by freckles, solar lentigines, and hypomelanotic macules. Clearly, melanization is highly affected by UVR, though it is not always clear as to whether melanocyte melanin production, epidermal uptake or packaging of melanocytes, or both are deranged. Histologically, alterations in melanin distribution within keratinocytes may be obvious.

An appearance and feel of surface roughness, dryness, or scaliness may be partially explained by abnormalities of keratinocyte production, adhesion, and separation. Alternating compact and basketweave patterns of the stratum corneum and cellular heterogeneity are the histological counterparts. Dryness of skin has generally not been substantiated by instrumental means, as discussed later. It may be a visual and tactile perception but reflective of surface irregularities rather than water content.

Wrinkles of various depth, length, and location are a reflection of underlying dermal damage to collagen, elastin, and ground substance and their incomplete repair. Orientation of deeper wrinkles according to lines of underlying muscular forces may be pronounced. Although the exact correlate of the wrinkle is not observed histologically, the pronounced abnormalities of collagen, elastin, and ground substance observed by standard H&E staining and by immunohistochemical means provide more than adequate explanation for the surface contour abnormalities.

The color of photoaged skin may be sallow in some instances but otherwise is variable due to the irregularity of surface and of reflected light as well as to the variability of total skin thickness, melanin content and distribution, and influence of saturated and unsaturated hemoglobin. This is most difficult to characterize and quantitate by instrumental methods. Conversely, skin thickness may be easily quantitated by instrumental methods but is not uniformly changed during photoaging. When skin of the dorsal hands becomes atrophic; however, it is also significantly and functionally impaired and is very susceptible to tears, bruises, and abrasion by even relatively modest trauma.

Finally, the profound changes wrought to epidermal cell DNA result in many benign and malignant neoplasms of the skin. These range from the benign seborrheic keratosis which has not been conclusively demonstrated to be related to photoaging to the actinic keratosis and squamous cell carcinoma which are related. Here, the UVR induced but incompletely repaired DNA mutations including those of p53 are no doubt of extreme importance.

There are frequent clinical dichotomies of carcinogenesis and other manifestations of photoaging. We have observed innumerable men of celtic background with much neoplasia and hardly a wrinkle to be found. We also noted the frequent pronounced wrinkles of females of mediterranean background with not a cancer in sight.

METHODS OF STUDY

The methods of study of photoaging range from the simple to the sophisticated. Without doubt, the various instrumental bioengineering techniques that have been gradually developed and refined over the past decades will become the future gold standard for assessment of the many diverse clinical and functional manifestations of photoaging (8). Some of the techniques, however, are a bit too susceptible to the "Midas touch" which overemphasizes parameters of little clinical but much commercial relevance. Furthermore, correlation of the results obtained with the clinical parameters is better with some techniques than others. A study of 71 men aged 30–70 living in the mediterranean area demonstrated that elastotic, that is, photoaged skin was less elastic, dryer, darker, more erythematous, and less yellowish than nonexposed skin (9).

Instrumentation

Image analysis techniques utilize a soft dental impression material, Silflo, placed onto the skin to obtain a "skin replica" which is analogous to a topographic map in reverse. The replica is essentially side illuminated in a standardized way and the shadows generated which correspond to peaks and valleys can be quantitated utilizing computer image analysis software to determine roughness and wrinkling (10). The technique has been widely and successfully utilized in many large clinical trials.

Ultrasound techniques utilize a variety of instruments and can easily and objectively measure epidermal and dermal thickness. Although it is a useful tool in objectively quantitating psoriasis lesion thickness, it is less useful in photoaging where there is no direct correlation of skin thickness with parameters which have been noted to change after effective therapy such as roughness, wrinkles, and pigmentary alterations.

Levarometry, twistometry, and ballistometry measure forces of lift, torque, and indentation of the skin, respectively, all manifestations of its mechanical function or, in a clinical sense, various aspects of its rigidity or elasticity. Clinically, the slowness of return to normal contour after deformation is most noticeable in photoaged skin.

Colorimetry is specifically useful to quantitate discrete areas of pigmentary alteration such as solar lentigines but is not otherwise helpful in estimating the overall sallow complexion frequently noted in photoaging.

Capacitance and conductance measurements utilizing instruments such as those of the skin reflect actual water content of the stratum corneum but as with evaporimetry these changes are not specific to aging or photoaging and thus the two methods are presently more of commercial interest than of scientific importance in these conditions.

Evaporimetry which measures transepidermal water loss (TEWL) has been frequently utilized in the study of efficacy of moisturizers. However, TEWL is not specifically changed in aging or photoaging and thus the method is of limited utility in studies of these conditions.

Clinical Methods

Clinical methods which have been widely utilized and affirmed relevant are available and applicable to study of cosmeceuticals, irrespective of whether the product is closer to the cosmetic or pharmaceutical pole. The time-honored standard of a double-blind clinical trial conducted according to a defined protocol at multiple investigative sites will most often suffice to evaluate efficacy and safety of the product. A clinical grading system, which describes the overall clinical severity, with approximately 5–10 grades of differentiation has been often and satisfactorily employed in studies of efficacy of retinoids in photoaging (11). One such scoring system allots $0 =$ none, $1-3 =$ mild, $4-6 =$ moderate, and $7-9 =$ severe. A large study of tazarotene successfully employed a 5 point scale of $0 =$ none, $1 =$ minimal, $2 =$ mild, $3 =$ moderate, and $4 =$ severe to evaluate specific signs of fine wrinkling, mottled hyperpigmentation, lentigines, elastosis, irregular pigmentation, tactile roughness, coarse wrinkling, and telangiectasia (12).

Clinical panel methods utilize standardized photographs which are graded in a randomly viewed manner by investigators experienced with photoaging and trained in the method (13). Thus, both overall appearance and specific clinical signs can be reproduceably graded.

Image analysis of Silflo skin replicas, described earlier, is a labor intensive but well-established method for grading fine wrinkling of the face and correlates well with the clinical presentation (14). A much more elaborate photographic system has been developed and occasionally utilized for the determination of wrinkles. Carefully obtained standardized photographs are digitized and color corrected. Areas of the facial photograph which will not be analyzed are masked and wrinkles of areas of interest such as the supraorbital, suborbital, and central cheek areas are analyzed with a sophisticated image analysis software (15).

For evaluation of the pigmentary abnormalities due to photoaging, no technique is more dramatic than fluorescent photography (16). The results may be compared before and after treatment sequences with image analysis techniques but the pretreatment images alone are sufficient to discourage the subject from any further sun exposure.

Consumer panels utilizing trained observers or naive observers are inherently different than clinical trials in their approach to product evaluation and are best suited to attributes of the product itself and to the more cosmetic aspects of the product. The commercially available DermatoSensory Profile evaluates such characteristics as the perceived rate of absorption of the product into the skin including its spreadability and stickiness. It is also useful in evaluation of how the skin feels after product application, that is, its immediate afterfeel in terms of shininess, greasiness, or oiliness of the product on the skin. The sensation of resistance to motion over the skin, that is, drag or sensation of perception of something remaining on the skin (residue) can be evaluated at set time points defined as delayed afterfeel. Then, the product itself can be described in terms of color, thickness, substantivity, consistency, grittiness, smoothness, and odor.

PREVENTION OF PHOTOAGING

Sun avoidance is by far the most effective prevention for photoaging but is seldom practiced in the necessary degree to prevent some damage. Even suberythemic exposures may produce DNA damage and contribute to photoaging and this dose is easily achieved in a few minutes of noonday sun at the latitudes of New York or Madrid. In the tropics, even a few minutes of sun exposure may be clearly erythmogenic as well but it is easily forgotten that even at higher latitudes, the everyday and suberythemic exposures to sunlight accumulate over time and contribute to damage. Scheduling of outdoor activities in periods of less intense irradiation is possible. Golf or tennis at 6 a.m. in the summer avoids the most intense UVR exposure of midday and is a more pleasant and cooler time in any case. When these are not feasible, protective clothing may provide an option. Wide brimmed hats will not work for tennis but will protect the face of the shopper or gardener. Long sleeves may not appeal to the golfer on a hot day but may be acceptable to the fisherman. A number of products are now available such as those from Solumbra and Coolbar with specific fiber weave which is more completely protective.

Sunscreens are frequently viewed by the consumer and seemingly by some practitioners as the only and the optimum sun protectant and they are in fact an extremely important part of the totality of sun protection (17,18). When sufficient amounts of appropriate sunscreens are carefully and evenly applied to all potentially exposed skin, their rated SPF may be approached in actual practice. As they are tested for SPF in the USA with an application of 2 mg/cm^2, this amount should logically be utilized clinically. Those products that rub off or wash off more easily must be applied more frequently after exercise or swimming. In practice, these stipulations are frequently imperfectly followed but perhaps more importantly, consumers falsely assume that once a sunscreen has been applied, they may spend the rest of the day in summer sun with impunity. As photodamage can occur at even one-tenth of a person's minimal erythema dose (MED), it must be assumed that these inordinately long exposures, even if they do not result in burning, are not without consequence in the long term (19). Additionally, products are tested for their UVB protection and it is usually unclear exactly how much UVA protection is achieved even by the common addition of UVA blockers. If these reservations are noted, however, sunscreens can be considered as an obligatory cosmeceutical in the overall regimen of photoaging prevention. The frequent lack of toleration of components such as oxybenzone, cinnamates, para amino benzoic acid, and so on may usually be circumvented by the use of another product which does not contain the offending ingredient or contains it at a lower concentration.

Antioxidants have been extensively studied *in vitro* and in animal models and innumerable claims have often been made for their protective effects. It is clear that in several metabolic systems, the generation of ROS such as superoxide anion, hydrogen peroxide, and singlet oxygen can be inhibited by antioxidants such as vitamins C and E and a number of other entities. Proof of significant effect in the human everyday situation, however, has been for the most part, elusive. There may be several reasons for this disparity, including the vastly simpler experimental conditions in which chemical interactions are uninfluenced by the complexity of the total organism. Additionally, the effects of UVR are a diverse and profoundly complex equation and this complexity may hide or vastly overcome the potentially real but modest effect of any single and simple component such as an antioxidant. As with enzymes, a certain amount is necessary for the reaction to proceed but more may not make it proceed faster or better.

PRODUCTS FOR PHOTOAGING

Surgical and laser treatments for photodamage abound, may be highly effective, and should not be forgotten in the overall discussion of treatment of photodamage; they are well discussed elsewhere. There are, however, a host of other products and preparations ranging from the purely cosmetic to the definitely pharmaceutical which can be considered in the overall cosmeceutical approach to photoaging.

Prevention Products

Sunscreens, discussed earlier, are regulated variously around the world but in any case are not usually considered pharmaceutical and do not appear to change structure or function of the skin in any appreciable way. The wide variety of blockers of UVB and UVA allow a generalization to the patient: "Avoid midday sun exposure and consistently use a sunscreen which is cosmetically agreeable, nonirritating and is labeled as containing both UVB and UVA blocks with an SPF of at least 15".

Iron chelators have been studied in photoprotection. Studies of 2-furilioxime in animal models and in humans demonstrated a sun protection factor of 3 measured by erythema, sunburn cell formation and induction of ornithine decarboxylase. A greater protection factor is needed for clinical use and commercial viability and as yet this interesting concept has not reached fruition.

Self tanning agents contain dihydroxyacetone (DHA), which reacts with amino acids in the outer stratum corneum to produce a temporary brown color resembling a tan. DHA is contained in a large number of self tanning preparations and the pigment produced provides minimal sun protection in the range of SPF of 2–5.

Aliphatic and alicyclic diols such as dimethanol, butanediol, cyclopentadiol, propanediol, and isobutyl-methylxanthine have been shown to induce melanogenesis in cultured normal human melanocytes and in guinea pig skin and may be candidates for study as tanning agents (20).

Thymidine dimers, thymidine dinucleotides (pTpT), are small DNA fragments (photoadducts) which result from DNA damage by UVR. They appear to play a role not only in signaling for upregulation of DNA repair enzymes but also in signaling melanocytes. A tanning response which also confers a degree of photoprotection has been demonstrated in guinea pig skin (21). This fascinating work deserves rapid investigation in human studies.

Antioxidants comprise an exceptionally diverse group of vitamins, trace metals, and other chemical entities which are normal components of most oxidative systems of metabolism. Anabolism and catabolism generate free radicals of various types including those of oxygen as an integral part of their metabolic processes. As these free radicals such as ROS are highly reactive and potentially damaging, they are in turn inactivated by antioxidants. A number of antioxidants of known importance in normal human metabolism have been proposed or studied for prevention or reversal of photoaging and the entire subject has recently been well-reviewed (22).

Vitamin C, ascorbic acid, is without doubt one of the most important of the antioxidants in human metabolism. Its deficiency state, scurvy, is legendary in maritime history after the explorers of the 15th and 16th centuries took to the sea for extended periods without fresh fruits and vegetables. Other valiant attempts have been more recently made to establish the utility of vitamin C in photoaging because of its known general antioxidant effect and its prominent role in collagen synthesis. This attempt is a conundrum in that excellent science and overwhelming marketing have not yet been reflected in convincing clinical results which might place it closer to a pharmaceutical than a cosmetic.

Vitamin E, however, presents the most frustrating problem of all. It comprises eight molecular forms of tocopherols and tocotrienols found in dietary sources, of which alpha tocopherol is predominantly utilized by humans as an antioxidant. A voluminous literature attests to the importance of vitamin E in antioxidative functions *in vitro*, in animals, and in some clinical settings (23). Convincing proof of efficacy in clinical settings comparable to clinical trials of retinoids has been elusive. Perhaps, only a small amount of the vitamin is needed for normal antioxidative effect and addition beyond certain levels is superfluous in the complicated *in vivo* setting. Alternately, one could theorize that the process of aging or photoaging is so complex and determined in a certain direction that much more than antioxidative effect is needed to halt or reverse the processes. In any case, the lack of conviction is not represented in the marketplace where tons of vitamin E are included as ingredients (for proven antioxidant effect on the formulation itself) or in cosmetics. In any case, other than the occasional sensitization to vitamin E, little harm appears to result from its widespread utilization.

Selenium, a trace metal, is essential in human metabolism as a cofactor for the enzyme glutathione peroxidase, a quencher of free radicals. Investigation of topical L-selenomethionine in photoaging demonstrated protection against erythema and blistering in the mouse and dose-dependant increase in MED and decreased tanning in nine human subjects (24).

Treatment Products

Moisturizers

Regulated nearly everywhere as cosmetic, and containing innumerable combinations of various substances including specific humectants, moisturizers may nonetheless affect structure and function of the skin and are extensively and effectively utilized in photoaging. Appearance and tactile feel of skin can be dramatically, though temporarily, altered by even a single application of many preparations due to simple surface changes and consequent alterations in light reflectance and corneocyte cohesion. Many attempts have been made to determine whether aged or photoaged skin is dry but the results have been inconclusive. Stratum corneum hydration is affected by intrinsic (general hydration status, perspiration) and extrinsic factors (especially ambient humidity), and even the most sophisticated instrumentation results of hydration status can be misleading. Under normal conditions, aged skin may not be dry but after disruption of barrier function by surfactants or solvents, recovery of normal hydration may be slowed (25). It is here especially that some moisturizers may act as more than just occlusive barriers to stratum corneum water loss but as true cosmeceuticals. Triceram, oil in water preparation containing a specific ratio of ceramides, free fatty acids, and cholesterol, has been demonstrated to be more effective in barrier repair than standard moisturizers.

Retinoids

Retinoids can be considered prototypic cosmeceuticals with profiles and efficacies ranging from cosmetic to pharmaceutical depending upon the particulars of molecule, concentration and vehicle or finished product. They are the perfect class with which to rekindle several previously raging debates about the significance of photoaging in general, cosmeceuticals in particular, and because of their potential for production of teratogenicity, a host of issues of ethics, safety and public policy.

Tretinoin, all-*trans* retinoic acid, vitamin A acid, definitively proven efficacious in several large clinical studies in the 1980s continues to be of central interest because of the vast literature associated with both its clinical and research studies and their implications for other retinoids of the class. It appears to be the biologically active molecule in most systems by which its precursor or related molecules of retinol (vitamin A alcohol), retinal palmitate (the usual dietary source of vitamin A), and isotretinoin (13-*cis* retinoic acid) function. Furthermore, it occupies a pivotal and temporally and developmentally intermediate position between retinol, the "parent" compound and the newer generations of retinoids especially those of the third generation such as tazarotene.

In treatment of photoaging, tretinoin has been repeatedly demonstrated to statistically and clinically significantly improve fine wrinkles, roughness, and mottled hyperpigmentation within a time frame of up to 6 months (26–28). Continued improvement in some parameters in up to 48 weeks of treatment has also been noted (29). A so called "rosy glow", that is, erythema, is frequently noted with its use and is felt by some but not all patients to be of pleasant appearance. The main drawbacks to treatment are the initial irritation which can be reduced by careful upward titration of concentration and dosing frequency and the long period before noticeable results. As with all treatments for photoaging, a rigorous regimen of sun avoidance and sunscreen use is advised.

Isotretinoin has been repeatedly demonstrated to have similar efficacy to tretinoin with some evidence of less irritation potential (30,31). From the standpoint of commercial development, the topical formulation appears to have been delayed by the controversy over the teratogenic potential of the systemic formulation, although there are no convincing data substantiating systemic absorption or toxicity of the topical product.

Retinol in low concentrations has found its way simply as one of many ingredients of a host of cosmetics, the marketing of which, however, then heavily capitalizes on its relationship to tretinoin. It in fact became so fashionable a claim that counterclaims of "retinol free" are now appearing. A study of 53 patients of at least 80 years of age demonstrated increased fibroblast growth and collagen synthesis and reduced levels of matrix-degrading metalloproteinase levels after 7 days of application of retinol (32). Although retinol is less active than tretinoin, it penetrates skin more readily. It is not clear whether activity of retinol is due to increased penetration and subsequent conversion to tretinoin, to the molecule itself, or to some combination of the two.

Retinaldehyde has demonstrated reduction of wrinkles and skin roughness in a 125 patient double-blind study comparing retinaldehyde, retinoic acid, and vehicle creams (33). A dose-ranging study of 0.5%, 0.1%, and 0.05% concentrations demonstrated significant and dose-dependant increases in facial skin epidermal thickness.

Beta carotene is a dietary retinoid precursor molecule, which when cleaved in its center, yields two molecules of retinol. It may function as an antioxidant. Although it has been claimed to be somewhat effective in reducing the UVR sensitivity of erythropoeitic protoporphyria, there has been no convincing recent work to substantiate this claim or the claim of photoprotection for normal skin.

Tazarotene is a third generation retinoid with rapid and comprehensive efficacy in treatment of photodamaged skin. In a double-blind, vehicle-controlled trial of 563 patients, fine and course wrinkles, mottled hyperpigmentation, lentigines, elastosis, pore size, irregular hypopigmentation, and tactile roughness were significantly improved after 24 weeks of treatment (34). Pigmentary changes and reduction of fine wrinkling were demonstrated after 2 and 12 weeks, respectively.

Alpha Hydroxy Acids

This large group of naturally occurring molecules including, among the most commonly utilized, lactic acid, glycolic acid, and citric acid could vie with the retinoids as prototypic cosmeceuticals. At their lower concentrations and generally in their regulatory status, alpha hydroxy acids (AHA) may be classed as ingredients or as cosmetics, but in higher concentrations and with increasing regulatory scrutiny they approach the pharmaceutical. For example, a double-blind, vehicle-controlled study of 41 patients treated with 50% glycolic acid peels demonstrated improvement in rough texture, fine wrinkling, and hyperpigmentation (35). However, even at much lower concentrations, a definite effect is demonstrable in photodamage. A study comparing 8% glycolic and 8% L-lactic demonstrated improvement in overall severity with both and statistical superiority of lactic acid to its vehicle in reduction of mottled hyperpigmentation, sallowness, and roughness (36). Finally, at lower concentrations of a few percent, numerous AHA appear as ingredients of undetermined utility in innumerable moisturizers and cosmetics.

Beta Hydroxy Acids

Beta hydroxy acids (BHA) represented by salicylic acid, although chemically unrelated to AHA, may be conveniently considered here. Topical application of salicylic acid reduces corneocyte adhesion possibly through solubilization of intercellular cement. Exfoliation of the skin surface may improve look and feel (irregularly adherent corneocytes). A large but uncontrolled study of 1.5% and 2% salicylic acid applied twice daily for 12 weeks demonstrated global improvement of appearance (37). There was also less stinging than with glycolic acid to which it was compared. More extensive use or investigation of salicylic acid in photoaging may be related to a general lack of interest due to its perceived age or lack of novelty. It has been used successfully for decades for treatment of acne, seborrheic dermatitis, psoriasis, and so on.

Vitamins

The various vitamin B deficiency states as manifested in skin such as the dermatitis of riboflavin deficiency and pellegra of niacin deficiency speaks to their importance in normal homeostasis. Vitamins are generally thought of as cofactors in a host of enzymatic processes many of which involve the skin. What is not clear is whether the deficiencies which have been noted in a number of skin diseases have anything to do with skin aging or photoaging. Furthermore, it has not been very convincingly demonstrated in clinical trials of photoaging that addition of any of these vitamins (except A) has any clinically relevant effect, although they are frequently touted as rejuvenating, and so on.

Vitamin D, calciferol, is not truly a vitamin but a hormone and acts on cells via classical receptor mechanisms. As with vitamin A, it has found utility far beyond its role as a simple "vitamin" and demonstrates convincing efficacy in treatment of psoriasis. Its effects on inhibition of epidermal proliferation and promotion of epidermal differentiation lead one to think that it should be investigated for a possible role in reversing some of the epidermal abnormalities of photoaging.

Hormones

As with vitamin deficiencies, various diseases of hormonal etiology can have pronounced effects upon skin. The effects of menopause and estrogen deficiency may be easily noted in thinned skin, periodic flushing, and changes in vaginal mucosa. One may also note the thickened coarse skin of growth hormone excess in acromegaly or the striae of Cushing's disease and myxedematous pretibial skin of hyperthyroidism. It is tempting especially in deficiency states to extrapolate these observations to a rationale for topical or systemic treatment with the putative hormone involved.

Hormone replacement therapy (HRT) for treatment of *estrogen* deficiency has recently fallen into substantial disfavor as a result of additional evidence of morbidity and mortality and cannot currently be recommended for treatment of aged skin only (38). However, there are a number of reasonably well-conducted studies reported in the past literature which indicate that systemic or topical estrogens are effective in improving skin texture, wrinkling, elasticity, and vascularization and additional study of topical estrogens for treatment of photoaged skin is worth consideration (39–41).

Androgens, by extrapolation from their mechanism of action in other tissues, should have a beneficial effect in photoaged skin but there is inadequate experimental information available, though the issue is worthy of study. The same query should be applied to human growth hormone and perhaps to some of the other anabolic hormones widely available for misuse but never adequately studied for appropriate use.

Depigmenting Agents

Melanocyte biology, keratinocyte melanization, and the many and varied types of hypopigmentation and hyperpigmentation are too complicated and need to be adequately simplified in discussion of several marketed hypopigmenting agents. Suffice it to say that some function as tyrosinase inhibitors, and some by other or unknown mechanisms.

Hydroquinone, an inhibitor of tyrosinase and other melanocyte metabolic processes and related compounds such as 4-hydroxyanisol (mequinol) demonstrate some effect in various conditions of hyperpigmentation. They are available as both prescription and OTC products, and can be useful in treatment of some of the pigmentary alterations associated with photodamage. A combination of 2% mequinol and 0.01% tretinoin (Solage) is effective in treatment of solar lentigines and is superior to either component alone (42).

Tri-Luma, a combination of 4% hydroquinone, 0.05% tretinoin, and 0.01% fluocinolone acetanide has demonstrated convincing efficacy in treatment of melasma (43). Its use in photoaging is logical given the known effects of retinoids in general and hydroquinone in pigmentation, but this application has not yet been studied systematically.

Azelaic acid and soy extract both demonstrated skin lightening after 3 weeks of topical application, possibly through interaction with a protease-activated receptor of keratinocytes (44).

Miscellaneous Agents

Our previous admonition to keep an open mind about claims for the possible utility of naturally occurring botanicals still partially pertains to hyaluronic acid, dead sea salts, ingested natural cartilage polysaccharides, and so on but becomes more difficult to globally defend as the extravagance of the commercial claims rises so much faster than substantial scientific evidence accrues (45–47). Some useful products will likely result from this unending search but most will disappear after their brief place in the sun.

FUTURE TRENDS

The enormous and accumulating volume of scientific and lay literature and the extensive education and public health efforts warning of photoaging have had, at best, modest success in dissuading the general public from their enjoyment of the sun. Like dieting, avoidance of the pleasure of the warmth of the sun and the cosmetic appeal of a youthful tan requires more will power than most of us can generate. The steady increase in availability of cosmeceutical products which can prevent or reverse photoaging is thus most welcome to patient and therapist even if occasional claims are less than credible. The boundless sea and limitless jungle will continue to yield new and rediscovered animals, vegetables, and minerals which will find their temporary place in the almost boundless and limitless creativity of claims for cosmetic benefit. However, even more significantly, the unstoppable rapid advances of science, particularly in the areas of gene regulation will continue to provide pharmaceutical and device products which will be of even greater utility than current cosmeceuticals.

REFERENCES

1. Yaar M, Gilcrest BA. Skin aging; possible mechanisms and consequent changes in structure and function. Clin Geriatr Med 2001; 17(4):617–630.
2. Kligman LH. Intensification of ultraviolet-induced dermal damage by infrared radiation. Arch Dermatol Res 1982; 272(3–4):229–238.
3. Lavker RM, Gerberick GF, Veres D et al. Cumulative effects from repeated exposures to suberythemal dose of UVB and UVA in human skin. J Am Acad Dermatol 1995; 32(1):53–62.
4. Kochevar IE. Molecular and cellular effects of UV radiation relevant to chronic photoaging. In: Gilcrest BA, ed. Photoaging. Cambridge: Blackwell Science, 1995:51–67.
5. Fisher GJ, Kang A, Varani J et al. Mechanisms of photoaging and chronological skin aging. Arch Dermatol 2002: 138(11):1462–1470.
6. Warren R, Gartstein V, Kligman AM et al. Age, sunlight, and facial skin: a histologic and quantitative study. J Am Acad Dermatol 1991; 25(5 Pt 1):751–760.
7. Fritschi L, Green A. Sun damage in teenagers' skin. Aust J Public Health 1995; 19(4):383–386.
8. Leveque JL. Quantitative assessment of skin aging. Clin Geriatr Med 2001; 17(4):673–689.
9. Adhoute H, de Rigal J, Marchand JP, Privat Y, Leveque JL. Influence of age and sun exposure on the biophysical properties of the human skin: an *in vivo* study. Photodermatol Photoimmunol Photomed 1992; 9:99–103.
10. Grove GL, Grove MJ. Effects of topical retinoids on photoaged skin as measured by optical profilometry. Methods Enzymol 1990; 190:360–371.
11. Griffiths CE, Wang TS, Hamilton TA et al. A photonumeric scale for the assessment of cutaneous photodamage. Arch Dermatol 1992; 128(3):347–351.
12. Kang S, Leyden JJ, Lowe NJ et al. Tazarotene cream for the treatment of facial photodamage: a multicenter, investigator-masked, randomized, vehicle-controlled, parallel comparison of 0.01%, 0.025%, 0.05%, and 0.1% tazarotene creams with 0.05% tretinoin emollient cream applied once daily for 24 weeks. Arch Dermatol 2001; 137(12):1597–1604.

13. Armstrong RB, Lesiewicz J, Harvey G et al. Clinical panel assessment of photodamaged skin treated with isotretinoin using photographs. Arch Dermatol 1992; 128(3):352–356.
14. Grove GL, Grove MJ, Leyden JJ et al. Skin replica analysis of photodamaged skin after therapy with tretinoin emollient cream. J Am Acad Dermatol 1991; 25(2 Pt 1):231–237.
15. Gartstein, V, Shaya SA. Image analysis of facial skin features. Proc Int Soc Optic Eng 1986; 626:284–288.
16. Kollias N, Gillies R, Cohen-Goihman C et al. Fluorescence photography in the evaluation of hyperpigmentation in photodamaged skin. J Am Acad Dermatol 1997; 36(2 Pt 1):226–230.
17. McLean DI, Gallager R. Sunscreens, use and misuse. Dermatol Clin 1998; 16(2):219–226.
18. DeBuys HV, Levy SB, Murray JC, Madey DL, Pinnell SR. Modern approaches to photoprotection. Dermatol Clin 2000; 18(4):577–590.
19. Soter N. Sunburn and suntan: immediate manifestations of photodamage. In: Gilcrest BA, ed. Photoaging. Cambridge: Blackwell Science, 1995:12–25.
20. Brown DA, Ren WY, Khorlin A, Lesiak K, Conklin D, Wananabe KA, Seidman MM, George J. Aliphatic and alicyclic diols induce melanogenesis in cultured ce and guinea pig skin. J Invest Dermatol 1998; 110(4):428–437.
21. Gilchrist BA, Eller MS. DNA photodamage stimulates melanogenesis and other photoprotective responses. J Invest Dermatol Symp Proc 1999; 4(1):35–40.
22. Pinnell S. Cutaneous photodamage, oxidative stress, and topical antioxidant protection. J Am Acad Dermatol 2003; 48(1):1–19.
23. Nachbar F, Korting HC. The role of vitamin E in normal and damaged skin. J Mol Med 1995; 73:7–17.
24. Burke KE, Bedford RG, Combs GF et al. The effect of topical L-selenomethionine on minimal erythema dose of ultraviolet irradiation in humans. Photodermatol Photoimmunol Photomed 1992; 9:52–57.
25. Elias PM, Ghadially R. Geriatric dermatology, Part II: the aged epidermal permeability barrier: basis for functional abnormalities. Clin Geriatr Med 2002; 18(1):103–120.
26. Cordero A. La vitamina A ácida en la piel senil. Actua Ter Dermatol 1983; 6:49–54.
27. Kligman AM, Grove GL, Hirose R et al. Topical tretinoin for photoaged skin. J Am Acad Dermatol 1986; 15(4 Pt 2):836–859.
28. Weiss JS, Ellis CN, Headington JT et al. Topical tretinoin improves photoaged skin: a double-blind vehicle-controlled study. J Am Med Assoc 1988; 259(4):527–532.
29. Olsen EA, Katz HI, Levine N et al. Tretinoin emollient cream for photodamaged skin: results of 48-week, multicenter, double-blind studies. J Am Acad Dermatol 1997; 37(2 Pt 1):217–226.
30. Cunningham WJ, Bryce GF, Armstrong RA et al. Topical isotretinoin and photodamage. In: Saurat J-H, ed. Retinoids: 10 Years On. Basel: Karger, 1991:182–190.
31. Sendagorta E, Lesiewicz J, Armstrong RB. Topical isotretinoin for photodamaged skin. J Am Acad Dermatol 1992; 27(6 pt 2):S15–S18.
32. Duell EA, Kang S, Voorhees JJ. Unoccluded retinol penetrates human skin *in vivo* more effectively than unoccluded retinyl palmitate or retinoic acid. J Invest Dermatol 1997; 109(3):301–305.

33. Saurat JH, Didierjean L, Masgrau E et al. Topical retinaldehyde on human skin: biologic effects and tolerance. J Invest Dermatol 1994; 103(6):770–774.
34. Kang S, Leyden JJ, Lowe NJ et al. Tazarotene cream for the treatment of facial photodamage: a multicenter, investigator-masked, randomized, vehicle-controlled, parallel comparison of 0.01%, 0.025%, 0.05%, and 0.1% tazarotene creams with 0.05% tretinoin emollient cream applied once daily for 24 weeks. Arch Dermatol 2001; 137(12):1597–1604.
35. Newman N, Newman A, Moy LS, Babapour R, Harris AG, Moy RL. Clinical improvement of photodamaged skin with 50% glycolic acid. Dermatol Surg 1996; 22:455–460.
36. Stiller MJ, Bartolone J, Stern R et al. Topical 8% glycolic acid and 8% L-lactic acid creams for the treatment of photodamaged skin: a double-blind vehicle-controlled clinical trial. Arch Dermatol 1996; 132(6):631–636.
37. Kligman AM. Salicylic acid: an alternative to alpha hydroxy acids. J Ger Dermatol 1997; 5(3):128–131.
38. Schairer C, Lubin J, Troisi R et al. Menopausal estrogen and estrogen–progestin replacement therapy and breast cancer risk. J Am Med Assoc 2000; 283(4):485–491.
39. Creidi P, Faivre B, Agache P, et al. Effect of conjugated oestrogen (Premarin®) cream on aging facial skin: a comparative study with a placebo cream. Maturitas 1994; 19:211–223.
40. Schmidt JB, Binder M, Demschik G et al. Treatment of skin aging with topical estrogens. Int J Dermatol 1996; 35(9):669–674.
41. Phillips TJ, Demircay Z, Sahu M. Geriatric dermatology, Part I: hormonal effects on skin aging. Clin Geriatr Med 2001; 17(4):661–672.
42. Fleischer AB, Schwartzel EH, Colby SI, Altman DJ. The combination of 2% 4-hydroxyanisole (mequinol) and 0.01% tretinoin is effective in improving the appearance of solar lentigines and related hyperpigmented lesions in two double-blind multicenter clinical studies. J Am Acad Dermatol 2000; 42(3):459–467.
43. Pezeshki S, Bell FE, Grummer S, McMichael AJ. Therapeutic options for melasma. Cosmet Dermatol 2003; 16(3):33–45.
44. Hermans JF, Petit L, Martalo O, Pierard-Franchimont C, Cauwenbergh G, Pierard GE. Unraveling the patterns of subclinical pheomelanin-enriched facial hyperpigmentation: effect of depigmenting agents. Dermatology 2000; 201(2):118–122.
45. Ghersetich I, Teofoli P, Benci M et al. Ultrastructural study of hyaluronic acid before and after the use of a pulsed electromagnetic field, electrorydesis, in the treatment of wrinkles. Int J Dermatol 1994; 33(9):661–663.
46. Ma'or Z, Magdassi S, Efron D et al. Dead Sea mineral-based cosmetics-facts and illusions. Isr J Med Sci 1996; 32:S28–S35.
47. Eskelinin A, Santalahti J. Natural cartilage polysaccharides for the treatment of sun-damaged skin in females: a double-blind comparison of Vivida and Imedeen. J Int Med Res 1992; 20(2):227–233.

14

Phytosterols

C. Bayerl
Department of Dermatology, Venerology and Allergology, Mannheim University Clinic

Plant Sterols	279
Animal Sterols in Plants	281
Sources of Phytosterols	281
Phytosterols in Membranes	282
Phytosterols and Cholesterol-Lowering Functional Foods	282
Phytosterols and the Immune System	283
Clinical Examples for the Use of Phytosterols in Medicine	284
Phytosterols and Cancer	284
Sterols/Phytosterols and the Skin	285
Phytosterols and Eczema	286
Phytosterols in Cosmeceuticals—The Future?	287
Are Risks Entailed in Using Phytosterols?	288
Trends—From Insect to Plant to Skin	289
References	289

PLANT STEROLS

Sterols are natural components of cell membranes. Both animals and plants produce them. Cholesterol is exclusively an animal sterol. Phytosterols play a role in plants similar to that of cholesterol in humans and mammals by forming cell membrane structures; they are consequently of importance for plant cell growth. Structurally, phytosterols resemble cholesterol except that they are always substituted at the C24 position in the sterol side chain (Fig. 1). Phytosterols differ substantially in their intestinal absorption and metabolic fate, as they are not synthesized in humans. They are also poorly absorbed and excreted faster from the liver than cholesterol. This explains their low abundance in

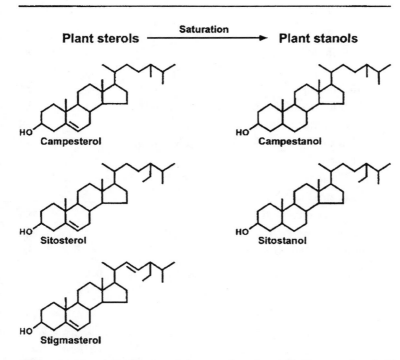

Figure 1 Chemical structure of plant sterols and stanols. Plant sterols, of which campesterol, beta-sitosterol, and stigmasterol are the most abundant in nature are structurally related to cholesterol, but they have a different side-chain configuration. Saturation of the sterols with hydrogen leads to the formation of plant stanols such as campestanol and sitostanol. [According to van Kerckhoffs et al. (7).]

human tissues. Over 40 phytosterols have been identified so far. The most common plant sterols are beta-sitosterol, campesterol, and stigmasterol, which are structurally very similar to cholesterol (Fig. 1). Plant stanols are the hydrogenated counterparts of the respective common plant sterols, for example, stigmastanol is the hydrogenated form of stigmasterol (1,2). The unsaturated form, called sterols, is common and present in many plants. The saturated form, called stanols, is found only in small amounts in cereals, fruits, and vegetables (3).

ANIMAL STEROLS IN PLANTS

Certain animal sterols were discovered in plant tissues. The human female sex hormone, estrone, has been found in trace amounts in the pollen and seeds of the date palm (*Phoenix dactylifera*), and the seeds of pomegranate (*Punica granatum*). Estradiol (beta-estradiol) occurs in the seeds of the French bean (*Phaseolus vulgaris*) and possesses considerably more estrogenic activity than estrone. Various phytoestrogens, lignans, and coumestans are present in linseed oil, lucerne, and whole grains (2). Isoflavones, the phytoestrogens from soybean, fruits, or vegetables, such as genistein and daidzein, manifest estrogenic effects on females. Even after topical application of phytoestrogen, postmenopausal skin shows a reduction of small wrinkles in a controlled multicenter study (4). The male hormone testosterone is present in the pollen of Scots pine, *Pinus sylvestris*, as well as in date palm and in marine red algae (*Rhodophyceae*) (3). In contrast to the animal sterols in plants, a sterol for membrane biosynthesis is not necessarily a sterol for the purposes of hormone biosynthesis (5). Therefore, this article focuses on phytosterols in plants and not on animal sterols in plants.

SOURCES OF PHYTOSTEROLS

Plant sterols are present in small quantities in fruits, vegetables, nuts, seeds, cereals, and legumes and in products made from these, for example, vegetable oils, pine tree oil from pine tree wood pulp, soybean oil, rice bran oil, and shea nut oil. Corn oil, for example, contains 0.77% phytosterols by weight, while processing reduces the phytosterol content. The typical human consumption of plant sterols is 200–400 mg/day. The following are some of the phytosterols and their occurrence in plants (2):

1. Campesterol and brassicasterol, found in rapeseed oil (*Brassica napus*);
2. Stigmasterol, found in higher plants such as soybeans (*Glycine max*), calabar beans (*Physostigma venenosum*);

3. Beta-sitosterol, found in wheat germ (*Triticum*), sweet corn (*Zea mays*), and in herbs such as saw palmetto (*Pygeum africanum*) and pumpkin seed oil.

Commercially, phytosterols are isolated from two major sources: pine tree oil and vegetable oils (soybean, canola, and sunflower). Sterols and stanols are esterified with fatty acids to make them soluble in food products, for example, cholesterol-lowering margarines.

PHYTOSTEROLS IN MEMBRANES

In evolution, there has been a clear correlation between cholesterol and the development of a nervous system as the brain biosynthesizes cholesterol. According to "Behring's conclusion" sterols cannot be synthesized by anaerobic bacteria because the formation of epoxysqualene is an aerobic process in which molecular oxygen is introduced in the molecule. The absence of sterols in anaerobic bacteria means that they have a less functional cytoplasmic envelope and have to utilize a fatty acid as an approximate substitute for a sterol. The 24-alkylsterols of plants are turned over much faster than cholesterol and the absorption through the intestinal wall is limited. Nevertheless, phytosterols have been shown to be growth-promoting sterols (5) (Table 1).

PHYTOSTEROLS AND CHOLESTEROL-LOWERING FUNCTIONAL FOODS

The structural similarity of phytosterols to cholesterol allows them to compete with cholesterol during its absorption in the digestive tract. However, phytosterols are absorbed only minimally in the digestive tract of humans. Plant sterols and stanols (hydrogenated form of sterols) are present in the average Western diet in small amounts, 250–500 mg/day for plant sterols and 20–60 mg/day for plant stanols. Both oral and parenteral administration of plant sterols and stanols results in reduced concentrations of plasma total and LDL cholesterol. LDL cholesterol levels were especially lowered in hypercholesterolemic subjects

Table 1 Sterols and Growth of *Mycoplasma arthritidis*

Growth promoting	Not growth promoting
Cholesterol	3-Epicholesterol
Sitosterol	Solanesol
Stigmasterol	Cholestane
Ergosterol	Squalene
Carotenol	Fatty acid esters of cholesterol

Source: Modified according to Nes (5).

and in subjects on a cholesterol-rich diet for 9–14% (6). The FDA has allowed food manufacturers to label phytosterol-enriched foods with the claim that they may reduce the risk of coronary heart disease (7). Up to now, only one potentially adverse effect with consumption of stanol esters arises, namely a dose-dependent decrease in plasma carotenoid levels. The reason is decreased carotenoid absorption that probably results from competition at the micelle level or additional mechanisms that have not been identified so far (2).

PHYTOSTEROLS AND THE IMMUNE SYSTEM

Beta-sitosterol is found in tissues and plasma of healthy individuals at a concentration 1000× lower than that of endogenous cholesterol. Its glucoside, beta-sitosterol glucoside, is found in even lower concentrations. However, immunomodulatory effects of these two compounds have been shown *in vivo* (1). TH1 lymphokines were enhanced, whereas TH2 helper cell lymphokines remained relatively unchanged (Fig. 2). Accordingly, the secretion of IL-2 and gamma interferon was enhanced, whereas the release of IL-4 remained unchanged. Anti-inflammatory properties became evident by an inhibition of the secretion of IL-6 and tumor necrosis factor alpha in endotoxin-activated human monocytes. The mixture has additional antiglucocorticoid activity as proved by its ability to abolish dexamethasone-induced endocrinological responses.

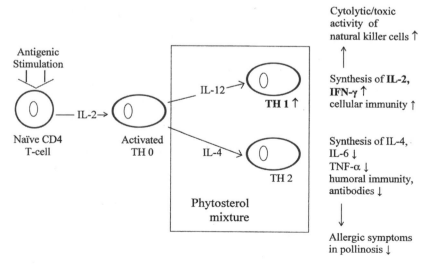

Figure 2 The effect of phytosterols on Th1/Th2 CD4 helper cells. [Modified according to Bouic (1).]

In clinical studies, the phytosterol/glucoside mixture group showed faster clinical recovery after tuberculosis and prevention of infectious episodes in endurance sport athletes. In a study with this mixture in HIV infected patients, the CD4 cell numbers that are attained in patients in times of relatively intact immunity could be maintained. Disease activity in rheumatoid arthritis and pollen allergic rhinitis was attenuated (1). These studies focused on the anti-inflammatory properties of the phytosterol/glucoside mixture and are based on the current theory that Th1 and Th2 CD4 helper cells need to be balanced (Fig. 2).

CLINICAL EXAMPLES FOR THE USE OF PHYTOSTEROLS IN MEDICINE

Phytosterols are thought to be responsible for the health benefits of a variety of medicinal plants. Experimental and clinical studies corroborated the use of plants with effects on steroid metabolism. Commission E of the BfArM (State Organization for Drug Licensing in Germany) releases monographs on phytotherapeutics with the appraisals "positive", "negative", and "null". These judgments have mostly been found to be congruent with ESCOP (European Scientific Cooperative on Phytotherapy) recommendations and WHO drug monographs. The Commission E has published positive monographs for benign prostata hyperplasia for saw palmetto, stinging nettle, and pumpkin seed, because of their anti-inflammatory, antiedematous, and immunomodulatory effects (8,9).

Saw palmetto (*Serenoa repens*, syn. *fructus sabalis serrulati*) contains delta-3- and delta-5-phytosterols, among these free and glycosylated beta-sitosterols. The fruit is used to improve symptoms of prostate hyperplasia, but does not reduce prostate hyperproliferation. Moreover, it is used in hair preparations and shampoos, where the antiandrogenic effect caused by a partial inhibition of 5-alpha-reductase in the hair follicle has been shown *in vitro*, but not proven in humans. Stinging nettle (*Urticae radix*) has shown *in vivo* inhibition of leucocyte elastasis that leads to a reduction in structure elements of the tissue as collagen and elastic fibers and to an inhibition of complement activation. Obstructive symptoms during prostata hyperplasia improve. The phytosterols delta-5- and delta-7-sterols are found in pumpkin (*Cucurbita pepo*) seeds. Placebo-controlled studies showed improvement of symptoms, objectively in uroflow, in patients with prostatic proliferation but without effect on the latter. Pumpkin seed reduces dihydrotestosterone and the dihydrotestosterone binding to cellular receptors (8,10).

PHYTOSTEROLS AND CANCER

Phytosterols are bioactive compounds (3). *In vivo* experiments have shown that the lytic activity of the natural killer cells close to a cancer cell line was enhanced, when they were preincubated with a mixture of beta-sitosterone together with beta-sitosterone gluconate (1). Clinical studies showed that beta-sitosterol has effects in benign prostatic hyperplasia (9). Moreover, there are reports on the beneficial effect on health, especially of beta-sitosterone in prostate cancer, in which it decreases tumor growth by 24% by induction of apotosis (11) and its positive effects on breast cancer cells *in vitro* (12). The effect of plant sterol intake on stomach cancer (13) and colorectal cancer (14) has been studied in a few epidemiologic trials in different populations, but more evidence is required.

STEROLS/PHYTOSTEROLS AND THE SKIN

Lipid synthesis is localized in the keratinocytes. The lamellar bodies located in keratinocytes secrete lipids into the intercellular spaces of the stratum corneum (15). The major human stratum corneum lipid classes are cholesterol sulfate, glucosylceramides, major ceramide fractions, free sterols, free fatty acids, triglycerides, sterol squalene, and *n*-alkanes (16). Lipids of the stratum corneum are implicated in cohesion, desquamation, and the maintenance of normal barrier function. Cholesterol synthesis is regulated by the enzyme HMG-CoA reductase and by the synthesis of other lipids (17). Changes in cholesterol homeostasis are regulated via the scavenger receptor class B, type I. This receptor is expressed in keratinocytes in the epidermis and regulated by cellular cholesterol requirements or barrier disruption (18). Acute disturbance of barrier function by acetone, for example, leads to an increase in cholesterol synthesis mainly in the stratum basale/stratum spinosum. Chronic disturbances induced by a chronic dietary deficiency of essential fatty acids result in increased cholesterol synthesis in the stratum granulosum (15). UV light therapy significantly increases the amount of skin surface lipids available for free-cholesterol synthesis (19).

In atopic dermatitis, lamellar ichthyosis, or otherwise diseased and dry skin, a reduction or structural alteration of ceramides has been found as well as differences in free fatty acid–cholesterol ratio that are responsible for the impaired barrier function in the skin (20–22). In recessive X-linked ichthyosis, cholesterol sulfate is accumulated and by this cholesterol is reduced to 50%. Interestingly, the functional and structural abnormalities in this disease can be corrected by topical application of cholesterol (23).

With the addition of plant sterols to the diet ($\sim$30 g/day), for example, beta-sitosterol reappeared in the skin by 12 days (^{3}H-radioactivity) and in the skin surface lipids at 20 days (mass spectroscopy). In contrast, cholesterol was measured earlier in the skin surface lipids, namely at 7 days. From this it was concluded that beta-sitosterol is incorporated only in epidermal basal cells after addition to the diet, whereas cholesterol is presumably incorporated into epidermal cells during differentiation. The accumulation of beta-sitosterol in epidermal basal cells may lead to its excretion in the skin surface lipids in conjunction with dead cells desquamated during the average time of about 20 days (24).

It can be concluded that part of the nutritional phytosterols are excreted through the skin of humans. Nutritional sterols are transferred from the plasma to the skin after their absorption from the diet in small quantities. The normal absorption is <5%. Fecal excretion of sterols from the body is the primary pathway. Excretion of plant sterols via the skin is the second pathway (24). Rare cases of lipid storage diseases have been described with plant sterols initiating the development of xanthomas with otherwise normal plasma cholesterol levels and without the formation of artherosclerotic plaques (25).

PHYTOSTEROLS AND ECZEMA

Phytosterols are becoming interesting in the topical treatment of eczema. It is thought that these substances stabilize damaged-cell membranes by reducing the increased release of arachidonic acid and the formation of prostaglandins and leucotrienes. It has been reported that phytosterols in an extract of avocado sprouts reduces itching, redness, vesiculation, and desquamation. However, a controlled study has not been conducted up to now.

Alcoholic extracts of deadly nightshade (*Dulcamara stipites*) definitely contains no phytosterols, but is mentioned here merely to accentuate the difference from steroid analogs. The extracts of deadly nightshade are rich in glycosidically bound steroid alkaloids and basic and neutral steroid saponins that show a mild steroid-like effect. An ointment containing deadly nightshade extract showed some effects on atopic dermatitis in a clinical study.

Balloon vine (*Cardiospermi herba*) contains, among other ingredients, beta-sitosterin, campesterin, and stigmasterin; it was shown to have anti-inflammatory and antipruritic effects in a study on atopic dermatitis (Fig. 3). It is

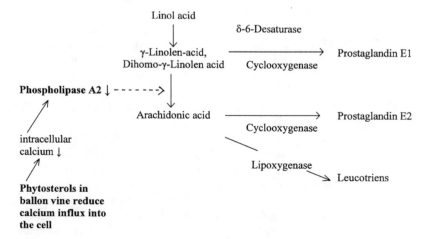

Figure 3 Indirect effect of balloon vine on phospholipase A2. [According to Schilcher and Kammerer (8).]

thought that phytosterols open ionic channels and reduce the immense calcium influx into the cell. That leads to a reduction of the activity of phospholipase A2, which is a key enzyme in inflammatory processes (8,10).

PHYTOSTEROLS IN COSMECEUTICALS—THE FUTURE?

Topically applied lipids have been studied for their effects on surfactant-irritated skin. For *barrier repair*, the optimal physiological lipid mixture comprising ceramides, cholesterol, and free fatty acids are essential, for example, in murine skin. Acrylceramides alone have shown to delay barrier recovery, whereas mixtures with cholesterol within a specific range of molar ratios improved barrier repair (26). In murine skin, an equimolar mixture of cholesterol, ceramides, and essential/nonessential fatty acids allowed normal recovery in chronologically aged mice, whereas a 3:1:1:1 mixture with cholesterol as the dominant lipid accelerated barrier recovery dramatically (27). Regarding phytosterols, a sterol-enriched fraction from canola oil showed beneficial effects on the skin barrier in murine skin (28). These studies imply the specific requirement for selected stratum corneum lipid mixtures including phytosterols for optimized barrier repair in human skin.

Chronological *aging*, hormone level, and environmental factors such as UV irradiation determine the condition of our skin. Among other factors, skin aging depends on lipid peroxidation, a process in which cellular membranes are damaged by oxidative stress. Sterols (mainly free cholesterol) with a concentration of up to 50 mol% in the lipid barrier of the stratum corneum effectively compete with the UV-induced peroxidation of the human skin lipids ceramides and free fatty acids (29). Up to now, there has been only one *in vitro* study showing that phytosterols decrease membrane lipid peroxidation (30).

Demand for plant-derived chemicals is growing year by year in the USA. The European soy market is expanding mostly because growth will be driven by nonplant-based pharmaceuticals. Nevertheless, botanical extracts will be the fastest growing segment. Slogans are "mother nature knows better". In the following, some more examples of plants containing phytosterol are cited, because there is increased interest in new botanical substances for phytonutrition as well as for cosmeceuticals.

The powder or ointment from the bark of *Mimosa tenuiflora* contains many ingredients, especially tannins, saponins, and some phytosterols. In Mexico, preparations for treating skin wounds and burns have been popular. In the cosmetic industry, diverse products of *M. tenuiflora* wood such as shampoos, creams, capsules, and soaps have been marketed as immunostimulants that are moreover able to increase the number of fibroblasts (31).

Ginseng (*Ginseng radix*) contains ginsenosides and phytosterols. It is only used orally and in teas, but might be of further interest by virtue of its antioxidative effects.

The seed of Jambul tree (*Syzygii cumini semen*) is an astringent but also contains beta-sitosterone. It is used for infections of the oral mucosa and to treat superficial skin inflammation.

Butcher's broom (*Rusci aculeati rhizoma*) has an anti-inflammatory effect and is used in venous insufficiency and to alleviate itching and burning in hemorrhoids.

Elder (*Sambucus nigra*) was used historically to dye hair black.

Extracts of guaijacum wood (*Guajaci lignum*) and dandelion (*Taraxaci radix cum herba*) root with leaves have anti-inflammatory effects.

Stargrass root or african potato (*Hypoxis rooperi radix*) is a mixture of beta-sitosterol, beta-sitosterol glucoside, campesterol, and other phytosterols with anti-inflammatory and anti-exudative effects, derives from Africa and has been used to treat prostate hyperplasia.

Horse chestnut (*Hippocastanei semen*) has proved its anti-exudative, anti-edematous, and tonic effects on the venous vessels in clinical studies.

Sandalwood (*Santali albi lignum*) acts antibacterially and spasmolytically, but mostly because of its ethereal oil content (8,10).

ARE RISKS ENTAILED IN USING PHYTOSTEROLS?

The root or the juice from the root of liquorice (*Glycyrrhiza glabra*) contains phytosterols, flavonoids, and isoflavonoids and has been used orally for its anti-inflammatory effect in the treatment of gastric ulcers with a semisynthetic ingredient carbenoxolone. It has mostly been used as an expectorant. Studies have shown that the pain can be reduced in peptic ulcers, whereas healing of the ulcer is not affected. In contrast it has been shown that liquorice might induce intoxication. The glycyrrhicic acid in liquorice interferes with corticosteroid metabolism, binds to the mineralocorticoid receptors in the spleen, and might induce pseudo-hyperaldosteronism with hypokalemia, hypertension, and edema (8,10).

Data on the safety of *Arnica montana*, the extract derived from dried flowerheads of the plant, are not sufficient at the moment with respect to UV photosensitization, the effects on the major organ systems associated with repeated dermal exposure, inhalation toxicity, or genotoxicity. The composition of this extract includes phytosterols, but also coumarins, triterpenoid alcohols, sesquiterpene lactones, and heavy metals. Until all data are available, the safety of this ingredient in cosmetic formulations cannot be confirmed (32).

The amount of phytosterols (113–265 mg/100 g oil) in extra virgin olive oil (*Olivum oleum*) depends on the cultivation and the degree of ripeness of the olives (33). As risks have been reported, such as allergies after topical application of olive oil, and studies have not been reported, a negative monograph was issued by Commission E of BfArM, even if this is quite astonishing for dermatologists who have applied olive oil topically for centuries without major complications.

Milk thistle (*Silybi marianae fructus, fructus cardui mariae*) contains silymarin, a mixture of different flavonolignans such as silybin, silchristin, and silydianin, flavonoids such as taxifolin, and phytosterols. The fruit is used for preparations that are intended to protect the cell membranes of the liver from toxic substances. It is given intravenously in intoxications with death cap (*Amanita phalloides*) as a cell-protective substance against the toxin alpha-amanitin. Milk thistle was issued a null monograph by BfArM Commission E because the beneficial effects are not adequately proven. The classification null means that milk thistle may be used as risks are not known (8).

TRENDS—FROM INSECT TO PLANT TO SKIN

Ecdysteroids are insect molting hormones. They regulate metamorphoses in insects, showing beneficial effects in humans and animals alike. Therefore medicinal plants have been subjected to meticulous investigations addressing the presence of phytoecdysteroids, for example, the herb *Silene otites*. Health improvement preparations are in the market that claim to make the body adaptogenic, possess anabolic actions, and shield the body from stress. In mice and rat, anti-inflammatory effects, immunostimulation, and pain relief have been shown for phytoecdysteroids. In humans, phytoecdyteroids have shown to favor skin regeneration (34).

REFERENCES

1. Bouic PJD. The role of phytosterols and phytosterolins in immune modulation: a review of the past 10 years. Curr Opin Clin Nutr Metab Care 2001; 4:471–475.
2. Kris-Etherton PM, Hecker KD, Bonamone A, Coval SM, Binkoski AE, Hilpert KF, Griel AE, Etherton TD. Bioactive compounds in foods: their role in the prevention of cardiocascular disease and cancer. Am J Med 2002; 113:71S–88S.
3. Orzechowski A, Ostazewski P, Jank M, Berwid SJ. Bioactive substances of plant origin in food—impact of genomics. Reprod Nutr Dev 2002; 42:461–477.
4. Bayerl C, Keil D. Isoflavonoids in the treatment of skin aging in postmenopausal women. Akta Dermatol 2002; 28:S14–S18.
5. Nes WR. Role of sterols in membranes. Lipids 1974; 9:596–612.
6. Jones PJ, McDougall DE, Ntanios F, Vanstone CA. Dietary phytosterols as cholesterol- lowering agents in humans. Can J Physiol Pharmacol 1997; 75:217–227.
7. van Kerckhoffs DAJM, Brouns F, Hornstra G, Mensink RP. Effects on the human serum lipoprotein profile of beta-glucan, soy protein and isoflavones, plant sterols and stanols, garlic and tocotrienols. J Nutr 2002; 132:2494–2505.
8. Schilcher H, Kammerer S. Leitfaden Phytotherapie. 1st ed. München, Jena: Urban and Fischer, 2000.
9. Wild T, Ishani A, MacDonald R, Stark G, Mulrow C, Lau J. Beta-sitosterol for benign prostatic hyperplasia. Cochrane Database Syst Rev 2000; 2:CD001043. Review.
10. Braun H, Frohne D. Heilpflanzenlexikon, Wirkungen, Verordnung, Selbstmedikation. 6th ed. Auflage: Gutav Fischer, 1994.

11. von Holtz RL, Fink CS, Awad AB. Beta-Sitosterol activates the shingomyelin cycle and induces apoptosis in LNCaP human prostate cancer cells. Nutr Cancer 1998; 32:8–12.
12. Awad AB, Fink CS. Phytosterols as anticancer dietary components: evidence and mechanism of action. J Nutr 2000; 130:2127–2130.
13. de Stefani E, Boffetta P, Ronco AL, Brennan P, Deneo-Pellegrini H, Carzoglio JC, Mendilaharsu M. Plant sterols and risk of stomach cancer: a case control study in Uruguay. Nutr Cancer 2000; 37:140–144.
14. Norman AL, Brandts HA, Voorips LE, Andersson HA, van den Brandt PA, Goldbohm RA. Plant sterol intakes and colorectal cancer risk in the Netherlands Cohort on Diet and Cancer. Am J Clin Nutr 2001; 74:141–148.
15. Proksch E. Regulation of the epidermal permeability barrier by lipids and hyperproliferation. Hautarzt 1992; 43:331–338.
16. Melnik BC, Hollmann J, Erler E, Verhoeven B, Plewig G. Micoranalytical screening of all major stratum corneum liquids by sequential high-performance thin-layer chromatography. J Invest Dermatol 1989; 92:231–234.
17. Siefken W, Höppner H, Harris IR. Regulation of cholesterol synthesis by oleic and plamitic acid in keratinocytes. Exp Dermatol 2000; 9:138–145.
18. Tsuruoka H, Khovidhunkit W, Brown BE, Fluhr JW, Elias PM, Feingold KR. Scavenger receptor class B type I is expressed in cultured keratinocytes and epidermis. Regulation in response to changes in cholesterol homeostasis an barrier requirements. J Biol Chem 2002; 277:2916–2922.
19. Gloor M, Karenfeld A. Effect of ultraviolet light therapy, given over a period of several weeks, on the amount and composition of the skin surface lipids. Dermatologica 1977; 154:5–13.
20. Yamamoto A, Serizawa S, Ito M, Sato Y. Stratum corneum lipid abnormalities in atopic dermatitis. Arch Dermatol Res 1991; 283:219–223.
21. Bouwstra JA, Gorris GS, Dubbelaar FE, Ponec M. Phase behaviour of stratum corneum lipid mixtures on ceramides. The role of natural and synthetic ceramide 1. J Invest Dermatol 2002; 118:606–617.
22. Lavrijsen AP, Bouwstra JA, Gorris GS, Weerheim A, Bodde HW, Boddé HE, Ponec M. Reduced skin barrier function parallels abnormal stratum corneum lipid organization in patients with lamellar ichthyosis. J Invest Dermatol 1995; 105:619–624.
23. Zettersten E, Man MQ, Sato J, Denda M, Farrell A, Ghadially R, Williams ML, Feingold KR, Elias PM. Recessive x-linked ichthyosis: role of cholesterol-sulfate accumulation in the barrier abnormality. J Invest Dermatol 1998; 111:784–790.
24. Bhattacharyya AK, Connor WE, Lin DS. The origin of plant sterols in the skin surface lipids in humans. From diet to plasma to skin. J Invest Dermtol 1983; 80:294–296.
25. Bhattacharyya AK, Connor WE. Beta-siterolemia and xanthomatosis. J Clin Invest 1974; 53:1033–1043.
26. Mao-Qiang M, Feingold KR, Thornfeldt CR, Elias PM. Optimization of physiological lipid mixtures for barrier repair. J Invest Dermatol 1996; 106:1096–1101.
27. Zettersten E, Ghadially R, Feingol KR, Crumrine D, Elias PM. Optimal ratios of topical stratum corneum lipids improve barrier recovery in chronologically aged skin. J Am Acad Dermatol 1997; 37:403–408.
28. Lodén M, Andersson AC. Effect of topically applied lipids on the surfactant-irritated skin. Br J Dermatol 1996; 1134:215–220.

29. Lasch J, Schonfelder U, Walke M, Zellner S, Beckert D. Oxidative damage of human skin lipids. Dependence of lipid peroxidation on sterol concentration. Biochem Biophys Acta 1997; 1349:171–181.
30. van Rensburg SJ, Daniels WM, van Zyl JM, Taljaard JJ. A comparative study of the effects of cholesterol, beta-sitosterol, beta-sitosterol glucoside, dehydroepiandrosterone and melatonin on *in vitro* lipid peroxidation. Metab Brain Dis 2000; 15:257–265.
31. Camargo-Ricalde SL. Descripción, distribución, composición químicy y usos de *Mimosa tenuiflora* (Fabaceae-Mimosoideae) en México. Rev Biol Trop 2000; 48:939–954.
32. Final report on the safety and assessment of *Arnica montana* extract and *Arnica montana*. Int J Toxicol 2001; 20:1–11.
33. Gutierrez F, Jiminez BB, Ruiz A, Albi MA. Effect of olive ripeness on the oxidative stability of virgin oil extracts from the varieties picuall and hojiblanca and on the components involved. K Agric Food Chem 1999; 47:121–127.
34. Báthori M. Phytoecdysteroids effects on mammalians, isolation and analysis. Mini Rev Med Chem 2002; 2:285–293.

15

Protective Creams

J. W. Fluhr, J. Praessler, and Peter Elsner
Department of Dermatology, Friedrich-Schiller University, Jena, Germany

Introduction	293
Specific Aspects of Topical Formulations	294
SC and Hydration	294
Role of Physiological Lipids	296
Barrier Protection and Barrier Recovery	297
Protective Creams with Special Ingredients	300
Application	300
Adverse Effects and Contraindications	301
Conclusion	301
References	302

INTRODUCTION

The *stratum corneum* (SC) is a very resilient tissue, resulting from the cornified envelope of individual corneocytes, which is highly resistant to both physical and chemical assaults, and from the interdigitation of adjacent corneocytes, as well as from the riveting of adjacent corneocytes via specialized desmosomes (corneodesmosomes). An interconnected network of structural proteins disperses the force of external physical insults laterally throughout the skin. SC elasticity (1) is also influenced by the extent of hydration of corneocyte cytosolic proteins, a variable that is regulated by the hygroscopic breakdown products of filaggrin (2), by the sebaceous gland-derived glycerol (3), resulting from high rates of triglyceride turnover (4), and by changes in external humidity (5,6). SC proteins, lipids (especially, ceramides), glycerol, and low molecular weight byproducts of keratohyalin (filaggrin) catabolism, known as natural moisturizing factors (NMF), bind and retain water in the SC, thereby maintaining its elasticity (4).

Prevention should be a major target of dermatological intervention of irritant contact dermatitis (ICD) and allergic contact dermatitis (ACD). Apart from elimination of cutaneous exposure to hazardous substances and the use of gloves or protective clothing, protective creams (PCs) are important tools in an integrated concept of preventive measures. Skin protection in the workplace consists of pre-exposure PCs, mild skin cleansers, and post-exposure skin care products. Although PCs are designed to prevent skin damage due to irritant contact, skin cleaning should remove aggressive substances from the skin, and skin care is intended to enhance epidermal barrier regeneration (7).

Research has shown that the composition of PCs is of great importance for their efficacy. In this review, a number of features of PCs will be presented, including composition, classification, and potential mechanisms of vehicle function including their role in epidermal barrier function. Beneficial effects of an oil-in-water (o/w) moisturizing cream on the permeability barrier function in ICD and ACD have been shown (8). The chosen vehicle should no longer be regarded simply as a drug carrier, vehicle, or delivery system, but as an essential component of successful topical treatment and protection. For example, a ceramide-dominant barrier repair lipid mixture in atopic dermatitis showed an increased barrier repair and SC hydration (9). Furthermore, it has been shown that the use of fatty acid-rich emollients prevents the development of atopic eczema (10). It may be of importance to adapt the type and composition of PCs to the SC properties, for example, hydration.

SPECIFIC ASPECTS OF TOPICAL FORMULATIONS

SC and Hydration

The classification of commercially available products is often difficult or impossible solely because of product labeling. For example, the listed specification for the emulsion systems is commonly abbreviated either as o/w, to delineate oil in water, or as w/o, to delineate water in oil. As a consequence, the amount of water, and conversely the lipid fraction, in the different emulsion systems are usually not specified.

Dermatological and protective creams exert a number of effects, in and on the skin, including skin hydration, skin cooling, and barrier effect. The relative cooling effect of PCs can be attributed to the amount of water and/or alcohol in the emulsion system(s) and to water "activity", more precisely, the amount of freely evaporating water that is liberated in the early phase after topical application. Moreover, the emulsion structure (e.g., liquid crystals) and the presence of hydrotopes determine the water-liberation properties. This effect is more pronounced when the vehicle is formed by an aqueous or hydro-alcoholic phase or when the vehicle is present within the external phase of the formulation, for example, lotions, hydrogels, or o/w emulsions. However, relatively nonstable w/o emulsions, like cold creams, also can exert mild cooling effect when applied topically to the skin. This is due to the special structure of these traditional emulsions. In modern times, some emulsifiers (like sucrose esters) or gelling polymers (e.g., taurates) also provide a cooling effect.

PCs are also well known to influence the hydration of the SC for which at least three different mechanisms have been proposed:

First, the cosmetic vehicle can exert a direct hydrating effect by liberating water from the formulation itself (11). In short-term applications, this hydrating effect is more pronounced with formulations containing a high percentage of free water when compared with lipid-rich and low free water-containing preparations (12). As expected, the hydrating effect of o/w systems in short-term applications depends primarily on the water activity (unbound water content) of the formulation, as only the presence of free (unbound) water ensures immediate hydration of the SC. In contrast, long-term applications of either w/o or o/w emulsions with different water contents revealed hydration of the SC with the w/o but not with the o/w emulsions (13,14). Thus, although a w/o emulsion may be cosmetically less acceptable (but this is true only with older formulations), such a formulation can be expected to achieve better SC hydration, especially with prolonged use.

Secondly, the occlusive effect of the formulation can influence SC hydration, especially in long-term applications. A standard model for this occlusion effect is petrolatum (15), for which the highest occlusive effect was detected (16). W/o emulsions with low water content may have occlusive effects similar to petrolatum, whereas w/o emulsions with high water content very rarely have occlusive properties and behave similarly to o/w emulsions (16). But, even o/w formulations with high water content can exert an occlusion effect after the unbound water has evaporated.

Thirdly, a mechanism by which PCs influence skin hydration, is evident when highly hygroscopic compounds like glycerol, or hydrotropes like hyaluronic acid or trimethylglycine are applied. By absorbing water either from the vehicle itself, from surface water, or from water evaporation, these agents are able to increase SC hydration (17,18). Recent publications have shown that the epidermal water/glycerol transporter aquaporin-3 (AQP3) plays an important role in SC hydration via glycerol content (19).

It should be noted that compounds with distinct dielectric constants have been shown to influence the electrophysical properties of the SC, as measured by capacitance- or conductance-based instruments (17). Thus, it is plausible that topically applied moisturizing creams might be a source of false positive results using these instruments (20). Although a good correlation between capacitance values and water content of the tested creams has been demonstrated (20), a sufficient time lag following application of compounds should be allotted before any such measurements are registered; moreover, the regression curve of vehicle effects should be studied as a function of time.

Role of Physiological Lipids

The barrier function of the skin is mediated by intercellular bilayers in the SC. Cholesterol, ceramides, and essential and non-essential fatty acids play a key role in the formation of these bilayers (21,22). SC lipids are composed of 40% ceramides, 25% cholesterol, and 20% free fatty acids (by weight) (22). Taking the average molecular weight of these three lipid classes into account, the normal SC has an approximately equimolar physiologic ratio of ceramides, cholesterol, and free fatty acids. Following barrier disruption in hairless mice, epidermal cholesterol and fatty acid syntheses are immediately increased, whereas increased ceramide production is evident ~6 h later (21,23–25). These key barrier lipids are delivered to the intercellular space of the SC as a mixture of precursors by the extrusion of lamellar body content at the SG–SC interface (26,27). Fusion of the extruded lamellar contents within the lower SC leads to continuous membrane sheets, which ultimately form mature membrane bilayer structures (27,28). The final membrane structural transformation correlates with changes in lipid composition; that is, the polar lipid precursors (glycosphingolipids, phospholipids, and cholesterol sulfate) are metabolized to more-nonpolar lipid products (21,26). The lipid bilayer maturation within the different depths of the SG and the SC is mediated by different classes of pH-dependent enyzmes, namely, secretory phospholipase A_2 and steroid sulfatase (both with a near-neutral pH-optimum) and sphingomyelinase and beta-glucocerebrosidase (both with an acidic pH-optimum). These enzymes are responsible for a coordinated maturation of the extruded lipid sheets from lamellar bodies to lamellar bilayers.

Topical application of physiologic lipids has effects distinct from those of nonphysiologic lipids, like petrolatum. Studies have shown that topical application of only one or two of the three physiologic lipids to a disrupted hairless mouse skin impedes rather than facilitates barrier recovery, as evidenced by changes in transepidermal water loss (25). However, if members of all three key lipid classes (i.e., cholesterol, ceramide, and free fatty acid or their precursors) are applied together to barrier-disrupted skin, normalized rates of barrier repair can be observed (25,29). The topically applied physiologic lipids are not only concentrated in the SC membrane domains, but also delivered to the nucleated layers of the epidermis (25,29). Depending on the composition of the lipid mixture, either normal or abnormal lamellar bodies are formed, ultimately resulting in either normal or abnormal lamellar membrane unit structures in the SC intercellular spaces (25,29). The process of passive lipid transport across the SC as well as the uptake into nucleated cells (SG) are important. It appears that the incorporation of applied physiologic lipids into barrier lipids follows two pathways: First, direct incorporation into SC membrane domains; second, lipids appear to traverse the intercellular route in the SC, and ultimately get incorporated into lower SG cells. The intercellular lipids then appear able to enter the nucleated cells, incorporate into the appropriate lipid metabolic pathway(s), and ultimately utilize the lamellar body delivery system to re-enter the intercellular membrane domains (29). Topically applied lipids to either intact or acetone-treated skin did not down-regulate the physiological lipid synthesis (29,30).

In contrast, nonphysiologic lipids like petrolatum appear to simply form a bulk hydrophobic phase in the SC intercellular spaces to restore the permeability barrier under similar conditions (29,31). The same studies showed further enhancement of barrier recovery if the proportion of one of the fatty acids (linoleic acid, palmitic acid, or stearic acid) or the other key species was augmented to threefold in a four-component system consisting of fatty acid, ceramide, cholesterol, and essential fatty acids in a 3:1:1:1 ratio (32). Interestingly, the structural requirements of this lipid mixture are not restricted to essential fatty acids; findings were confirmed in similarly disrupted human barrier (32). Acylceramides applied as a single agent delayed barrier recovery. However, acylceramides in a mixture with cholesterol (optimum ratio of 1.5:1 or 1:2) also revealed accelerated barrier recovery after acute barrier disruption (32). These findings were confirmed as accelerated barrier repair was noted using a similar formulation after tape stripping, solvent treatment, and some types of detergent treatment (33). Specifically, topical application of the physiologic lipids cholesterol, ceramide, palmitate, and linoleate in the ratio of 4.3:2.3:1:1.08 showed enhanced barrier recovery. However, it must be noted that, in barrier repair vs. hydration studies, correlations between moisturizing properties and barrier repair mechanism of applied lipid mixtures are not always evident. Actually, the best hydrating lipid composition is often different from the optimal barrier repair formulation (34).

Barrier Protection and Barrier Recovery

A number of factors are involved in the determination of the effectiveness of dermatological and PCs to protect skin barrier. Commonly used barrier creams, which are either w/o emulsions or PCs with strongly lipophilic character, are claimed to protect against hydrophilic irritants. On the other hand, barrier creams that are o/w emulsion systems, or act like hydrophilic systems, are mistakenly thought to protect against lipophilic irritants. Dermatological skin protection (especially in work conditions) is based on different product groups in situations where barrier or PCs are employed. For example, pre-exposure skin care includes the use of o/w and w/o emulsions, tannery substances, zinc oxide, talcum, perfluorpolyethers, chelating agents, and UV protectors (35). However, cleansing products and post-exposure skin care are two other important components of skin protection. The post-exposure skin care is based on dermatological and PCs, long-term moisturizers, fast humectants, and lipid-rich formulations. Although, protective effects have been shown using specific test conditions, double-blinded, placebo-controlled, randomized trials are still lacking, especially under conditions that approximate real workplace situation(s) (35). In fact, cumulative stress tests with repetitive application of irritants appear to be the best methods for approximating work conditions (35–41).

The distinction between skin protection and skin care is not always clear. For example, in nurses, a barrier cream was compared with its vehicle for effects on clinical improvement. Interestingly, both clinical skin status as well as SC hydration improved significantly in each treatment group, without evidence of a difference between the vehicle and the barrier cream groups (42). Thus, Berndt and colleagues (42) proposed to abolish the distinctions between skin care and skin protection products. Correct instructions for the consumer use should be stressed with regard to regular and frequent application of a protection product in order to be effective (43). In addition, a recent study discussed whether claims could be made with respect to protective and preventive properties of topically applied body lotions and barrier creams (44). In this particular study, enhanced SC hydration, improved barrier function, as well as a faster barrier recovery were reported after sodium lauryl sulfate (SLS)-barrier disruption (44).

Exposure to tensides represents a common potential workplace irritant. Protection against tensides seems to be more effective with lipid-enriched, lipid external-phase emollient, such as w/o emulsions (36). In contrast, Held and colleagues (45) showed that a 4 week pretreatment of normal skin with some w/o protective creams increases susceptibility to detergents (SLS). Incorporation of high amounts of emulsifiers into the vehicle and subsequently emulsifying the intercorneocyte lipids could be the reason for the controversial results. Moreover, emulsifiers can act as carrier of aggressive substances, enhancing their penetration into the skin. Alternatively, the deposited lipids can function as traps (solvents) for tensioactive molecules. Thus, the long-term application of barrier creams in working conditions where detergents are present should be carefully evaluated.

Clinical observations have established the fact that skin irritants are more harmful in dry skin conditions. Therefore, vehicles often are used to increase the water content of the SC (46) as a preventive measure (47). Moisturizer-containing PCs prevent irritant skin reactions induced by detergents, and may also accelerate the regeneration of permeability barrier function in irritated skin (48). PCs with moisturizing properties, usually contain either single or in combination humectants, such as ammonia, lactic, citric, and pyrrolidone carboxylic acids and their salts, urea, glycerol, sorbitol, and amino acids. Most of these agents belong to a group considered NMF, as they are similar to the blend of hydrosoluble ingredients found in the SC. Their common properties include the increase of hydration and the enhancement of water-binding capacity in the upper SC. Reduced NMF content in the SC can diminish water-absorption capacity and may result in perturbation of corneodesmolysis leading to hyperkeratosis (49). It has been shown that dry environmental conditions increase epidermal DNA synthesis and amplifies the hyperproliferative response to barrier disruption (50–52). Furthermore, changes in environmental humidity contribute to the seasonal exacerbations/amelioration of cutaneous disorders, such as atopic dermatitis and psoriasis, the diseases which are characterized by a defective barrier, epidermal hyperplasia, and inflammation (50). Application of topical glycerol prevented the epidermal hyperplasia, and dermal mast cell hypertrophy, and degranulation induced by exposure to low humidity (53).

PCs with barrier properties also can prevent certain types of epidermal damage. For example, Fartasch and colleagues (54) have shown that alterations in the lower part of SC and damage to the nucleated layers of the epidermis are induced by SLS. In this model, formation of lamellar lipid membrane structures was disturbed in the lower SC. In contrast, the upper SC showed intact intercellular lipid bilayers. The barrier disruption effect of SLS was prevented by the application of a barrier cream with diminished SLS penetration as the likely mechanism (54).

Since Suskind (55) introduced the "slide test" to evaluate PCs in the 1950s various *in vitro* techniques and *in vivo* tests on animal or human skin were developed to investigate the efficacy of PCs as pre-exposure skin protectors (56–58). In recent years, noninvasive biophysical measurements have achieved great importance, especially for clinically weak reactions. Mahmoud and Lachapelle (59,60) showed PCs to have some effects against the acute irritative and locally toxic action of solvents using skin biopsies and Doppler flowmetry. Also, using a guinea pig model, Frosch et al. (40,61) carried out cumulative irritation by SLS, sodium hydroxide, and TOL. Irritation was measured by a visual score and biophysiological techniques (evaporimetry and Doppler velocimetry).

Considering human models for PC evaluation, Frosch et al. (39) proposed the model of a repetitive irritation test to examine efficacy of barrier creams in a human test model. Thirty minutes after treatment with two different products, SLS was applied to the ventral forearm of healthy volunteers daily for 2 weeks. Cutaneous irritation was evaluated by a visual score, evaporimetry, laser-Doppler velocimetry, and colorimetry. The authors observed a significant suppression of irritancy with one of the tested creams. In a subsequent paper, Frosch and Kurte (41) reported on the RIT with a set of four standard irritants (10% SLS, 1% NaOH, 30% lactic acid and undiluted TOL) using the mid-back as a larger area than the forearm. Thus, three products could be compared simultaneously to a nonpretreated control site. The irritant cutaneous reactions were quantified by erythema score, transepidermal water loss, blood flow volume, and SC hydration. The tested products demonstrated a specific profile of efficacy against the four irritants used. Using the RIT, our group showed that four products tested were very effective against 10% SLS and three products showed a partial protective effect against all ionic irritants (62). However, the necessity of a 2 week period of cumulative irritation is still discussed and a model with a repeated irritation at the forearms has been evaluated for further testings (38,63). Grunewald et al. (36) developed a repetitive washing procedure with SLS on the forearms for 7 days, demonstrating protection of skin function for the tested creams. Zhai and Maibach (64) presented an *in vivo* method using cyanoacrylate strips of protected skin samples to measure the effectiveness of PCs against two dye-indicator solutions: methylene blue in water and oil red O in ethanol, representatives of model hydrophilic and lipophilic compounds. One formulation was protective against the permeation of methylene blue and oil red O, whereas the other was protective against oil red O only.

Protective Creams with Special Ingredients

Some ingredients are claimed to have special protective properties such as natural or synthetic tannery substances, zinc oxide, talcum, chelating agents, or other substances that can bind metal ions or reduce the penetration through the skin. Zinc oxide exerts a covering effect. Tannin is supposed to act as an astringent to the skin increasing the mechanical resistance of the skin surface against micro traumas. Additionally, tannery agents cause a local decrease of perspiration as it seems to be helpful while wearing gloves (65). The decrease of corneocyte swelling is caused by direct binding of the tanning substance to keratin. Chelating agents are used in order to protect against sensitizing substances. Tartaric acid and glycine chelate chromate reduce chrome VI to chrome III, which is less allergenic (66). DPTA has shown to significantly decrease the number and the severity of patch test reactions in subjects with contact dermatitis due to nickel sulfate (67). EDTA can bind nickel ions as well and prevent them from penetration into the skin, but its own allergenic potency limits the therapeutical use (68).

Perfluorpolyethers have some benefit in the prevention of irritation due to hydrophilic and lipophilic substances (69). As petrolatum is effective against water-soluble and water-insoluble irritants, it was recommended as a standard substance against which PCs may be compared (70). Although PCs have been shown to reduce ACD in sensitized individuals under experimental conditions (71,72), their use in the prevention of ACD has been disappointing under practical conditions. However, recent publications indicate a benefit for some PCs used as "active" creams in the prevention of ACD like nickel dermatitis or poison oak dermatitis (66,73–77).

APPLICATION

PCs should be applied before contact to irritants which includes an application after each break. It is clear that for PCs to be effective, they must be applied frequently enough in adequate amounts and to all skin areas that need protection. Particularly, proper application with attention to the interdigital spaces should be performed. In a recent study, a simple method is described to determine and quantify how exactly self-application of a PC was performed at the workplace. Using a fluorescence technique, it could be visualized that the application was mostly incomplete in different professional groups (43), especially in the dorsal aspects of the hands and wrists (78). These findings indicate that in washing their hands many people miss certain areas. Also in the application of PCs, these misses are frequent. Individuals should apply the cream systematically in anatomic regions, ensuring that each region is adequately covered. To improve the daily application, instructive brochures may be given to the workers but they are usually not very successful. It was shown that the fluorescence technique is also a useful tool in the educational demonstration of the most common mistakes compared with the use of an instructive videotape (79).

ADVERSE EFFECTS AND CONTRAINDICATIONS

Some authors reported a satisfactory protective action of PCs, whereas others found no protection from or even aggravation of ICD. A foamy "skin protector" was not convincing in a guinea pig model; moreover, it had an aggravating effect of the irritation due to NaOH (61). Also, using a guinea pig model, Goh (80) showed that treatment with PC increases skin irritation induced by cutting oil fluids. Bomann and Mellström (81) showed that absorption of butanol through stripped skin treated with PC was higher than absorption through skin not treated this way. Recently, a PC was shown to cause an amplification of inflammation by TOL (62) and the protective properties against systemic absorption of solvents are less than adequate (81–83).

Besides less efficacy against irritants or even amplification of barrier damage, the creams themselves can induce ICD or ACD (84,85). Preservatives, cream bases such as woolwax alcohols, emulsifiers, and fragrances are potential allergens. Preparations marketed as "invisible glove" may feign a seeming protection that causes workers at risk to be careless of contact to irritants. Additionally, it is of utmost importance to apply PCs on intact skin only. They are not intended to be used on diseased skin, because of some irritant properties of many formulations (86–88).

CONCLUSION

Current PCs are still not perfect. Much effort is necessary to develop products that will give more protection and few side effects. Efficacy and cosmetical acceptance are both important qualities of PCs to be used for protective success at the workplace but the knowledge of how they are used correctly is a basic factor. Their benefit in the prevention of ICD and ACD has to be evaluated in controlled studies. Results of animal experiments may not be valid for humans, particularly when dealing with irritants, in view of their complex action mechanisms and the high interindividual variability in susceptibility of human skin (64). Thus, confirmatory studies of animal data in humans are necessary. Regarding the various models to investigate the efficacy of PCs, the validation of a sensitive, standardized, and widely accepted model proved by interlaboratory standardization or controlled clinical studies at the workplace seems to be necessary. Studies both under experimental conditions and in the workplace situation are needed in order to allow a rational recommendation for product safety and effective skin protection. The benefit of various PCs cannot be extensive and complete in all cases but only against individual irritants. The data of *in vitro* and *in vivo* tests underline the importance of careful selection of PCs for specific workplaces. Choosing the wrong preparation may well worsen the effect of an irritant. On the basis of the presented data, PCs should be used critically according to the noxious substances used at the workplace and complete labeling of the ingredients of PCs should be given on the packages.

REFERENCES

1. Leveque JL et al. Are corneocytes elastic? Dermatologica 1988; 176(2):65–69.
2. Engelke M, et al. Effects of xerosis and ageing on epidermal proliferation and differentiation. Br J Dermatol 1997; 137(2):219–225.
3. Fluhr JW et al. Glycerol regulates stratum corneum hydration in sebaceous gland deficient (Asebia) mice. J Invest Dermatol 2003; 120(5):728–737.
4. Jokura Y et al. Molecular analysis of elastic properties of the stratum corneum by solid-state 13C-nuclear magnetic resonance spectroscopy. J Invest Dermatol 1995; 104(5):806–812.
5. Denda M et al. Low humidity stimulates epidermal DNA synthesis and amplifies the hyperproliferative response to barrier disruption: implication for seasonal exacerbations of inflammatory dermatoses. J Invest Dermatol 1998; 111(5):873–878.
6. Sato J et al. Water content and thickness of the stratum corneum contribute to skin surface morphology. Arch Dermatol Res 2000; 292(8):412–417.
7. Wigger-Alberti W, Elsner P. Preventive measures in contact dermatitis. Clin Dermatol 1997; 15(4):661–665.
8. De Paepe K et al. Beneficial effects of a skin tolerance-tested moisturizing cream on the barrier function in experimentally-elicited irritant and allergic contact dermatitis. Contact Dermatitis 2001; 44(6):337–343.
9. Chamlin SL et al. Ceramide-dominant barrier repair lipids alleviate childhood atopic dermatitis: changes in barrier function provide a sensitive indicator of disease activity. J Am Acad Dermatol 2002; 47(2):198–208.
10. Billmann-Eberwein C et al. Modulation of atopy patch test reactions by topical treatment of human skin with a fatty acid-rich emollient. Skin Pharmacol Appl Skin Physiol 2002; 15(2):100–104.
11. Blichmann CW, Serup J, Winther A. Effects of single application of a moisturizer: evaporation of emulsion water, skin surface temperature, electrical conductance, electrical capacitance, and skin surface (emulsion) lipids. Acta Dermatol Venereol 1989; 69(4):327–330.
12. Loden M. The increase in skin hydration after application of emollients with different amounts of lipids. Acta Dermatol Venereol 1992; 72(5):327–330.

13. Fluhr JW, Vrzak G, Gloor M. Hydratisierender und die Steroidpenetration modifizierender Effekt von Harnstoff und Glycerin in Abhängigkeit von der verwendeten Grundlage. Z Hautkr 1998; 73:210–214.
14. Gloor M, Gehring W. Increase in hydration and protective function of horny layer by glycerol and a w/o emulsion: are these effects maintained during long-term use? Contact Dermatitis 2001; 44(2):123–125.
15. Loden M, Barany E. Skin-identical lipids versus petrolatum in the treatment of tape-stripped and detergent-perturbed human skin. Acta Dermatol Venereol 2000; 80(6):412–415.
16. Lehmann L et al. Stability and occlusitivity of dermatological ointments. H & G Zeitschrift für Hautkrankheiten 1997; 8:585–590.
17. Fluhr JW et al. Glycerol accelerates recovery of barrier function in vivo. Acta Dermatol Venereol 1999; 79(6):418–421.
18. Batt M, Fairhust E. Hydration of the stratum corneum. Int J Cosmet Sci 1986; 8:253–264.
19. Hara M, Ma T, Verkman AS. Selectively reduced glycerol in skin of aquaporin-3-deficient mice may account for impaired skin hydration, elasticity, and barrier recovery. J Biol Chem 2002; 277(48):46616–46621.
20. Jemec GB, Na R, Wulf HC. The inherent capacitance of moisturising creams: a source of false positive results? Skin Pharmacol Appl Skin Physiol 2000; 13(3–4):182–187.
21. Elias PM, Feingold KR. Lipids and the epidermal water barrier: metabolism, regulation, and pathophysiology. Semin Dermatol 1992; 11(2):176–182.
22. Schurer NY, Elias PM. The biochemistry and function of stratum corneum lipids. Adv Lipid Res 1991; 24:27–56.
23. Feingold KR et al. Cholesterol synthesis is required for cutaneous barrier function in mice. J Clin Invest 1990; 86(5):1738–1745.
24. Holleran WM et al. Regulation of epidermal sphingolipid synthesis by permeability barrier function. J Lipid Res 1991; 32(7):1151–1158.
25. Mao-Qiang M, Elias PM, Feingold KR. Fatty acids are required for epidermal permeability barrier function. J Clin Invest 1993; 92(2):791–798.
26. Elias PM, Menon GK. Structural and lipid biochemical correlates of the epidermal permeability barrier. Adv Lipid Res 1991; 24:1–26.
27. Menon GK, Feingold KR, Elias PM. Lamellar body secretory response to barrier disruption. J Invest Dermatol 1992; 98(3):279–289.
28. Fartasch M, Bassukas ID, Diepgen TL. Structural relationship between epidermal lipid lamellae, lamellar bodies and desmosomes in human epidermis: an ultrastructural study. Br J Dermatol 1993; 128(1):1–9.
29. Mao-Qiang M et al. Exogenous nonphysiologic vs. physiologic lipids. Divergent mechanisms for correction of permeability barrier dysfunction. Arch Dermatol 1995; 131(7):809–816.
30. Menon GK et al. *De novo* sterologenesis in the skin. II. Regulation by cutaneous barrier requirements. J Lipid Res 1985; 26(4):418–427.
31. Ghadially R, Halkier-Sorensen L, Elias PM. Effects of petrolatum on stratum corneum structure and function. J Am Acad Dermatol 1992; 26(3 Pt 2):387–396.
32. Man MM et al. Optimization of physiological lipid mixtures for barrier repair. J Invest Dermatol 1996; 106(5):1096–1101.

33. Yang L et al. Topical stratum corneum lipids accelerate barrier repair after tape stripping, solvent treatment and some but not all types of detergent treatment. Br J Dermatol 1995; 133(5):679–685.
34. Thornfeldt CR. Critical and optimal molar ratios of key lipids. In: Loden M, Maibach HI, eds. Dry Skin and Moisturizers: Chemistry and Function. Boca Raton: CRC Press LLC, 2000:337–348.
35. Wigger-Alberti W, Krebs A, Elsner P. Experimental irritant contact dermatitis due to cumulative epicutaneous exposure to sodium lauryl sulphate and toluene: single and concurrent application. Br J Dermatol 2000; 143(3):551–556.
36. Grunewald A et al. Efficacy of skin barrier creams. In: Elsner P, Maibach HI, eds. Irritant Dermatitis: New Clinical and Experimental Aspects. Basel: Karger, 1995:187–197.
37. Wigger-Alberti W, Hinnen U, Elsner P. Predictive testing of metalworking fluids: a comparison of 2 cumulative human irritation models and correlation with epidemiological data. Contact Dermatitis 1997; 36(1):14–20.
38. Wigger-Alberti W et al. Efficacy of protective creams in a modified repeated irritation test. Methodological aspects. Acta Dermatol Venereol 1998; 78(4):270–273.
39. Frosch PJ, Kurte A, Pilz B. Efficacy of skin barrier creams (III). The repetitive irritation test (RIT) in humans. Contact Dermatitis 1993; 29(3):113–118.
40. Frosch PJ et al. Efficacy of skin barrier creams (I). The repetitive irritation test (RIT) in the guinea pig. Contact Dermatitis 1993; 28(2):94–100.
41. Frosch PJ, Kurte A. Efficacy of skin barrier creams (IV). The repetitive irritation test (RIT) with a set of 4 standard irritants. Contact Dermatitis 1994; 31(3):161–168.
42. Berndt U et al. Efficacy of a barrier cream and its vehicle as protective measures against occupational irritant contact dermatitis. Contact Dermatitis 2000; 42(2):77–80.
43. Wigger-Alberti W et al. Self-application of a protective cream. Pitfalls of occupational skin protection. Arch Dermatol 1997; 133(7):861–864.
44. De Paepe K, et al. Incorporation of ceramide 3B in dermatocosmetic emulsions: effect on the transepidermal water loss of sodium lauryl sulphate-damaged skin. J Eur Acad Dermatol Venereol 2000; 14(4):272–279.
45. Held E, Sveinsdottir S, Agner T. Effect of long-term use of moisturizer on skin hydration, barrier function and susceptibility to irritants. Acta Dermatol Venereol 1999; 79(1):49–51.
46. Gloor M et al. Triclosan, a topical dermatologic agent. *In vitro* and *in vivo* studies on the effectiveness of a new preparation in the New German Formulary. Hautarzt 2002; 53(11):724–729.
47. Zhai H, Maibach HI. Moisturizers in preventing irritant contact dermatitis: an overview. Contact Dermatitis 1998; 38(5):241–244.
48. Ramsing DW, Agner T. Preventive and therapeutic effects of a moisturizer. An experimental study of human skin. Acta Dermatol Venereol 1997; 77(5):335–337.
49. Watkinson A et al. Water modulation of stratum corneum chymotryptic enzyme activity and desquamation. Arch Dermatol Res 2001; 293(9):470–476.
50. Denda M et al. Low humidity stimulates epidermal DNA synthesis and amplifies the hyperproliferative response to barrier disruption: implication for seasonal exacerbations of inflammatory dermatoses. J Invest Dermatol 1998; 111(5):873–878.

51. Sato J, et al. Drastic decrease in environmental humidity decreases water-holding capacity and free amino acid content of the stratum corneum. Arch Dermatol Res 2001; 293(9):477–480.
52. Sato J, et al. Abrupt decreases in environmental humidity induce abnormalities in permeability barrier homeostasis. J Invest Dermatol 2002; 119(4):900–904.
53. Denda M, et al. Exposure to a dry environment enhances epidermal permeability barrier function. J Invest Dermatol 1998; 111(5):858–863.
54. Fartasch M, Schnetz E, Diepgen TL. Characterization of detergent-induced barrier alterations—effect of barrier cream on irritation. J Invest Dermatol Symp Proc 1998; 3(2):121–127.
55. Suskind RR. The present status of silicone protective creams. Ind Med Surg 1955; 24:413–416.
56. Marks R, Dykes PJ, Hamami I. Two novel techniques for the evaluation of barrier creams. Br J Dermatol 1989; 120(5):655–660.
57. Treffel P, Gabard B, Juch R. Evaluation of barrier creams: an *in vitro* technique on human skin. Acta Dermatol Venereol 1994; 74(1):7–11.
58. Tronnier H. Methodische Ansätze zur Prüfung von Hautschutzmitteln. Dermatosen 1993; 41:100–107.
59. Mahmoud G, Lachapelle JM, van Neste D. Histological assessment of skin damage by irritants: its possible use in the evaluation of a 'barrier cream'. Contact Dermatitis 1984; 11(3):179–185.
60. Mahmoud G, Lachapelle JM. Evaluation of the protective value of an antisolvent gel by laser Doppler flowmetry and histology. Contact Dermatitis 1985; 13(1):14–19.
61. Frosch PJ et al. Efficacy of skin barrier creams (II). Ineffectiveness of a popular "skin protector" against various irritants in the repetitive irritation test in the guinea pig. Contact Dermatitis 1993; 29(2):74–77.
62. Schluter-Wigger W, Elsner P. Efficacy of 4 commercially available PCs in the repetitive irritation test (RIT). Contact Dermatitis 1996; 34(4):278–283.
63. Wigger-Alberti W et al. Experimentally induced chronic irritant contact dermatitis to evaluate the efficacy of protective creams in vivo. J Am Acad Dermatol 1999; 40(4):590–596.
64. Zhai H, Maibach HI. Effect of barrier creams: human skin in vivo. Contact Dermatitis 1996; 35(2):92–96.
65. Jepsen JR, Sparre Jorgensen A, Kyst A. Hand protection for car-painters. Contact Dermatitis 1985; 13(5):317–320.
66. Romaguera C et al. Formulation of a barrier cream against chromate. Contact Dermatitis 1985; 13(2):49–52.
67. Wohrl S et al. A cream containing the chelator DTPA (diethylenetriaminepenta-acetic acid) can prevent contact allergic reactions to metals. Contact Dermatitis 2001; 44(4):224–228.
68. Kimura M, Kawada A. Contact dermatitis due to trisodium ethylenediaminetetra-acetic acid (EDTA) in a cosmetic lotion. Contact Dermatitis 1999; 41(6):341.
69. Elsner P, Wigger-Alberti W, Pantini G. Perfluoropolyethers in the prevention of irritant contact dermatitis. Dermatology 1998; 197(2):141–145.
70. Wigger-Alberti W, Elsner P. Petrolatum prevents irritation in a human cumulative exposure model in vivo. Dermatology 1997; 194(3):247–250.
71. Blanken R, Nater JP, Veenhoff E. Protective effect of barrier creams and spray coatings against epoxy resins. Contact Dermatitis 1987; 16(2):79–83.

72. Schuppli R, Ziegler G. New possibilities of skin protection against metals. Z Haut Geschlechtskr 1967; 42(10):345–348.
73. Gawkrodger DJ, Healy J, Howe AM. The prevention of nickel contact dermatitis. A review of the use of binding agents and barrier creams. Contact Dermatitis 1995; 32(5):257–265.
74. Fullerton A, Menne T. In vitro and in vivo evaluation of the effect of barrier gels in nickel contact allergy. Contact Dermatitis 1995; 32(2):100–106.
75. Menne T. Prevention of nickel allergy by regulation of specific exposures. Ann Clin Lab Sci 1996; 26(2):133–138.
76. Grevelink SA, Murrell DF, Olsen EA. Effectiveness of various barrier preparations in preventing and/or ameliorating experimentally produced toxicodendron dermatitis. J Am Acad Dermatol 1992; 27(2 Pt 1):182–188.
77. Marks JG Jr et al. Prevention of poison ivy and poison oak allergic contact dermatitis by quaternium-18 bentonite. J Am Acad Dermatol 1995; 33(2 Pt 1):212–216.
78. Bankova L et al. Influence of the galenic form of a skin-protective preparation on the application pattern assessed by a fluorescence method. Exogen Dermatol 2003; 1:313–318.
79. Wigger-Alberti W et al. Training workers at risk for occupational contact dermatitis in the application of PCs: efficacy of a fluorescence technique. Dermatology 1997; 195(2):129–133.
80. Goh CL. Cutting oil dermatitis on guinea pig skin (I). Cutting oil dermatitis and barrier cream. Contact Dermatitis 1991; 24(1):16–21.
81. Boman A, Mellstrom G. Percutaneous absorption of 3 organic solvents in the guinea pig. (III). Effect of barrier creams. Contact Dermatitis 1989; 21(3):134–140.
82. Lauwerys RR, et al. The influence of two barrier creams on the percutaneous absorption of m-xylene in man. J Occup Med 1978; 20(1):17–20.
83. Boman A, Wahlberg JE, Johansson G. A method for the study of the effect of barrier creams and protective gloves on the percutaneous absorption of solvents. Dermatologica 1982; 164(3):157–160.
84. Gupta BN et al. Safety evaluation of a barrier cream. Contact Dermatitis 1987; 17(1):10–12.
85. Pinola A et al. Occupational allergic contact dermatitis due to coconut diethanolamide (cocamide DEA). Contact Dermatitis 1993; 29(5):262–265.
86. Lapachelle J. Efficacy of protective creams and/or gels. In: Elsner P et al., eds. Prevention of Contact Dermatitis. Basel: Karger, 1996:182–192.
87. Fowler JF Jr. Treatment of occupational dermatitis. In: Hogan DJ, ed. Occupational Skin Disorders. New York: Igaka-Shoin, 1994:104–111.
88. Hogan DJ. The prognosis of hand eczema. In: Menné T, Maibach HI, eds. Hand Eczema. Boca Raton: CRC Press, 1993:285–292.

16

Sebum

Philip W. Wertz
University of Iowa, Iowa City, IA, USA
Bozena B. Michniak
New Jersey Center for Biomaterials, Newark, NJ, USA

Sebaceous Glands	307
Anatomy	307
Distribution	308
Sebum Secretion	308
Methods for Measurement	308
Hormonal Control	309
Variation with Age and Gender	310
Sebum Composition	310
Human	310
Lipid Class Composition	310
Fatty Chains	311
Other Species	313
Sebum in Health	313
Sebum in Disease—Acne	314
References	315

SEBACEOUS GLANDS

Anatomy

Sebaceous glands are multilobular holocrine glands generally associated with hair follicles (1). The basal sebocytes sit on a basal membrane at the outer limits of the lobes, and as cells move from the basal layer toward the lumen of the gland they synthesize lipids, which accumulate as intracellular lipid droplets. As they synthesize lipid, the cells become larger, and the nucleus and other internal organelles are degraded. Ultimately, the entire mass of the cell is converted into a viscous liquid phase lipid mixture. In most pilosebaceous units, sebum passes from the sebaceous gland into the hair follicle via the short sebaceous duct and outward onto the skin surface through the follicle. Generally, the hair follicle is large compared with the associated sebaceous gland; however, large sebaceous glands are associated with vellous hairs. These units are called sebaceous follicles and predominate on the forehead and cheeks.

Distribution

Pilosebaceous units are found over the entire surface of the skin except for the palmar and plantar regions (2). The density of follicles is greatest on the head, neck, and shoulders. In adults, the density of follicles on the scalp and face is in the range of 310–900 per cm^2 (1,3,4). On the torso and limbs, the density of follicles is generally <100 per cm^2 (3). Large sebaceous glands are present in the submucosal connective tissue of the lip and buccal mucosa (5,6). These sebaceous glands in the oral mucosa often appear as slightly raised yellow spots and are called Fordyce spots. Specialized sebaceous glands are also present on the edge of the eyelid (7) and the areolae of the nipples (3).

Sebum Secretion

Methods for Measurement

Early attempts to measure sebum secretion rates involved removal of lipid from the skin surface, followed by protection of a defined area of skin for a standard time (8,9). At the end of the timed interval, lipids were collected by extraction and analyzed either gravimetrically or chromatographically. These extraction-based methods tended to remove sebum from the follicles as well as some of the epidermal lipid from the stratum corneum. Therefore, methods based on direct extraction invariably overestimated the amount of lipid on the skin surface.

More recent investigations of sebum secretion have been based on adsorption of sebum as it is secreted. The adsorbents used for this purpose have included cigarette paper (10,11), bentonite gel (12), and Sebutape (Cuderm Corporation, Dallas, TX; 13,14). Sebutape turns translucent at the sites where sebum is secreted. This enables one to qualitatively assess sebum secretion rates by visual inspection (13). The sebutape is placed on a black background and compared with a set of reference patterns provided by the manufacturer. Five qualitative patterns are recognized. These include prepubescent, adolescent, acne, adult, and elderly. Alternatively, a more quantitative assessment can be achieved by image analysis (15), although the calibration and accuracy of the method have not been rigorously established. It is also possible to extract lipids from the sebutape and to quantitate them using thin-layer chromatography (14). With all three methods, the most frequent site of measurement has been the forehead, and the skin surface is depleted of sebum at the outset of measurement.

With the cigarette paper method, the paper is delipidized by extraction with ethyl ether. After thorough drying, the paper is held in contact with the skin surface by means of a gauze strip. After a defined standardized collection time, the paper is removed, adsorbed lipids are extracted into ethyl ether and analyzed. Total lipid can be determined by evaporating the solution onto a tared aluminum planchet or by thin-layer chromatography in conjunction with photodensitometry (16). The latter analytical method gives composition in addition to total amount. Although the cigarette paper method has been useful, it tends to overestimate the sebum secretion because the paper tends to deplete sebum from the follicular reservoir in addition to that which would have been secreted in the absence of an adsorbent.

The complications introduced by the follicular reservoir were most effectively addressed by the bentonite method (12). In this method, bentonite gel is applied to the forehead 14 h before the start of the measurement period, and this bentonite coating is replaced after 6 h. This pretreatment completely depletes the follicular reservoir of excess sebum. At the beginning of the measurement period, two small dacron disks are imbedded in freshly applied bentonite near the center of the depleted region. After 3 h, the disks are removed, and the lipids are extracted into ethyl ether and analyzed by quantitative thin-layer chromatography. This method yields the sustainable sebum secretion rate, which should reflect the rate at which sebum is synthesized. Although this method has been used in several studies of great importance which are cited below, it has not been widely used. This is, at least in part, because the suitability of bentonite for this application varies from one batch to another.

The currently most widely used method for studying sebum secretion is based on a porous polymeric tape called Sebutape. This material is coated with a weak adhesive sufficient to hold it in contact with the skin. As sebum is secreted from the orifice of a follicle, it is adsorbed into the pores in the polymer, and this turns the appearance of the tape from opaque to transparent. Densitometric and computer assisted image analysis methodology can yield information on the sebum secretion rate per unit area of skin or per follicle as well as a follicle density (15).

A more extensive review of the discussed methods as well as several variant methods based on the decrease in light scattering of a rough surface when it becomes coated with lipid has recently been published (17).

Hormonal Control

Sebaceous glands are stimulated by androgenic hormones produced by the testes, ovaries, and adrenal glands (3,18–20). Testosterone and androstenediol are produced by the testes. The ovaries also produce some testosterone, androstenediol, and dehydroepiandrosterone; however, the significance of these steroidal hormones in regulation of female sebaceous gland activity is uncertain. Dehydroepiandrosterone and dehydroepiandrosterone sulfate produced by the adrenal glands are the major circulating androgens in women and are also significant in men. In the sebocytes, the androgenic hormone binds to a cytosolic receptor, which then translocates to the nucleus and modulates gene expression (21–23).

Variation with Age and Gender

Sebaceous gland activity is high *in utero*, and this is responsible for production of the vernix caseosa, a coating of sebaceous lipid and exfoliated stratum corneum material that coats the newborn (24). By 1 year after birth, the sebum secretion rate is extremely low and remains so until the onset of puberty (25). At that time, the increased concentrations of androgenic hormones cause a rapid increase in sebum secretion rates. Although there is great individual variation in sebum secretion rates, on average sebum secretion rates begin to decline in the late teen years (26). This decline continues for the remainder of life. Although there is considerable overlap, the average sebum secretion rate at any given age is greater for men than for women (26).

SEBUM COMPOSITION

Human

Lipid Class Composition

Human sebum from isolated sebaceous glands consists mainly of squalene, wax esters, and triglycerides with small proportions of cholesterol and cholesterol esters (27). As this viscous liquid flows outward through the follicle, lipases of both microbial and epithelial origin hydrolyze some of the triglycerides (28). Thus, sebum collected from the skin surface has a reduced proportion of triglycerides compared with sebum from the lumen of the gland, and free fatty acids are now present. The extent of triglyceride hydrolysis varies widely. Representative compositions of sebum expressed from isolated glands and from the skin surface are summarized in Fig. 1. The large error bars associated with the triglyceride and fatty acid fractions from the skin surface lipid reflect the variability in triglyceride hydrolysis. Representative structures of the major sebaceous lipids are illustrated in Fig. 2. Squalene is normally an intermediate in the synthesis of cholesterol (31); however, in differentiating sebocytes the enzymes beyond this point in the biosynthetic pathway are not expressed. The small proportions of cholesterol and cholesterol esters present in sebum are derived from the original basal sebocyte membranes. It is also noteworthy that the wax ester fraction consists of fatty acids ester-linked to primary fatty alcohols.

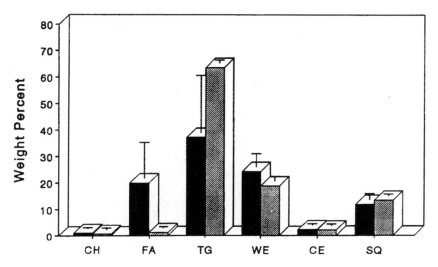

Figure 1 Composition of neutral, nonpolar lipids from the skin surface (solid bars) and isolated sebaceous glands (shaded bars). Error bars indicate 1 standard deviation. CH, cholesterol; FA, fatty acid; TG, triglyceride; WE, wax ester; CE, cholesterol ester; SQ, squalene. [Data from Downing et al. (29) and Stewart et al. (30).]

Fatty Chains

Unsaturated Species: The proportions of saturated and unsaturated fatty acids vary markedly among the several ester lipid classes in human sebum (24,27). The wax ester fraction contains ~60% monounsaturated and 40%

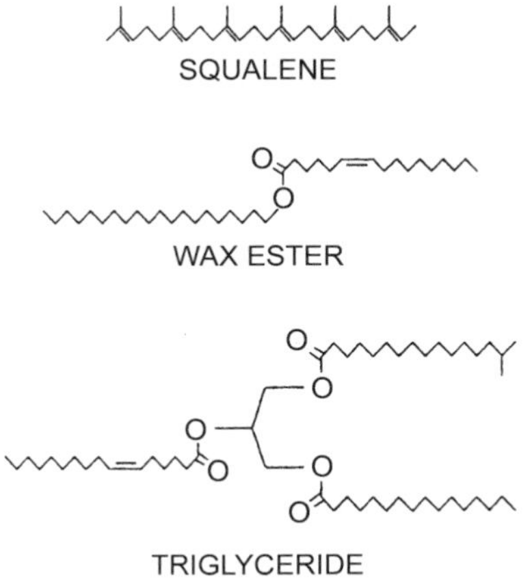

Figure 2 Representative structures of the major lipid classes of human sebum.

saturated fatty acids (24); whereas, in the cholesterol ester fraction 65% of the fatty acids are saturated and 30% are monounsaturated (24). Small proportions of dienoic acids are present in sebum (24,32). Both linoleic acid (C18:2 Δ9,12) and the Δ5,8 isomer of linoleic acid have been identified (32). The Δ9,12 isomer is derived from the diet (33); whereas, the Δ5,8 isomer is synthesized in the gland. Interestingly, the proportion of the Δ5,8 isomer relative to Δ9,12 is increased in acne patients (32). In the triglyceride fraction, the saturated and monounsaturated fatty acids comprise 70% and 30%, respectively (34). Most of the monounsaturated fatty acids are derived from C16:1 Δ6, or to a much lesser extent 18:1 Δ9, by extension or removal of 2-carbon units, and a small percentage of the monounsaturated fatty chains have iso or anteiso methyl branches (24,27). The chain lengths of the monounsaturates are almost entirely within the range of 14 through 18 carbons with C16:1 Δ6, called sapienic acid, being the most abundant. Sapienic acid is shown in Fig. 3.

Saturated Species: The saturated fatty acids are almost entirely in the range of 12 through 18 carbons in length with palmitic acid (C16:0) being the most abundant (24,27). Generally, the straight-chain species predominate, but the proportions of methyl branched species can be highly variable (35). The methyl branched species include iso and anteiso branches as shown in Fig. 3. There are also a wide variety of other mono- and multi-methyl branched saturated chains (36), but for a given individual the pattern of methyl branching appears to be constant (35). In addition, identical twins appear to have identical sebaceous fatty acid compositions including the pattern of methyl branching, whereas nonidentical twins have, although generally having similar branching patterns, sometimes differed as much as nontwin groups (37). All of this supports the contention that sebum composition is largely under genetic control.

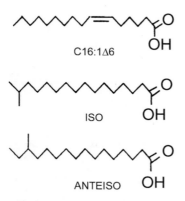

Figure 3 Fatty acids found in human sebum.

Other Species

All terrestrial mammals produce sebum, and in all cases the lipid mixture is a viscous liquid consisting of several types of nonpolar lipids (38,39). The lipid class composition is species specific. Among the most widely distributed sebaceous lipids are sterols and sterol esters. In addition to the wax monoesters as found in the human, the sebum from many species contains type I wax diesters in which a normal fatty acid is ester-linked to the hydroxyl group of an α-hydroxyacid, which in turn is ester-linked to a fatty alcohol or type II wax diesters in which two fatty acids are esterified to 1,2-diols. Sebum from the cow also contains triesters which contain 1,2-diols with an α-hydroxyacid esterified to one of the hydroxyls and a normal fatty acid ester-linked to the other (40). A second normal fatty acid is ester-linked to the α-hydroxyl group.

Members of closely related species tend to have similar sebum compositions. For example, sebum specimens from the members of the genus *Equus* all contain cholesterol, cholesterol esters, type II wax diesters, and giant ring ω-lactones (41,42). The lactones constitute from $\sim$50% to 70% of the total sebum mass and are formed by cyclization of 30- through 36-carbon ω-hydroxyacids. In general, the degree of unsaturation and methyl branching of the giant ring lactones from the different species of the equidae are in accord with the taxonomic relationships among these species (42). *Equus caballus*, the common domestic horse, produced lactones that predominantly contained one double bond and a methyl branch on the penultimate carbon. The lactones of the donkey, *Equus asinus*, were made from 30-, 32-, and 34-carbon straight-chained ω-hydroxyacids. The lactones of the mule, *E. caballus*/*E. asinus*, were monounsaturated, and 50% of the chains had the methyl branch whereas the other 50% were straight (42). Again, this observation indicates genetic control of sebum composition.

SEBUM IN HEALTH

In hairy mammals, sebum serves two clear functions. First, it serves as a water repellant on the fur which is clearly advantageous for aquatic mammals and for mammals living in moist environments. Second, 7-dehydrocholesterol secreted from the sebaceous glands onto the skin surface is photochemically converted to pre-vitamin D, which is then converted to vitamin D in a temperature dependent, nonenzymatic reaction (43). When the animal licks its fur during grooming, the vitamin D is recovered by means of a salivary vitamin D binding protein (44). In humans, a function for sebum is less well established, and it is possible that sebum production is a functionless vestige of our ancestors. One clue in this regard comes from the species known to produce squalene as a component of their sebum. In addition to human sebum, squalene is found in the sebum of the otter, beaver, kinkajou, and mole, *Scalopus aquaticus* (45,46). The otter and beaver are aquatic. The kinkajoo lives in the canopies of tropical rain forests, and *Scalopus aquaticus* lives in moist-wet soil. Could it be that our ancestors spent a great deal of their time in water along coasts or rivers and benefited from the waterproofing afforded by a coating of squalene?

Sebum no doubt contributes a degree of lubrication to the skin surface, and it has sometimes been suggested that dry skin results from insufficient sebum production. However, two lines of evidence argue against this. First, as has been pointed out, prepubertal children produce almost no sebum but most do not suffer dry skin or other skin problems (47). Second, in one study in which the sebum secretion rate was measured and subjects were surveyed about the condition of their skin, no correlation could be found between the occurrence of xerosis and sebum production (48).

Sebum definitely does not contribute to the permeability barrier function of the skin. In fact, if human sebum is applied to neonatal rodent skin barrier function is decreased (49).

One possible function of sebum is a contribution to the antimicrobial defense of the skin. It has long been known that fatty acids produced by sebaceous triglyceride hydrolysis have antibacterial properties (50), and it has more recently been demonstrated that sebaceous lipids can interfere with the adherence of yeast to the stratum corneum (51). In addition to a decline in function of the immune system, the decline in sebum secretion with age could contribute to the increased incidence of bacterial and fungal infections of the skin in the elderly (52). The fact that prepubertal children do not have a high incidence of skin infections may be attributed to their healthy immune systems. So sebum is clearly not essential for the avoidance of skin infections, but it may be helpful in this regard in some individuals.

Although it is not synthesized in the sebaceous glands and represents an insignificant proportion of the secreted material, it has been recognized in recent years that vitamin E is delivered to the skin surface through sebum secretion (53,54). This may be significant in protection of unsaturated sebaceous lipids and stratum corneum components against oxidation.

SEBUM IN DISEASE—ACNE

There is a clear positive correlation between the occurrence and severity of acne and the sebum secretion rate (55,56). In one study comparing age and gender matched subjects with moderate, mild, or no acne, the subjects with moderate acne had the highest sebum secretion rates, whereas those with mild acne had sebum secretion rates intermediate between those measured for subjects without acne and those with moderate acne (55). The average sebum secretion rate for all subjects with acne was three times that for the subjects without acne, and in no case did a subject with acne have a sebum secretion rate that was not greater than the sebum secretion rate of the matched control.

The development of an inflammatory acne lesion is a multistep process (3). The initiating event is the formation of a keratinous plug, or comedo, that blocks the pore of the follicle. Then, bacteria within the follicle grow, and the follicle becomes distended. The follicular epithelium becomes thin, and an inflammatory response is induced as bacterial products diffuse into the surrounding tissue.

It has been suggested that the development of acne may result from essential fatty acid deficiency localized to the follicular epithelium (57). In experimental systemic essential fatty acid deficiency, the skin becomes scaly and more permeable (33,58). If sebaceous fatty acids were to penetrate into the follicular epithelial cells and compete with linoleic acid from the circulation for incorporation into lipids, a localized essential fatty acid deficiency could be produced. The resulting scaling could lead to comedo formation, and the defective barrier function would facilitate exchange of materials between the follicle and surrounding tissue. This would include an influx of water and nutrients into the follicle to support bacterial growth as well as the eflux of inflammatory mediators.

Reduction of the sebum secretion rate is therapeutic for acne. This can be achieved by oral administration of retinoids (59,60), estrogen (61,62), or antiandrogens (62,63). Estrogen is thought to act by reducing production of testosterone, and antiandrogens act by blocking the androgenic receptors on sebocytes, thereby preventing binding of androgens.

Orally administered 13-*cis* retinoic acid is an effective treatment for moderate to severe acne vulgaris (59,60). Although the retinoids probably act through specific receptors (64,65), many details of their mechanisms of action remain uncertain (66). It has been established that 13-*cis* retinoic acid undergoes isomerization to the all-*trans* isomer within sebocytes (67). A subsequent chapter in this book deals with retinoids, so further discussion will not be included here.

REFERENCES

1. Montagna W. The sebaceous gland in man. In: Montagna W, Ellis RA, Silver AS, eds. Advances in Biology of Skin: the Sebaceous Glands, IV. Oxford: Pergamon Press, 1963:19–31.
2. Downing DT, Stewart ME, Wertz PW, Strauss JS. Lipids of the epidermis and sebaceous glands. In: Fitzpatrick TB, Eisen AZ, Wolff K, Freedberg IM, Austen KF, eds. Dermatology in General Medicine. Vol. 1. 4tj ed. New York: McGraw-Hill Inc, 1993:210–221.
3. Leyden JJ. New understandings of the pathogenesis of acne. J Am Acad Dermatol 1995; 32:S15–25.
4. Pagnoni A, Kligman AM, el Gammal S, Stoudemayer T. Determination of density of follicles on various regions of the face by cyanoacrylate biopsy: correlation with sebum output. Br J Dermatol 1994; 131:862–865.
5. Dreher A, Grevers G. Fordyce spots. A little regarded finding in the area of lip pigmentation and mouth mucosa. Laryngol Rhinol Otol 1995; 74:390–392.
6. Daley T. Pathology of intraoral sebaceous glands. J Oral Path 1993; 22:241–245
7. Tiffany JM. The lipid secretion of the meibomian glands. Advan Lipid Res 1987; 22:1–62.

8. Greene RS, Downing DT, Pochi PE, Strauss JS. Anatomical variation in the amount and composition of human skin surface lipid. J Invest Dermatol 1970; 54:240–247.
9. Saint-Leger D, Leveque JL. Les Methodes d'evaluation quantitative des lipides de surface chez l'homme: Presentation d'une nouvelle procedure. Int J Cosmet Sci 1980; 2:283–294.
10. Strauss JS, Pochi PE. The quantitative gravimetric determination of sebum production. J Invest Dermatol 1961; 36:293–298.
11. Cotteril JA, Cunliff WJ, Williamson B, Bulusu L. Age and sex variation in skin surface lipid composition and sebum excretion rate. Br J Dermatol 1972; 87:333–340.
12. Downing DT, Stranieri AM, Strauss JS. The effect of accumulated lipids on measurement of sebum secretion in human skin. J Invest Dermatol 1982; 79:226–228.
13. Kligman AM, Miller DL, McGinley K. Sebutape: a device for visualization and measuring human sebaceous secretion. J Soc Cosmet Chem 1986; 37:369–374.
14. Nordstrom KM, Schmus HG, McGinley KJ, Leyden JJ. Measurement of sebum output using a lipid absorbant tape. J Invest Dermatol 1986; 87:260–263.
15. Piérard GE. Rate and topography of follicular sebum excretion. Dermatologica 1986; 173:61–65.
16. Downing DT. Photodensitometry in the thin-layer chromatographic analysis of neutral lipids. J Chrom 1968; 38:91–99.
17. Clarys P, Barel A. Quantitative evaluation of skin surface lipids. Clin Dermatol 1995; 13:307–321.
18. Downing DT, Stewart ME, Strauss JS. Changes in sebum secretion and the sebaceous gland. Clin Gen Med 1989; 5:109–114.
19. Pierard G, Pierard-Franchimont C. The sebutape technique for monitoring androgen dependent disorders. Eur J Med 1992; 1:109–112.
20. Thiboutot D. Hormones and acne: pathophysiology, clinical evaluation, and therapies. Semin Cutan Med Surg 2001; 20:144–153.
21. Takayasu S. Metabolism and action of androgen in the skin. Int J Dermatol 1979; 18:681–692.
22. Roy AK, Chatterjee B. Androgen action. Crit Rev Eukaryot Gene Express 1995; 5:157–176.
23. Chang C, Saltzman A, Young W, Keller E, Lee HJ, Wang C, Mizokami A. Androgen receptor: an overview. Crit Rev Eukaryot Gene Express 1995; 5:97–125.
24. Nicolaides N, Fu HC, Ansari MNA, Rice GR. The fatty acids of wax esters and sterol esters from vernix caseosa and from human skin surface lipid. Lipids 1972; 7:506–517.
25. Pochi PE, Strauss JS. Endocrinologic control of the development and activity of the human sebaceous gland. J Invest Dermatol 1974; 62:191–201.
26. Jacobsen E, Billings JK, Frantz RA, Kinney CK, Stewart ME, Downing DT. Age-related changes in sebaceous wax ester secretion rates in men and women. J Invest Dermatol 1985; 85:483–485.
27. Downing DT, Stewart ME. Analysis of sebaceous lipids. In: Skerrow D, Skerrow CJ, eds. Methods in Skin Research. New York: John Wiley & Sons Ltd., 1985:349–379.
28. Shalita AR. Genesis of free fatty acids. J Invest Dermatol 1974; 62:332–335.
29. Downing DT, Strauss JS, Pochi PE. Variability in the chemical composition of human skin surface lipids. J Invest Dermatol 1969; 53:322–327.
30. Stewart ME, Downing DT, Strauss JS. The fatty acids of human sebaceous gland phosphatidylcholine. Biochim Biophys Acta 1978; 529:380–386.

31. Bloch K. The biological synthesis of cholesterol. Science 1965; 150:19–28.
32. Krakow R, Downing DT, Strauss JS, Pochi PE. Identification of a fatty acid in human skin surface lipids apparently associated with acne vulgaris. J Invest Dermatol 1973; 61:286–289.
33. Holman RT. Essential fatty acid deficiency. Prog Chem Fats Other Lipids 1968; 9:275–348.
34. Downing DT, Strauss JS. Synthesis and composition of surface lipids of human skin. J Invest Dermatol 1974; 62:228–244.
35. Green SC, Stewart ME, Downing DT. Variation in sebum fatty acid composition among adult humans. J Invest Dermatol 1984; 83:114–117.
36. Nicolaides N, Apon JMB. Further studies of the saturated methyl branched fatty acids of vernix caseosa lipid. Lipids 1976; 11:781–790.
37. Stewart ME, McDonnell MW, Downing DT. Possible genetic control of the proportions of branched-chain fatty acids in human sebaceous wax esters. J Invest Dermatol 1986; 86:706–708.
38. Nicolaides N, Fu HC, Rice GR. The skin surface lipids of man compared with those of eighteen species of animals. J Invest Dermatol 1968; 51:83–89.
39. Lindholm JS, McCormick JM, Colton SW 6th, Downing DT. Variation of skin surface lipid composition among mammals. Comp Biochem Physiol 1981; 69B:75–78.
40. Downing DT, Lindholm JS. Skin surface lipids of the cow. Comp Biochem Physiol 1982; 73B:327–330.
41. Downing DT, Colton SW 6th. Skin surface lipids of the horse. Lipids 1980; 15:323–327.
42. Colton SW 6th, Downing DT. Variation in skin surface lipid composition among the equidae. Comp Biochem Physiol 1983; 75B:429–433.
43. Holick MF. Environmental factors that influence the cutaneous production of vitamin D. Am J Clin Nut 1995; 61(3 suppl):638S–645S.
44. Krayer JW, Emerson DL, Goldschmidt-Clermont PJ, Nel AE, Werner PA, Galbraith RM. Qualitative and quantitative studies of Gc (vitamin D-binding protein) in normal subjects and patients with periodontal disease. J Periodent Res 1987; 22:259–263.
45. Lindholm JS, Downing DT. Occurrence of squalene in the skin surface lipids of the otter, the beaver and the kinkajou. Lipids 1980; 15:1062–1063.
46. Downing DT, Stewart ME. Skin surface lipids of the mole *Scalopus aquaticus*. Comp Biochem Physiol 1987; 86B:667–670.
47. Kligman AM, Shelley WB. An investigation of the biology of the human sebaceous gland. J Invest Dermatol 1958; 30:99–125.
48. Frantz RA, Kinney CK. Variables associated with skin dryness in the elderly. Nursing Res 1986; 35:98–100.
49. Squier CA, Wertz PW, Williams DM, Cruchley AT. Permeability of oral mucosa and skin with age. In: Squire CA, Hill MW, eds. The Effect of Aging in Oral Mucosa and Skin. Boca Raton: CRC Press, 1994:91–98.
50. Burtenshaw JM. The mechanisms of self disinfection of the human skin and its appendages. J Hyg 1942; 42:184–209.
51. Law S, Fotos PG, Wertz PW. Skin surface lipids inhibit adherence of *Candida albicans* to stratum corneum. Dermatology 1997; 195:220–223.
52. Kligman AM. Perspectives and problems in cutaneous gerontology. J Invest Dermatol 1979; 73:39–46.

53. Thiele JJ, Schroeter C, Hsieh SN, Podda M, Packer L. The antioxidant network of the stratum corneum. Current Prob Dermatol 2001; 29:26–42.
54. Passi S, De Pita O, Puddu P, Littarru GP. Lipophilic antioxidants in human sebum and aging. Free Rad Res 2002; 36:471–477.
55. Harris HH, Downing DT, Stewart ME, Strauss JS. Sustainable rates of sebum secretion in acne patients and matched normal control subjects. J Am Acad Dermatol 1983; 8:200–203.
56. Toyoda M, Morohashi M. Pathenogenesis of acne. Med Electron Micros 2001; 34:29–40.
57. Downing DT, Stewart ME, Wertz PW, Strauss JS. Essential fatty acids and acne. J Am Acad Dermatol 1986; 14:221–225.
58. Melton JL, Wertz PW, Swartzendruber DC, Downing DT. Effects of essential fatty acid deficiency on epidermal O-acylsphingolipids and transepidermal water loss in young pigs. Biochim Biophys Acta 1987; 921:191–197.
59. Shalita AR, Armstrong RB, Leyden JJ, Pochi PE, Strauss JS. Isotretinoin revisited. Cutis 1988; 42:1–19.
60. Jansen T, Plewig G. Advances and perspectives in acne therapy. Eur J Med Res 1997; 2:321–334.
61. Ebling FJ. Steroids and the skin: a general review. Biochem Soc Trans 1976; 4:597–602.
62. Shaw JC. Antiandrogen and hormonal treatment of acne. Dermatol Clinics 1996; 14:803–811.
63. Sawaya ME, Hordinsky MK. The antiandrogens. When and how they should be used. Dermatol Clinics 1993; 11:65–72.
64. Fisher GJ, Voorhees JJ. Molecular mechanisms of retinoid actions in skin. FASEB J 1996; 10:1002–1013.
65. Kim MJ, Ciletti N, Michel S, Reichert U, Rosenfield RL. The role of specific retinoid receptors in sebocyte growth and differentiation in culture. J Invest Dermatol 2000; 114:349–353.
66. Geiger JM. Retinoids and sebaceous gland activity. Dermatology 1995; 191:305–310.
67. Tsukada M, Schroder M, Roos TC, Chandraratna RA, Reichert U, Merk HF, Orfanos CE. 13-cis retinoic acid exerts its specific activity on human sebocytes through selective intracellular isomerization to all-trans retinoic acid and binding to retinoid acid receptors. J Invest Dermatol 2000; 115:321–327.

17

Topical Retinoids

Ai-Lean Chew, Saqib J. Bashir, and Howard I. Maibach
University of California, San Francisco, CA, USA

Overview	319
Historical Background	322
Cosmeceuticals	322
Retinol	322
Penetration, Absorption, and Cutaneous Metabolism of Topical Retinoids	323
Cellular Uptake of Retinol	324
Cutaneous Metabolism	325
Pharmacological Effects of Retinol *In Vitro* and *In Vivo*	326
Tretinoin Therapy in Photoaging	327
Toxicity	329
The Future	330
References	330

OVERVIEW

The retinoids are a diverse class of pharmacological compounds, consisting of vitamin A (retinol) and its naturally occurring and synthetic derivatives, which possess biological vitamin A activity (Tables 1 and 2). Vitamin A generically encompasses retinol (vitamin A alcohol), retinal (vitamin A aldehyde), and

Table 1 Classification of Retinoids

Generation	Retinoid
First generation	Tretinoin (all-*trans*-retinoic acid)
	Isotretinoin (13-*cis*-retinoic acid)
Second generation	Etretinate (Ro 10-9359)
	Etretin (Ro 10-1670)
Third generation	Arotinoid (Ro 15-0778)
	Arotinoid ethylester (Ro 13-6298)
	Arotinoid methyl sulfone (Ro 14-9706)
	Adapalene (CD271)
Naturally occurring in humans	Retinol (vitamin A)
	Retinal (vitamin A aldehyde)
	Retinoic acid

retinoic acid (vitamin A acid) (Fig. 1). In clinical use, retinoids have established their effectiveness in treating acneiform eruptions (e.g., isotretinoin), disorders of keratinization, such as psoriasis (e.g., acitretin), as well as some neoplastic processes (e.g., tretinoin for leukemia, isotretinoin for squamous cell carcinomas). Additional retinoids are currently being investigated, as novel uses of retinoids already established in clinical practice. The main focus of retinoid usage in cosmeceuticals has been its role as the mythical "fountain of youth" (i.e., reversal of photoaging) (Table 3). Retinoids, like all drugs, have adverse effects, the most infamous one being teratogenicity. Over 2000 derivatives have been developed in the hope of finding retinoids with increased therapeutic efficacy coupled with diminished local and systemic toxicity. The recent focus of retinoids has been on topical delivery systems, as this route not only provides a safer adverse effect profile, but also delivers a higher dose to a targeted area (i.e., the skin).

Table 2 The Roles of Naturally Existing Retinoids

Retinoid	Role
Retinol	Growth promotion, differentiation/maintenance of epithelia, reproduction
Retinal	Vision
Retinoic acid	Growth promotion, differentiation/maintenance of epithelia

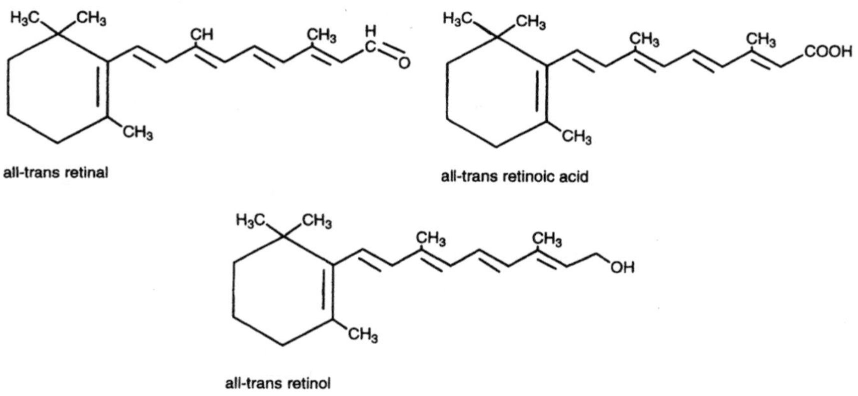

Topical Retinoids

Figure 1 Structure of retinoids.

This chapter provides a review of topical retinoids, focusing on the potential cosmeceutical applications of this class of drug. Oral retinoids with no significant cosmeceutical activity, such as acitretin, will not be covered. Not that the definition of drug vs. cosmeceutical for this class is regulatory (man made) and not biological.

Table 3 Uses of Topical Retinoids

Retinoid	Proprietary name	Uses	
Tretinoin	Retin-A	Acne vulgaris	Primary
(all-*trans*-retinoic acid)	Renova	Photoaging	indication
		Actinic keratoses	
		Lichen planus	Secondary
		Melasma	indication
		Postinflammatory hyperpigmentation	
Isotretinoin		Acne vulgaris	
Alitretinoin	Panretin	Kaposi's sarcoma	
(9-*cis*-retinoic acid)			
Retinol		Cosmetic ingredient	
Retinyl palmitate		Cosmetic ingredient	
Retinyl aldehyde		Cosmetic ingredient	
Adapalene		Acne vulgaris	
Tazarotene		Psoriasis	
		Acne vulgaris	
Motretinide		Acne vulgaris	

HISTORICAL BACKGROUND

The ancient Egyptians recognized the importance of vitamin A activity as early as 1500 BC, as evidenced by early writings in "Eber's Papyrus" describing the benefits of liver in treating night blindness (1). However, it was not until the early 20th century that definitive knowledge of this substance was discovered. In 1909, a fat-soluble extract from egg yolk was found to be essential for life (2). This substance, initially termed "fat-soluble A" (3) and later named "vitamin A" (4), was also found in butter fat and fish oils, demonstrating growth-promoting activity (5). Synthesis of vitamin A was achieved in the 1940s and from then on an upsurge of interest in the therapeutic uses of vitamin A became apparent.

Topical tretinoin was first used successfully by Stüttgen to treat disorders of epidermal keratinization in the 1960s (6). However, the irritation produced by the concentrations and formulations used in these studies inhibited widespred acceptance. Subsequently, Kligman proved the therapeutic efficacy of topical tretinoin in acne vulgaris (7), and went on to pioneer and popularize the use of retinoids in cosmetic dermatology by demonstrating its effects on photoaged skin (8).

COSMECEUTICALS

The major forms of retinoids that may be of significant interest to the cosmeceutical industry are retinol, retinal, and, possibly, retinoic acid. The main role of retinoids in cosmeceuticals are in extrinsic aging (photoaging). Currently, topical retinoic acid is FDA-approved for the treatment of acne, and in the adjunct treatment of fine skin wrinkling, skin roughness, and hyperpigmentation due to photoaging, as well as reducing the number of senile lentigines (liver spots) (9–11). At present, retinol is becoming an increasingly utilized ingredient in cosmetic preparations, such as moisturizers and hair products. One reason for this is that retinol is a nonprescription preparation. It has also been demonstrated to be less irritating topically than retinoic acid (12), which makes retinol a more favorable cosmetic ingredient than retinoic acid. It is therefore necessary to review the scientific basis for use of retinoids and their purported efficacy.

RETINOL

Vitamin A is a necessary dietary nutrient, required for growth and done development, vision, reproduction, and the integrity of mucosal and epithelial surfaces. Vitamin A deficiency results in visual problems, such as xerophthalmia and nyctalopia (night blindness), hyperkeratosis of the skin, epithelial metaplasia of the mucous membranes, and decreased resistance to infections. Vitamin A is fat-soluble, and occurs as various stereoisomers. Retinol (vitamin A1) is present in esterified form in dairy products, meat, liver, kidney, and oily saltwater fish.

For clinical purposes, vitamin A is available as retinol (vitamin A alcohol) or esters of retinol formed from edible fatty acids, primarily acetic and palmitica acid.

PENETRATION, ABSORPTION, AND CUTANEOUS METABOLISM OF TOPICAL RETINOIDS

Any active substance administered to the skin must penetrate the skin in sufficient amounts in order to have a pharmacological effect. This section presents evidence that the topical retinoids can be utilized effectively. Several methods have been utilized, including enzyme induction as a marker of effective penetration, radiolabeling, and high-pressure liquid chromatography (HPLC).

Duell et al. (13) studied the penetration characteristics of all-trans-retinol (ROL), all-trans-retinoic acid (RA), all-trans-retinaldehyde (RAL), and retinyl palmitate (ROL palm) in human skin *in vivo*. An enzyme marker was utilized to demonstrate that penetration had occurred and to measure the potency of each retinoid. As the enzyme, cytochrome P-450-dependent RA 4-hydoxylase, is induced by retinoic acid, its induction can identify whether sufficient ROL, RAL, and ROL palm penetration and metabolism to RA occur. Therefore, this enzyme can qualitatively reflect penetration and potency in the epidermis.

Utilizing microsomal preparations from human skin biopsies, a significant induction in this enzyme was noted following topical application to human skin *in vivo*. After 48 h of occlusion, ROL ($\geq 0.025\%$) increased the enzyme activity significantly; however, lower concentrations did not cause significant induction. The increase in enzyme induction was nonlinear, with the higher doses only causing a small increase in acitvity.

RAL also caused a significant induction of enzyme activity after 48 h of occlusive application. Similarly to ROL, induction was seen at concentrations $>0.025\%$, but not lesser. Enzyme activity increased in a dose-related manner, with similar peak activity to equivalent concentrations of ROL. At lower doses (0.01% and 0.025%), RAL was a greater inducer than ROL, but at higher concentrations (0.05%, 0.25%, 0.5%, 1%), ROL and RAL were equally effective inducers.

RA itself was a more potent inducer of the hydroxylase enzyme than ROL and RAL. Induction was seen in RA after 24 h of occlusion, compared with 48 h for ROL and RAL, and the degree of induction was much greater.

ROL palm applied under occlusion also induced enzyme activity. The 0.6% ROL palm significantly induced the enzyme, whereas lower concentrations, vehicle, or equivalent concentrations of palmitate alone did not. However, ROL palm was applied for 4 days, in contrast to the 24 and 48 h studies outlined earlier (Table 4).

The effect of occlusion on the ability of ROL, RA, and ROL palm was also assessed. Although unoccluded RA significantly induced RA-hydroxylase, a significantly greater induction occurred under occlusion. A similar effect was seen

Table 4 Assaying Retinoid Effects Utilizing Cutaneous Markers

Compound	Marker	Time to induction (under occlusion)	Minimum inducing concentration (%)	Does occlusion enhance induction?
ROL	cP450-OHase	48 h	0.025	No
RA	cP450-OHase	24 h	0.001	Yes
ROL palm	cP450-OHase	4 days	0.6	Yes
RAL	cP450-OHase	48 h	0.025	N/A

Source: Duell et al. (13).

for ROL palm. However, this occlusive effect was not seen with ROL: both occluded and unoccluded sites produced a similar significant increase in enzyme induction compared with vehicle. Enzyme activity induced by 0.25% ROL (either unoccluded or occluded) was similar to that induced by 0.025% RA (under occlusion).

Whether the induction of this or other enzyme markers in the skin reflects the ability of retinoids to produce a pharmacological effect is not clear. However, cosmetic-type preparations mandate sufficient retinoid concentrations to allow adequate penetration for a pharmacological effect. As a threshold level could be identified for enzyme induction in the above study, there may also be a threshold for a pharmacological effect. An insufficient concentration in the cosmetic, or inadquate application by the consumer, may render the formulation relatively ineffective.

Cellular Uptake of Retinol

In addition to sufficient delivery of the retinoid to the skin, the retinoid should be delivered in the correct form to allow cellular uptake and metabolism. Retinoids occur in human plasma bound to proteins: retinoic acid is bound to albumin and ROL to retinol-binding protein (RBP) (14). Therefore, the possibility that protein binding can determine the ability of a cell to take up retinoids has been considered. (The influence of protein binding on metabolism is discussed later.)

Hodam and Creek (15) studied the uptake of retinol, either free (in ethanol) or bound to RBP, in cultured human keratinocytes. Utilizing radiolabeled compounds, they demonstrated that the retinol uptake was much greater in the free than in the bound form. Free retinol added to the culture medium had a maximum uptake of 35% of the applied dose within 3 h of incubation, falling to 20% by 12 h. In contrast, RBP retinol had a peak uptake of 7.5% of the applied dose, detected at 24 h. Therefore, keratinocytes demonstrated a much slower uptake of RBP retinol compared with free retinol.

Cutaneous Metabolism

The metabolism of vitamin A and its derivatives in the skin is considered important for the understanding of their pharmacological effect. It has been hypothesized that the effects of ROL and RAL may result from their cutaneous metabolism to RA. Although some investigators have shown that this metabolism may occur, pharamacological effects have also been seen in the absence of measurable RA. This section discusses the evidence that RA is an essential metabolite in the activity of ROL and RAL.

In vitro, metabolism of ROL, RAL, and RA was studied utilizing human skin and dermal fibroblasts (16). Radiolabeled ROL, RAL, and RA were applied either topically to the skin biopsies or to the culture media of the fibroblast suspensions, and the metabolites were identified by HPLC after 24 h of incubation. The skin cultures demonstrated a gradient distribution of the retinoids within the skin: 75% of absorbed activity was in the epidermis, 20% in the dermis, and 2–6% in the culture medium for the three retinoids tested. Of the epidermal extracts, 60% of applied ROL remained unmetabolized. The main ROL metabolites in the epidermis were retinyl esters (18.5%), a finding that has also been demonstrated in keratinocyte cultures. RA (2%), RAL (1.6%), 13-*cis*-retinoic acid (1%), and polar compounds were also found. The dermis yielded similar metabolites, but a higher proportion of polar compounds.

RAL was also metabolized in the epidermis: 43% of the absorbed radioactivity was RAL, 9% retinyl esters, 14% ROL, and 0.8% RA. When RA itself was applied, 66% of the epidermal radioactivity was from RA, 17% from 13-*cis*-RA, and 10% from polar compounds. RA was not metabolized to ROL or RAL. Dermal fibroblasts also metabolized ROL, RAL, and RA in culture medium, but the significance of this *in vivo* is not yet clear. It is possible that these cells may contribute to the role of the dermis in the kinetics and dynamics of these substances.

These skin studies demonstrate the capacity for topical ROL, RAL, and RA to penetrate the skin in a gradient manner from the epidermis to the dermis. The activity in the epidermis was five times greater than that in the dermis, suggesting an accumulation of compounds in the layer. Although a proportion of the absorbed compound remains unchanged within the skin, significant metabolism was seen. ROL and RAL were metabolized to RA, which may play a role in the pharmacology of these substances.

Randolph and Simon (17) utilized ROL and RA bound to their endogenous binding proteins in their *in vitro* study: retinol was bound to RBP and retinoic acid was bound to albumin, as has been found in human plasma (14,18). Dermal fibroblasts, cultured either in collagen gel or on plastic dishes, were exposed to radiolabeled ROL or RA, and metabolites were detected by HPLC. In contrast to Bailey et al. (16), ROL was not metabolized by the dermal fibroblasts, although their findings for RA metabolism did concur. This may have been because of decreased availability of ROL to the dermal fibroblasts because of its protein binding. It was therefore suggested that the metabolism of ROL might only occur under pharmacological conditions. Supporting this explanation are the findings of Hodam and Creek (15) described previously, which demonstrate decreased uptake of RBP retinol compared with free ROL in cultured keratinocytes. However, the role of protein binding in uptake of ROL in dermal fibroblasts requires further elucidation.

As certain cell types preferentially metabolize different forms of retinoids, the cell content of a tissue may influence the availability of retinol and its metabolites to the surrounding tissue. The significance of this finding in cosmetic use is not yet clear. Hodam and Creek (15), in addition to determining the effect of protein binding on cellular uptake metabolism of the retinoids once intracellular. In both cases, retinyl esters were the major metabolite and the percentage of ROL cell-associated radioactivity that was converted to retinyl esters was independent of the mode of delivery.

Several studies have therefore demonstrated a metabolic capacity for topical ROL and RAL. Retinyl esters appear to be the major metabolite, whereas the formation of RA from these substances constitutes a small proportion of the metabolites formed. However, this conversion may be sufficient for pharmacological activity. *In vivo* studies may better quantify both metabolism and dose–response relationships.

Pharmacological Effects of Retinol *In Vitro* and *In Vivo*

In vitro and *in vivo* studies of retinol and its derivatives have demonstrated several pharmacological effects on the skin. However, whether these effects are caused by RA as a derivative of ROL or RAL applied to the skin is not clear. The evidence is discussed below.

Kang et al. (12) found that epidermal changes could be demonstrated *in vivo* following topical application of ROL, without measurable retinoic acid levels. This suggests that ROL itself is active in the skin. Following 4 days of occlusive application of ROL, epidermal thickness increased significantly compared with vehicle control. This increase was dose-dependent: a significant increase was seen with 0.05% ROL, and the maximum concentration used (1.6% ROL) caused an increase similar in magnitude to 0.025% RA applied over the same period. Further evidence of the pharmacological activity of ROL in the epidermis was an increase in the number of mitotic figures and in epidermal spongiosis (ranked on an ordinal scale).

Interestingly, the authors were not able to detect RA, or found only trace amounts, in the time points tested (0–96 h). Reverse-phase HPLC yielded ROL, 13-*cis*-ROL, and retinyl esters (RE) in the samples, which had been tape stripped to remove the stratum corneum prior to biopsy. These results differ from those presented earlier where RA was found *in vitro* utilizing human skin. Nevertheless, cellular retinoic acid binding protein (CRABP-II) mRNA was increased, indicating *CRABP-II* gene activation, which supports the idea of ROL conversion to RA. The same laboratory also demonstrated an increase in a retinoic-specific hydroxylase enzyme *in vivo* in a previous study (REFS). However, it is possible that ROL may indirectly mediate *CRABP-II* gene expression by an unidentified mechanism, other than conversion to RA.

Goffin et al. (19) compared a retinol cream with a vitamin E preparation on humans *in vivo* utilizing bioengineering methods. In this crossover study, subjects were exposed to environmental insults, such as ultraviolet (UV) irradiation and a topical surfactant (sodium lauryl sulfate), and assessed utilizing squamometry, corneosurfametry, and optical profilometry. The authors suggest that the retinol preparation may provide some beneficial effects against these insults and also reduce the trend in shallow wrinkling induced by the irradiation. However, these data are difficult to interpret because of the crossover study design, and also because the retinol preparation was a complex cosmetic formulation. Therefore, the effects seen cannot be attributed to the effect of retinol alone. Additionally, no vehicle control was utilized.

TRETINOIN THERAPY IN PHOTOAGING

Chronic exposure to sunlight causes a characteristic collection of signs presumed to be due to aging in the past, but are now recognized primarily as the consequences of solar and other environmental injury. This is termed photoaging or dermatoheliosis. This familiar stigmata of photoaged skin are rough, leathery skin with coarse wrinkles and yellow or mottled complexion. Histologically, the dermis exhibits changes known as solar elastosis; the collagenous connective tissue in the upper dermis is replaced by fragmented, disorganized elastic fibers (20). Ultraviolet radiation stimulates collagenases (UV-responsive matrix metalloproteinases), thereby enhancing collagen degradation and resulting in this deficiency of dermal collagen (21). Irregular epidermal thickening is seen in photoaged skin, sometimes accompanied by irregularities in cell and nuclear size, shape, and staining reactions. Melanocytic hyperplasia is a frequent feature in chronically sun-exposed skin, seen diffusely as a background of increased pigmentation, or focally as "senile lentigines" (22). A telangiectatic network is often seen in photodamaged skin as the disorganized dermis fails to support vessel walls, allowing them to dilate passively (23).

Topical tretinoin (all-*trans*-retinoic acid), used for the past two decades as antiacne therapy, has also been found effective in the treatment of photoaging. Its role in photoaging was first described and subsequently popularized by Kligman (24). He observed that women treated with tretinoin described smoother skin with less wrinkles. This clinical observation prompted him to perform clinical trials comparing the effects of tretinoin on photoaging with an inert cream. In the first of these studies, 0.05% tretinoin in a cream base was applied twice daily for 3 months on dorsal forearms of elderly volunteers, and the results were compared with similar application of an inert cream to the opposite forearms. Punch biopsy specimens, taken before and after treatment, were examined using light and electron microscopy. Skin bioengineering data were also obtained. In the second study, 0.05% tretinoin cream was applied to photodamaged facial skin and specimens obtained and analyzed in a similar fashion. A third, uncontrolled study consisted of long-term facial application of 0.05% or 0.1% tretinoin cream in over 400 healthy females. The studies demonstrated significant beneficial effects on photodamaged skin, including reversal of epidermal atropy, dysplasia, and atypia, eradication of microscopic actinic keratoses, uniform dispersion of melanin granules, new collagen formation in the papillary dermis, and angiogenesis (8). Kligman reinforced this work with animal studies using the photodamaged hairless mouse model (24).

These results were consolidated by Weiss et al. (25), who similarly demonstrated in a 4 month randomized, blinded, vehicle-controlled study that 0.1% tretinoin improved photodamaged skin, both histologically and ultrastructurally. Volunteers in the tretinoin-treated group showed significant reduction in lentigines, epidermal thickening, compaction of the stratum corneum with presence of glycosaminoglycan-like substance, increased mitoses in keratinocytes, and increased number 3 of anchoring fibrils at the dermoepidermal junction. Ellis et al. (9) then extended the tretinoin therapy in an open-label trial, utilizing the same subjects for up to 22 months, indicating that clinical improvement was sustained during long-term tretinoin therapy. They found that 71% of discrete lentigines had disappeared after this prolonged period. Further, the problems of dryness, erythema, and flaking of the skin associated with retinoid use had diminished or declined after the 22 month period, with maintenance of clinical benefit.

The findings in these earlier studies have now been reinforced by a solid background of formal clinical trials (26–28). [Tretinoin reverses photoaging by epidermal and dermal effects. The epidermal effects include epidermal thinning, reduction in corneocyte adhesion, decreased melanin production, and increased Langerhans cells. The dermal effects include increased collagen production, increased angiogenesis, and decreased collagenase and glycosaminoglycans (25).]

More recently, the emphasis on research in tretinoin has branched out, for instance, fine-tuning the optimum conditions for tretinoin therapy and new uses. In a recent double-blinded, vehicle-controlled comparison of 0.1% and 0.025% tretinoin creams in patients with photoaged skin, tretinoin 0.025% showed similar efficacy to 0.1%, while showing significantly less irritation.

Having more than proved its efficacy in the reversal of photoaging, the logical question is: Can retinoid therapy also improve intrinsically aged skin? The answer to this may be on the horizon. Varani et al. (29) completed an *in vitro* study utilizing cell culture techiniques to investigate the effects of tretinoin on skin. Retinoic acid stimulated growth of keratinocytes and fibroblasts and stimulated extracellular matrix production by fibroblasts. Adult skin from sun-exposed and sun-protected sites responded equally well, whereas neonatal skin responded minimally. The implications are that retinoids may be able to repair intrinsically aged skin as well as photoaged skin, and that retinoids may modulate skin cell function in a manner that is age-related, not simply a response to photo-damage.

TOXICITY

The adverse effects of retinoids are legion, and are mostly associated with hypervitaminosis A (acute or chronic). Fetal malformations, spontaneous abortions, hyperlipidemia (particularly elevated triglycerides), bone abnormalities, skin and mucosal dryness, retinoid dermatitis, pruritus, hair loss, pseudotumor cerebri, arthralgias, myalgias, and abnormal liver function tests (increased liver transaminases and alkaline phosphatase) are among the myriad potential adverse effects of retinoid therapy (30). Most of the above effects are reversible upon discontinuation of the retinoid, although some serious effects, such as fetal malformations and bone abnormalities, are not. We do not have sufficient case population data to be certain of cause and effect and no true double-blind studies exist. Recently, two classes of nuclear receptors, the retinoic acid receptors and the RXRs (retinoid x receptors) have been identified, which are thought to play an important role in mediating retinoid-induced toxicity. The details of this mechanism are beyond the scope of this chapter and the reader is directed toward a recent review for elucidation (31).

Topical application has the benefit of a significantly better adverse effect profile. The most common sequelae are mucocutaneous effects, characterized by skin and mucosal dryness (xerosis, cheilitis, conjunctivitis), desquamation, erythema, and pruritus. These effects typically start after several days of therapy, peak within the first few weeks, then wane as tolerance develops (32). They are easily treatable—frequent application of emollients and other precautionary measures (such as avoidance of harsh soaps, astringents, abrasives, and excessive bathing) will ameliorate the situation. The mucocutaneous effects are dose-dependent and reversible upon discontinuation of the retinoid.

Teratogenicity, well documented as the most serious side effect of oral retinoids (33), is logically the potential concern with topical retinoids. With oral retinoids, most aromatic retinoids cross the placenta; *in utero* exposure results in limb and craniofacial deformities, as well as cardiovascular and central nervous system abnormalities. Systemic absorption of topical retinoids, however, is thought to be negligible (34). A large retrospective study of birth defects in off-spring born to mothers exposed to topical tretinoin (all-*trans*-retinoic acid) during pregnancy has demonstrated no significant risk (35). Animal studies by Willhite et al. (36) support these data, suggesting that the drug would not be expected to cross the placenta unless present at extremely high concentrations. Even in light of this evidence, many clinicians feel strongly about avoiding topical retinoids in pregnancy (37).

Reports of enhanced photocarcinogenicity in experimental mice exist (38), but no evidence exists of a comparable process with humans (39). Conversely, topical retinoids appear to have a protective effect against ultraviolet-induced premalignant and malignant lesions. However, skin treated with topical retinoids is more reactive to chemical and physical stresses (including ultraviolet light), because of the thinner horny layer and amplified vasculature. The concomitant use of sunscreens is therefore a necessary precaution.

THE FUTURE

Retinoids have revolutionized dermatological and cosmeceutical therapeutics for the past two decades. The successful trials of topical tretinoin have inspired the pursuit of other topical retinoids that could be effective in photoaging with fewer adverse effects. Undoubtedly, newer derivatives with safer adverse effect profiles will be forthcoming. Specifically, two new retinoids, adapalene and tazarotene, licensed for the treatment of acne and psoriasis, respectively, will almost certainly be investigated for photodamage.

REFERENCES

1. Mandel HG, Cohn VH. Fat-soluble vitamins. In: Gilman AG, Goodman LS, Gilman A, eds. The Pharmacological Basis of Therapeutics, 6th ed. New York: Macmillan, 1980:1583–1592.
2. Stepp W. Versuche über Fütterung mit lipoidfreier Nahrung. Biochem Z 1909; 22:452.
3. McCollum EV, Kennedy C. The dietary factors operating in the production of polyneuritis. J Biol Chem 1916; 24:491–502.
4. Drummond JC. The nomenclature of the so-called accessory food factors (vitamins). Biochem J 1920; 14:660.
5. McCollum EV, Davis M. The necessity of certain lipins in the diet during growth. J Biol Chem 1913; 15:167–175.
6. Stüttgen G. Zur Lokalbehandlung von Keratosen mit Vitamin-A Säure. Dermatologica 1962; 124:65–80.
7. Kligman AM, Fulton JE, Plewig G. Topical vitamin A acid in acne vulgaris. Arch Dermatol 1969; 99:469–476.
8. Kligman AM, Grove GL, Hirose R, Leyden JJ. Topical tretinoin for photoaged skin. J Am Acad Dermatol 1986; 15:836–859.
9. Ellis CN, Weiss JS, Hamilton TA, Headington JT, Zelickson AS, Voorhees JJ. Sustained improvement with prolonged topical tretinoin (retinoic acid) for photoaged skin. J Am Acad Dermatol 1990; 23(4 Pt 1):629–637.
10. Misiewicz J, Sendagorta E, Golebiowska A et al. Topical treatment of multiple actinic keratoses of the face with arotinoid methyl sulfone (Ro 14-9706) cream versus tretinoin cream: a double blind, comparative study. J Am Acad Dermatol 1991; 24(3):448–451.
11. Kligman AM. Guidelines for the use of topical tretinoin (retin-A) for photoaged skin. J Am Acad Dermatol 1989; 21(3 Pt 2):650–654.
12. Kang S, Duell EA, Fisher GJ, Datta SC, Wang Z-Q, Reddy AP, Tavakkol A, Yi JY, Griffiths CEM, Elder JT, Voorhees JJ. Application of retinol to human skin in vivo

induces epidermal hyperplasia and cellular retinoid binding proteins characteristic of retinoic acid, but without measurable retinoic acid levels or irritation. J Invest Dermatol 1995; 105(4):549–556.
13. Duell EA, Derguini F, Kang S, Elder JT, Voorhees JJ. Extraction of human epidermis treated with retinol yields retro-retinoids in addition to free retinol and retinyl esters. J Invest Dermatol 1996; 107(2):178–182.
14. Blaner WS, Olson JA. Retional and retinoic acid metabolism. In: Sporn MB, Roberts AB, Goodman DS, eds. The Retinoids: Biology, Chemistry and Medicine, 2nd ed. New York: Raven Press, 1994:283–318.
15. Hodam JR, Creek KE. Comparison of the metabolism of retinol delivered to human keratinocytes either bound to serum retinol-binding protein or added directly to the culture medium. Exp Cell Res 1998; 238(1):257–264.
16. Bailly J, Cretaz M, Schifflers MH, Marty JP. In vitro metabolism by human skin and fibroblasts of retinol, retinal and retinoic acid. Exp Dermatol 1998; 7:27–34.
17. Randolph RK, Simon M. Dermal fibroblasts actively metabolize retinoic acid but not retinol. J Invest Dermatol 1998; 111(3):478–484.
18. Soprano DR, Balner WS. Plasma retinol-binding protein. In: Sporn MB, Roberts AB, Goodman DS, eds. The Retinoids: Biology, Chemistry, and Medicine, 2nd ed. New York: Raven, 1994:257–282.
19. Goffin V, Henry F, Pirard-Franchimont C, Pirard GE. Topical retinol and the stratum corneum response to an environmental threat. Skin Pharmacol 1997; 10:85–89.
20. Matsuoka LY, Uitto J. Alterations in the elastic fibers in cutaneous aging and solar elastosis. In: Balin AK, Kligman Am, eds. Aging and the Skin. New York: Raven Press, 1989, Ch. 7.
21. Kang S, Fisher G, Voorhees JJ. Photoaging and topical tretinoin. Arch Dermatol 1997; 133:1280–1284.
22. Gilchrest BA, Blog FB, Szabo G. Effects of aging and chronic sun exposure on melanocytes in human skin. J Invest Dermatol 1979; 73:77–83.
23. Braverman IM. Elastic fiber and microvascular abnormalities in aging skin. In: Kligman AM, Talase Y, eds. Cutaneous Aging. Tokyo: University of Tokyo Press, 1988:369.
24. Kligman LH. Effects of all-trans-retinoic acid on the dermis of hairless mice. J Am Acad Dermatol 1986; 15:779–785.
25. Weiss JS, Ellis CN, Headington JT et al. Topical tretinoin improves photoaged skin. JAMA 1988; 259:527–532.
26. Leyden JJ, Grove GL, Grove MJ et al. Treatment of photodamaged facial skin with topical tretinoin. J Am Acad Dermatol 1989; 21:638–644.
27. Lever L, Kumar P, Marks R. Topical retinoic acid in the treatment of solarelastotic degeneration. Br J Dermatol 1990; 122:91–98.
28. Olsen EA, Katz I, Levine N et al. Tretinoin emollient cream: a new therapy for photodamaged skin. J Am Acad Dermatol 1992; 26:215–224.
29. Varani J, Fisher GJ, Kang S, Voorhees JJ. Molecular mechanisms of intrinsic skin aging and retinoid-induced repair and reversal. Symposium Proceedings, J Invest Dermatol 1998; 3(1):57–60.
30. Silverman AK, Ellis CN, Voorhees JJ. Hypervitaminosis A syndrome: a paradigm of retinoid side effects. J Am Acad Dermatol 1987; 16(5):1027–1039.

31. Doran TI, Cunningham WJ. Retinoids and their mechanisms of toxicity. In: Marzulli FN, Maibach HI, eds. Dermatotoxicology, 5th ed. Washington DC: Taylor & Francis, 1996:289–298.
32. Kligman AM, Dogadkna D, Lavher RM. Effects of topical tretinoin on non-sun-exposed protected skin of the elderly. J Am Acad Dermatol 1993; 29:25–33.
33. Lammer EJ, Chen DT, Hoar RM, Agnish ND, Benke PJ, Braun JT, Curry CJ, Fernhoff PM, Grix AW, Lott IT, Richard JM, Sun SC. Retinoic acid embryopathy. N Engl J Med 1985; 313:837–841.
34. Worobec SM, Wong FGA, Tolman EL et al. Percutaneous absorption of 3H-tretinoin in normal volunteers. J Invest Dermatol 1991; 96:574A.
35. Jick SS, Terris BZ, Jick H. First trimester topical tretinoin congenital disorders. Lancet 1993; 341:1181–1182.
36. Willhite CC, Sharma RP, Allen PV, Berry DL. Percutaneous retinoid absorption and embryotoxicity. J Invest Dermatol 1990; 95:523–529.
37. Martinez-Frias ML, Rodriguez-Pinila E. First-trimester exposure to topical tretinoin: its safety is not warranted. Teratology 1999; 60:5.
38. Forbes PD, Urbach F, Davies RE. Enhancement of experimental photocarcinogenesis by topical retinoic acid. Cancer 1979; 7:85–90.
39. Epstein JH. Photocarcinogenesis and topical retinoids. In: Marks R, ed. Retinoids in Cutaneous Malignancy. Oxford: Blackwell Scientific Publications, 1991:171–182.

18

UV Care

Kumi Arakane
Research & Development Division, KOSE Corporation, Azusawa Itabashi, Tokyo, Japan

Introduction	333
Acute UV-Induced Skin Damage	334
Chronic UV-Induced Skin Damage	336
Reactive Oxygen Species Generated by UV Irradiation and Skin Damage	336
Superoxide Anion, Hydrogen Peroxide, and Hydroxyl Radical	337
Singlet Oxygen	338
Nitric Oxide	339
Prevention of Skin Damage by Scavenging of Reactive Oxygen Species	341
Antioxidants	341
Iron Chelators	343
Conclusion	345
References	346

INTRODUCTION

Living organisms are protected from harmful ultraviolet (UV) rays and UV irradiation by the ozone layer surrounding the earth. However, depletion of the ozone layer, which plays an important role in shielding the earth from UV rays, and an increase in the amount of UV rays in sunlight reaching the earth's surface have been recently reported. As a result, social concerns over the effects of UV on living organisms have been increasing year by year. Especially, an increase in skin cancer incidence has emerged as a serious problem.

UV rays are generally electromagnetic waves with wavelengths of 100–400 nm, and are classified as vacuum UV (100–190 nm), UVC (190–290 nm), UVB (290–320 nm), and UVA (320–400 nm) according to their biological action. Vacuum UV and UVC do not reach the surface of the earth, whereas about half of UVB and all of UVA reach the surface. UV (UVB + UVA) energy accounts for about 6% of the total energy of the sun's rays, whereas visible light and infrared rays account for about 52% and 42%, respectively.

Because the skin covers the outer surface of the body, it is most vulnerable to UV. Regarding transmission of UV rays reaching the earth's surface to the skin, light of shorter wavelengths (UVB) is scattered on the skin surface and absorbed in the epidermis, and light of longer wavelengths (UVA) penetrates deep into the skin (1). Substances that absorb UVB in the epidermis include DNA, protein, and lipid. These molecules are damaged by UV rays, causing various cellular functional changes. The wavelengths of UV rays and substances in the skin that absorb UV energy are related to skin damage induced by UV irradiation, which is very important in understanding the characteristics of skin damage caused by UV rays.

ACUTE UV-INDUCED SKIN DAMAGE

Skin responses to UV irradiation can largely be classified as acute and chronic damages. An acute reaction, browning of the skin resulting from exposure to the sun's rays, generally includes "sunburn" (inflammation of the skin) and "suntan" (pigmentation that occurs following sunburn). Sunburn is a normal acute response of skin exposed to UVB. In sunburned skin UVB-induced erythema is observed. UVB-induced erythema is caused by the dilation of dermal blood vessels resulting from the exposure to UV rays, and starts to appear a few hours after UV exposure and reaches its peak 12–24 h after exposure.

Minimum erythema dose (MED) is used as an index to express the sensitivity of the skin to UV. MED is the minimum dose of UVB that will produce an erythema reaction in the skin observable with the naked eye 24 h after exposure. The higher the sensitivity to UVB, the smaller the amount of UVB required to induce an erythema reaction. The minimum dose of UVB that will produce an erythema reaction in the skin depends on the wavelength and can be expressed as a curve, the so-called "erythema action spectrum". The relative intensity curve of the erythema reaction obtained from the action spectrum for erythema in human skin and the spectral distribution of sunlight indicates that sunlight of about 310 nm is most likely to cause an erythema reaction. This indicates that cutting-out light at around 310 nm is effective to protect the skin from sunburn. Accordingly, sunscreen agents containing various UV-scattering agents and UV absorbers are being developed.

In a series of acute responses, histological changes, including formation of sunburn cells (considered to be a type of apoptosis) and thickening of the epidermis, are observed in addition to pigmentation and exfoliation following erythema formation. Formation of sunburn cells is one of the histological changes, characteristic of skin damage induced by UV, especially UVB. Sunburn cells are defined as apoptotic keratinocytes within the epidermis exhibiting an eosinophilic cytoplasm and hematoxilinophilic condensed nucleus by hematoxylin and eosin staining (2,3). Sunburn cells start to appear a few hours after UVB irradiation and the number of cells reaches its peak 24–48 h after irradiation. Because formation of sunburn cells correlates with the amount of UV rays, it is used as a quantitative indicator to measure damage to the epidermis induced by UV. Although cells at the same distance from the skin surface are exposed to the same amount of UV rays, not all cells become sunburn cells, and neighboring keratinocytes show no morphological changes. Because formation of sunburn cells is reduced when the cell cycle is suppressed (4), the sensitivity of a keratinocyte to UV is considered to vary depending on the cell cycle (5).

Acute damages such as skin inflammation, erythema, and sunburn cell formation caused by UV can be considered as protective functions of the skin to minimize damage induced by UV irradiation and provide further protection against subsequent UV exposure. In other words, acute damage serves as a trigger that activates protective functions of keratinocytes and melanocytes against UV and induces various protective responses.

It is widely known that UVB accelerates melanogenesis in melanocyte. Endothelin, α-melanocyte-stimulating hormone, and diacylglycerol have been considered to induce melanogenesis. A study has shown that DNA damage following UVB irradiation and repair of the damaged DNA are the signals generated by UV irradiation to stimulate pigmentation in human skin (6). This finding indicates that DNA damage is strongly related not only to sunburn, but also to suntan.

After UVB irradiation damages the barrier function of the epidermis, destroys the intercellular lamellar structure, and increases transepidermal water loss, biosynthesis of epidermal lipids, such as cholesterol, free fatty acids, and sphingolipid, rapidly progresses to repair the barrier functions of the skin. Because the activity of transglutaminase, an enzyme that catalyzes the formation of the cornified envelope at the final differentiation of keratinocytes, increases after UVB irradiation, differentiation of keratinocytes is also considered to be temporarily enhanced (7).

A recent report demonstrated that p53 (a protein of tumor suppressor gene)-mediated cell cycle arrest, in other words, p53-dependent induction of the cell cycle inhibitor p21, might potentially play a central role in a defense mechanism to protect the skin from UV (8).

CHRONIC UV-INDUCED SKIN DAMAGE

UV damages essential elements, including collagen and elastin which maintain elasticity and firmness of the skin, and also damages the function of fibroblasts producing these elements. People who have been engaged often in outdoor activities and exposed to sunlight over long periods of time have atrophic, shriveled, and pigmented skin. This is called actinic elastosis. Severe cases of actinic elastosis include Favre–Racouhot syndrome and farmer's skin. In farmer's skin, rhomboidal wrinkles (deep grooves crossing obliquely to form rhombus-shaped wrinkles) are observed. Because these features are prominently observed only in sun-exposed areas, they are apparently caused by chronic damage due to accumulated UV exposure and are called photoaging to distinguish them from normal intrinsic aging.

In addition to a change in appearance (large deep wrinkles) histological changes, including thickening of the epidermis and dermis, elastin fiber deposition, and decreased collagen fibers, are observed as a result of continuous UV (UVB or UVB + UVA) irradiation (9). Because an increase in tissue iron content associated with a chronic increase in permeability of skin vasculature is observed in sun-exposed sites in the skin, involvement of ferric ion-mediated action of reactive oxygen species is suggested in photoaging (10).

Recently, localization of advanced glycation endproducts (AGEs), end products of the Maillard reaction, was found in areas of actinic elastosis. This finding suggests involvement of AGEs in photoaging (11). As AGEs produce reactive oxygen species when exposed to UVA irradiation, it is also speculated that reactive oxygen species are involved in the processes of AGEs production and acceleration of elastic fiber degeneration by AGEs (12).

UVB damages Langerhans cells in the epidermis, as well as keratinocytes and fibroblasts, destroying the dendricity of Langerhans cells and decreasing the Langerhans cell population. Observation of morphological damage revealed that a considerable amount of time is necessary to repair UVB-induced damage (13). If the same amount of UVB is irradiated, repeated UVB irradiation of sub-erythema dose can cause more damage than a single high-dose irradiation (Fig. 1) (14). A decrease in the Langerhans cell population in chronically UV-exposed skin has also been reported (15,16).

Damage in the epidermis caused by UV-induced immunosuppression leads to dysfunction of immune responses, the host defense mechanism. This is markedly different from other damage in the epidermis.

REACTIVE OXYGEN SPECIES GENERATED BY UV IRRADIATION AND SKIN DAMAGE

It has already been shown that reactive oxygen species are responsible for many diseases. Recently, involvement of reactive oxygen species in UV-induced skin damages, such as sunburn, phototoxicity, and photoallergy, and skin diseases,

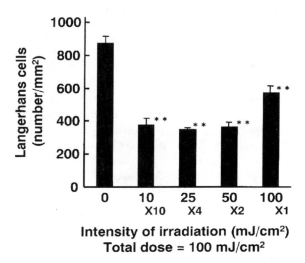

Figure 1 Number of Langerhans cells in UVB-irradiated epidermal specimens. Repeated irradiation with low-dose UVB. The total energy of each irradiation was 100 mJ/cm². Langerhans cells in specimens irradiated four times with 25 mJ/cm² are markedly fewer than in specimens irradiated once with 100 mJ/cm². The data are presented as mean $\pm$ S.D. ($n = 12$). **$P < 0.01$ vs. no irradiation, Student's t-test.

such as atopic dermatitis and psoriasis, was suggested (17–19). Because reactive oxygen species are highly reactive, they react with various neighboring *in vivo* substances and cause oxidative damages such as lipid peroxidation, protein modification, and DNA damage, inducing cellular damage and dysfunction. Accumulation of these oxidative damages lead to aging.

The skin is exposed to the air and is unique organ in terms of oxygen stress. Continuously exposed to oxygen and UV, the skin is a primary target of reactive oxygen species generated by UV irradiation and plays a protective role against toxicity of reactive oxygen species.

Superoxide Anion, Hydrogen Peroxide, and Hydroxyl Radical

Reactive oxygen species generated by UV irradiation include singlet oxygen ($^1O_2$), superoxide anion (O_{2-}), hydrogen peroxide (H_2O_2), hydroxyl radical (·OH), and nitric oxide (NO). A number of reports indicate that reactive oxygen species generated by UV irradiation are responsible for the formation of sunburn cells and a decrease in Langerhans cells (20–22).

Measurement of reactive oxygen species, generated when UV rays in the wavelength range of UVB and UVA are irradiated, has recently been started. In UVB-irradiated dermal fibroblasts in mice and humans, ·OH was detected when the ESR spectrum was measured. Accumulated H_2O_2 in cells following UVB irradiation is considered to be transformed into the ·OH in the presence of metal ions (23). Highly reactive ·OH nonspecifically reacts with neighboring substances and causes cellular damage via DNA strand breakage and protein fragmentation (24).

When fibroblasts are treated with a specific inhibitor of catalase, 3-amino-1H-1,2,4-triazole, a similar increase in H_2O_2 concentration and aggravation of cellular damage are observed, as with UVB irradiation. This fact indicates that catalase plays an important role in the H_2O_2-scavenging systems in cells (25). UVA irradiation specifically decreases only catalase activity among antioxidant enzymes in the skin (26). Such a decrease in catalase activity naturally causes a rapid increase in H_2O_2 concentration in cells.

It is also reported that H_2O_2 generated by UVA irradiation induces DNA mutation (27). It is important to note that H_2O_2 is a precursor of ·OH and induces cell damage.

Singlet Oxygen

Photosensitivity caused by erythropoietic protoporphyria and pheophorbide is a major disease induced by UV irradiation. Because oral administration of a $^1O_2$ quencher, β-carotene, markedly relieves symptoms of photosensitivity, it is speculated that $^1O_2$ generated during the photosensitization process is a causative agent of photosensitivity.

Tetracyclines are representative drugs that induce phototoxicity as an adverse reaction. It has been shown that members of the tetracycline family generate $^1O_2$ during UV irradiation, and the amount of generated $^1O_2$ and degree of phototoxicity are well correlated (28). This result demonstrates that $^1O_2$ is a major reactive intermediate that induces tetracycline phototoxicity.

$^1O_2$ has been only determined as one of the reactive oxygen species that induce these specific skin diseases. Although it is suggested that $^1O_2$ is the main reactive intermediate responsible for damaging living organisms, there are few studies clearly demonstrating the generation and reactivity of $^1O_2$ in living organisms. However, recently, directly measurement of the near-infrared emission spectrum corresponding to $^1O_2$ (1268 nm) has shown that a metabolite of *Propionibacterium acnes* (*P. acnes*), coproporphyrin, existing on the skin surface generates $^1O_2$ when the skin was irradiated with UV rays (Fig. 2) (29).

The fact the porphyrins, produced by *P. acnes* and constantly existing on the skin, generate $^1O_2$ when the skin was irradiated with UV rays suggests that $^1O_2$ potentially induces reactions in the skin to cause various skin damage, not only in special cases such as photosensitivity as in erythropoietic protoporphyria, but also in healthy skin under physiological conditions.

Recent reports indicate that the reactive oxygen species responsible for UV-induced peroxidation of skin surface lipids is $^1O_2$ (Fig. 3) (30). $^1O_2$ induces cross-linking of collagen, one of the main components of the dermis (Fig. 4) (31), and the reactive oxygen species responsible for cellular aging by chronic UVA irradiation of human dermal fibroblasts is $^1O_2$ (32).

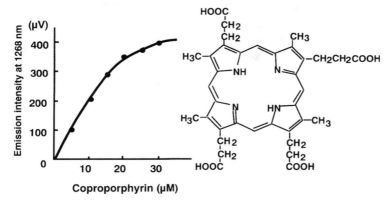

Figure 2 Singlet oxygen emission photosensitized by coproporphyrin. Singlet oxygen generation in coproporphyrin methanol solution (5–30 μM) excited by Ar laser light at UVA region with 100 mW output power was monitored by measuring the emission intensity at 1268 nm. [From Ref. (29).]

Nitric Oxide

In 1987, NO was found to be synthesized in the body and NO itself was an endothelium-derived relaxing factor. NO is synthesized by nitric oxide synthase (NOS) from arginine (a substrate for NOS). The main roles of NO synthesized by NOS are considered to be signaling and cytotoxicity.

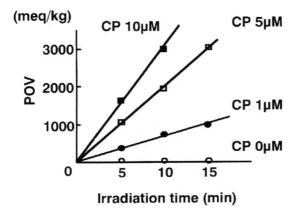

Figure 3 Peroxidation of skin surface lipid (squalene) by singlet oxygen produced by coproporphyrin. Squalene (5 mM) chloroform/methanol solution was irradiated with UVA by solar simulator with coproporphyrin (0–10 μM) and POV was measured at the indicated time. [From Ref. (30).]

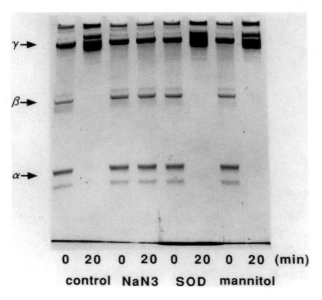

Figure 4 Effect of various quenchers on cross-linking of collagen by reactive oxygen species. Collagen solutions in 50 mM Tris–HCl buffer (pH 7.5) with various quenchers of reactive oxygen species (100 mM NaN$_3$, 10 mg/mL SOD, or 10 mg/mL mannitol) were irradiated by UVA for 10 min with 20 μM hematoporphyrin. [From Ref. (31).]

Recently, the relation between NO and skin diseases has been extensively studied. Reflecting its physiological action, NO is closely related to hyperproliferative skin diseases, inflammatory skin diseases, and immune-mediated skin diseases. There is concrete evidence suggesting that psoriasis, atopic dermatitis, sunburn erythema, allergic contact dermatitis, cutaneous lupus erythematosus, rosacca, and skin cancer are associated with NO (33–37). Especially, a number of reports indicate that NO is related to atopic dermatitis. In infected skin sites in patients with atopic dermatitis, expression of inducible nitric oxide synthase (iNOS) is about 100–1000 times that in normal skin. Regarding the relation between NO generation in the skin and UV irradiation, many studies demonstrated a correlation between UV-induced erythema in the skin and NO production. First, it was found that NOS or NO was possibly involved in the vasodilator response in the skin induced by UV irradiation (38,39). Then, it became clear that NO released from human keratinocytes following UVB irradiation played a major role in erythema production (40,41).

Studies have reported that not only NO, but also peroxynitrite is involved in the inflammatory process of erythema production, based on the relation between induction of NOS and activity of xanthine oxidase, a superoxide-generating system, in UVB-irradiated human keratinocytes, and on the correlation between an increase in NOS activity and the amount of generated peroxynitrite, a reaction product of superoxide and NO (42,43).

Romero-Graillet et al. (44,45) reported that NO produced by UVA or UVB-irradiated keratinocytes stimulated melanogenesis. NOS activity following UV irradiation is increased nearly threefold only 30 min after UVA or UVB irradiation, and its increased activity is maintained for 24 h after irradiation. Therefore, it is suggested that UVA and UVB stimulate melanogenesis by increasing the release of NO via stimulation of NOS in keratinocytes. As a mechanism of stimulation of melanogenesis, an increase in cGMP generated by stimulation of guanylate cyclase has been reported.

PREVENTION OF SKIN DAMAGE BY SCAVENGING OF REACTIVE OXYGEN SPECIES

Antioxidants

Many reports indicate that formation of sunburn cells, which is used as an index of UV-induced epidermal damage, can be prevented by various antioxidants. Major antioxidants include vitamin C (46) and superoxide dismutase (SOD) (47,48). A study reported that an SOD-containing cream was effective in preventing an increase in lipid peroxide (49).

It is known that the transcription factor NF-κB, which plays an important role in suppressing expression of genes involved in inflammatory and immune responses, is activated by UVB irradiation. Cysteine derivatives and DL-α-lipoic acid are reported to suppress its activation (50).

$^1O_2$ quenchers are effective in the treatment of UVA-induced damage. Increased production of matrix metalloprotease-1 (MMP-1) caused by UVA irradiation of fibroblasts and activation of activator protein-1 (a transcription factor which regulates MMP-1 expression) can be suppressed by $^1O_2$ quenchers (51). $^1O_2$ quenchers are effective against the shortened cell life span by chronic UVA irradiation of human dermal fibroblasts, early expression of senescence markers, and overexpression of extracellular matrix (32).

In addition to histological and biochemical analyses of human skin receiving UV irradiation for a long period of time, effective protection methods against photoaging are being investigated using photoaging models (hairless mice receiving UV irradiation over an extended time period). It goes without saying that application of UV-absorbing agents is effective in preventing changes associated with photoaging. It is also reported that antioxidants, such as vitamins C and E, tea polyphenols, and concomitant use of antioxidants and anti-inflammatory agents are effective (52,53).

Although the involvement of $^1O_2$ in photoaging remains unknown, we were able to demonstrate that $^1O_2$ quenchers play an important role in repair of photoaging, using a carotenoid, astaxanthin, which has no pro-vitamin A activity unlike β-carotene (which has high pro-vitamin A activity and is converted to vitamin A

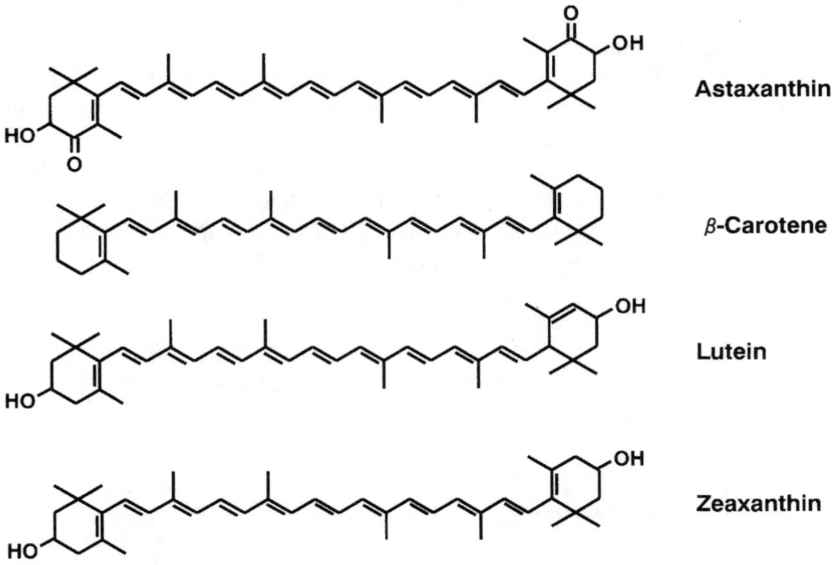

Figure 5 Structure of carotenoids.

in the body) (Fig. 5). The $^1O_2$-quenching ability of astaxanthin was extremely high compared with vitamin E or β-carotene (Fig. 6), and astaxanthin significantly reduced wrinkles in hairless mice as a model of photoaging (Fig. 7). Electron micrographs of the ultrastructure of dermal collagen and elastin fiber bundles showed that application of astaxanthin yielded marked maintenance of the bundle structures of dermal collagen and elastin fibers destroyed by UVB irradiation over a long period of time.

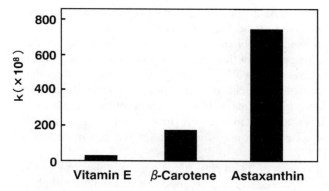

Figure 6 Rate constant of reaction of astaxanthin, β-carotene, and vitamin E with singlet oxygen.

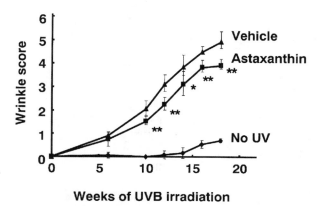

Figure 7 Inhibitory effect of astaxanthin on UVB-induced skin aging. Grading score for visible changes of mice skin by vehicle (▲), astaxanthin (■), and no UVB (◆). The data are expressed as mean ± S.D. ($n = 6$). Asterisk (*) indicates the significantly different values (*$P < 0.05$, **$P < 0.01$) from vehicle and UVB.

Iron Chelators

In the production of reactive oxygen species or free radicals, the ferric ion plays an important role as a catalyst (Fig. 8). The amount of ferric ion in the skin is increased by UVB irradiation over a long period of time. When the amount of iron found in sun-exposed skin of the human body and nonexposed skin was compared, sun-exposed skin such as the neck, forehead, and cheek had two to four times as much iron as nonexposed skin such as the thigh and buttock. This finding suggests that ferric ions serve as a causative agent of skin damage and

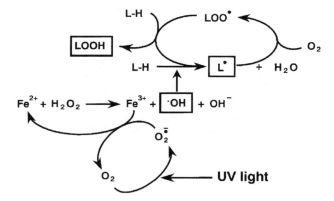

Figure 8 Role of ferrous/ferric iron in generation of reactive oxygen species induced by UVB irradiation.

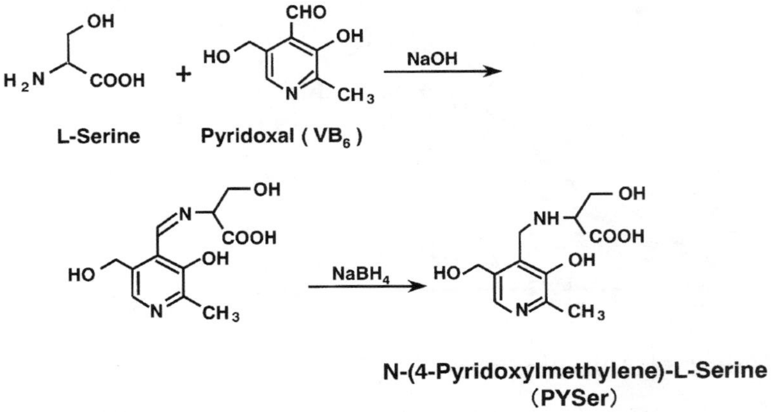

Synthesis of PYSer

L-Serine + Pyridoxal (VB$_6$) →(NaOH) N-pyridoxylidene-L-serine →(NaBH$_4$) **N-(4-Pyridoxylmethylene)-L-Serine (PYSer)**

Figure 9 Synthesis of PYSer. PYSer was prepared by condensation of L-serine with pyridoxal in an alkaline solution to form *N*-pyridoxylidene-L-serine and its direct catalytic reduction.

photoaging induced by UV irradiation (10). On the basis of these findings, topically applied iron chelators including 2,2-dipyridylamine, 1,10-phenannthroline, and 2-furildioxime are considered to be effective in minimizing acute damage or wrinkle formation by UVB irradiation (10,54). Development of new iron chelators using biomimetic molecules has been underway taking biocompatibility into account. *N*-(4-pyridoxylmethylene)-L-serine (PYSer) consists of a stabilized conjugate molecule of pyridoxal (vitamin B$_6$) and L-serine (amino acid). PYSer is created using compounds existing in the living body so that it can mimic the

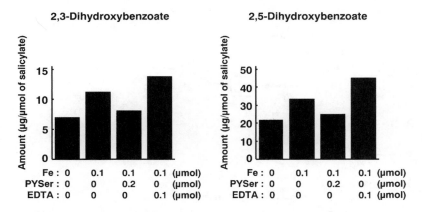

Figure 10 Inhibitory effect of PYSer on iron-induced hydroxyl radical formation in a salicylate hydroxylation assay. Influence on iron-induced formation of (left) 2,3-dihydroxybenzoate and (right) 2,5-dihydroxybenzoate by PYSer and EDTA. [From Ref. (50).]

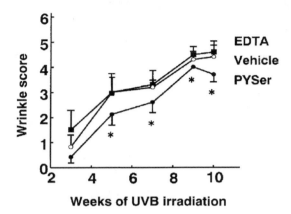

Figure 11 Inhibitory effect of PYSer on UVB induced skin aging. Grading score for visible changes of mice skin by vehicle (○), PYSer (●), and EDTA (■). The data are expressed as mean ± S.D. ($n = 5$). Asterisk (*) indicates significantly different value ($P < 0.05$) from vehicle and UVB. [From Ref. (50).]

coordinated bonding and stabilization of the chelate structure of iron-sequestering proteins in the living body and effectively suppress the production of ·OH (Fig. 9) (55).

PYSer decreases iron-catalyzed production of ·OH. On the other hand, EDTA increases the production of ·OH although it is a potent iron chelator (Fig. 10). Therefore, creation of iron chelators for the purpose of decreasing the production of ·OH must be performed very carefully. PYSer, which decreases iron-catalyzed production of ·OH, significantly suppressed wrinkle formation in hairless mice as a photoaging model (Fig. 11).

CONCLUSION

Acute and chronic skin damages caused by UV irradiation place a significant burden on the maintenance of homeostasis and the host-defense system. As a result, histological and biochemical changes occur in the skin, leading to changes in appearance such as pigmentation and wrinkle formation. Protecting the skin not only from intense UV exposure in the mountains or at the beach, but also from daily UV exposure is important to maintain our host-defense systems responsible for maintaining healthy, beautiful, and younger looking skin.

We believe that protection against UV continues to be the most important function of cosmetics. To increase the efficacy of cosmetics and provide more visible results, studies on skin science need to be further advanced and conducted thoroughly, so that effective materials or cosmetics will be developed for UV protection.

REFERENCES

1. Harber LC, Bickers DR. Photosensitivity Diseases. 2d ed. Toronto: BC Decker, 1989.
2. Daniels F, Brophy D, Lobitz W. Histochemical responses of human skin following ultraviolet irradiation. J Invest Dermatol 1961; 37:351–357.
3. Olson RL, Gaylor J, Everett MA. Ultraviolet-induced individual cell keratinization. J Cutan Pathol 1974; 1:120–125.
4. Danno K, Takigawa M, Horio T. Relationship of the cell cycle to sunburn cell formation. Photochem Photobiol 1981; 34:203–206.
5. Danno K, Horio T. Formation of UV-induced apoptosis relates to the cell cycle. Br J Dermatol 1982; 107:423–428.
6. Eller MS, Gilchrest BA. Tanning as part of the eukaryotic SOS response. Pigment Cell Res 2000; 13(suppl 8):94–97.
7. Asano H, Masunaga T, Takemoto Y. Effect of single challenge of UVB on corneocytes in $vivo$. Photomed Photobiol 1997; 19:123–124.
8. Hall PA, Mckee PH, Menage HD, Dover R, Lane DP. High-levels of p53 protein in UV-irradiated normal human skin. Oncogene 1993; 8:203–207.
9. Kligman AM, Takase Y, Gilchrest BA, Nordlund JJ, Pinnell SR. Cutaneous Aging. Tokyo: University of Tokyo Press, 1988.
10. Bissett DL, Chatterjee R, Hannon DP. Chronic ultraviolet radiation-induced increase in skin iron and the photoprotective effect of topically applied iron chelators. Photochem Photobiol 1991; 54:215–223.
11. Mizutari K, Ono T, Ikeda K, Kayashima K, Horiuchi S. Photo-enhanced modification of human skin elastin in actinic etastosis by N-(carboxymethyl)lysine, one of the glycoxidation products of the maillard reaction. J Invest Dermatol 1997; 108:797–802.
12. Masaki H, Okano Y, Sakurai H. Generation of active oxygen species from advanced glycation end products (AGEs) during ultraviolet light A (UVA) irradiation and a possible mechanism for cell damaging. Biochem Biophys Acta 1999; 1428:45–56.
13. Hatao M, Mark R, Stoudemayer T, Gabriel K. Recovery process of Langerhans cells in human skin following ultraviolet B irradiation. J Toxicol-Cut Ocular Toxicol 1993; 12:293–301.
14. Ishitsuka Y, Masunaga T, Koide C, Arakane K. Repeated irradiation with suberythemal ultraviolet B reduces the number of epidermal Langerhans cells. Arch Dermatol Res 2003; 295:155–159.
15. Thiers BH, Maize JC, Spicer SS, Cantor AB. The effect of aging and chronic sun exposure on human Langerhans cell population. J Invest Dermatol 1982; 82:223–226.
16. Hatao M, Stoudemayer T, Lichtin JL, Sakr A, Kligman AM. Effect of chronic actinic exposure on epidermal Langerhans cells of different ethnic groups. J Soc Cosmet Chem 1996; 47:117–128.
17. Matsuo I, Ohkido M. Effect of skin surface lipid peroxidation on photosensitivity. J Jpn Cosmet Sci Soc 1986; 10:138–140.
18. Hayaishi O, Imamura S, Miyachi Y. The Biological Role of Reactive Oxygen Species in Skin. Tokyo: University of Tokyo Press, 1987.
19. Carbonare MD, Pathak MA. Skin photosensitizing agents and the role of reactive oxygen species in photoaging. J Photochem Photobiol 1992; 14:105–124.
20. Horio T, Okamoto H. Oxygen intermediates are involved in ultraviolet radiation-induced damage of Langerhans cells. J Invest Dermatol 1987; 88:699–702.

21. Danno K, Horio T. Histochemical staining of sunburn cells for sulphhydryl disulphide groups: a time course study. Br J Dermatol 1980; 102:535–539.
22. Gilchrest BA, Soter NA, Stoff JS, Mihm MC Jr. The human sunburn reaction: histologic and biochemical studies. J Am Acad Dermatol 1981; 5:411–422.
23. Masaki H, Atsumi T, Sakurai H. Detection of hydrogen peroxide and hydroxyl radicals in murine skin fibroblasts under UVB irradiation. Biochem Biophys Res Commum 1995; 206:474–479.
24. Kawanishi S, Hiraku T. Sequence-specific DNA damage induced by UVA radiation in the presence of endogenous and exogenous photosensitizers. In: Thiele J, Elsner P, eds. Oxidants and Antioxidants in Cutaneous Biology. Curr Probl Dermatol. Basel: Karger, 2001, Vol. 29:74–82.
25. Masaki H, Sakurai H. Increased generation of hydrogen peroxide possibly mitochondrial respiratory chain after UVB irradiation of murine fibroblasts. J Dermatol Sci 1997; 14:207–216.
26. Takisada M, Arakane K, Kaji K. Fluctuation of antioxidant enzymes in skin by UV-A irradiation. J Soc Cosmet Chem Jpn 1997; 31:396–402.
27. Cadet J, Odin F, Mouret JF, Polverelli M, Audic A, Giacomoni P, Favier A, Richard MJ. Chemical and biochemical postlabeling methods for singling out specific oxidative DNA lesions. Mutat Res 1992; 275:343–354.
28. Hasan T, Khan AU. Phototoxicity of the tetracyclines: photosensitized emission of singlet delta dioxygen. Proc Natl Acad Sci USA 1986; 83:4604–4606.
29. Arakane K, Ryu A, Hayashi C, Masunaga T, Shinmoto K, Mashiko S, Nagano T, Hirobe M. Singlet oxygen ($^1\Delta g$) generation from coproporphyrin in *Propionibacterium acnes* on irradiation. Biochem Biophys Res Commun 1996; 223:578–582.
30. Ryu, A, Arakane K, Hayashi C, Masunaga T, Shinmoto K, Nagano T, Hirobe M, Mashiko S. Peroxidation of skin surface lipids by singlet oxygen produced by *Propionibacterium acnes*. J Jpn Cosmet Sci Soc 1995; 19:1–6.
31. Ryu A, Naru E, Arakane K, Masunaga T, Shinmoto K, Nagano T, Hirobe M, Mashiko S. Cross-linking of collagen by singlet oxygen generated with UV-A. Chem Pharm Bull 1997; 45:1243–1247.
32. Naru E, Moriyama M, Inomata K, Hayashi A, Arakane K, Kaji K. Functional changes induced by chronic UV-A irradiation to human dermal fibroblasts. J Jpn Cosmet Sci Soc 2002; 26:79–85.
33. Kolb-Bachofen V, Fehsel K, Michel G, Ruzicka T. Epidermal keratinocyte expression of inducible nitric oxide synthase in skin lesions of psoriasis vulgaris. Lancet 1994; 344:139.
34. Sirsjo A, Karlsson M, Gidlof A, Rollman O, Torma H. Increased expression of inducible nitric oxide synthase in psoriatic skin and cytokine-stimulated cultured keratinocytes. Br J Dermatol 1996; 134:643–648.
35. Ormerod AD, Weller R, Copeland P, Benjamin N, Ralston SH, Grabowksi P, Herriot R. Detection of nitric oxide and nitric oxide synthase in psoriasis. Arch Dermatol Res 1998; 290:3–8.
36. Kuhn A, Fehsel K, Lehmann P, Krutmann J, Ruzicka T, Kolb-Bachofen V. Aberrant timing in epidermal expression of inducible nitric oxide synthase after UV irradiation in cutaneous lupus erythematosus. J Invest Dermatol 1998; 111:149–153.
37. Bruch-Gerharz D, Ruzicka T, Kolb-Bachofen V. Nitric oxide and its implications in skin homeostasis and disease—a review. Arch Dermatol Res 1998; 290:643–651.

38. Warren JB, Loi RK, Coughlan ML. Involvement of nitric oxide synthase in the delayed vasodilator response to ultraviolet light irradiation of rat skin in vivo. Br J Pharmacol 1993; 109:802–806.
39. Warren JB. Nitric oxide and human skin blood flow responses to acetylcholine and ultraviolet light. FASEB J 1994; 8:247–251.
40. Deliconstantinos G, Villiotou V, Stavrides JC. Release by ultraviolet B radiation of nitric oxide from human keratinocytes: a potential role for nitric oxide in erythema production. Br J Pharmacol 1995; 114:1257–1265.
41. Deliconstantinos G, Villiotou V, Stavrides JC. Inhibition of ultraviolet B-induced skin erythema by N-nitro-L-arginine and N-monomethyl-L-arginine. J Dermatol Sci 1997; 15:23–35.
42. Deliconstantinos G, Villiotou V, Stavrides JC. Alterations of nitric oxide synthase and xanthine oxidase activities of human keratinocytes by ultraviolet B radiation. Potential role for peroxynitrite in skin inflammation. Biochem Pharmacol 1996; 51:1727–1738.
43. Deliconstantinos G, Villiotou V, Stavrides JC. Increase of particulate nitric oxide synthase activity and peroxynitrite synthesis in UVB-irradiated keratinocyte membranes. Biochem J 1996; 320:997–1003.
44. Romero-Graillet C, Aberdam E, Biagoli N, Massabni W, Ortonne JP, Ballotti R. Ultraviolet B radiation acts through the nitric oxide and cGMP signal transduction pathway to stimulate melanogenesis in human melanocytes. J Biol Chem 1996; 271:28052–28056.
45. Romero-Graillet C, Aberdam E, Clement M, Ortonne JP, Ballotti R. Nitric oxide produced by ultraviolet-irradiated keratinocytes stimulates melanogenesis. J Clin Invest 1997; 99:635–642.
46. Darr D, Combs S, Dunston S, Manning T. Topical vitamin C protects porcine skin from ultraviolet radiation induced damage. Br J Dermatol 1992; 127:247–253.
47. Miyachi Y, Horio T, Imamura S. Sunburn cell formation is prevented by scavenging oxygen intermediates. Clin Exp Dermatol 1983; 8:305–310.
48. Danno K, Horio T, Takigawa M, Imamura S. Role of oxygen intermediates in UV-induced epidermal cell injury. J Invest Dermatol 1984; 83:166–168.
49. Ogura R, Sugiyama M. Active oxygen species and free radicals formed in the epidermis exposed to ultraviolet light. J Act Oxyg Free Rad 1992; 3:270–277.
50. Kitazawa M, Iwasaki K, Sakamoto K, Saliou C, Packer L. Redox system regulates UV induced-inflammation in human epidermal cells. J Jpn Cosmet Sci Soc 2000; 24:168–171.
51. Kitazawa M, Iwasaki K, Sakamoto K, Saliou C, Packer L. Influence on AP-1 activation and MMP-1 expression by UV irradiation to human normal dermal fibroblasts. J Jpn Cosmet Sci Soc 2001; 25:125–129.
52. Pinnell SR. Cutaneous photodamage, oxidative stress, and topical antioxidant protection. J Am Acad Dermatol 2003; 48:1–19.
53. Bissett DL, Chatterjee R, Hannon DP. Protective effect of a topically applied antioxidant plus an anti-inflammatory agent against ultraviolet radiation-induced chronic skin damage in the hairless mouse. J Soc Cosmet Chem 1992; 43:85–92.
54. Bissett DL, McBride JF. Synergistic topical photoprotection by a combination of the iron chelator 2-furildioxime and sunscreen. J Am Acad Dermatol 1996; 35:546–549.
55. Kitazawa M, Iwasaki K, Ishitsuka Y, Kobayashi M, Arakane K. Molecular design of a novel antioxidant for suppression of photoaging. J Soc Cosmet Chem Jpn 2001; 35:149–154.

19

Use of Growth Factors in Cosmeceuticals

Richard E. Fitzpatrick
Dermatology Associates of San Diego County, Inc., Encinitas, California, USA

Introduction	349
Pathology of Photoaged Skin	350
Cosmetic Approaches to Photoaged Skin	350
Growth Factors: What Are They?	351
Growth Factors and Wound Healing	351
Growth Factors in Cosmetic Applications	353
Combination Approaches: Laser Plus Topical Growth Factors	356
Risks Associated with Growth Factors	357
Conclusions	358
Acknowledgment	359
References	359

INTRODUCTION

The pathology of photoaged (sun exposed) skin has been likened to that of a chronic wound in which remodeling is incomplete because of the extensive surface area involved and the complication of ongoing photodamage (sun exposure) (1). Indeed, healing wounds serve well as a physiologic "system" by which factors affecting skin renewal can be studied. Recently, the cosmetics and aesthetics industries have sought to achieve a rational approach to skin care by the use of "cosmeceutical" preparations with known physiologic activities. For example, vitamin A derivatives (retinoids) and vitamin C are common ingredients in cosmeceuticals, and are known to have activities beneficial to skin repair. An emerging trend in cosmeceuticals is the modulation of aging changes by the use of naturally occurring cell regulatory proteins called growth factors. Growth factors are normally present in tissues to stimulate cell growth, modulate immunity, and orchestrate cell development. They have been studied in wound healing systems (*in vitro* and *in vivo*) for many years and definitive evidence of proregenerative effects in wound healing have been demonstrated. Thus, it is reasonable to consider that they would have similar benefits in skin care applications. This chapter provides the rationale for the use of growth factors for the modulation of aged and photodamaged skin and includes some recent clinical trials evidence to support this assumption.

PATHOLOGY OF PHOTOAGED SKIN

Cumulative exposure to the sun, both ultraviolet A and B wavelengths (UVA and UVB), results in epidermal changes that include changes in keratinocyte proliferation and keratin production; increased, irregular pigmentary patterns; and disruption of the dermal–epidermal junction, with flattening of the dermal papillary layer (2–4). Changes in the dermal matrix include accelerated degeneration of collagen and elastin, resulting in loss of structural integrity, and dilated surface capillaries (telangiectases). Chronic inflammatory activity and degenerative processes result in the unchecked production of oxygen-free radicals, which perpetuate the catabolic environment. These cellular events translate to external characteristics such as fine wrinkles (loss of collagen and elastin), sagging, thinner skin (loss of adipose tissue in the subcutis as well as dermal changes), deepened lines of expression, dry skin (reduced keratinocyte turnover and sebum production), and age spots (solar lentigines) (4).

COSMETIC APPROACHES TO PHOTOAGED SKIN

Traditionally, the cosmetic response to photoaging changes has been (1) removal of the superficial layers of the affected skin with chemical peels, dermabrasion, or by pulsed laser technology, followed by regeneration of healthy tissue (5–9), and/or (2) application of topical products that include ingredients known to augment cellular regenerative processes. The synthetic vitamin A derivative, tretinoin (Retin-A, Renova), has been on the market for more than 30 years and has well-substantiated collagen-promoting and epithelial cell-stimulating effects (10). Milder forms of vitamin A, such as retinol and retinyl palmitate, have epidermal activity as a result of their conversion to retinoic acid in the skin (11–14).

Vitamin C is essential for collagen production and is a known antioxidant, characteristics that are advantageous in promoting skin repair (15–20). Most recently the search for a scientifically rational approach to skin renewal has embraced a group of naturally occurring soluble proteins known to be essential for cell growth and communication processes. These proteins are called growth factors.

GROWTH FACTORS: WHAT ARE THEY?

Growth factors are cytokines, proteins produced by a variety of cell types, which function to regulate cell growth, development, and activation. Many cytokines play a significant role in the mediation of the immune response, which is highly active during disease and trauma conditions. Nevertheless, as cellular communications are necessary in all tissues for the maintenance of general homeostasis, cytokine activity is ongoing during all phases of physiologic process. Growth factors are capable of acting on different cell types and are redundant in the functions they perform. This makes categorization by functional class difficult. Some growth factors, transforming growth factor beta (TGF-β) for example, are capable of stimulating cells from a variety of different tissues. Thus, the regulation of tissue repair and immune response are interconnected and highly complex.

Over the past 25 years, the participation of growth factors in wound healing has been extensively studied and more completely defined, although much remains to be known of this extremely complex process. The roles of certain growth factors in the restoration of an intact epithelium and the re-establishment of a structurally intact connective tissue dermis are well established. The cellular activity necessary to achieve restoration of the intact integument is extraordinarily complex and involves, once again, both tissue repair and regulation of immune response. It is of utmost importance to recognize that tissue repair is the result of the *interaction* of many cytokines and growth factors working together to re-establish a balanced homeostatic tissue environment.

GROWTH FACTORS AND WOUND HEALING

Understanding the four phases of wound healing: hemostasis, inflammation, proliferation (granulation), and remodeling, provides a better understanding of the roles of some individual growth factors and their interrelationships.

During hemostasis, platelets release various cytokines and other growth factors at the wound site to stimulate chemotaxis and mitogenesis, with resultant clot formation (21). In the inflammatory stage, neutrophils and monocytes (macrophages) called to the wound site in response to platelet-derived cytokines, initiate phagocytosis and release additional enzymes and growth factors [collagenase, interleukins, tumor necrosis factor (TNF), among others] that attract fibroblasts, promote vascular ingrowth (angiogenesis), and stimulate keratinocytes, marking the transition to the reconstructive (proliferative) phase of wound repair.

Epithelialization, angiogenesis, and granulation tissue formation (collagen, elastin, and matrix glycoprotein deposition) are orchestrated by a milieu of growth factors (Table 1) as reconstruction efforts proceed, while the final stages of inflammation are completed (22). During proliferation, keratinocytes restore barrier function to the skin and secrete additional growth factors that stimulate the expression of new keratin proteins (EGF and KGF). Fibroblasts produce collagen that is deposited in the wound bed [fibroblast growth factor (FGF), TGF-β, platelet-derived growth factor (PDGF)]. This cycle of collagen production and growth factor secretion continues in a type of autocrine feedback loop of continuous wound repair.

Once inflammation is resolved and substantial proliferation of viable new tissue is established, the remodeling phase of wound healing can begin. This phase is the final step in the wound repair process and typically lasts several months. It is during remodeling that the extracellular matrix is reorganized,

Table 1 Phases of Wound Healing and Growth Factor Involvement

Phase	Activities	Growth factors involved
Hemostasis	Neutrophils, platelets, and plasma proteins infiltrate the wound and initiate vasoconstriction	TGF-α, TGF-β, PDGF, EGF, IGF-1, VEGF
	Platelets release clotting factors to initiate coagulation	
	Platelets then release cytokines and other growth factors that attract neutrophils, macrophages, monocytes, and other cells necessary for cutaneous healing	
Inflammation	Neutrophils initiate phagocytosis and attract macrophages	PDGF, IL-1, IL-8, TNF-α, G-CSF, GM CSF
	Macrophages continue phagocytosis and release additional growth factors and cytokines, which attract fibroblasts to the wound, promote angiogenesis, and stimulate keratinocyte growth	
Proliferation (also known as granulation)	Fibroblasts synthesize collagen	EGF, PDGF, TGF-β
	New collagen fibers begin to form a matrix, or scaffold, for additional fibroblast attachment	
Remodeling (also known as maturation)	Collagen fibers are remodeled, or crosslinked, into an organized matrix	TFG-β, KGF, PDGF, HGF
	Additional collagen fibers attach to the matrix and are assembled into new tissue	
	Wound contraction and tissue strengthening occurs	

scar tissue is formed, and the wound is strengthened. Type III collagen deposited during the proliferation phase is gradually replaced by type I collagen, which is more tightly crosslinked and provides more tensile strength to the matrix than type III collagen.

Historically, growth factor products have found application and enthusiastic acceptance as a treatment of burns and chronic wounds, such as diabetic and stasis ulcers. The human fibroblast-derived temporary skin substitute TransCyte™ (Smith and Nephew Wound Care, La Jolla, CA) is a tissue-engineered product currently marketed (since 1997) for use as a wound covering for third-degree and partial-thickness burns. TransCyte™ is produced by growing human fibroblasts on a three-dimensional scaffold that allows the cells to actively proliferate and generate an extracellular matrix composed of naturally produced collagen, growth factors, and cytokines. TransCyte™ significantly improves the management and healing rate of partial thickness burns compared with human cadaver allograft, and produces less hypertrophic scarring compared with wounds treated with standard burn ointments (23–25).

A similar product, Dermagraft™ (Smith and Nephew, Wound Management) is a cryopreserved human fibroblast-derived dermal substitute composed of fibroblasts, extracellular matrix, and a bioabsorbable scaffold, indicated for use in chronic diabetic ulcers. This product actually delivers metabolically active dermal components to the wound bed to accelerate healing (26).

GROWTH FACTORS IN COSMETIC APPLICATIONS

Sun-exposed skin undergoes changes much like that of a chronic wound wherein tissue degeneration overwhelms tissue regeneration. Of primary importance is the loss of structural integrity of the dermal matrix resulting in clinical features: generalized thinning of the skin, softening and sagging, loss of elasticity, fine wrinkles, and deepening of lines of expression.

The fibroblast is the cell with the most important role in production of the dermal matrix. Fibroblasts express both PDGF and TGF-β, both of which have profound effects on the matrix components. Both PDGF and TGF-β are potently chemotactic for inflammatory cells (27–33). They stimulate glycosaminoglycan (GAG) and proteoglycan production by fibroblasts (34.). The secretion of proteases and protease inhibitors is modulated by PDGF, EGF, FGF2, and TGF-β (35–37). Most importantly, TGF-β stimulates collagen synthesis and regulates the production of matrix ground substance elements, fibronectin, and hyaluronic acid. TGF-β is probably the most broadly acting growth factor, as nearly all cells express TGF-β receptors.

Growth factors used in cosmetic formulations are derived from either natural animal or plant sources or produced synthetically. Epidermal growth factor is widely incorporated into lotions and creams and is derived from various sources including plants, yeast, and recombinant genetic technologies. Some products contain extracts of placenta and bovine colostrum said to contain specific growth factors [Interleukin 1 (IL-1), TGF(α and β)] or to contain factors generally identified as "proteins". Though all of these products claim growth factor activity, little scientific evidence is found to support such contentions. In addition, it is difficult to ascertain if concentrations of growth factors in these products are sufficient to render a tissue response.

Much of the knowledge of the biochemical roles of growth factors has been learned through *in vitro* studies, and indeed, this "artificial" environment is a well-controlled laboratory in which specific activities of single growth factors can be tested. *In vivo* research has primarily focused on the roles of growth factors in wounds and has also generally sought to define the unique characteristics of single growth factors. Likewise, the single growth factor approach is widely employed in cosmeceutical product formulations, although "complex" or combination products may include less active ingredients typically used in the industry, such as botanical extracts or moisturizers.

A product currently receiving much attention is TNS Recovery Comple® with Nouricel-MD™ (SkinMedica, Carlsbad, CA). This product contains a concentrated, naturally-derived human growth factor solution (containing amino acids, vitamins, antioxidants, and several cytokines/growth factors), which appears to have clinically measurable effects on photoaged skin (Table 2). Nouricel-MD™, the growth factor component of TNS Recovery Complex®, is obtained from the growth medium of cultured neonatal foreskin fibroblasts, grown on an artificial three-dimensional matrix (the same process by which TransCyte™ is produced). This product capitalizes on the physiological advantage of interaction among active cytokines in order to maximally stimulate tissue repair. Early *in vitro* studies with Nouricel-MD™ demonstrated stimulation of keratinocyte and fibroblast cell proliferation and stimulation of collagen production (38). Preliminary studies using unformulated Nouricel-MD™ twice daily to the forearm for 4 weeks resulted in a 38% increase in fibroblast nuclei and a 22% increase in epidermal thickness. Once daily applications of formulated product for 4 weeks demonstrated a 15–78% improvement in upper dermal collagen (38).

Subsequent research targeted the reversal of photodamaged facial skin (1). Fourteen patients with at least Class II wrinkling classification applied TNS Recovery Complex® with Nouricel-MD™ [a gel containing 10× concentrated

Table 2 TNS Recovery Complex Growth Factors and Cytokines

Angiogenic	VEGF (vascular endothelial growth factor)
	HGF (Hepatocyte growth factor)
	PDGF (platelet-derived growth factor)
Anti-inflammatory	Interleukins
Matrix deposition	TGF-β-1 (transforming growth factor β-1)
	PDGF

Table 3 Fitzpatrick Wrinkling Score (Mean ± SD, $n = 14$)

	Periorbital	Perioral	Cheeks	Forehead
Before TNS	7.07 ± 1.14	5.86 ± 1.0	5.64 ± 1.5	5.79 ± 1.12
After TNS	6.21 ± 1.05	5.36 ± 1.4	5.21 ± 1.4	5.43 ± 1.5
% Decrease	12.2	8.5	7.6	6.2
p-value[a]	0.0003	0.08	0.29	0.21

[a]Two-tailed paired t-test.
Source: Adapted from Fitzpatrick and Rostan (1).

growth factor solution (85%) and a lipid-based gel (15%)] on the face twice daily for 2 months. Clinical grading according to the Fitzpatrick wrinkling classification, 3 mm punch biopsies of the lateral cheek, and optical profilometry of the upper lateral cheek below the lateral canthus were measured. Subjective patient assessments were also recorded. Eleven of the fourteen patients showed clinical improvement in at least one facial area. A 12% decrease in periorbital wrinkling score was highly statistically significant ($p = 0.0003$), though 8.5% decrease in the perioral measurement was considered meaningful, albeit not statistically significant (Table 3). Figure 1 depicts a before and after comparison of the periorbital area of one patient. Optical profilometry measurements showed statistically significant changes in the shadowing measurements (50% in east–west, $p = 0.01$; 32% in north–south, $p = 0.02$) and 14% decrease in RAEW measurement ($p = 0.04$), indicating an improvement in the depth and number of textural irregularities and fine lines (Table 4).

Biopsies revealed a 37% increase in Grenz Zone thickness and a 27% increase in epidermal thickness. Eight patients felt their wrinkles were improved and twelve patients reported an improvement in skin texture.

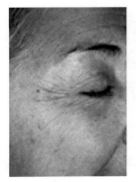 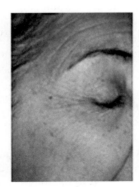 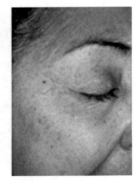

Figure 1 Periorbital lines in a 60-year-old woman at baseline, after 3 months TNS Recovery Complex BID, and after 6 months TNS Recovery Complex BID (left to right).

Table 4 Optical Profilometry (Mean ± SD, $n = 11$)

	East–west measurements		
	RAEW	RZEW	SHEW
Before TNS	12.16 ± 3.50	67.35 ± 16.60	2.36 ± 2.01
After TNS	10.45 ± 2.74	61.94 ± 17.50	1.18 ± 1.40
% Decrease	14.06	8.03	50.0
p-value[a]	0.04	0.4	0.01
	North–south measurements		
	RANS	RZNS	SHNS
Before TNS	17.58 ± 6.50	86.02 ± 17.03	7.27 ± 5.90
After TNS	15.53 ± 5.27	81.09 ± 16.70	4.90 ± 5.05
% Decrease	11.67	5.7	32.6
p-value[a]	0.10	0.27	0.02

[a]Two-tailed paired t-test.
Source: Adapted from Fitzpatrick and Rostan (1).

This study provides the first scientific evidence that the effects of topically applied growth factors may penetrate the epidermal barrier and deliver regenerative effects that are clinically measurable. As previously stated, penetrability and adequate concentration must be considered when formulating a cosmeceutical for active effects. The nature of the formulation is critical when large proteins, such as growth factors and cytokines, are to be delivered to the appropriate site of action. Lipid-soluble carrier systems have vastly facilitated this potential hindrance. Studies have shown that growth factor quantities as little as 1–2 ng have long-lasting effects on acute wounds. If so little is required, then concentrating the growth factors in the formulation would improve the potential for delivery of appropriate physiologic amounts.

To summarize, the "ideal" cosmeceutical growth factor product would provide a concentrated milieu of several growth factors formulated such that the natural tissue conditions could be restored and enhanced.

COMBINATION APPROACHES: LASER PLUS TOPICAL GROWTH FACTORS

Use of growth factors following ablative and nonablative procedures is a logical application of the technology, given the history of growth factor use in wounds. Positive reports of the results of this type of application are to date, anecdotal, but may be reasonably substantiated with reliance upon well-established evidence for the beneficial effects of growth factors in wound healing applications.

Aestheticians and dermatologists have experimented with various cosmeceutical products to facilitate postpeel tissue resurfacing and reduce irritation. Some have reported superior success with growth factor products, citing reductions in postpeel erythema and dryness. Clinical correlation may be made to the human fibroblast-derived temporary skin substitute (TransCyte™) previously discussed in Growth Factors and Wound Healing. Study of the use of fibroblast-derived temporary skin after CO_2 laser resurfacing produced faster healing and less pain and inflammation than traditional postoperative measures (unpublished data). For noninvasive, nonablative laser resurfacing, the posttreatment application of growth factors in a topical formulation may provide benefit in accelerated or improved wound healing. A study is currently underway to evaluate the efficacy of a mixture of growth factors compared with platelet-rich plasma applied topically after CO_2 laser resurfacing.

RISKS ASSOCIATED WITH GROWTH FACTORS

Topical application of growth factors to wounds has not been associated with adverse reactions proven to be related to these agents. However, the potential for allergic reaction in patients with hypersensitivity must be kept in mind. Once again, the interplay of these cytokines is very complex and still incompletely understood. Research efforts are ongoing to discern the discrete interactive roles of cytokines in tissue growth and differentiation. Thus, some theoretical concerns are currently under investigation. These are (1) the potential for growth factors to perpetuate tumor growth and (2) the role of growth factors in hypertrophic scarring.

Concerns regarding the potential for growth factors to stimulate the development or increase aggressiveness of certain tumor types are based on the presence of receptors for some growth factors, such as VEGF, TGF-β, and EGF, known to be expressed by neoplastic cells (39–43). Functionally, growth factors may affect neoplastic cell proliferation directly or by modification of the environment around cancerous cells to promote tumor growth. For example, VEGF, which is a key factor in tumor neoangiogenesis, is expressed by some types of skin tumors. Whether increased VEGF expression contributes to tumor growth is uncertain, however. Exogenous VEGF added to melanoma cells was shown in one study to increase cell proliferation (44), but increased expression of VEGF in another study did not result in melanoma cell proliferation (45). In contrast, VEGF expression in squamous cell carcinomas of the head and neck was shown to produce a significant inhibitory effect on cell proliferation and tumor cell migration (46). Whether VEGF contributes to tumor cell proliferation or is produced in response to the growth of a tumor is unknown.

Epidermal growth factor *receptor* is also known to be overexpressed in certain epithelial cell malignancies, among them are nonsmall cell lung cancer, bladder cancer, squamous cell carcinoma, and colon cancer. Much research is currently underway to investigate the potential benefits of EGF receptor inhibitory agents as stand-alone and adjunct chemotherapies (42,47,48).

Studies of the association of growth factors with tumors have focused on the production of growth factors or expression of growth factor receptors by neoplastic cells. This research does not support the theory that exogenous application of growth factors to wounds or intact skin would initiate a neoplastic process. As with VEGF, TGF-β has been alternately reported to decrease or promote cancer progression (40,49). Generally, this growth factor has been found to have inhibitory effects on tumor growth (49), but the activity of TGF-β in cancerous tissue is complex and has not been fully elucidated.

The concern about the contribution of growth factors to hypertrophic scarring is, as yet, scientifically unfounded. Elevated levels of TGF-β at the site of dermal injury has led to the postulation that this growth factor may increase scarring potential as a result of its fibroblast activating activity and collagen stimulatory effects, but this hypothesis has not been borne out by research. Polo et al. (50) suggested that the abnormal response of proliferative scar fibroblasts to TGF-β stimulation might contribute to the development of keloid and burn scars. In fact, evaluation of patients with a genetic proclivity for the development of keloid scars failed to demonstrate a relationship between TGF-β plasma levels and keloid formation (51). Recall also that the biological covering containing growth factors (TransCyte^{TM}), used in patients with partial-thickness wounds, showed significantly less hypertrophic scarring at 6 and 12 months postburn than silver sulfadiazine-treated counterparts (25).

CONCLUSIONS

Study of the role of growth factors in cutaneous wound healing has led to research demonstrating positive clinical and cosmetic outcomes in photodamaged skin. Although the topical use of growth factors is an emerging treatment approach, initial studies suggest that dermal collagen production and clinical improvement in photodamage appearance are substantial. Further, the increase in dermal collagen produced by topical growth factors can be measured quantitatively by biopsy. Although the functions of growth factors in the natural wound healing process are complex and incompletely understood, it appears that wound healing is dependent on the synergistic interaction of many growth factors. Currently, most studies of single growth factors provide limited understanding within a narrow scope. The most promising research suggests that multiple growth factors used in combination may stimulate the growth of collagen, elastin, and GAGs. The use of a multiple-growth factor topical formulation appears to provide a promising first-line treatment for mild to moderate photodamaged skin. Combination with laser therapy for more severe damage has not been studied but may provide additional benefit.

ACKNOWLEDGMENT

The author wishes to thank Peggy Beatty, DVM, MS of Bryan and Klein, Inc., for assistance in manuscript preparation.

REFERENCES

1. Fitzpatrick RE, Rostan EF. Reversal of photodamage with topical growth factors: a pilot study. J Cosmet Laser Ther 2003; 5:25–34.
2. Gilchrest BA. Skin aging and photoaging. Dermatol Nurs 1990; 2:79–82.
3. Warren R, Gartstein V, Kligman AM et al. Age, sunlight, and facial skin: a histologic and quantitative study. J Am Acad Dermatol 1991; 25:751–760.
4. Shai A, Maibach HI, Baran R. Handbook of Cosmetic Skin Care. 1st ed. London, England: Martin Dunitz Ltd, 2001.
5. Winton GR, Salasche SJ. Dermabrasion of the scalp as a treatment for actinic damage. J Am Acad Dermatol 1986; 14:661–668.
6. Fitzpatrick RE, Goldman MP, Satur NM, Tope WD. Pulsed carbon dioxide laser resurfacing in photodamaged skin. Arch Dermatol 1996; 132:395–402.
7. Kauvner ANB, Waldorf HA, Geronemus RG. A histopathological comparison of "char-free" carbon dioxide lasers. Dermatol Surg 1996; 22:343–348.
8. Cotton J, Hood AF, Gonin R, Beesen WH, Hanke CW. Histologic evaluation of preauricular and postauricular human skin after high-energy, short-pulse carbon dioxide laser. Arch Dermatol 1996; 132:425–428.
9. Stuzin JM, Baker TJ, Baker TM, Kligman AM. Histologic effects of the high energy pulsed CO_2 laser on photodamaged facial skin. Plast Reconstr Surg 1997; 99(7):2036–2050.
10. Kligman AM, Grove GL, Hirose R, Leyden JJ. Topical tretinoin for photoaged skin. J Am Acad Dermatol 1986; 15:836–859.
11. Kang S, Duell EA, Fisher GJ, Datta SC, Wang Z-Q, Reddy AP, Tavakkol A, Yi JY, Griffiths CEM, Elder JT, Voorhees JJ. Application of retinol to human skin *in vivo* induces epidermal hyperplasia and cellular retinoid binding proteins characteristic of retinoic acid, but without measurable retinoic acid levels or irritation. J Invest Dermatol 1995; 105(4):549–556.
12. Duell EA, Derguini F, Kang S, Elder JT, Vorhees JJ. Extraction of human epidermis treated with retinol yields retro-retinoids in addition to free retinol and retinyl ester. J Invest Dermatol 1996; 107(2):178–182.
13. Hodam JR, Creek KE. Comparison of the metabolism of retinol delivered to human keratinocytes either bound to serum retinol-binding protein or added directly to the culture medium. Exp Cell Res 1998; 238(1):257–264.
14. Bailly J, Cretaz M, Schifflers MH, Marty JP. *In vitro* metabolism by human skin and fibroblasts of retinol, retinal and retinoic acid. Exp Dermatol 1998; 7:27–34.
15. Darr D, Combs SB, Pinnell SR. Ascorbic acid and collagen synthesis: rethinking a role for lipid peroxidation. Arch Biochem Biophys 1993; 307(2):331–335.
16. Phillips CL, Combs SB, Pinnell SR. Effects of ascorbic acid on proliferation and collagen synthesis in relation to the donor age of human dermal fibroblasts. J Invest Dermatol 1994; 103(2):228–232.

17. Phillips CL, Tajima S, Pinnell SR. Ascorbic acid and transforming growth factor-$\beta1$ increase collagen biosynthesis via different mechanisms: coordinate regulation of pro alpha 1(I) and pro alpha 1(III) collagens. Arch Biochem Biophys 1992; 295(2):397–403.
18. Pinnel SR, Murad S, Darr D. Induction of collagen synthesis by ascorbic acid: a possible mechanism (Review). Arch Dermatol 1987; 123(12):1684–1686.
19. Niki E. Action of ascorbic acid as a scavenger of active and stable oxygen radicals. Am J Clin Nutr 1991; 54(6 Suppl):1119S–1124S.
20. Frei B, England L, Ames B. Ascorbate is an outstanding antioxidant in human blood plasma. Proc Natl Acad Sci USA 1989; 86:6377–6381.
21. Moulin V. Growth factors in skin wound healing. Eur J Cell Biol 1995; 68(1):1–7.
22. Rosenberg L, de la Torre J. Wound healing, growth factors. http://www.emedicine.com/plastic/topic457.htm. Accessed: 04/17/04.
23. Purdue GF, Hunt JL, Still JM Jr et al. A multi-centre clinical trial of biosynthetic skin replacement, Dermagraft-TC, compared with cryopreserved human cadaver skin for temporary coverage of burn wounds. J Burn Care Rehabil 1997; 18(1–1): 52–57.
24. Demling RH, DeSanti L. Management of partial thickness facial burns (comparison of topical antibiotics and bioengineered skin substitutes). Burns 1999; 25:256–261.
25. Noordenbos J, Dore C, Hansbrough JF. Safety and efficacy of TransCyte for the treatment of partial thickness burns. Journal Burn Care Rehabil 1999; 20(4):275–281.
26. Smith and Nephew, Wound Management US. http://www.dermagraft.com/Diabetes/Tissue2.html. Accessed: 4/21/04.
27. Antoniades HN, Galanopoulos T, Neville-Golden J et al. Injury induces *in vivo* expression of PDGF and PDGF receptor MRNAs in skin epithelial cells and PDGF mRNA in connective tissue fibroblasts. Proc Natl Acad Sci USA 1991; 88:565–569.
28. Messadi DV, Berg S, Shung-Cho K et al. Autocrine TGFβ1 activity and glycosaminoglycan synthesis by human cutaneous scar fibroblasts. Wound Repair Regen 1994; 2:284–291.
29. Tsuboi R, Sato C, Kurita Y et al. KGF (FGF-7) stimulates migration and plasminogen activator activity of normal human keratinocytes. J Invest Dermatol 1993; 101:49–53.
30. Bronson RE, Bertolami CN, Seibert EP. Modulation of fibroblast growth and GAG synthesis by interleukin-1. Coll Relat Res 1987; 7:323–332.
31. Ignotz RA, Endo T, Massague J. Regulation fibronectin and type I collagen mRNA levels by TGFβ. J Biol Chem 1987; 262:6443–6446.
32. Pierce GF, Mustoe TA, Lingelbach J et al. Platelet derived growth factor and transforming growth factor-beta enhance tissue repair activities by unique mechanisms. J Cell Biol 1989; 190:429–440.
33. Deuel TF. Polypeptide growth factors: roles in normal and abnormal cell growth. Annu Rev Cell Biol 1987; 3:443–492.
34. Heldin P, Laurent TC, Heldin CH. Effect of growth factors on hyaluronan synthesis in cultured human fibroblasts. Biochem J 1989; 257:919–922.
35. Taylor CR, Stern RS, Leyden JJ et al. Photoaging/photodamage and photoprotection. J Am Acad Dermatol 1990; 22:1–15.
36. Buckley-Sturrock A, Woodward SC, Senior RM et al. Differential stimulation of collagenase and chemotactic activity in fibroblasts derived from rat wound repair tissue and human skin by growth factors. J Cell Physiol 1989; 138:70–78.

37. Chua CC, Geiman DE, Keller GH, Ladda RL. Induction of collagenase secretion in human fibroblast cultured by growth promoting factors. J Biol Chem 1985; 260:5213–5216.
38. Naughton GK, Pinney E, Mansbridge J, Fitzpatrick RE. Tissue-engineered derived growth factors as a topical treatment for rejuvenation of photodamaged skin. Soc Invest Dermatol Poster, 05/12/01.
39. Lazar-Molnar E, Hegyesi H, Toth S, Falus A. Autocrine and paracrine regulation by cytokines and growth factors in melanoma. Cytokine 2000; 12(6):547–554.
40. Lewis MP, Lygoe KA, Nystrom ML et al. Tumour-derived TGF-beta1 modulates myofibroblast differentiation and promotes HGF/SF-dependent invasion of squamous carcinoma cells. Br J Cancer 2004; 90(4):822–832.
41. Waksal HW. Role of an anti-epidermal growth factor receptor in treating cancer. Cancer Metastasis Rev 1999; 18(4):427–436.
42. Ciardello F, Tortora G. Anti-epidermal growth factor receptor drugs in cancer therapy. Expert Opin Investig Drugs 2002 Jun; 11(6):755–768.
43. Baselga J. Why the epidermal growth factor receptor? The rationale for cancer therapy. Oncologist 2002; 7(Suppl 4):2–8.
44. Liu B, Earl HM, Baban D et al. Melanoma cell lines express VEGF receptor KDR and respond to exogenously added VEGF. Biochem Biophys Res Commun 1995; 217(3):721–727.
45. Graeven U, Fiedler W, Karpinski S et al. Melanoma-associated expression of vascular endothelial growth factor and its receptors FLT-1 and KDR. J Cancer Res Clin Oncol 1999; 125(11):621–629.
46. Herold-Mende C, Steiner HH, Andl T et al. Expression and functional significance of vascular endothelial growth factor receptors in human tumor cells. Lab Invest 1999; 79(12):1573–1582.
47. Janmaat ML, Giaccone G. The epidermal growth factor receptor pathway and its inhibition as anticancer therapy. Drugs Today. 2003; 39(Suppl C):61–80.
48. Modi S, Seidman AD. An update on epidermal growth factor receptor inhibitors. Curr Oncol Rep 2002 Jan; 4(1):47–55.
49. Ramont L, Pasco S, Hornebeck W, Maquart FX, Monboisse JC. Transforming growth factor-beta1 inhibits tumor growth in a mouse melanoma model by down-regulating the plasminogen activation system. Exp Cell Res 2003; 291(1):1–10.
50. Polo M, Smith PD, Kim YJ, Wang X, Ko F, Robson MC. Effect of TGF-beta2 on proliferative scar fibroblast cell kinetics. Ann Plast Surg 1999; 43(2):185–190.
51. Bayat A, Bock O, Mrowietz U et al. Genetic susceptibility to keloid disease and hypertrophic scarring: transforming growth factor beta1 common polymorphisms and plasma levels. Plast Reconstr Surg 2003; 111(2):535–543.

Substances

20

Dimethylaminoethanol

Rachel Grossman, Christiane Bertin, and Nathalie Issachar
Johnson&Johnson Consumer Products Co., Skillman, New Jersey, USA and Issy les Moulineaux, France

Introduction	365
Chemical Structure	366
Biological and Pharmacological Actions	366
Nicotinic Receptors	367
Muscarinic Receptors	368
Possible Roles of DMAE	369
Anti-inflammatory	369
Free-Radical Scavenger	369
Skin Firmness	369
Sagging	370
Safety	370
Conclusion	371
References	371

INTRODUCTION

Dimethylaminoethanol (DMAE), a new anti-aging firming ingredient used in the cosmetic skin care market, has a long history of investigation in the treatment of mood and hyper-kinetic disorders (1), enhancement of memory (2) and learning, and behavioral disorders in children (3,4) thanks to its activity as a precursor of choline and cholinergic neurotransmitter acetylcholine (ACh). Dr. N. Perricone first utilized it for a cosmetic application due to its firming and anti-aging benefits (5). Moreover, it was patented in 1999 as a skin permeation enhancer (6). Recent evidence suggests a nonneuronal role for DMAE, since ACh has been shown to act as an autocrine and paracrine factor, regulating basic cellular functions such as mitosis, differentiation, cell–cell contact, cytoskeletal organization, secretion, absorption, trophic and locomotor functions, as well as barrier and immune functions (7,8).

Chemical Structure

2-DMAE or deanol is a simple amine base [$C_4H_{11}NO/(CH_3)_2NCH_2CH_2OH$], with a molecular weight of 89.1 (Fig. 1). It has structural similarity to choline.

BIOLOGICAL AND PHARMACOLOGICAL ACTIONS

Several biological and pharmacological actions of DMAE are described in the literature.

ACh plays a role in memory, skeletal and smooth muscle contraction, relaxation, heart activity, glandular secretion, and cell division, adherence, and mobility.

DMAE doses of 3 mmol/kg (267.3 mg/kg) administered intraperitoneally induced an increase in choline concentration, as well as an inhibition of the oxidation and phosphorylation of [^{3}H]methylcholine in the kidneys. Moreover, intraperitoneal administration of 2.4 mmol/kg (213.8 mg/kg) DMAE in rats has been shown to increase ACh content in the brain tissues, because it is converted to choline and then to ACh (9,10).

In the liver, DMAE inhibited the rate of phosphorylation of [^{3}H]methylcholine but neither affected its oxidation nor increased its levels in this tissue.

Systemic administration of DMAE to mice showed an increase of the concentration and of the turnover rate of free choline in blood and in kidneys, and an inhibition of the rate of oxidation and phosphorylation of IV administered [^{3}H]methylcholine; this increase of choline concentration being attributed to an inhibition of its metabolism in tissues (11).

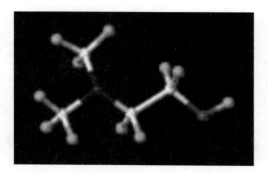

Figure 1 Chemical structure of 2-DMAE.

The cutaneous influx of choline or increase of ACh in skin following topical application of DMAE has not yet been documented.

ACh synthesis and degradation:

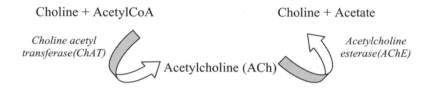

At a molecular level (12):

[Reaction 1: Choline + Acetyl CoA → (Choline acetyltransferase) → Acetylcholine + Coenzyme A]

[Reaction 2: Acetylcholine + H₂O → (Cholinesterase) → Choline + Acetic acid]

Free nonneuronal ACh has been shown to be present in significant amount in the skin and ChAT activity has been localized to the epidermis, indicating that ACh synthesis can occur in the skin (13). In the skin, ACh regulates eccrine sweat gland secretion, pigmentation, blood flow, vascular permeability, and mast cell activity (13).

ACh does not cross lipid membranes conversely to DMAE because of its highly polar, positively charged ammonium group. It is the reason why it generates its biological effects within cells by activating two different classes of cholinergic cell-surface receptors, the nicotinic and muscarinic ACh receptors. Cholinergic cell-surface receptors modulate a wide variety of cellular activities including proliferation, differentiation, migration, and viability.

Human epidermal keratinocytes possess cholinergic enzymes, which synthesize and degrade ACh and express both nicotinic and muscarinic cholinergic receptors on their surface (13). It was shown that addition of cholinergic agents to cultured human keratinocytes modifies their viability, proliferation, shape, and mobility.

Nicotinic Receptors

Nicotinic receptors are pentameric transmembrane proteins belonging to the superfamily of ligand-gated ion channels (Fig. 2). They are constituted by an association of five polypeptides forming a channel for ions.

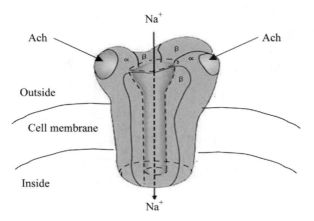

Figure 2 Nicotinic receptor.

Muscarinic Receptors

There is a high density of muscarinic ACh receptors on the cell surface of intact human keratinocytes. The muscarinic ligands have the ability to regulate the adhesion and mobility of these cells. Monoclonal antibodies have also identified muscarinic ACh receptors on the cell surfaces of human skin fibroblasts (10). Indeed, human skin fibroblasts express the m2, m4, and m5 molecular subtypes of muscarinic ACh receptors (13,14).

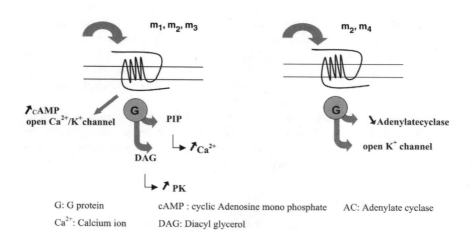

POSSIBLE ROLES OF DMAE

Anti-inflammatory

DMAE appears to have moderate anti-inflammatory activity as documented in a peripheral blood lymphocyte (PBL) assay (15). Human PBLs were stimulated with phytohemagglutinin *in vitro* to induce the clonal expression and secretion of cytokines by T cells. The addition of DMAE to this system was shown to strongly inhibit interleukin (IL)-2 secretion and to moderately inhibit IL-6 and IL-10 secretion. All those three cytokines are important in the regulation of humoral immunity, antibody responses, and allergic reactions. IL-2 can additionally mediate macrophage activation and delayed hypersensitivity reactions. DMAE was also shown to moderately inhibit proliferation of and to exhibit stimulatory activity against tumor necrosis factor α. No activity was documented against the remaining cytokines tested (IL-1α, IL-4, IL-12, and interferon-γ).

The cutaneous anti-inflammatory activity of DMAE remains to be documented.

Free-Radical Scavenger

Excessive formation of free radicals during the aging process can have damaging effects, particularly at the cell membrane.

DMAE seems to reduce protein cross-linking, a characteristic of cellular aging, by acting as a free-radical scavenger (16). Indeed, electron spin resonance spectroscopic method demonstrates that DMAE is a free-radical scavenger (17,18). An *in vitro* experiment showed that it prevented the polymerization of bovine serum albumin induced by OH free radicals (16). Antiaging therapies should therefore increase the number of available electrons on the inside of the plasma membrane to scavenge the OH free radicals and stabilize cell membranes. Moreover, DMAE has long been known as a precursor of phosphatidylcholine, the primary phospholipid of cell membranes. Thus, it may also serve to stabilize cell membranes via phosphatidylcholine formation.

Skin Firmness

A double blind randomized study vs. placebo was performed to assess the efficacy of a facial gel containing 3% DMAE on skin elasticity and firmness by measuring shear wave propagation with a Reviscometer™. An increased shear wave velocity was observed in the direction where mechanical anisotropy of skin showed looseness. In this context, DMAE seemed to act on skin firmness by increasing contractility and cell adhesion of epidermal and dermal cells. The mechanism of action remains unclear, but one hypothesis is that it may act by an ACh pathway at the level of neuromuscular junction, or by increasing the contractility of nonmuscular epidermal and dermal cells, or by changing the partitioning of water between cellular membranes and matrix macromolecules of the dermis which could enhance the water retention in the superficial connective tissue (19).

Sagging

With age, subcutaneous muscles lengthen and give a sagging appearance to the skin, because underlying muscle is looser (the degree of contraction relaxes in the resting state, particularly in the face) (6).

In order for a muscle to contract, a message is sent from the brain to the spinal cord, and then from the spinal cord to skeletal muscles. This is accomplished by an action potential, which travels down the axon of the nerve. The nerve ends at an area called the synaptic knob, and this action potential causes the synaptic knob to release small diffusible chemical neurotransmitters into the synaptic cleft. The synaptic knob is rich in tiny vesicles containing ACh. ACh has receptors on the muscle surface, which causes the muscle to become permeable to sodium ions and results in membrane potential increases (about 75 mV), which induces muscle contraction. Once this contraction takes place, the remaining ACh is destroyed by cholinesterase enzyme. The choline is then reabsorbed to be used again to synthesize ACh. Thus, it is at this neuromuscular junction where ACh causes its effect.

The aging process results in damage to presynaptic knobs, and therefore, fewer neurotransmitters become available to a muscle for contraction. Receptor sites on muscle also deteriorate and are unable to respond to the level of ACh present. Muscle tone maintained by the release of ACh by nerve fibers is decreased inducing sagging appearance (6).

Topical application of a catecholamine precursor or topical products containing DMAE acting as an ACh precursor may increase muscle tone causing a slight shortening of the muscle. A shorter muscle results in a lifting of overlying skin, with the cosmetic appearance of a decrease in sagging (20).

SAFETY

A gel containing 3% of DMAE was used in a multicenter, double blind, and placebo-controlled study (21). The study included 156 subjects who were randomized to receive the DMAE gel or placebo gel, every day, for 16 weeks. The overall incidence of adverse effects was 40% in the DMAE group and 47% in the placebo group. None of these side effects were considered by the investigator as definitely or probably related to the applications. At the end of 16 weeks, patients were eligible to enter an open-label 8-month extension of the study. The incidence of erythema and irritation was reduced compared with baseline, suggesting that irritation attenuated over time. Thus, DMAE facial gel has been studied for long-term use, with documented safety up to 12 months of continuous use among subjects. No adverse events were related to the DMAE gel.

In human modified repeated-insult patch tests (sensitization), 3% DMAE facial gel did not elicit any sensitization ($N = 382$).

The potential genotoxicity of DMAE has been evaluated *in vitro*, including bacterial and mammalian cell gene mutation essays. Negative findings were obtained in those studies. Additionally, a negative result was obtained in a mouse bone marrow micronucleus study *in vivo*. These findings indicate that DMAE is not genotoxic.

CONCLUSION

DMAE has a wide range of benefits on various parts of the body, including skin. Although its mechanism of action is not completely understood, it seems that as a precursor of choline and neurotransmitter ACh, it acts as an autocrine and paracrine factor triggering effects on skin cells such as keratinocytes and fibroblasts. This may explain its activity on skin aging signs such as wrinkles and sagging.

REFERENCES

1. Ré O. 2-Dimethylaminoethanol (deanol): a brief review of its clinical efficacy and postulated mechanism of action. Current Ther Res 1974; 16(11):1238–1242.
2. Flood JF, Smith GE, Cherkin A. Memory retention: potentiation of cholinergic drug combinations in mice. Neurobiol Aging 1983; 4(1):37–43.
3. Saccar CL. Drug therapy in the treatment of minimal brain dysfunction. Am J Hosp Pharm 1978; 35(5):544–552.
4. Lewis JA, Young R. Deanol and methylphenidate in minimal brain dysfunction. Clin Pharmacol Ther 1975; 17(5):534–540.
5. Patent 5.554.647.
6. Patent 5.879.690.
7. Wessler I, Kirkpatrick CJ, Racké K. Non-neuronal acetylcholine, a locally acting molecule, widely distributed in biological system: expression and function in humans. Pharmacol Ther 1998; 77(1):59–79.
8. Wessler I, Kirkpatrick CJ, Racké K. The cholinergic 'pitfall': acetylcholine, a universal cell molecule in biological systems, including humans. Clin Exp Pharmacol Physiol 1999; 26(3):198–205.
9. DMAE (Dimethylaminoethanol). Life Link. Biosupplements from around the world for better bodies and minds (Lifelinknet.com).
10. Haubrich DR, Wang PF, Clody DE. Increase in rat brain acetylcholine induced by choline or deanol. Life Sci 1975; 17:975–980.
11. Haubrich DR, Gerber NH, Pflueger AB. Deanol affects choline metabolism in peripheral tissues of mice. J Neurochem 1981; 37(2):476–482.
12. Feldman RS, Quenzer LF. Fundamentals of Neuropsychopharmacology, Sinauer Associates: Sunderland, MA, 1997.
13. Grando SA, David A, Kist DA, Qi M, Dahl MV. Human keratinocytes synthesize, secrete, and degrade acetylcholine. J Invest Dermatol 1993; 101(1).
14. Buchli R, Ndoye A, Rodriguez JG, Zia S, Webber RJ. Human skin fibroblasts express m2, m4, and m5 subtypes of muscarinic acetylcholine receptors. J Cell Biochem 1999; 74:264–277.

15. Data on file, Johnson & Johnson, 2000.
16. Nagy I, Nagy K. On the role of cross-linking of cellular proteins in aging. Mech Ageing Dev 1980; 14(1–2):245–251.
17. Nagy I, Floyd RA. Electron spin resonance spectroscopic demonstration of the hydroxyl free radical scavenger properties of dimethylaminoethanol in spin trapping experiments confirming the molecular basis for the biological effects of centrophenoxine. Arch Gerontol Geriatr 1984; 3(4):297–310.
18. Nagy K, Dajko G, Uray I. Comparative studies on the free radical scavenger properties of two nootropic drugs, CPH and BCE-001. Ann N Y Acad Sci 1994; 717:115–121.
19. Uhoda I, Faska N, Robert C, Cauwenbergh G, Pierard GE. Split face study on the cutaneous tensile effect of 2-dimethylaminoethanol (deanol) gel. Skin Res Technol 2002; 8:164–167.
20. Patent 5.643.586.
21. Davies C, Maidment S, Hanley P, Griffin P, Evans S, Ogunbiyi AO. Dimethylaminoethanol (DMAE) Risk assessment document HSE Book.

21

Hyaluronan: The Natural Skin Moisturizer

Birgit A. Neudecker, Howard I. Maibach, and Robert Stern
University of California, San Francisco, CA, USA

Introduction	374
Historical Perspective	375
The "Ground Substance" Era	375
"Mucopolysaccharide" Period	376
Discovery of HA (Hyaluronan)	376
The Modern Era	376
The Postmodern Period	377
Biology of Hyaluronan	377
Overview	377
Structure and Terminology	378
Function	379
General	379
Embryonic Development	380
Wound Healing	381
Carcinogenesis	381
Aging	381
Hyaladherins	382
Hyaluronan in the ECM	383
Intracellular Hyaluronan	383
Hyaluronan Receptors	384
CD44	384
RHAMM	385

Hyaluronan in Skin	385
Artifacts of Hyaluronan Histolocalization in Skin	385
Epidermal Hyaluronan	386
Dermal Hyaluronan	387
Aging Skin	387
Photoaging of Skin	388
Acute and Chronic Inflammation	388
Hyaluronan in Skin Substitutes	389
Hyaluronan Synthases	390
Hyaluronan Catabolism	390
The Hyaluronidases	390
Non-enzymatic Degradation	391
Hyaluronidase Inhibitors	391
Macromolecular Inhibitors	391
Low Molecular Weight Inhibitors	392
Oxidative Stress and Skin Hyaluronan	393
Enhancing Skin Moisture by Modulating Hyaluronan	394
Alpha-Hydroxy Acids	394
Retinoic Acid and Its Derivatives	394
Steroids	395
General Comments from Dermatology and Cosmetic Perspectives	395
Future Developments	396
References	396

INTRODUCTION

Skin is a large and complex tissue, with a vast range of functions that interfaces with a hostile environment. The mechanisms that underlie the resilience of skin to the harsh outside world, and the extraordinary ability of the skin to also protect underlying tissues are just beginning to be understood. Skin retains a large amount of water, and much of the external trauma to which it is constantly subjected, in addition to the normal process of aging, causes loss of moisture. The key molecule involved in skin moisture is hyaluronan (hyaluronic acid, HA) with its associated water-of-hydration. Understanding the metabolism of HA, its reactions within skin, and the interactions of HA with other skin components will facilitate the ability to modulate skin moisture in a rational manner, different from the empirical attempts that have been utilized up to now.

    Recent progress in the details of the metabolism of HA has also clarified the long appreciated observations that chronic inflammation and sun damage caused by ultraviolet light cause premature aging of skin. These processes as well as normal aging utilize similar mechanisms that cause loss of moisture and changes in HA distribution.

In the past several decades, the constituents of skin have become better characterized. The earliest work on skin was devoted predominantly to the cells that make up the layers of skin: epidermis, dermis, and underlying subcutis. Now it is beginning to be appreciated that the materials that lie between cells, the matrix components, have major instructive roles for cellular activities. This extracellular matrix (ECM) endows skin with its hydration properties. The components of ECM, though they appear amorphous by light microscopy, form a highly organized structure of glycosaminoglycans (GAGs), proteoglycans, glycoproteins, peptide growth factors, and structural proteins such as collagen and to a lesser extent, elastin. However, the predominant component of ECM of skin is HA. It is the primordial and the simplest of GAGs, and the first ECM component to be elaborated in the developing embryo. It is the water-of-hydration of HA that forms the blastocyst, the first recognizable structure in embryonic development. Attempts to enhance the moisture content of skin, in the most elemental terms, require increasing the level and the length of time HA is present in skin, preserving optimal chain length of this sugar polymer, and inducing expression of the best profile of HA-binding proteins to decorate the molecule.

HISTORICAL PERSPECTIVE

The "Ground Substance" Era

The term "ground substance" was first attributed to the amorphous-appearing material between cells by the German anatomist Henle in 1841 (1). It is a mistranslation of the German "Grundsubstanz", which would be better translated as "basic", "fundamental", or "primordial" substance. By 1855, sufficient information had accumulated for "Grundsubstanz" to be included in a textbook of human histology by Kölliker (2).

The study of ground substance began in earnest in 1928, with the discovery of a "spreading factor" by Duran-Reynals (3–7). A testicular extract was shown to stimulate the rapid spreading of materials injected subcutaneously, and to function by causing a dissolution of ground substance. Thus, a new field of research was founded. The active principle in the extract was later shown to be a hyaluronidase, one of the class of enzymes that degrade HA (8,9). The observed dissolution of "ground substance" stimulated Duran-Reynals to write the following (10), which is just as applicable today:

> "If the importance of a defensive entity is to be judged by the magnitude of the measures taken against it, nature is certainly pointing its finger to the ground substance, as if no invite us to learn more about it."

"Mucopolysaccharide" Period

"Ground substance" was subsequently renamed "mucopolysaccharides", a term first proposed by Karl Meyer (11) to designate the hexosamine-containing polysaccharides that occur in animal tissues, referring to the sugar polymers alone, as well as when bound to proteins. However, the term "ground substance" persisted for many years afterwards, and could be found in textbooks of Biochemistry, Dermatology, and Pathology as late as the 1970s. It is now established that HA is the predominant mucopolysaccharide of skin, and the major component of the ground substance.

Discovery of HA (Hyaluronan)

Hyaluronan, the major constituent of ground substance or mucopolysaccharide component, and the substrate for the "spreading factor" was identified in 1938 by Karl Meyer (12) as a hexuronic acid-containing material that also provided the turgor for the vitreous of the eye. The name hyaluronic acid was proposed from the Greek *hyalos* (glassy, vitreous) and uronic acid. However, it required 20 years before the chemical structure of HA was established (13). It was later found to be a polymer present throughout the body, identified in virtually every vertebrate tissue, the highest concentrations occurring in the vitreous of the eye, in the synovial fluid in the joint capsule, and in the umbilical cord as Wharton's jelly. However, over 50% of total body HA is present in skin (14).

The Modern Era

The modern era of HA biology began with the realization that HA is a critical regulator of cell behavior, with profound effects on cellular metabolism, and not merely a passive structural component of ECM. This was brought into focus by a number of observations:

1. HA is prominent in embryogenesis, in maintenance of the undifferentiated state, with its removal required prior to the onset of differentiation, as was established by the pioneering work of Brian Toole (15).
2. HA has a dynamic turnover rate. In the circulation, HA has a half-life of 3–5 min (16).
3. HA is prominent in the earliest stages of adult wound healing (17), whereas elevated levels occur over a long period during scar-free repair (18–20). The prolonged presence of HA is invoked as the mechanism of such scar-free repair.
4. HA is involved in malignant progression (21), and the aggressiveness of tumors correlates with levels of HA on the cancer cell surface (22).
5. HA is a signaling molecule, and fragmented HA has major influences on angiogenesis (23,24) and inflammation (25–27).
6. HA has receptors on cell surfaces. The predominant HA receptors CD44 (28–30) and RHAMM (31,32) have complex variant isoforms,

and these receptors have the ability to confer motility upon cells with signaling to the cytoskeleton (33–35).
7. These receptors themselves are regulated and are the substrates for phosphokinases (36).
8. HA is found intracellularly, and has intracellular modes of action (35,37,38).

The Postmodern Period

The growth of molecular genetics and progress in the human genome project have facilitated rapid development in the understanding of HA metabolism. The enzymes that synthesize HA, HA synthases (HAS), as well as the enzymes that catalyze the catabolic reaction, the hyaluronidases, are all multigene families of enzymes with distinct patterns of tissue expression. The HA receptors, which also come in a myriad of forms, owe their diversity to both variant exon expression and posttranslational modifications. The multiple sites for the control of HA synthesis, deposition, cell- and protein-association, and degradation are a reflection of the complexity of HA metabolism. Their relationships are becoming clarified through the ability to sequence rapidly using the new techniques of molecular genetics. There promises to be an enormous increase in information, and in the understanding of HA biology, as the genes for these enzymes and proteins becomes sorted out.

BIOLOGY OF HYALURONAN

Overview

Hyaluronan is a high molecular weight, very anionic polysaccharide that promotes cell motility, adhesion, and proliferation, processes requiring cell movement and tissue organization (39). The tight regulation required of HA expression under such conditions is modulated in part by association of HA with cell surface receptors.

Despite the monotony of its composition, without branch points or apparent variations in sugar composition, HA has an extraordinarily high number of functions. Physicochemical studies indicate that the polymer can take on a vast number of shapes and configurations, dependent on polymer size, pH, salt concentration, and associated cations. Hyaluronan also occurs in a number of physiological states, circulating freely, tissue-associated by way of electrostatic interactions but easily dissociated, and in equilibrium with the HA in the rest of the body.

Hyaluronan may be bound to proteins termed hyaladherins (40,41). HA can be very tightly associated with hyaladherins through electrostatic interactions. HA in ECM of cartilage is an organizer of the matrix, the proteoglycan aggrecan and link proteins decorating the HA in a bottlebrush configuration.

The K_m of such associations are of such magnitude that HA is not easily dissociated and is not in equilibrium with the HA of the surrounding loose connective tissues. HA also occurs covalently bound to proteins such as inter-alpha inhibitor, a plasma protein that also functions as a stabilizer of HA-rich structures (42).

Tissues that contain high molecular weight HA are unusually resistant to invasion and penetration (43). Blood vessels are unable to penetrate joint synovium, cartilage, and the vitreous of the eye. It is also unusual for tumor metastases to develop in these structures. It may be the large size of the HA polymer that also protects such structures from invasion by parasites. The mechanism by which such high molecular weight structures resist hyaluronidase degradation, and avoid the rapid HA turnover characteristic of the rest of the body is not known. Potent hyaluronidase inhibitors may be involved, a class of molecules about which little is known.

Structure and Terminology

Hyaluronan is composed of repeating alternating units of glucuronic acid and N-acetylglucosamine, all connected by β-linkages, GlcAβ(1 $\rightarrow$ 3)GlcNAcβ(1 $\rightarrow$ 4). The β-linkage is of more than passing interest and not merely a curiosity relevant only to carbohydrate chemists. Glycogen is a polymer of α-linked glucose. Changing to a β-linkage converts the polymer to cellulose. A high molecular weight chain of β-linked N-acetylglucosamine is the structure of chitin. Chitin and cellulose are the most abundant sugar polymers on the surface of the earth. Yet, such β-linked sugar polymers are rare in vertebrate tissues, and require unusual reactions for their catabolic turnover.

Hyaluronan is the simplest of GAGs, the only one neither covalently linked to a core protein nor synthesized by way of a Golgi pathway, and it is the only nonsulfated GAG. The current terminology refers to: (1) GAGs, the straight chain hexosamine sugars and (2) proteoglycans, referring to GAG chains together with the core protein to which they are covalently bound. Hyaluronan is thus the only GAG that is not also a component of a proteoglycan.

Existing models suggest that for high molecular mass HA, super molecular organization consists of networks in which molecules run parallel for hundreds of nanometers, giving rise to flat sheets and tubular structures which separate and then join again into similar aggregates. There is strong evidence that an H_2O bridge between the acetamido and carboxyl groups is involved in the secondary structure. The hydrogen-bonded secondary structure also shows large arrays of contiguous–CH groups, giving a hydrophobic character to parts of the polymer that may be significant in the lateral aggregation or self-association and for interaction with membranes (44). This same hydrophobic character is perhaps involved in the extrusion of newly synthesized HA chains from the cytoplasmic surface of the plasma membrane where the HA synthases are located, through the membrane to the exterior of the cell (45). The unusually stiff tertiary polymeric structure is also stabilized by such hydrophobic interactions.

GAGs and proteoglycans must be distinguished from "mucins", the branch-chained sugars and their associated proteins. These occur more often on cell surfaces, though they also accumulate in the intercellular ground substance, particularly in association with malignancies. The terms are used carelessly, particularly among pathologists and histologists, and "mucin", "mucinous", "myxomatous", "myxoid", or "acid mucoproteins" unless they have been defined biochemically, may or may not refer to the HA-containing materials. This problem has arisen in part because of the ill-defined or unknown nature of histochemical color reactions. A recent example of this ambiguity is the incorrect assumption that the stain Alcian blue has some specificity for HA at pH 3.0 and for the sulfated GAGs at pH 1.5 (46).

By electron microscopy, HA is a linear polymer (47). It is polydisperse, but usually has a molecular mass of several million Daltons. In solution at physiological pH and salt concentrations, HA is an expanded random coil with an average diameter of 500 nm. The molecular domain encompasses a large volume of water, and even at low concentrations, solutions have very high viscosity. The HA in high concentrations, as found in ECM of the dermis, regulates water balance, osmotic pressure, functions as an ion exchange resin, and regulates ion flow. It functions as a sieve, to exclude certain molecules, to enhance the extracellular domain of cell surfaces, particularly the lumenal surface of endothelial cells, to stabilize structures by electrostatic interactions, and can also act as a lubricant.

Hyaluronan also acts as an organizer of ECM, the central molecule around which other components of ECM distribute and orient themselves (48). The avidity of HA for certain ECM moieties, such as the NH_2-terminal of the proteoglycan aggrecan, approaches that of avidin-biotin. The anomalous ability of HA to be both hydrophobic and hydrophilic, to associate with itself, with cell surface membranes, with proteins, or with other GAGs speaks to the versatility of this remarkable molecule.

Function

General

The large volume that HA occupies including its cloud of solvent, the water-of-hydration under physiological conditions, underlies its ability to distend and maintain the extracellular space, and preserve tissue hydration. Hyaluronan content increases whenever rapid tissue proliferation, regeneration, and repair occur (15). Its ability to organize ECM and its voluminous water-of-hydration, and its interaction with other macromolecules explain only a portion of the functions with which it is associated.

For example, bursts of HA deposition correlate with mitosis (49–51). Elevated levels promote cell detachment, in preparation for mitosis, as cells leave tissue organization, and enter the transient autonomy required for the mitotic event to occur. Cells must then degrade that HA after mitosis has occurred, to regain adhesiveness, and to reenter the "social contract". The prediction is that HA synthesis occurs as cells enter mitosis, and that a hyaluronidase activity is activated as cells leave mitosis. To date, such experiments have not been carried out in synchronized cells. The persistent presence of HA also inhibits cell differentiation (52,53), creating an environment that instead promotes cell proliferation. The elevated levels of anti-adhesive surface HA that promotes cell detachment, also permit the embryonic cell to migrate (54) or the tumor cell to move and metastasize (21,22). The water-of-hydration also opens up spaces creating a permissive environment for cell movement.

Hyaluronan is generally produced in the interstitium, in the mesenchymal connective tissue of the body, and is largely a product of fibroblasts. It reaches the blood through the lymphatics. Most of the turnover of HA, ~85%, occurs in the lymphatic system. This remaining 15% that reaches the blood stream has a rapid turnover, with a $t_{1/2}$ of 3–5 min, being rapidly eliminated by receptors in the liver and, by unknown mechanisms in the kidney (16,55,56). When the hepatic or renal arteries are ligated, there is an immediate rise in the level of circulating HA (57). Thus, humans synthesize and degrade several grams of HA daily.

During acute stress, such as in shock or with septicemia, there is a rapid rise in circulating HA (58–61). Such HA may function as a volume expander, as a survival mechanism to prevent circulatory collapse. Some of this rapid rise in HA represents HA recruited from interstitial stores and from lymphatics, and not entirely a reflection of increased synthesis or decreased degradation (62). However, higher plasma levels of HA do correlate with decreased turnover rates, the $t_{1/2}$ reaching 20–45 min in situations of acute stress.

The mean serum and plasma level in healthy young people is 20–40 μg/L (63,64). This value increases with age (65,66) and probably reflects slower clearance, and decreased HA degradative capacity, though this has not been carefully investigated. Hyaluronan also increases in the circulation in liver disease, particularly cirrhosis, and in renal failure reflecting aberrant degradation (65–69), in rheumatoid arthritis (70) and consistently in some malignancies as a result of increased tumor tissue synthesis (71).

Embryonic Development

The developing embryo is rich in HA. HA creates the spaces permissive for fetal cell migration and proliferation. The HA concentration is high not only in fetal circulation, but also in amniotic fluid (72), fetal tissues, fetal membranes, and placenta. The HA levels reach a maximum of 20 μg/mL at approximately 20 weeks of gestation, and then drop until, at 30 weeks gestation, they reach the 1 μg/mL adult-like levels. This corresponds approximately to the time when a "switch" from the scar-free fetal wound healing to the adult-like wound healing with scarring occurs (73). The factors in the fetal circulation that support such high levels of HA synthesis have been explored and partially characterized (74), but have not yet been isolated nor fully identified.

The neural crest cells as they pinch off from the neuroectoderm migrate through the embryonic body in a sea of HA (54). When these cells reach their particular destination, hyaluronidases remove HA, and cell migration then ceases. In embryology, as parenchymal glands develop, HA can be found in the stroma immediately ahead of the arborizing tips, creating the spaces into which the growing glands can grow (75,76).

The classic studies of Bryan Toole and his laboratory separate embryology into two stages, a model that can be superimposed on the development of virtually all parenchymal organs and vertebrate structures: (1) a primary HA-rich phase in which undifferentiated stem cells involved proliferate and migrate, followed by (2) removal of HA and the onset of cellular differentiation and morphogenesis (15).

Wound Healing

ECM in the earliest stages of wound healing is rich in HA. There is also an abundance of inflammatory cells, a necessary component for the normal process of wound healing. In the adult, HA levels rapidly reach a maximum and then drop rapidly (20), reminiscent of the stages in embryology. Decrease in HA levels is followed by increase in amounts of chondroitin sulfate, the appearance of fibroblasts, and then deposition of a collagen-rich ECM. In the adult, wound healing often results in scar formation. In the fetus, however, wound repair is associated with levels of HA that remain elevated, and the final result is a wound free of scar. Such observations are made in both the experimental fetal rabbit and sheep models, and clinically, in term infants following mid-gestational *in utero* surgery. It is on this basis that elevated HA in the wound matrix is invoked as a key to decreased scarring, contractures, and adhesions in adult wound repair. Aspects of wound healing appear to be a strategic retreat to an embryonic situation, followed by a rapid recapitulation of ontogeny.

Carcinogenesis

In malignancy, HA also appears to play a critical role (21,77). Levels of HA on the surface of tumor cells correlate with their aggressiveness (22). In a study of tumor cell-associated HA, the proportion of tumor HA-positive cells, and intensity of HA staining are unfavorable prognostic factors in colorectal cancer (78). However, overexpression of hyaluronidase also correlates with disease progression, as shown in bladder (79,80) and in breast tumor metastases (81,82). These apparently diverse scenarios may indicate that HA and hyaluronidase are required at different stages in the multistep progression of cancer.

Aging

HA levels are high in the fetal circulation and fall shortly after birth. After maintaining a steady level for several decades, circulating levels of HA then begin to increase again in old age (63,66,83). Elevated levels of circulating

HA are also found in the syndromes of premature aging, in progeria (84) and in Werner's Syndrome (85).

Increased HA levels in the bloodstream decrease immune competence (86). Various mechanisms have been invoked. An HA coating around circulating lymphocytes may prevent ligand access to lymphocyte surface receptors (87–90). The increased HA may represent one of the mechanisms for the immuno-suppression in the fetus. The reappearance of high levels of HA in old age may be one of the mechanisms of the deterioration of the immune system in the elderly. The increasing levels of HA with aging may be a reflection of the deterioration of hydrolytic reactions, including the hyaluronidases that maintain the steady state of HA. This is a far more likely mechanism than an increase in HA synthase activity.

The increased HA that is often found in malignancy in the bloodstream (91–94) as well as on the surface of tumor cells (22) may be one of the techniques of cancer for compromising host immune function. It is the probable basis of the failure to rosette in the classic sheep red blood cell rosette test, a former laboratory procedure used to diagnose malignancy (95,96). The rosetting failure may have been due to the HA coating on the cancer patients' lymphocyte surfaces.

Hyaladherins

Hyaluronan exists in a number of states in the vertebrate body. Within ECM, it can be firmly intercalated within proteoglycans and binding proteins in a bottle-brush-like configuration. It can be bound to cells by means of cell surface receptors. Some of the HA exists in a free-form circulating in the lymphatic or cardiovascular system. However, even in this relatively free-from, there are a number of binding proteins that decorate HA. These are referred to collectively as hyaladherins, a term coined by Bryan Toole (40). The hyaladherins associate with HA through electrostatic or covalent bonds (42). It is likely that some of the unique properties attributed to HA are in fact a function of the hyaladherins that are bound to HA. Growth factors, collagen (96) and a myriad of other proteins have been identified.

One of the major challenges and opportunities in dermatology is to identify the profile of hyaladherins specific for the HA of epidermis and dermis, to characterize these proteins, and to understand their function in relation to age-related changes. In an examination of skin as a function of age, the levels of HA did not decrease, as would be expected, but rather the binding of HA to tissue proteins became more tenacious, and HA became increasingly more difficult to extract (97,98). Another challenge is to understand how HA as a substrate for degradation by hyaluronidases is effected by associated hyaladherins. It is also reasonable to assume that the secondary structure of the HA polymer is modulated, in part, by the hyaladherins bound to it.

Hyaluronan in the ECM

ECM that surrounds cells and occupies the variable spaces between cells is composed predominantly of structural proteins such as collagen and elastin, as well as proteoglycans, and a number of glycoproteins. The basal lamina or basement membrane that separates dermis and epidermis is composed of similar materials, and is therefore also considered an ECM structure.

A number of growth factors are embedded in ECM, concentrated by ECM components where they are protected from degradation. Such factors are presented to cells as mechanisms for growth control and modulators of cell function. Heparan sulfate-containing proteoglycans bind members of the FGF and EGF families (99), whereas HA can bind growth factors such TGF-β (100). A complex picture is emerging suggesting that the two classes of GAGs, HA and heparan sulfate, have opposing functions. An HA-rich environment is required for the maintenance of the undifferentiated, pluripotential state, facilitating motility and proliferation, whereas the heparan sulfate proteoglycans promote differentiation. However, the concentration of HA in ECM can vary widely. Even when the levels are decreased, as in areas of marked fibrosis, HA functions as an organizer of ECM, as a scaffold about which other macromolecules of ECM orient themselves. Diameters of collagen fibers can be modulated by levels of HA, the thinner more delicate fibers being favored in regions of high HA concentrations. In fibroblast cultures, the addition of exogenous HA to the medium decreases the diameter of the collagen fibers that accumulate (unpublished observations).

The ability of HA to promote cell proliferation is dependent in part on the concentration of the HA molecule (101), opposite effects being achieved at high and low concentrations. Size is also important. High molecular weight HA is antiangiogenic (43), whereas lower molecular weight HA moieties are highly angiogenic, stimulating growth of endothelial cells (22), attracting inflammatory cells, and also inducing expression of inflammatory cytokines in such cells (25–27). Partially degraded HA may have the opposite effect, possibly because it is no longer able to retain and release growth factors such as TGF-β (100).

The intense staining for HA in psoriatic lesions may in part be due to partially degraded HA, and may be the mechanisms for the marked capillary proliferation and inflammation that characterize these lesions (101–104). Attempts to stimulate HA deposition for purposes of promoting skin hydration must use caution that the HA deposited is of high molecular weight, by preventing free radical-catalyzed chain breaks and by carefully restricting the catabolic reactions of the hyaluronidases.

Intracellular Hyaluronan

The most recent development is the realization that HA and associated hyaldherins are intracellular, and have major effects on cellular metabolism. Much of the recent advance comes from the ability to remove ECM of cultured cells using the highly specific Streptomyces hyaluronidase. Permeabilizing such cells and using confocal microscopy then make it possible to use localization techniques for the identification of intracellular HA and its associated proteins (35,37,38). Such HA complexes also appear to be a component of the nuclear matrix in a wide variety of cells (105,106). They also have importance in regulating the cell cycle and gene transcription. A vertebrate homolog of the cell cycle control protein CDC37 was recently cloned and found to be an hyaladherin (107), as was a protein that copurified with the splicing factor SF2 (108). An intracellular form of the HA receptor RHAMM was demonstrated to regulate erk kinase activity. Changes in function of these intracellular hyaladherins, depending on whether or not they have HA molecules attached, confers another layer of complexity dependent on intracellular hyaluronidase enzymes.

In the HA-rich vertebrate embryo and fetal tissues, there is minimal intercellular ECM. Most of HA is intracellular, and the role of such intracellular HA in development is unknown. The HA-rich germinal epithelium and pluripotential basal cells of the bone marrow as well as basal epithelium keratinocytes contain large amounts of HA that are involved in cell physiology. Such HA should be separated from the HA of the ECM, presumably the more important compartment when dealing with skin moisture.

HYALURONAN RECEPTORS

CD44

There are a variety of HA-binding proteins that are broadly distributed, and with wide variations in locations: ECM, cell surface-associated, intracellular, both cytoplasmic and nuclear. The same molecule may occur in multiple locations. However, it is those that attach HA to the cell surface that constitute receptors. The most prominent among these is CD44, a transmembrane glycoprotein that occurs in a wide variety of isoforms, products of a single gene with variant exon expression (28–30). CD44 is coded for by 10 constant exons, plus from 0 to 10 variant exons, all inserted into a single extracellular position near the membrane insertion site (109). Additional variations in CD44 can occur as a result of posttranslational glycosylation, addition of various GAGs, including chondroitin sulfate and heparan sulfate. CD44 is able to bind a variety of other ligands, some of which have not yet been identified. CD44 has been shown, however, to interact with fibronectin, collagen, and heparin-binding growth factors. CD44 is distributed widely, being found on virtually all cells except red blood cells. It plays a role in cell adhesion, migration, lymphocyte activation and homing, and cancer metastasis.

The appearance of HA in dermis and epidermis parallels the histolocalization of CD44. The nature of the CD44 variant exons in skin at each location has not been described. The ability of CD44 to bind HA can vary as a function of differential exon expression. It would be of intrinsic interest to establish whether modulation occurs in CD44 variant exon expression with changes in the state of skin hydration. Changes in the profile of CD44 variant exon expression as a result of skin pathologies also await description.

Only one of many possible examples of the importance of CD44–HA interactions in normal skin physiology is given here. HA in the matrix surrounding keratinocytes serves as an adhesion substrate for the Langerhans cells with their CD44-rich surfaces, as they migrate through the epidermis (110,111). In skin pathophysiology, the effect of local and systemic immune disorders on such interactions between Langerhans cells and keratinocytes awaits explication (111,112).

RHAMM

The other major receptor for HA is RHAMM (Receptor for HA-Mediated Motility) (113,114), discovered and characterized by Eva Turley. This receptor is implicated in cell locomotion, focal adhesion turnover, and contact inhibition. It is also expressed in a number of variant isoforms. The interactions between HA and RHAMM regulate locomotion of cells by a complex network of signal transduction events and interaction with the cytoskeleton of cells. It is also an important regulator of cell growth (115).

The TGF-β stimulation of fibroblast locomotion utilizes RHAMM. TGF-β is a potent stimulator of motility in a wide variety of cells. In fibroblasts, TGF-β triggers the transcription, synthesis, and membrane expression of not only RHAMM, but also the synthesis and expression of the HA, all of which occurs coincident with the initiation of locomotion (116).

Both RHAMM and CD44 may be among the most complex biological molecules ever described, with locations in an unusually wide variety of cell compartments, and associated with a spectrum of activities involving signal transduction, motility, and cell transformation. The apparent inconsistency of observations between different laboratories regarding the receptors CD44 and RHAMM (117) reflects the subtle ways HA exerts its broad spectrum of biological effects and the myriad of mechanisms for controlling levels of HA expression and deposition. Particularly in the experimental laboratory situation, minor changes in culture conditions, differences in cell passage number, length of time following plating, variations in growth factors contained in lots of serum, or differences in stages of cell confluence have major repercussions in expression of HA, its receptors or the profile of hyaladherins that decorate the HA molecule.

HYALURONAN IN SKIN

Artifacts of Hyaluronan Histolocalization in Skin

Hyaluronan occurs in virtually all vertebrate tissues and fluids, but skin is the largest reservoir of body HA, containing >50% of the total. Earlier studies on the distribution of HA in skin, using histolocalization techniques, seriously underestimated HA levels. Formalin is an aqueous fixative, and much of the soluble tissue HA is eluted by this procedure. The length of time the tissue is in the formalin is a variable that may explain the conflicting results that are often encountered. Acidification and addition of alcohol to the fixative cause HA to become more avidly fixed, so that subsequent aqueous steps are unable to elute HA out of the tissue (46).

Comparisons have been made of HA localization in skin sections fixed with acid-formalin/ethanol and conventional formalin fixation. Much of the HA, particularly in the epidermis, is eluted during the process of formalin fixation. This suggests that epidermal HA is more loosely associated with cell and tissue structures than is dermal HA. A further incubation of 24 h in aqueous buffer further increases the disparity between the acid-formalin/alcohol and the conventional fixation technique. Once the tissue has been exposed to the acid-formalin/alcohol, the HA association with tissue becomes tenaciously fixed, with little loss of apparent HA observed following additional aqueous incubation, whereas the formalin-fixed tissues demonstrates progressive loss of HA.

Epidermal Hyaluronan

Until recently, it was assumed that only cells of mesenchymal origin were capable of synthesizing HA, and HA was therefore restricted to the dermal compartment of skin. However, with the advent of the specific techniques for the histolocalization of HA, the biotinylated HA-binding peptide (118), evidence for HA in the epidermis became apparent (98,119–122). In addition, techniques for separating dermis and epidermis from each other permitted accurate measurement of HA in each compartment, verifying that epidermis does contain HA (123).

Hyaluronan is most prominent in the upper spinous and granular layers of the epidermis, where most of it is extracellular. The basal layer has HA, but it is predominantly intracellular, and is not easily leeched out during aqueous fixation. Presumably, basal keratinocyte HA is involved in cell cycling events, whereas the secreted HA in the upper outer layers of the epidermis are mechanisms for disassociation and eventual sloughing of cells.

Cultures of isolated keratinocytes have facilitated the study of epithelial HA metabolism. Basal keratinocytes synthesize copious quantities of HA. When Ca^{2+} of the culture medium is increased, from 0.05 to 1.20 mM, these cells begin to differentiate, HA synthesis levels drop (124), and there is the onset of hyaluronidase activity (125). This increase in calcium that appears to stimulate in culture the natural *in situ* differentiation of basal keratinocytes parallels the increasing calcium gradient observed in the epidermis. There may be intracellular stores of calcium that are released as keratinocytes mature.

Alternatively, the calcium stores may be concentrated by lamellar bodies from the intercellular fluids released during terminal differentiation. The lamellar bodies are thought to be modified lysosomes containing hydrolytic enzymes, and a potential source of the hyaluronidase activity. The lamellar bodies fuse with the plasma membranes of the terminally differentiating keratinocytes, increasing the plasma membrane surface area. Lamellar bodies are also associated with proton pumps that enhance acidity. The lamellar bodies also acidify, and their polar lipids become partially converted to neutral lipids, thereby participating in skin barrier function.

Diffusion of aqueous material through the epidermis is blocked by these lipids synthesized by keratinocytes in the stratum granulosum, the boundary corresponding to the level at which HA-staining ends. This constitutes part of the barrier function of skin. The HA-rich area inferior to this layer may obtain water from the moisture-rich dermis. In addition, the water contained therein cannot penetrate beyond the lipid-rich stratum granulosum. The HA-bound water in both the dermis and the vital area of the epidermis is critical for skin hydration. In addition, the stratum granulosum is essential for maintenance of that hydration, not only for the skin, but also for the body in general. Profound dehydration is a serious clinical problem in burn patients with extensive losses of the stratum granulosum.

Dermal Hyaluronan

The HA content of the dermis is far greater than that of the epidermis, and accounts for most of the 50% of total body HA present in skin (14). The papillary dermis has the more prominent levels of HA than does reticular dermis (98). HA of the dermis is in continuity with both the lymphatic and vascular systems, whereas epidermal HA is not. Exogenous HA is cleared from the dermis and rapidly degraded (55).

The dermal fibroblast provides the synthetic machinery for dermal HA, and should be the target for pharmacological attempts to enhance skin hydration. The fibroblasts of the body, the most banal of cells from a histologic perspective, are probably the most diverse of all vertebrate cells with the broadest repertoire of biochemical reactions and potential pathways for differentiation. Much of this diversity is site specific. What makes the papillary dermal fibroblast different from other fibroblasts is not known. However, these cells have an HA synthetic capacity similar to that of the fibroblasts that line joint synovium, responsible for the HA-rich synovial fluid (Stern, unpublished experiments).

Aging Skin

Though dermal HA is responsible for most skin HA, epidermal cells are also able to synthesize HA. The most dramatic histochemical change observed in senescent skin is the marked decrease in epidermal HA (98). In senile skin, HA is still present in the dermis, whereas HA of the epidermis has disappeared entirely. The proportion of total GAG synthesis devoted to HA is greater in epidermis than in dermis, and the reasons for the precipitous fall with aging is unknown. The synthesis of epidermal HA is influenced both by the underlying dermis and by topical treatments, such as with retinoic acids, indicating that epidermal HA is under separate controls from dermal HA.

In contrast with previous *in vitro* (126,127) and *in vivo* (128,129) observations, recent studies document that the total level of HA remains constant in the dermis with aging. The major age-related change is the increasing avidity of HA with tissue structures with the concomitant loss of HA extractability. Such intercalated HA may have diminished ability to take on water-of-hydration. This decreased volume of water-of-hydration of HA is obviously a loss in skin moisture. An important study for the future would be to define precisely the hyaldherins, the HA-binding proteins, that decorate the HA in senile skin, and to compare that profile with the hyaladherins of young skin, in both the dermal and epidermal compartments. Progressive loss in the size of the HA polymer in skin as a function of age has also been reported (130).

The increased binding of HA with tissue as a function of age parallels the progressive cross-linking of collagen and the steady loss of collagen extractability with age. Each of these phenomena contributes to the apparent dehydration, atrophy, and loss of elasticity that characterizes aged skin.

Photoaging of Skin

Repeated exposure to UV radiation from the sun causes premature aging of skin (131,132). UV damage causes initially a mild form of wound healing, and is associated first with elevated dermal HA. As little as 5 min of UV exposure in nude mice causes enhanced deposition of HA (Thiele and Stern, unpublished experiments), indicating that UV-induced skin damage is an extremely rapid event. The initial "glow" after sun exposure may be a mild edematous reaction induced by the enhanced HA deposition. But the transient sense of well being in the long run extracts a high price, particularly with prolonged exposure. Repeated exposures ultimately simulate a typical wound healing response with deposition of scar-like type I collagen, rather than the usual types I and III collagen mixture that gives skin resilience and pliability. The biochemical changes that distinguish photoaging and chronological aging have not been identified.

The abnormal GAGs of photoaging are those also found in scars, in association with the changes found late in the wound healing response, with diminished HA and increased levels of chondroitin sulfate proteoglycans. There is also an abnormal pattern of distribution (132). The GAGs appear to be deposited on the elastotic material that comprises "elastosis" and diffusely associated with the actinic-damaged collagen fibers. These appear as "smudges" on H&E sections of sun-damaged skin, rather than between the collagen and elastin fibers as would be observed in normal skin.

Acute and Chronic Inflammation

Chronic inflammation causes premature aging of the skin, as observed in patients with atopic dermatitis. The constant inflammatory process leads to decreased function of the skin barrier, accompanied by loss of skin moisture. Presumably, the skin of such patients contains decreased levels of HA. Alternatively, HA may reflect that found in chronological aging, with a change in the ability to take on water-of-hydration with enhanced association with tissue structures and loss of extractability. Demonstration of such changes and the precise histolocalization of this decreased HA deposition would be of intrinsic interest, a study that has not been performed yet.

The acute inflammatory process is associated initially with increased HA levels, the result of the cytokines released by the polymorphonuclear leukocytes, the predominant cells of the acute inflammatory process. The erythema, swelling, and warmth of the acute process are followed later by the characteristic dry appearance and the formation of wrinkles. The precise mechanisms are unknown, but may relate to the differences between acute and chronic inflammatory cells and the attendant chemical mediators released by such cells. Alternatively, initiation of a wound healing response, with collagen deposition, may be a mechanism invoked for the premature aged appearance of the skin in chronic inflammation.

Hyaluronan in Skin Substitutes

There is a requirement for skin substitutes in a great number of clinical situations. In patients with extensive burns, insufficient skin is available for autologous split-thickness skin grafts. Resurfacing of the burned area can occur with autologous cultured epidermal cell autografts. However, this is dependent on a functioning dermal support, a problem that has given rise to a number of reasonable approaches. Cadaver skin dermis has the problem of possible contamination and potential infection. A synthetic dermis has the requirement for an HA content that will support epithelial migration, angiogenesis, and differentiation. Various methods have been examined for modifying natural HA to provide materials with properties similar to the native polymer. Many derivatives of HA have been formulated (133–135). Such materials could provide flat dressings that can be seeded with fibroblasts. These same artificial dressings could also be seeded with cultured autologous keratinocytes, and with laser-drilled microperforations, the keratinocytes can migrate through the membrane onto the wound bed. Such applications are already in use and result in complete healing with a minimum of scarring.

It is anticipated that in the coming years, a number of HA-derivatives will appear for clinical application in dermatology, which contain cross-linked HA polymers as well as HA-ester derivatives obtained by the conjugation of the carboxylic acid of HA with various drugs in their alcohol forms. The HA polymer, because of its intrinsic biocompatibility, reactivity, and degradability, will have many uses in the rapidly expanding field of tissue engineering and in the tissue substitutes of the future.

HYALURONAN SYNTHASES

Single protein enzymes are now recognized as being able to synthesize HA, utilizing the two UDP-sugar substrates. In eukaryotes, the enzyme resides on the cytoplasmic surface of the plasma membrane, and the HA product is extruded by some unknown mechanism through the plasma membrane into the extracellular space, permitting unconstrained polymer growth (45). Such growth could not occur in the Golgi or on the endoplasmic reticulum where most sugar polymers are synthesized, without destruction of the cell. Recent work has demonstrated that the HA synthases are a multigene family with at least three members, HAS-1, -2, and -3 (136,137), which are differentially regulated.

In situ expression of the HAS-1 and -2 genes is up-regulated in skin by TGF-β, in both dermis and epidermis, but there are major differences in the kinetics of the TGF-β response between HAS-1 and HAS-2, and between the two compartments, suggesting that the two genes are independently regulated. This also suggests that HA has a different function in dermis and epidermis.

Stimulation of HA synthesis also occurs following phorbol ester (PMA) and PDGF treatment, though a direct effect on HAS has not been demonstrated (138). Glucocorticoids induce a nearly total inhibition of HAS mRNA in both dermal fibroblasts and osteoblasts. Extracts of dermal fibroblasts indicate that HAS-2 is the predominant HA synthase therein. This may be the molecular basis of the decreased HA in glucocortcoid-treated skin. However, an additional effect on rates of HA degradation has not been examined.

The parallels between chitin, cellulose, and HA structures, all being β-chains of hexose polymers, are reflected in the striking similarity in sequence between the HA synthases from vertebrates, cellulose synthases from plants, and chitin synthases from fungi. A primordial ancestral gene must have existed from which all of these enzymes evolved, which are involved in the biosynthesis of all polymers that contain β-glycoside linkages, an ancient β-polysaccharide synthase.

HYALURONAN CATABOLISM

The Hyaluronidases

Hyaluronan is very metabolically active, with a half-life 3–5 min in the circulation, <1 day in skin, and even in an inert tissue as cartilage, HA turns over with a half-life of 1–3 weeks (16,55,56). This catabolic activity is primarily the result of hyaluronidases, endoglycolytic enzymes with a specificity in most cases for the β 1–4 glycosidic bond.

The hyaluronidase family of enzymes have, until recently, been neglected (139–141), in part because of the great difficulty in measuring their activity. They are difficult to purify and characterize, are present at exceedingly low concentrations, and have very high, and in the absence of detergents, unstable specific activities. New assay procedures have now facilitated their isolation and characterization (125,142). The human genome project has also promoted explication at the genetic level, and a virtual explosion of information has ensued.

An entire family of hyaluronidase-like genes has been identified (143). There are seven hyaluronidases in the human genome, a cluster of three on chromosome 3p, and a similar cluster of three on chromosome 7q31. This arrangement suggests that an original ancient sequence arose, followed by two tandem gene duplication events. This was followed by a more recent *en masse* duplication and translocation. From divergence data, it can be estimated that these events occurred over 300 million years ago, before the emergence of modern mammals. A seventh and nonhomologous hyaluronidase gene occurs on chromosome 10q (144). All of the hyaluronidase-like genes have unique tissue-specific tissue patterns.

The biology of hyaluronidases in skin has not been investigated, nor has it been established which of the various hyaluronidases participate in the turnover of HA in dermis and epidermis.

In vertebrate tissues, total HA degradation occurs by the concerted effort of three separate enzymatic activities, hyaluronidase, and the two exoglycosidases that remove the terminal sugars, a β-glucuronidase, and a β-N-acetyl glucosaminidase. Endolytic cleavage by the hyaluronidase generates ever increasing substrates for the exoglycosidases. The relative contribution of each to HA turnover in either dermis or epidermis has yet to be established. But each of these classes of enzymes as well as the hyaluronidases represent an important potential target for the pharmacological control of HA turnover in skin.

Non-enzymatic Degradation

The HA polymer can be degraded non-enzymatically by a free radical mechanism (145), particularly in the presence of reducing agents such as thiols, ascorbic acid, ferrous or cuprous ions. This mechanism of depolymerization requires the participation of molecular oxygen. The use of chelating agents in pharmaceutical preparations to retard free radical-catalyzed scission of HA chains has validity. However, a carefully monitored effect of such agents on HA chain length in human epidermis has not been attempted. Whether such agents can also affect the integrity of dermal HA in protecting them from free radical damage, and whether these agents have any substantial effect on the moisturizing properties of skin HA remain important questions to be answered.

HYALURONIDASE INHIBITORS

Macromolecular Inhibitors

The extraordinarily rapid turnover of HA in tissues suggests that tightly controlled modes exist for modulating steady-state levels of HA. HA of the vertebrate body is of unique importance, and rapid increases are required in situations of extreme stress. Rapid turnover of HA in the normal state indicates constant synthesis and degradation. Inhibition of degradation would provide a far swifter response to the sudden demand for increased HA levels than increasing the rate of HA synthesis. The ability to provide immediate high HA levels is a survival mechanism for the organism. This might explain the apparent inefficiency of rapid rates of HA turnover that occur in the vertebrate animal under basal conditions. It can be compared to the need to suddenly drive an automobile much faster in the case of an emergency, not by stepping on the accelerator, but by taking a foot off the break.

If inhibition of HA degradation by hyaluronidase occurs, then a class of molecules that have not been explored, the hyaluronidase inhibitors, are very important. It can be postulated that with extreme stress, hyaluronidase inhibitors would be found in the circulation as acute phase proteins, the stress response products synthesized by the liver. These would prevent the ever present rapid destruction and allow levels of HA to quickly increase.

Circulating hyaluronidase inhibitor activity has been identified in human serum over half a century ago (146,147). Modifications in levels of inhibitor activity have been observed in the serum of patients with cancer (148,149), liver disease (150), and with certain dermatological disorders (151). This area of biology is unexplored, and though some early attempts were made (152–154), and even though a review appeared (155), these hyaluronidase inhibitors have never been isolated nor characterized at the molecular level.

Inhibitors of mammalian origin, such as the serum inhibitor or heparin, are far more potent than the relatively weak inhibitors of plant origin. Hyaluronidase inhibitors of animal origin would provide a means for enhancing levels of HA in skin, and represent an important research area in attempting to enhance skin moisture.

Low Molecular Weight Inhibitors

Classes of lower molecular weight inhibitors of hyaluronidase have been identified, some of which come from folk medicines, from the growing field of ethnopharmacology. Some anti-inflammatories as well as some of the ancient beauty aids and practices for freshening of the skin may have some of these compounds as the basis of their mechanism of action.

Those that have been identified in recent times include flavonoids (156–158), aurothiomalate (159), hydrangenol (160), occurring in the leaves of Hydrangea, tannins (161), derivatives of tranilast (162), curcumin (163), an extract of the spice turmeric, glycyrrhizin (164), found in the roots and rhizomes of licorice (*Glycyrrhiza glabra*), used as an effective anti-inflamatory agent in Chinese medicine.

Clinically, heparin used as an anticoagulant, has potent antihyaluronidase activity (165), as does indomethacin (166,167), a classic nonsteroidal anti-inflammatory agent, and salicylates (168).

OXIDATIVE STRESS AND SKIN HYALURONAN

Reactive oxygen species or free radicals are a necessary component of the oxygen combustion that drives the metabolism of living things. Though they are important for generating the life force, they simultaneously are extraordinarily harmful. Organisms thus had to evolve protective mechanisms against oxidative stress. Over the course of evolution, different enzymatic and non-enzymatic anti-oxidative mechanisms were developed, such as various vitamins, ubiquinone, glutathione, and circulating proteins such as hemopexin. Hyaluronan may also be one such mechanism, acting also as a free radical scavenger (169).

Sunlight (UV light) is an additional generator of harmful oxygen-derived species such as hydroxyl radicals. Such radicals have the ability to oxidize and damage other molecules such as DNA causing cross-linking and chain scission. These hydroxyl radicals may also be destructive for proteins and lipid structures, as well as ECM components such as HA. After a very few minutes of UV exposure, disturbance in HA deposition can be detected (Thiele and Stern, unpublished experiments). Therefore, the anomalous situation exists that HA can be both protective as a free radical scavenger, and at the same time a target of free radical stress. This paradox may be understood by a hypothetical model in which HA protects the organism from the free radical stress generated by the oxygen-generated internal combustion, but is itself harmed by the more toxic free radicals generated by the external world, by UV irradiation.

The generation of HA fragments by UV may underlie some of the irritation and inflammation that often accompany long-term or intense sun exposure (170–173). As discussed above, HA fragments are themselves highly angiogenic and inflammatory, inducing the production of a cascade of inflammatory cytokines. Further complications have occurred in this assembly of metabolic-attack and counter-attack reactions that have been compiled in the selective forces of evolution. Unusually high levels of antioxidants are present in skin, such as vitamins C and E, as well as ubiquinone and glutathione. However, these precious compounds are depleted by exposure to sunlight (174–176).

To prevent this sun-induced cascade of oxidative injuries, topical preparations containing anti-oxidants have been developed in the past several decades. Initially, such anti-oxidants were added as stabilizers to various dermatologic and cosmetic preparations. In particular, lipophilic vitamin E has been a favorite as a stabilizing agent. However, following oxidation, vitamin E is degraded into particularly harmful pro-oxidative metabolites (177).

In the past several years, increasing concentrations of anti-oxidants have been used in such skin preparations, in an attempt to create complementary combinations, or to create constant recycling pairs that alternatingly oxidize and reduce each other (178). Finally, molecules such as HA should be protected by topical anti-oxidants, to prevent degradation. Topical anti-oxidants, protecting against free radical damage as well as maintaining HA integrity, may have major effects against natural aging and photo-aging (179,180).

ENHANCING SKIN MOISTURE BY MODULATING HYALURONAN

Alpha-Hydroxy Acids

Fruit compresses have been applied to the face as beauty aids for millennia. The alpha-hydroxy acids contained in fruit extracts, tartaric acid in grapes, citric acid in citrus fruits, malic acid in apples, mandelic acid in almond blossoms and apricots are thought to be active principles for skin rejuvenation. Such alpha-hydroxy acids do stimulate HA production in cultured dermal fibroblasts (unpublished experiments). The results of such alkaline preparations may depend more on their peeling effects rather than on the ability of alpha-hydroxy acids to stimulate HA deposition.

Lactic acid (181,182) citric acid (181,183), and glycolic acid (181,184–186), in particular, though frequent ingredients in alpha-hydroxy-containing cosmetic preparations, have widely varying HA-stimulating activity in the dermal fibroblast assay. Some of these mildly acidic (pH 3.7–4.0) preparations may owe their effectiveness to their traumatic peeling, astringent properties, with constant wounding of the skin. The cosmetic effects of these preparations of alpha-hydroxy acids, including lactic acid, involve increased skin smoothness with the disappearance of lines and fine wrinkles.

Long-term use, however, results in thickening of the skin, in both the epidermal and papillary dermal layers, because of a mild fibrous reaction. This results from a reaction similar to diffuse wound healing, and explains the increased thickness and firmness of both dermis and epidermis. The increased collagen deposition documented in skin after prolonged use is consistent with a wound healing effect (187). Preparations of alpha-hydroxy acids, as would have been found in the fruit compresses of the ancients, have yet to find current cosmetic equivalents, though such vehicles are actively being sought (188).

Upon examining the structure, it is obvious that ascorbic acid is similar in structure to an alpha-hydroxy acid. This is generally not appreciated. However, ascorbic acid is also present in fruit, and may underlie some of the effects attributed to fruit extracts. It has pronounced HA-stimulating effects in the fibroblast assay. But its antioxidant activity confounds the effects it may induce.

Retinoic Acid and Its Derivatives

Topical applications of retinoic acid derivatives reduce the visible signs of aging and of photodamage (189) though there is little correlation between the histologic changes and the clinical appearance of the skin. Initial improvement in fine wrinkling and skin texture correlates with the deposition of HA in the epidermis.

Although vitamin D is considered the "sunshine vitamin", vitamin A has been accepted as an apparent antidote for the adverse effects of sun exposure, and assumed to prevent and repair cutaneous photodamage (189). Application of vitamin A derivatives do reverse some of the sun damage to skin, roughness, wrinkling, and irregular pigmentation (190,191). For the over-40 generation, brought up in an era of "suntan chic", appropriate preparations to restore or to prevent further deterioration of skin are critically important.

Impairment of the retinoid signal transduction pathways occurs as a result of prolonged UV exposure. Down regulation of nuclear receptors for vitamin A occurs (192), resulting in a functional deficiency of vitamin A. Application of vitamin A derivatives would appear to be an obvious treatment modality. Topical application of vitamin A does increase the HA in the epidermal layer, increasing the thickness of the HA meshwork after prolonged treatment (193).

Steroids

Topical and systemic treatment with glucocorticoids induces atrophy of skin, bone, as well as a number of other organs, with a concomitant decrease in GAGs, in particular HA. In human skin organ cultures, hydrocortisone has a bimodal effect. At low physiological concentrations, 10^{-9} M, hydrocortisone maintains active synthesis and turnover of HA in the epidermis; whereas at high concentrations, 10^{-5} M, hydrocortisone reduces epidermal HA content. The effect is achieved through both decreased synthesis and decreased rates of degradation (194). The high concentrations of cortisone also enhance terminal differentiation of keratinocytes and reduces rates of cell proliferation.

Hydrocortisone is also a potent inhibitor of HA synthesis in fibroblasts. HAS-2 is the predominant synthase of dermal fibroblasts, of the three HA synthase genes. Glucocorticoids induce a rapid and near total suppression of HAS-2 mRNA levels. The inhibition of HA deposition thus appears to occur at the transcriptional level. Progesterone inhibits HA synthesis in fibroblasts cultured from the human uterine cervix (195). The steroid effect on HA appears to be system-wide.

Edema is one of the four cardinal signs of acute inflammation. The ability of glucocorticoids to suppress inflammation occurs in part by their ability to suppress the deposition of HA, the primary mechanism of edematous swelling that occurs during the inflammatory response.

GENERAL COMMENTS FROM DERMATOLOGY AND COSMETIC PERSPECTIVES

The natural moisture of skin is attributed to its HA content. The critical property of HA is its ability to retain water, more than any known synthetic or naturally occurring compound. Even at very low concentrations, aqueous solutions of HA have very high viscosity.

The advantage of using HA in cosmetic preparations was recognized very soon after its discovery. Difficulties in preparing large enough amounts of HA free of contaminating glycoproteins, lipids, and other issue materials prevented its convenient use in commercial preparations including its use in cosmetics.

Initially, HA was isolated from rooster combs. This HA was highly purified, and used in ophthalmology as a visco-elastic to replace fluid loss following cataract surgery. The revolution in biotechnology and molecular genetics made it possible more recently to engineer bacteria with augmented HA production, by amplifying the HA synthase genes. This generates a material much lower in molecular weight that has the additional disadvantage of frequent contamination by residual bacterial pyrogens. Such HA, processed from vast fermentation of engineered bacteria, has reduced the price of HA drasticaly, bringing the price into a range that is reasonable for its use in cosmetics. However, this genetically engineered HA of bacterial origin is not of sufficient purity for injectional use.

Many of the cosmetic preparations that contain HA have a concentration of 0.025–0.050%, sufficient to give the preparations a very smooth and viscous feel. Such solutions, applied to the skin, form hydrated films that hold water for considerable periods, and confer the properties of a moisturizer.

Currently, research is underway to modify HA in such a way as to make it more stabile and to confer very specific properties. Another direction in such research is to combine it with other materials, such as chondroitin sulfate and modified sugar polymers, to simulate more closely the associations that HA has in its natural state in vertebrate tissues. As the low molecular size HA fragments are highly angiogenic, defining the optimal size of the HA polymer for cosmetic purposes should be a major goal of such research.

FUTURE DEVELOPMENTS

Currently, the biology of HA and its metabolic cycle is in its infancy. The enzymatic steps that constitute extracellular and intracellular HA cycles are beginning to be sorted out. The goals that lie before us are the identification of such reactions, and new modes of modulating these reactions, in order to enhance skin appearance and to increase the moisture content of photo-damaged and aging skin.

REFERENCES

1. Henle F. Vom Knorpelgewebe, Allgemeine Anatomielehre, Von den Mischungsund Formbestandteilen des Menschlichen Koerpers. Leipzig: Leopold Voss Verlag, 1841:791.
2. Kölliker A. Von den Geweben, Handbuch der Gewebelehre des Menschen, Leipzig: Wilhelm Engelmann Verlag, 1852:51.
3. Duran-Reynals F. Exaltation de l'activité du virus vaccinal par les extraits de certains organs. Compt Rend Soc Biol 1928; 99:6.
4. Duran-Reynals F, Suner Pi J. Exaltation de l'activité du Staphylocoque par les extraits testiculaires. Compt Rend Soc Biol 1929; 99:1908.
5. Duran-Reynals F. The effect of extracts of certain organs from normal and immunized animals on the infecting power of virus vaccine virus. J Exp Med 1929; 50:327.

6. Duran-Reynals F, Stewart FW. The action of tumor extracts on the spread of experimental vaccinia of the rabbit. Am J Cancer 1933; 15:2790.
7. Duran-Reynals F. Studies on a certain spreading factor existing in bacteria and its significance for bacterial invasiveness. J Exp Med 1933; 58:161.
8. Chain E, Duthie ES, Identity of hyaluronidase and spreading factor. Br J Exp Pathol 1940; 21:324.
9. Hobby GL, Dawson MH, Meyer K, Chaffee E. The relationship between spreading factor and hyaluronidase. J Exp Med 1941; 73:109.
10. Casals J. Significance and transcendence of the scientific work of Duran–Reynals, viruses and cancer. In: Stanley WM, Casals J, Oro J, Segura R, eds. Span Biochem Soc Press, 1971:416.
11. Meyer K. The chemistry and biology of mucopolysaccharides and glycoproteins. Sympos Quant Biol 1938; 6:91.
12. Meyer K, Palmer JW. The polysaccharide of the vitreous humor. J Biol Chem 1934; 107:629.
13. Rapport MM, Weissman B, Linker A, Meyer K. Isolation of a crystalline disaccharide, hyalobiuronic acid, from hyaluronic acid. Nature 1951; 168:996.
14. Reed RK, Lilja K, Laurent TC. Hyaluronan in the rat with special reference to the skin. Acta Physiol Scand 1988; 134:405.
15. Toole BP. Proteoglycans and hyaluronan in morphogenesis and differentiation. In: Hay ED, ed. Cell Biology of Extracellular Matrix. New York: Plenum Press, 1991:14.
16. Fraser JR, Laurent TC, Pertoft H, Baxter E. Plasma clearance, tissue distribution and metabolism of hyaluronic acid injected intravenously in the rabbit. Biochem J 1981; 200:415.
17. Weigel PH, Fuller GM, LeBoeuf RD. A model for the role of hyaluronic acid and fibrin in the early events during the inflammatory response and wound healing. J Theor Biol 1986; 119:219.
18. DePalma RL, Krummel TM, Durham LA, Michna BA, Thomas BL, Nelson JM, Diegelmann RF. Characterization and quantitation of wound matrix in the fetal rabbit. Matrix 1989; 9:224.
19. Mast BA, Flood LC, Haynes JH, DePalma RL, Cohen IK, Diegelmann RF, Krummel TM. Hyaluronic acid is a major component of the matrix of fetal rabbit skin and wounds: implications for healing by regeneration. Matrix 1991; 11:63.
20. Longaker MT, Chiu ES, Adzick NS, Stern M, Harrison MR, Stern R. Studies in fetal wound healing. V. A prolonged presence of hyaluronic acid characterizes fetal wound fluid. Ann Surg 1991; 213:292.
21. Knudson W. Tumor-associated hyaluronan. Providing an extracellular matrix that facilitates invasion. Am J Pathol 1996; 148:1721.
22. Zhang L, Underhill CB, Chen L. Hyaluronan on the surface of tumor cells is correlated with metastatic behavior. Cancer Res 1995; 55:428.
23. West DC, Kumar S. The effect of hyaluronate and its oligosaccharides on endothelial cell proliferation and monolayer integrity. Exp Cell Res 1989; 183:179.
24. Rooney P, Kumar S, Ponting J, Wang M. The role of hyaluronan in tumour neovascularization. Int J Cancer 1995; 60:632.
25. Horton MR, McKee CM, Bao C, Liao F, Farber JM, Hodge-DuFour J, Purae E, Oliver BL, Wright TM, Noble PW. Hyaluronan fragments synergize with interferon-gamma to induce the C-X-C chemokines mig and interferon-inducible protein-10 in mouse macrophages. J Biol Chem 1998; 273:35088.

26. Horton MR, Burdick MD, Strieter RM, Bao C, Noble PW. Regulation of hyaluronan-induced chemokine gene expression by IL-10 and IFN-gamma in mouse macrophages. J Immunol 1998; 160:3023.
27. Slevin M, Krupinski J, Kumar S, Gaffney J. Angiogenic oligosaccharides of hyaluronan induce protein tyrosine kinase activity in endothelial cells and activate a cytoplasmic signal transduction pathway resulting in proliferation. Lab Invest 1998; 78:987.
28. Underhill C. CD44: the hyaluronan receptor. J Cell Sci 1992; 103:293.
29. Lesley J, Hyman R. CD44 structure and function. Front Biosci 1998; 3:616.
30. Naor D, Sionov RV, Ish-Shalom D. CD44: structure, function, and association with the malignant process. Adv Cancer Res 1997; 71:241.
31. Pilarski LM, Masellis-Smith A, Belch AR, Yang B, Savani RC, Turley EA. RHAMM, a receptor for hyaluronan-mediated motility, on normal human lymphocytes, thymocytes and malignant B cells: a mediator in B cell malignancy? Leuk Lymphoma 1994; 14:363.
32. Hall CL, Turley EA. Hyaluronan: RHAMM mediated cell locomotion and signaling in tumorigenesis. J Neurooncol 1995; 26:221.
33. Bourguignon LY, Lokeshwar VB, Chen X, Kerrick WG. Hyaluronic acid-induced lymphocyte signal transduction and HA receptor. J Immunol 1993; 151:6634.
34. Entwistle J, Hall CL, Turley EA. HA receptors: regulators of signalling to the cytoskeleton. J Cell Biochem 1996; 61:567.
35. Collis L, Hall C, Lange L, Ziebell M, Prestwich R, Turley EA. Rapid hyaluronan uptake is associated with enhanced motility: implications for an intracellular mode of action. FEBS Lett 1998; 440:444.
36. Formby B, Stern R. Phosphorylation stabilizes alternatively spliced CD44 mRNA transcripts in breast cancer cells: inhibition by antisense complementary to casein kinase II mRNA. Mol Cell Biochem 1998; 187:23.
37. Evanko SP, Wight TN. Intracellular localization of hyaluronan in proliferating cells. J. Histochem. Cytochem. 1999; 47:1331.
38. Laurent TC, Fraser JR. Hyaluronan. FASEB J 1992; 6:2397.
39. Laurent TC, ed. The Chemistry, Biology and Medical Applications of Hyaluronan and its Derivatives. London: Portland Press, 1998.
40. Toole BP. Hyaluronan and its binding proteins. The hyaladherins. Curr Opin Cell Biol 1990; 2:839.
41. Knudson CB, Kundson W. Hyaluronan-binding proteins in development, tissue homeostasis, and disease. FASEB J 1993; 7:1233.
42. Zhao M, Yoneda M, Ohashi Y, Kurono S, Iwata H, Ohnuki Y, Kimata K. Evidence for the covalent binding of SHAP, heavy chains of inter-alpha-trypsin inhibitor, to hyaluronan. J Biol Chem 1995; 270:26657.
43. Feinberg RN, Beebe DC. Hyaluronate in vasculogenesis. Science 1983; 220:1177.
44. Scott JE. Secondary structures in hyaluronan solutions: chemical and biological implications. In: Evered D, Whelan J, eds. The Biology of Hyaluronan. Chichester: John Wiley & Sons, 1989:16.
45. Prehm P. Hyaluronate is synthesized at plasma membranes. Biochem J 1984; 220:597.
46. Lin W, Shuster S, Maibach HI, Stern R. Patterns of hyaluronan staining are modified by fixation techniques. J Histochem Cytochem 1997; 45:1157.
47. Fessler JH, Fessler LI. Electron microscopic visualization of the polysaccharide hyaluronic acid. Proc Natl Acad Sci USA 1966; 56:141.

48. Wight TN, Heinegard DK, Hascall VC. Proteoglycans structure and function. In: Hay ED, ed. Cell Biology of the Extracellular Matrix. New York: Plenum Press, 1991:45.
49. Tomida M, Koyama H, Ono T. Hyaluronate acid synthetase in cultured mammalian cells producing hyaluronic acid: oscillatory change during the growth phase and suppression by 5-bromodeoxyuridine. Biochim Biophys Acta 1974; 338:352.
50. Mian N. Analysis of cell-growth-phase-related variations in hyaluronate synthase activity of isolated plasma-membrane fractions of cultured human skin fibroblasts. Biochem J 1986; 237:333.
51. Brecht M, Mayer U, Schlosser E, Prehm P. Increased hyaluronate synthesis is required for fibroblast detachment and mitosis. Biochemistry 1986; 239:445.
52. Kujawa MJ, Pechak DG, Fiszman MY, Caplan AI. Hyaluronic acid bonded to cell culture surfaces inhibits the program of myogenesis. Dev Biol 1986; 113:10.
53. Kujawa MJ, Tepperman K. Culturing chick muscle cells on glycosaminoglycan substrates: attachment and differentiation. Dev Biol 1983; 99:277.
54. Pratt RM, Larsen MA, Johnston MC. Migration of cranial neural crest cells in a cell-free hyaluronate-rich matrix. Dev Biol 1975; 44:298.
55. Reed RK, Laurent UB, Fraser JR, Laurent TC. Removal rate of [3H]hyaluronan injected subcutaneously in rabbits. Am J Physiol 1990; 259:H532.
56. Laurent UB, Dahl LB, Reed RK. Catabolism of hyaluronan in rabbit skin takes place locally, in lymph nodes and liver. Exp Physiol 1991; 76:695.
57. Engstroem-Laurent A, Hellstroem S. The role of liver and kidneys in the removal of circulating hyaluronan. An experimental study in the rat. Connect Tissue Res 1990; 24:219.
58. Onarheim H, Reed RK, Laurent TC. Elevated hyaluronan blood concentrations in severely burned patients. Scand J Clin Lab Invest 1991; 51:693.
59. Onarheim H, Missavage AE, Gunther RA, Kramer GC, Reed RK, Laurent TC. Marked increase of plasma hyaluronan after major thermal injury and infusion therapy. J Surg Res 1991; 50:259.
60. Ferrara JJ, Reed RK, Dyess DL, Townsley MI, Onarheim H, Laurent TC, Taylor AE. Increased hyaluronan flux from skin following burn injury. J Surg Res 1991; 50:240.
61. Berg S, Brodin B, Hesselvik F, Laurent TC, Maller R. Elevated levels of plasma hyaluronan in septicaemia. Scand J Clin Lab Invest 1988; 48:727.
62. Onarheim H, Reed RK, Laurent TC. Increased plasma concentrations of hyaluronan after major thermal injury in the rat. Circ Shock 1992; 37:159.
63. Engstroem-Laurent A, Laurent UB, Lilja K, Laurent TC. Concentration of sodium hyaluronate in serum. Scand J Clin Lab Invest 1985; 45:497.
64. Chichibu K, Matsuura T, Shichijo S, Yokoyama MM. Assay of serum hyaluronic acid in clinical application. Clin Chim Acta 1989; 181:317.
65. Lindqvist U, Laurent TC. Serum hyaluronan and aminoterminal propeptide of type III procollagen: variation with age. Scand J Clin Lab Invest 1992; 52:613.
66. Yannariello-Brown J, Chapman SH, Ward WF, Pappas TC, Weigel PH. Circulating hyaluronan levels in the rodent: effects of age and diet. Am J Physiol 1995; 268:C952.
67. Haellgren R, Engstroem-Laurent A, Nisbeth U. Circulating hyaluronate. A potential marker of altered metabolism of the connective tissue in uremia. Nephron 1987; 46:150.

68. Lindqvist U, Engstroem-Laurent A, Laurent U, Nyberg A, Bjeorklund U, Eriksson H, Pettersson R, Tengblad A. The diurnal variation of serum hyaluronan in health and disease. Scand J Clin Lab Invest 1988; 48:765.
69. Cooper EH, Rathbone BJ. Clinical significance of the immunometric measurements of hyaluronic acid. Ann Clin Biochem 1990; 27:444.
70. Smedegeard G, Bjeork J, Kleinau S, Tengblad A. Serum hyaluronate levels reflect disease activity in experimental arthritis models. Agents Actions 1989; 27:356.
71. Frebourg T, Lerebours G, Delpech B, Benhamou D, Bertrand P, Maingonnat C, Boutin C, Nouvet G. Serum hyaluronate in malignant pleural mesothelioma. Cancer 1987; 59:2104.
72. Dahl L, Hopwood JJ, Laurent UB, Lilja K, Tengblad A. The concentration of hyaluronate in amniotic fluid. Biochem Med 1983; 30:280.
73. Longaker MT, Whitby DJ, Adzick NS, Crombleholme TM, Langer JC, Duncan BW, Bradley SM, Stern R, Ferguson MW, Harrison MR. Studies in fetal wound healing, VI. Second and early third trimester fetal wounds demonstrate rapid collagen deposition without scar formation. J Pediatr Surg 1990; 25:63.
74. Decker M, Chiu ES, Dollbaum C, Moiin A, Hall J, Spendlove R, Longaker MT, Stern R. Hyaluronic acid-stimulating activity in sera from the bovine fetus and from breast cancer patients. Cancer Res 1989; 49:3499.
75. Bernfield MR, Banerjee SD, Cohn RH. Dependence of salivary epithelial morphology and branching morphogenesis upon acid mucopolysaccharide-protein. J Cell Biol 1972; 52:674.
76. Gakunga P, Frost G, Shuster S, Cunha G, Formby B, Stern R. Hyaluronan is a prerequisite for ductal branching morphogenesis. Development 1997; 124:3987.
77. Delpech B, Girard N, Bertrand P, Courel MN, Chauzy C, Delpech A. Hyaluronan: fundamental principles and applications in cancer. J Intern Med 1997; 242:41.
78. Ropponen K, Tammi M, Parkkinen J, Eskelinen M, Tammi R, Lipponen P, Agren U, Alhava E, Kosma VM. Tumor cell-associated hyaluronan as an unfavorable prognostic factor in colorectal cancer. Cancer Res 1998; 58:342.
79. Lokeshwar VB, Obek C, Soloway MS, Block NL. Tumor-associated hyaluronic acid: a new sensitive and specific urine market for bladder cancer. Cancer Res 1997; 57:773.
80. Lokeshwar VB, Soloway MS, Block NL. Secretion of bladder tumor-derived hyaluronidase activity by invasive bladder tumor cells. Cancer Lett 1998; 131:21.
81. Bertrand P, Girard N, Duval C, d'Anjou J, Chauzy C, Maenard JF, Delpech B. Increased hyaluronidase levels in breast tumor metastases. Int J Cancer 1997; 73:327.
82. Madan AK, Yu K, Dhurandhar N, Cullinane C, Pang Y, Beech DJ. Association of hyaluronidase and breast adenocarcinoma invasiveness. Oncol Rep 1999; 6:607.
83. Engstroem-Laurent A. Changes in hyaluronan concentration in tissues and body fluids in disease states. In: Evered D, Whelan J, eds. The Biology of Hyaluronan. Chichester: John Wiley & Sons, 1989:233.
84. Brown WT. Progeria: a human-disease model of accelerated aging. Am J Clin Nutr 1992; 55:1222S.
85. Kieras FJ, Brown WT, Houck GE Jr, Zebrower M. Elevation of urinary hyaluronic acid in Werner's syndrome and progeria. Biochem Med Metabl Biol 1986; 36:276.
86. Laurent TC, Laurent UB, Fraser JR. Serum hyaluronan as a disease marker. Ann Med 1996; 28:241.

87. Delmage JM, Powars DR, Jaynes PK, Allerton SE. The selective suppression of immunogenicity by hyaluronic acid. Ann Clin Lab Sci 1986; 16:303.
88. McBride WH, Bard JB. Hyaluronidase-sensitive halos around adherent cells. Their role in blocking lymphocyte-mediated cytolysis. J Exp Med 1979; 149:507.
89. Forrester JV, Wilkinson PC. Inhibition of leukocyte locomotion by hyaluronic acid. J Cell Sci 1981; 48:315.
90. Dick SJ, Macchi B, Papazoglou S, Oldfield EH, Kornblith PL, Smith BH, Gately MK. Lymphoid cell-glioma cell interaction enhances cell coat production by human gliomas: novel suppressor mechanism. Science 1983; 220:739.
91. Manley G, Warren C. Serum hyaluronic acid in patients with disseminated neoplasm. J Clin Pathol 1987; 40:626.
92. Wilkinson CR, Bower LM, Warren C. The relationship between hyaluronidase activity and hyaluronic acid concentration in sera from normal controls and from patients with disseminated neoplasm. Clin Chim Acta 1996; 256:165.
93. Delpech B, Chevallier B, Reinhardt N, Julien JP, Duval C, Maingonnat C, Bastit P, Asselain B. Serum hyaluronan in breast cancer. Int J Cancer 1990; 46:388.
94. Hasselbalch H, Hovgaard D, Nissen N, Junker P. Serum hyaluronan is increased in malignant lymphoma. Am J Hematother 1995; 50:231.
95. Gross RL, Levin AG, Steel CM, Singh S, Brubaker G, Peers FG. In vitro immunological studies on East African cancer patients. II. Increased sensitivity of blood lymphocytes from untreated Burkitt lymphoma patients to inhibition of spontaneous rosette formation. Int J Cancer 1975; 15:132.
96. Gross RL, Latty A, Williams EA, Newberne PM. Abnormal spontaneous rosette formation and rosette inhibition in lung carcinoma. N Engl J Med 1975; 292:169.
97. Burd DA, Siebert JW, Ehrlich HP, Garg HG. Human skin and postburn scar hyaluronan: demonstration of the association with collagen and other proteins. Matrix 1989; 9:322.
98. Meyer LJ, Stern R. Age-dependent changes of hyaluronan in human skin. J Invest Dermatol 1994; 102:385.
99. Piepkorn M, Pittelkow MR, Cook PW. Autocrine regulation of keratinocytes: the emerging role of heparin-binding, epidermal growth factor-related growth factors. J Invest Dermatol 1998; 111:715.
100. Locci P, Marinucci L, Lilli C, Martinese D, Becchetti E. Transforming growth factor beta 1-hyaluronic acid interaction. Cell Tissue Res 1995; 281:317.
101. Goldberg RL, Toole BP. Hyaluronate inhibition of cell proliferation. Arthritis Rheum 1987; 30:769.
102. Kumar S, West DC. Psoriasis, angiogenesis and hyaluronic acid. Lab Invest 1990; 62:664.
103. Tammi R, Paukkonen K, Wang C, Horsmanheimo M, Tammi M. Hyaluronan and CD44 in psoriatic skin. Intense staining for hyaluronan on dermal capillary loops and reduced expression of CD44 and hyaluronan in keratinocyte–leukocyte interfaces. Arch Dermatol Res 1994; 286:21.
104. Gustafson S, Wikstreom T, Juhlin L. Histochemical studies of hyaluronan and the hyaluronan receptor ICAM-1 in psoriasis. Int J Tissue React 1995; 17:167.
105. Eggli PS, Graber W. Association of hyaluronan with rat vascular endothelial and smooth muscle cells. J Histochem Cytochem 1995; 43:689.
106. Evanko SP, Wight TN. Intracellular localization of hyaluronan in proliferating cells. J Histochem Cytochem 1999; 47:1331.

107. Grammatikakis N, Grammtikakis A, Yoneda M, Yu Q, Banerjee SD, Toole BP. A novel glycosaminoglycan-binding protein is the vertebrate homologue of the cell cycle control protein, Cdc37. J Biol Chem 1995; 270:16198.
108. Deb TB, Datta K. Molecular cloning of human fibroblast hyaluronic acid-binding protein confirms its identity with P-32, a protein co-purified with splicing factor SF2. Hyaluronic acid-binding protein as P-32 protein, co-purified with splicing factor SF2. J Biol Chem 1996; 271:2206.
109. Screaton GR, Bell MV, Jackson DG, Cornelis FB, Gerth U, Bell JI. Genomic structure of DNA encoding the lymphocyte homing receptor CD44 reveals at least 12 alternatively spliced exons. Proc Natl Acad Sci USA 1992; 89:12160.
110. Weiss JM, Sleeman J, Renkl AC, Dittmar H, Termeer CC, Taxis S, Howells N, Hofmann M, Keohler G, Scheopf E, Ponta H, Herrlich P, Simon JC. An essential role for CD44 variant isoforms in epidermal Langerhans cell and blood dendritic cell function. J Cell Biol 1997; 137:1137.
111. Weiss JM, Renkl AC, Sleeman J, Dittmar H, Termeer CC, Taxis S, Howells N, Scheopf E, Ponta H, Herrlich P, Simon JC. CD44 variant isoforms are essential for the function of epidermal Langerhans cells and dendritic cells. Cell Adhes Commun 1998; 6:157.
112. Seiter S, Schadendorf D, Tilgen W, Zeoller M. CD44 variant isoform expression in a variety of skin-associated autoimmune diseases. Clin Immunol Immunopathol 1998; 89:79.
113. Turley EA. Hyaluronan and cell locomotion. Cancer Metastasis Rev 1992; 11:21.
114. Turley E, Harrison R. RHAMM, a member of the hyaladherins. http://www.glycoforum.gr.jp, 1999.
115. Mohapatra S, Yang X, Wright JA, Turley EA, Greenberg AH. Soluble hyaluronan receptor RHAMM induces mitotic arrest by suppressing Cdc2 and cyclin B1 expression. J Exp Med 1996; 183:1663.
116. Samuel SK, Hurta RA, Spearman MA, Wright JA, Turley EA, Greenberg AH. TGF-beta 1 stimulation of cell locomotion utilizes the hyaluronan receptor RHAMM and hyaluronan. J Cell Biol 1993; 123:749.
117. Hofmann M, Assmann V, Fieber C, Sleeman JP, Moll J, Ponta H, Hart IR, Herrlich P. Problems with RHAMM: a new link between surface adhesion and oncogenesis? Cell 1998; 95:591.
118. Ripellino JA, Bailo M, Margolis RU, Margolis RK. Light and electron microscopic studies on the localization of hyaluronic acid in developing rat cerebellum. J Cell Biol 1988; 106:845.
119. Tammi R, Ripellino JA, Margolis RU, Tammi M. Localization of epidermal hyaluronic acid using the hyaluronate binding region of cartilage proteoglycan as a specific probe. J Invest Dermatol 1988; 90:412.
120. Wang C, Tammi M, Tammi R. Distribution of hyaluronan and its CD44 receptor in the epithelia of human skin appendages. Histochemistry 1992; 98:105.
121. Bertheim U, Hellstroem S. The distribution of hyaluronan in human skin and mature, hypertrophic and keloid scars. Br J Plast Surg 1994; 47:483.
122. Tammi R, Tammi M. Hyaluronan in the epidermis. http://www.glycoforum.gr.jp, 1998.
123. Tammi R, Seaeameanen AM, Maibach HI, Tammi M. Degradation of newly synthesized high molecular mass hyaluronan in the epidermal and dermal compartments of human skin in organ culture. J Invest Dermatol 1991; 97:126.

124. Lamberg SI, Yuspa SH, Hascall VC. Synthesis of hyaluronic acid is decreased and synthesis of proteoglycans is increased when cultured mouse epidermal cells differentiate. J Invest Dermatol 1986; 86:659.
125. Frost GI, Stern R. A microtiter-based assay for hyaluronidase activity not requiring specialized reagents. Analt Biochem 1997; 251:263.
126. Schachtschabel DO, Wever J. Age-related decline in the synthesis of glycosaminoglycans by cultured human fibroblasts. Mech Aging Dev 1978; 8:257.
127. Sluke G, Schachtschabel DO, Wever J. Age-related changes in the distribution pattern of glycosaminoglycans synthesized by cultured human diploid fibroblasts. Mech Aging Dev 1981; 16:19.
128. Breen M, Weinstein HG, Blacik LJ, Borcherding MS. Microanalysis and characterization of glycosaminoglycans from human tissue via zone electrophoresis. In: Whistler RL, BeMiller JN, eds. Methods in Carbohydrate Chemistry. New York: Academic Press, 1976:101.
129. Poulsen JH, Cramers MK. Determination of hyaluronic acid, dermatan sulphate, heparan sulphate and chondroitin 4/6 sulphate in human dermis, and a material of reference. Scand J Clin Lab Invest 1982; 42:545.
130. Longas MO, Russell CS, He XY. Evidence for structural changes in dermatan sulfate and hyaluronic acid with aging. Carbohydr Res 1987; 159:127.
131. Gilchrest BA. A review of skin aging and its medical therapy. Br J Dermatol 1996; 135:876.
132. Bernstein EF, Underhill CB, Hahn PJ, Brown DB, Uitto J. Chronic sun exposure alters both the content and distribution of dermal glycosaminoglycans. Br J Dermatol 1996; 135:255.
133. Prestwich GD, Marecak DM, Marecek JF, Vercruysse KP, Ziebell MR. Controlled chemical modification of hyaluronic acid: synthesis, applications, and biodegradation of hydrazide derivatives. J Control Release 1998; 53:93.
134. Vercruysse KP, Prestwich GD. Hyaluronate derivatives in drug delivery. Crit Rev Ther Drug Carrier Syst 1998; 15:513.
135. Duranti F, Salti G, Bovani B, Calandra M, Rosati ML. Injectable hyaluronic acid gel for soft tissue augmentation. A clinical and histological study. Dermatol Surg 1998; 24:1317.
136. Itano N, Kimata K. Molecular cloning of human hyaluronan synthase. Biochem Biophys Res Commun 1996; 222:816.
137. Weigel PH, Hascall VC, Tammi M. Hyaluronan synthases. J Biol Chem 1997; 272:13997.
138. Asplund T, Brinck J, Suzuki M, Briskin MJ, Heldin P. Characterization of hyaluronan synthase from a human glioma cell line. Biochem Biophys Acta 1998; 1380:377.
139. Kreil G. Hyaluronidases—a group of neglected enzymes. Protein Sci 1995; 4:1666.
140. Frost GI, Csoka T, Stern R. The hyaluronidases: a chemical, biological and clinical overview. Trends Glycosci Glycotechnol 1996; 8:419.
141. Csoka TB, Frost GI, Stern R. Hyaluronidases in tissue invasion. Invasion Metastasis 1997; 17:297.
142. Guntenheoner MW, Pogrel MA, Stern R. A substrate-gel assay for hyaluronidase activity. Matrix 1992; 12:388.
143. Csoka TB, Scherer SW, Stern R. Expression analysis of paralogous human hyaluronidase genes clustered on chromosomes 3p21 and 7q31. Genomics 1999; 15:356.

144. Heckel D, Comtesse N, Brass N, Blin N, Zang KD, Meese E. Novel immunogenic antigen homologous to hyaluronidase in meningioma. Hum Mol Genet 1998; 7:1859.
145. Lapcik L Jr, Chabreacek P, Staasko A. Photodegradation of hyaluronic acid: EPR and size exclusion chromatography study. Biopolymer 1991; 31:1429.
146. Haas E. On the mechanism of invasion. I. Antivasin I, an enzyme in plasma. J Biol Chem 1946; 163:63.
147. Dorfman A, Ott ML, Whitney R. The hyaluronidase inhibitor of human blood. J Biol Chem 1948; 223:621.
148. Fiszer-Szafarz B. Demonstration of a new hyaluronidase inhibitor in serum of cancer patients. Proc Soc Exp Biol Med 1968; 129:300.
149. Kolarova M. Host-tumor relationship XXXIII. Inhibitor of hyaluronidase in blood serum of cancer patients. Neoplasma 1975; 22:435.
150. Snively GG, Glick D. Mucolytic enzyme systems. X. Serum hyaluronidase inhibitor in liver disease. J Clin Invest 1950; 29:1087.
151. Grais ML, Glick D. Mucolytic enzyme systems. II. Inhibition of hyaluronidase by serum in skin diseases. J Invest Dermatol 1948; 257:259.
152. Moore DH, Harris TN. Occurrence of hyaluronidase inhibitors in fractions of electrophoretically separated serum. J Biol Chem 1949; 179:377.
153. Newman JK, Berenson GS, Mathews MB, Goldwasser E, Dorfman A. The isolation of the non-specific hyaluronidase inhibitor of human blood. J Biol Chem 1955; 217:31.
154. Mathews MB, Moses FE, Hart W, Dorfman A. Effect of metals on the hyaluronidase inhibitor of human serum. Arch Biochem Biophys 1952; 35:93.
155. Mathews MB, Dorfman A. Inhibition of hyaluronidase. Physiol Rev 1955; 35:381.
156. Kuppusamy UR, Khoo HE, Das NP. Structure–activity studies of flavonoids as inhibitors of hyaluronidase. Biochem Pharmacol 1990; 40:397.
157. Kuppusamy UR, Das NP. Inhibitory effects of flavonoids on several venom hyaluronidases. Experientia 1991; 47:1196.
158. Li MW, Yudin AI, VandeVoort CA, Sabeur K, Primakoff P, Overstreet JW. Inhibition of monkey sperm hyaluronidase activity and heterologous cumulus penetration by flavonoids. Biol Reprod 1997; 56:1383.
159. Perreault S, Zaneveld LJ, Rogers BJ. Inhibition of fertilization in the hamster by sodium aurothiomalate, a hyaluronidase inhibitor. J Reprod Fertil 1980; 60:461.
160. Kakegawa H, Matsumoto H, Satoh T. Inhibitory effects of hydrangenol derivatives on the activation of hyaluronidase and their antiallergic activities. Plant Med 1988; 54:385.
161. Kakegawa H, Mitsuo N, Matsumoto H, Satoh T, Akagi M, Tasaka K. Hyaluronidase-inhibitory and anti-allergic activities of the photo-irradiated products of tranilast. Chem Pharm Bull 1985; 33:3738.
162. Kakegawa H, Matsumoto H, Endo K, Satoh T, Nonaka G, Nishioka I. Inhibitory effects of tannins on hyaluronidase activation and on the degranulation from rat mesentery mast cells. Chem Pharm Bull 1985; 33:5079.
163. Tonnesen HH. Studies on curcumin and curcuminoids. XIV. Effect of curcumin on hyaluronic acid degradation in vitro. Int J Pharm 1989; 50:91.
164. Furuya T, Yamagata S, Shimoyama Y, Fujihara M, Morishima N, Ohtsuki K. Biochemical characterization of glycyrrhizin as an effective inhibitor for hyaluronidases from bovine testis. Biol Pharm Bull 1997; 20:973.

165. Wolf RA, Glogar D, Chaung LY, Garrett PE, Ertl G, Tumas J, Braunwald E, Kloner RA, Feldstein ML, Muller JE. Heparin inhibits bovine testicular hyaluronidase activity in myocardium of dogs with coronary artery occlusion. Am J Card 1984; 53:941.
166. Szary A, Kowalczyk-Bronisz SH, Gieldanowski J. Indomethacin as inhibitor of hyaluronidase. Arch Immun Ther Exp 1975; 23:131.
167. Kushwah A, Amma MK, Sareen KN. Effect of some anti-inflammatory agents on lysosomal & testicular hyaluronidases. Indian J Exp Biol 1978; 16:222.
168. Guerra F. Hyaluronidase inhibition by sodium salicylate in rheumatic fever. Science 1946; 103:686.
169. Foschi D, Castoldi L, Radaelli E, Abelli P, Calderini G, Rastrelli A, Mariscotti C, Marazzi M, Trabucchi E. Hyaluronic acid prevents oxygene free-radical damage to granulation tissue: a study in rats. Int J Tissue React 1990; 12:333.
170. Takahashi Y, Ishikawa O, Okada K, Kojima Y, Igarashi Y, Miyachi Y. Disaccharide analysis of human skin glycosaminoglycans in sun-exposed and sun-protected skin of aged people. J Dermatol Sci 1996; 11:129.
171. Uchiyama V, Dobashi Y, Ohkouchi K, Nagasawa K. Chemical change involved in the oxidative reductive depolymerisation of hyaluronic acid. J Biol Chem 1990; 265:7753.
172. Saari H. Oxygen derived free radicals and synovial fluid hyaluronate. Ann Rheum Dis 1991; 50:389.
173. Greenwald RA, Moy WW. Effect of oxygen-derived free radicals on hyaluronic acid. Arthritis Rheum 1980; 23:455.
174. Thiele JJ, Trabber MG, Packer L. Depletion of human stratum corneum viamin E: an early and sensitive in vivo marker of UV photooxidation. J Invest Dermatol 1998; 110:756.
175. Kagan V, Witt E, Goldman R, Scita G, Packer L. Ultraviolett light-induced generation of vitamin E radicals and their recycling. A possible photosensitizing effect of vitamin E in skin. Free Radic Res Commun 1992; 16:51.
176. Fuchs J, Milbradt R. Antioxidant inhibition of skin inflammation induced by reactive oxidants: evaluation of the redox couple dihydrolipoate/lipoate. Skin Pharmacol 1994; 7:278.
177. Buettner GR. The pecking order of free radicals and antioxidants: lipid peroxidation, alpha-tocopherol, and ascorbate. Arch Biochem Biophys 1993; 300:535.
178. Kagan V, Serbinova E, Packer L. Antioxidant effects of ubiquinones in microsomes and mitochondria are mediated by tocopherol recycling. Biochem Biophys Res Commun 1990; 169:851.
179. Darr D, Dunston S, Faust H, Pinell S. Effectiveness of antioxidants (vitamin C and E) with and without sunscreens as topical photoprotectans. Acta Dermatol Venerol 1996; 76:264.
180. Fuchs J. Oxidative Injury in Dermatopathology. Berlin: Springer-Verlag, 1992.
181. Ditre CM, Griffin TD, Murphy GF, Sueki H, Telegan B, Johnson WC, Yu RJ, Van Scott EJ. Effects of alpha-hydroxy acids on photoaged skin: a pilot clinical, histologic, and ultrastructural study. J Am Acad Dermatol 1996; 187:34.
182. Smith WP. Epidermal and dermal effects of topical lactic acid. J Am Acad Dermatol 1996; 35:388.
183. Bernstein EF, Underhill CB, Lakkakorpi J, Ditre CM, Uitto J, Yu RJ, Scott EV. Citric acid increases viable epidermal thickness and glycosaminoglycan content of sun-damaged skin. Dermatol Surg 1997; 23:689.

184. Newman N, Newman A, Moy LS, Babapour R, Harris AG, Moy RL. Clinical improvement of photoaged skin with 50% glycolic acid. A double-blind vehicle-controlled study. Dermatol surg 1996; 22:455.
185. Ash K, Lord J, Zukowski M, McDaniel DH. Comparison of topical therapy for striae alba. Dermatol Surg 1998; 24:849.
186. Bergfeld W, Tung R, Vidimos A, Vellanki L, Remzi B, Stanton-Hicks U. Improving the cosmetic appearance of photoaged skin with glycolic acid. J Am Acad Dermatol 1997; 36:1011.
187. Kim SJ, Park JH, Kim DH, Won YH, Maibach HI. Increased in vivo collagen synthesis and in vitro cell proliferative effect of glycolic acid. Dermatol Surg 1998; 24:1054.
188. Wolf BA, Paster A, Levy SB. An alpha hydroxy acid derivative suitable for sensitive skin. Dermatol Surg 1996; 22:469.
189. Edward M. Effects of retinoids on glycosaminoglycan synthesis by human skin fibroblasts grown as monolayers and within contracted collagen lattices. Br J Dermatol 1995; 133:223.
190. Gilchrest B. Anti-sunshine vitamin A. Nat Med 1999; 5:376.
191. Bhawan J. Short- and long-term histologic effects of topical tretinoin on photodamaged skin. Int J Dermatol 1998; 37:286.
192. Lundin A, Berne B, Michaeelsson G. Topical retinoic acid treatment of photoaged skin: its effects on hyaluronan distribution in epidermis and on hyaluronan and retinoic acid in suction blister fluid. Acta Dermato-Venere 1992; 72:423.
193. Wang Z, Boudjelal M, Kang S, Voorhees JJ, Fisher GJ. Ultraviolet irradiation of human skin causes functional vitamin A deficiency, preventable by all-trans retinoic acid pre-treatment. Nat Med 1999; 5:418.
194. Agren UM, Tammi M, Tammi R. Hydrocortisone regulation of hyaluronan metabolism in human skin organ culture. J Cell Phys 1995; 164:240.
195. Tanaka K, Nakamura T, Takagaki K, Funahashi M, Saito Y, Endo M. Regulation of hyaluronate metabolism by progesterone in cultured fibroblasts from the human uterine cervix. FEBS Lett 1997; 402:223.

22

Kinetin

Stanley B. Levy

University of North Carolina School of Medicine at Chapel Hill, Chapel Hill, North Carolina, USA and Revlon Research Center, Edison, New Jersey, USA

Introduction	407
Chemistry	408
Biology	408
Mechanism of Action	410
Clinical Studies	410
Conclusion	411
References	411

INTRODUCTION

The success of retinoids and hydroxy acids as active ingredients in skin care products designed to improve the appearance of aging skin, has stimulated the search for additional compounds. The use of both retinoids and hydroxy acids may be associated with skin irritation, further stimulating interest in alternatives. A recent addition to this armamentarium is kinetin (N6-furfuryladenine). Kinetin is a plant hormone known for growth-promoting and anti-aging effects in plants. It has been incorporated into several cosmeceuticals prompting a more detailed review.

CHEMISTRY

Kinetin was first isolated from autoclaved Herring sperm DNA in 1955 (1,2). It is a derivative of one of the nucleic acid purine bases, adenine. Kinetin has been reported to be present in various plants (3,4) and human cell extracts (5). It has been identified as a naturally occurring base modification of DNA (6). The chemical structure of kinetin suggests that it can be formed from adenine and furfuryl (Fig. 1). The latter is a primary oxidation product of the deoxyribose moiety of DNA (7). It is not known if DNA repair enzymes remove this modified base from the DNA and make it available as free kinetin.

BIOLOGY

Kinetin was the first cytokinin identified (1,2). Cytokinins are plant growth substances that promote cell division and may play roles in cell differentiation. Most of the data for the biological properties of kinetin come from plant studies. Kinetin has been shown in plant systems to stimulate tRNA synthesis (8) and cell cycle progression (9). Calcium influx through the plasma-membrane calcium channel in plant cells is stimulated by low levels of kinetin (10) "anti-stress effects". More directly linked or related to anti-aging, kinetin is known to prevent yellowing and senescence of leaves and slow down overripening and degeneration of fruits (11).

Rattan and Clark (12) have reported the anti-aging effect of kinetin on human skin cells and fruitflies. As little as 10–20 ppm of kinetin delay the onset of some biochemical and cellular changes associated with cellular aging in cell culture. Human skin fibroblast cell cultures of both young cells that had completed <20% of their potential *in vitro* life span and older cells that had completed ≥90% of their life span were studied. Results were compared with cell cultures receiving no treatment (Table 1). Cytological manifestations of *in vitro* aging including cell enlargement, presence of multinucleated giant cells, accumulation of cellular debris and lipofuscin, and changes in actin filaments and microtubules were attenuated by the addition of kinetin. The number of cells per unit area in a confluent layer also markedly diminishes as a function of age. Kinetin treatment significantly diminished the age-associated reduction in

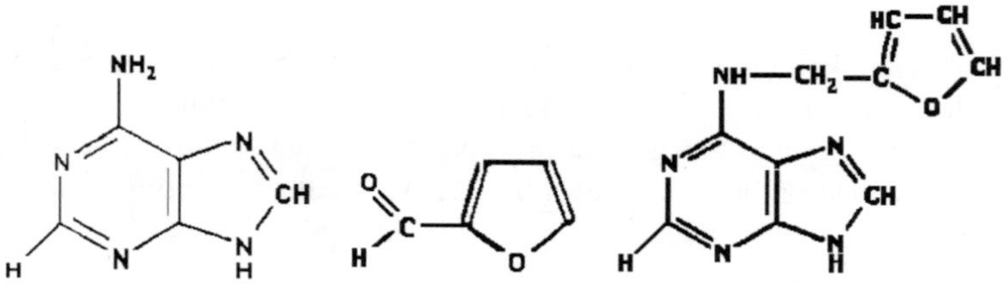

Figure 1 (Left) Adenine; (Middle) furfuryl; (Right) N6-furfuryl adenine.

Table 1 Kinetin's Effects on the Cytological Manifestations of *In Vitro* Aging

Characteristic	Untreated		Kinetin	
	Young	Old	Young	Old
Cell enlargement	None	Significant	None	Insignificant
Multinucleate cells	None	Present	None	None
Cellular debris	Minimal	Significant	Minimal	Minimal
Lipofuscin	Low	High	Low	Low
Actin filaments	Low	Highly polymerized	Diffuse	Less polymerized
Microtubules	Orderly	Disorganized	Orderly	Orderly

Source: Reproduced from Ref. (12).

cell yield (Fig. 2). Kinetin did not effect the longevity of culture cells or their ability to multiply.

A diet containing 20–50 ppm kinetin fed to fruitflies slowed down aging and development and prolonged average and maximum lifespan by 65% and 35%, respectively (13). The increase in lifespan was accompanied by a 55–60% increase in the anti-oxidant enzyme catalase (14). Catalase breaks down hydrogen peroxide associated with cell toxicity.

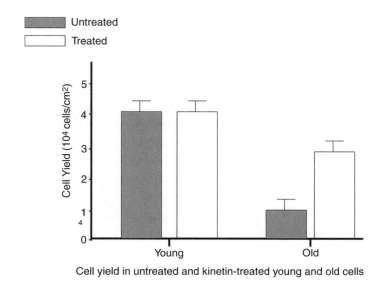

Figure 2 Cell yield in untreated and kinetin-treated young and old cells.

Recently, kinetin has been demonstrated to have inhibitory activity on free radical formation of active platelets *in vitro* and thrombus formation *in vivo* (15). Kinetin may therefore be a potential therapeutic agent for arterial thrombosis.

MECHANISM OF ACTION

The exact mechanism by which kinetin acts to exert its effects is unknown. Kinetin may act directly as a signaling molecule, involved in signal transduction, stimulating defense pathways such as DNA repair (16). Kinetin may also act indirectly as a natural anti-oxidant (17), preventing the formation of reactive oxygen species, or as a direct free radical scavenger (18). Oxygen radicals could abstract hydrogen from the alpha carbon of the amine bond N6-furfuryladenine (19). Oxygen radicals undergo a faster dismutation reaction when kinetin is complexed with copper. A direct effect of kinetin on superoxide dismutase activity has been observed in plants (17). Kinetin has also been shown to protect against oxidative and glycoxidative protein damage generated *in vitro* by sugars and an iron/ascorbate system (18).

The biological significance of kinetin's interaction with DNA or its antioxidant properties remains unknown. However, pluripotency may be a necessary prerequisite for effective anti-aging activity (20).

CLINICAL STUDIES

Percutaneous absorption studies of kinetin with human cadaver skin demonstrate significant skin penetration (McCullough, unpublished study). A dose–response was shown with 0.01% vs. 0.05% kinetin with tissue levels for both serum and lotion formulations. There was no significant difference in transdermal absorption with the two test formulations.

Thirty subjects with mild to moderate photodamaged facial skin were treated with topical kinetin 0.1% twice daily for 24 weeks (21). Significant improvements were seen in tactile roughness, mottled hyperpigmentation, and fine wrinkles at both 12 and 24 weeks. Overall photodamage was reported to be improved by both self-assessment and dermatologist grading. Transepidermal water loss decreased after 24 weeks consistent with skin barrier function improvement. Other than some initial contact folliculitis, no significant skin irritation was seen.

Ninety-eight subjects with mild to moderate photodamaged facial skin each applied a kinetin containing lotion and creams for 10 weeks (Revlon Research Center, unpublished studies). All subjects were assessed at baseline 4, 8, and 10 weeks for photodamage parameters. Statistically significant improvements were noted in all parameters, greatest with texture, skin clarity, discrete and mottled pigmentation, fine wrinkling, and global appearance. No significant irritation was noted.

Forty female subjects, aged 22–57, having mild to moderate facial skin photodamage, underwent a 12 week split face, double-blind, controlled and randomized study comparing a topically applied kinetin containing lotion twice daily on one side and retinol-containing lotion on the other (Almay Research, poster exhibit American Academy of Dermatology Meeting, New Orleans, LA, February 2002). Evaluations at 4 week intervals demonstrated significant improvements for all attributes graded including discrete and mottled pigmentation, fine wrinkling, and overall photodamage. The kinetin lotion produced greater improvements in texture and clarity.

Nine kinetins containing products in 200 subjects each were subject to modified Draize repeat insult patch tests. No instances of sensitization were seen in the challenge phase. In addition, controlled use testing for up to 6 weeks demonstrated no significant irritation (Almay Research, unpublished studies). Six kinetin-containing products were tested on 10 subjects each with skin phototypes I–III for UV sensitivity with a solar simulator (unpublished study, Ivy Research Laboratory, Philadelphia, PA). Panelists were treated with once daily applications of 2 mg/cm^2 to the mid-back for 2 weeks at six sites. After the final applications, no difference in minimal erythema dose was noted between untreated control and treated sites. These studies and clinical experience to date would suggest that kinetin has minimal or no potential to cause irritation, allergy, or photosensitization.

CONCLUSION

Kinetin (N6-furfuryladenine), a plant growth regulator, has been demonstrated to delay a range of cellular changes associated with the aging of human skin cells *in vitro*. In addition, kinetin has anti-oxidant properties formed as a response to free radical damage in human DNA. Before and after clinical studies have demonstrated improvements in photodamaged skin. As is generally the case with new cosmeceutical ingredients, active to vehicle comparison studies are not available (22). Studies have clearly shown that the use of kinetin is not associated with significant irritation and a potential alternative for individuals sensitive to retinoids and hydroxy acids.

REFERENCES

1. Miller CO, Skoog F, Von Saltza MH, Strong FM. Kinetin, a cell division factor from deoxyribonucleic acid. J Am Chem Soc 1955; 77:1392.
2. Miller CO, Skoog F, Okumura FS, Von Saltza MH, Strong FM. Isolation, structure, and synthesis of kinetin, a substance promoting cell division. J Am Chem Soc 1956; 78:1375–1380.
3. Ramman N, Elumalai S. Presence of cytokinin in the root nodules of *Casuarina equisetifolia*. Ind J Exp Biol 1996; 34:577–579.

4. Ratti N, Janardhanan KK. Effect on growth of and cytokinin contents of palmrosa (*Cymbopogon martinii var. motia*) by Glomus inoculation. Ind J Exp Biol 1996; 34:1126–1128.
5. Barciszewski J, Siboska GE, Pedersen BO, Clark BFC, Rattan SIS. Evidence for the presence of kinetin in DNA and cell extracts. FEBS Lett 1996; 393:197–200.
6. Barciszewski J, Siboska GE, Pedersen BO, Clark BFC, Rattan SIS. A mechanism for the *in vivo* formation of N6-furfuryladenine, kinetin as a secondary oxidative damage product in DNA. FEBS Lett 1997; 414:457–460.
7. Kahn QA, Hadi SM. Effect of furfural on plasmid DNA. Biochem Mol Bio Int 1993; 29:1153–1160.
8. Guadino RJ, Pikaard CS. Cytokinin induction of RNA polymerase I transcription in *Arabidopsis thaliana*. J Biol Chem 1997; 272:6799–6804.
9. Zhang KK, Letham DS, John PC. Cytokinin controls the cell cycle of at mitosis by stimulating the tyrosine dephosphorylation and activation of p34cdc-2-like H1 histone kinase. Planta 1996; 200:2–12.
10. Shumaker KS, Gizinski MJ. Cytokinin stimulates dihydropyridine-sensitive calcium uptake in moss protoplasts. Proc Natl Acad Sci USA 1993; 90:10937–10941.
11. McFarland GA, Holliday R. Retardation of the senescence of cultured human diploid fibroblasts. Exp Cell Res 1994; 212:167–175.
12. Rattan SIS, Clark BFC. Kinetin delays the onset of ageing characteristics in human fibroblasts. Biochem Biophys Res Commun 1994; 201:665–672.
13. Sharma SP, Kaur P, Rattan SIS. Plant growth hormone kinetin delays ageing, prolongs the lifespan and slows down development of the fruitfly *Zaprionus paravittiger*. Biochem Biophys Res Commun 1995; 216:1067–1071.
14. Sharma SP, Kaur J, Rattan SIS. Increased longevity of kinetin-fed *Zaprionus* fruitflies is accompanied by their reduced fecundity and enhanced catalase activity. Biochem Mol Biol Int 1997; 41:869–875.
15. Hsiao G, Shen MY, Lin KH, Chou CY, Tzu NH, Lin CH, Chou DS, Chen TF, Sheu JR. Inhibitory activity of kinetin on free radical formation of active platelets in vitro and on thrombus formation *in vivo*. Eur J Pharmacol 2003; 465(3):281–287.
16. Barciszewski J, Rattan SIS, Siboska G, Clark BFC. Kinetin-45 years on. Plant Sci 1999; 148:37–45.
17. Olsen A, Siboska GE, Clark BFC, Rattan SIS. N6-furfuryladenine, kinetin protects against Fenton reaction-mediated oxidative damage to DNA. Biochem Biophys Res Commun 1999; 265:499–502.
18. Verbeke P, Siboska GE, Clark BFC, Rattan SIS. Kinetin inhibits protein oxidation and glyoxidation *in vitro*. Biochem Biophys Res Commun 2000; 276:1265–1270.
19. Rattan SIS. N6-furfuryladenine (kinetin) as a potential anti-aging molecule. J Anti-Aging Med 2002; 5:113–116.
20. Hipkiss AR. On the "struggle between chemistry and biology during aging"— implications for DNA repair, apoptosois and proteolysis, and a novel route of intervention. Biogerontolgy 2001; 2(3):173–178.
21. McCullough JL, Weinstein GD. Clinical study of safety and efficacy of using topical kinetin 0.1% (Kinerase) to treat photodamaged skin. Cosmet Derm 2002; 15(9):29–32.
22. Kligman D. Cosmeceuticals. Dermatol Clin 2000; 18:609–615.

23

Melatonin: A Hormone, Drug, or Cosmeceutical

Tobias W. Fischer and Peter Elsner
Department of Dermatology and Allergology, Friedrich-Schiller University, Jena, Germany

Introduction	413
Melatonin and UV Protection	414
Melatonin: A "Hair Growth Inducer"	416
Melatonin: A Natural Product in Edible Plants	416
Melatonin: A Food Supplement	417
Conclusion	417
References	418

INTRODUCTION

Melatonin (*N*-acetyl-5-methoxytryptamine) is a phylogenetically very old molecule, which is produced by the pineal gland of mammals including the human being and primarily defined as a hormone. In this function, melatonin is active via three receptors, Mel 1, Mel 2, and Mel 3 (1,2). Melatonin regulates the day and night rhythm dependent on light perception of the retina, seasonal rhythm concerning reproduction and hair growth in animals, aging, and immunoregulation (3,4). Apart from the receptor-mediated hormonal function, melatonin is a strong antioxidative substance acting pharmacologically by directly scavenging free radicals as a nonreceptor dependent substance. It also stimulates antioxidative enzymes such as superoxiddismutase. In 1993, Reiter and Tan discovered the antioxidative potential of melatonin describing its strong affinity to the hydroxyl radical, one of the most damaging radicals involved in photoinduced oxidative stress (5). In different organ systems, numerous effects ascribed to the antioxidative capacities of melatonin have been reported and investigated: melatonin protects the stomach by inhibition of the gastral peroxidase and stimulation of the mitochondrial superoxiddismutase (6). Melatonin is used to protect the heart against oxidative damage induced by chemotherapeutics and is able to reduce the overall toxicity of chemotherapeutic agents in the body (7,8). Melatonin reduces the oxidative damage in the skin in disturbances of heme metabolism in porphyria. UVA light-induced toxic free radicals in the skin lead to oxidation of guanin-bases and lipid peroxidation which is suppressed by melatonin (9). Concerning the skin, melatonin is able to increase cell viability in fibroblasts challenged by UVB irradiation and ionizing irradiation (10,11). In this chapter, we review the results of *in vitro* and *in vivo* studies on melatonin, as well as its current therapeutic and possible future applications.

MELATONIN AND UV PROTECTION

Owing to its radical scavenging properties, melatonin is able to suppress free radical formation following UV irradiation. These antioxidative effects were investigated in an *in vitro* model with native human leukocytes and HaCaT-keratinocytes. Dose–response studies with different doses of UV irradiation and constant melatonin concentration were performed compared to nonmelatonin treated cell solutions, and different concentrations of melatonin were tested under constant doses of UV irradiation to find a dose–response relationship. With increasing doses of an UVA/UVB spectrum (280–360 nm, Waldmann UV 800, maximum 310 nm), a linear increase of radical formation was found in non-melatonin-treated cell solutions (75–150–300 mJ/cm^2), and radical formation was significantly suppressed in cell solutions incubated with 2 mM melatonin before irradiation. The radical formation was measured by the lucigenin-dependent chemiluminescence technique (LB 953 Bertold, Germany) (12).

In the same model, different melatonin concentrations ranging from 0.1 nM to 1 mM were chosen to find the concentration with optimal biologic effect. Under a constant UV irradiation, a significant suppression of free radical formation was observed in cell solutions incubated with 10 nM ($p < 0.01$) and 1 mM ($p < 0.001$) melatonin. The suppression of radical formation by 1 mM melatonin was 17-fold compared with nonmelatonin treated irradiated controls. A linear dose–response relationship was found in concentrations between 100 µM and 2 mM (Fig. 1) (13). Compared with vitamin C and trolox, melatonin revealed the strongest radical suppressive potency (14). Analogous experiments were conducted with HaCaT-keratinocytes at a lower irradiation dose of

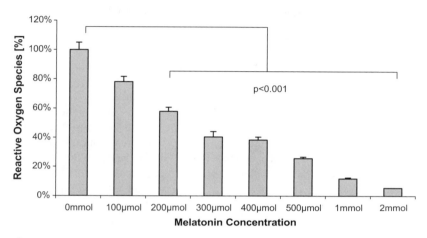

Figure 1 Linear dose–response relationship of melatonin in concentrations between 100 μM and 2 mM with significant suppression of free radicals >200 μM under the influence of UV irradiation (wavelength: 280–360 nm; 750 mJ/cm^2).

30 mJ/cm^2. In concentrations between 500 pM and 10 μM, the suppression of radical formation was significant with $p < 0.0001$ (unpublished personnel data, Fig. 2).

Clinically, the topical application of melatonin in a nanocolloid gel on the back skin of healthy volunteers leads to a significant suppression of UV erythema

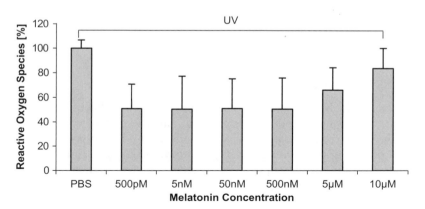

Figure 2 Nonlinear dose–response relationship of melatonin when given to HaCaT-keratinocytes in concentrations between 500 pM and 10 μM melatonin. The suppression of free radicals was significant in all concentrations ($p < 0.0001$). The UV irradiation was performed at a dose of 30 mJ/cm^2.

24 h after exposure compared with nontreated areas of the skin or when nanocolloid gel was applied after the UV exposure (15).

MELATONIN: A "HAIR GROWTH INDUCER"

Melatonin is widely used for the textile industry in Australia and New Zealand as a hair growth inducer and enhancer in fur producing animals such as sheep, cashmere goats, and New Zealand goats. These animals are fed with enriched melatonin starting from late winter to early spring to increase hair growth in springtime after the change of the winter coat. It has been shown that the growth activity of secondary follicles of cashmere goats is increased in springtime when melatonin is given orally (16). In New Zealand goats, histology investigations of hair follicles from skin biopsies of goat fed with 70 mg melatonin per day over a time period of 14 days revealed earlier transition of telogen phase follicles into the proanagen phase, which means earlier induction of springtime hair growth (17). Increased DNA-synthesis was found in cashmere goat follicles kept in hair organ culture over a time period of 120 h. The increase was dose dependent on the amount of melatonin given (50–150–300–600 ng/L). Consequently, the increase of the hair-shaft elongation was significantly higher compared with nonmelatonin-treated controls (18). In our own investigations, melatonin was used to stimulate human hair growth in hair organ culture. We have found out that in a low concentration of 30 μM melatonin, there was a significant increase of hair-shaft elongation compared with follicles incubated with higher concentrations of melatonin between 1 and 5 mM (19). In a clinical placebo-controlled pilot-study of 40 women with alopecia diffusa or alopecia androgenetica, we investigated the effects of daily application of 0.1% melatonin solution. Results of 6 months treatment were assessed by trichograms and there was an increase in occipital anagen hair of women with androgenetic alopecia. Similarly, in women with alopecia diffusa, frontal hair counts showed a significant increase of anagen hairs after 6 months of melatonin treatment (20).

MELATONIN: A NATURAL PRODUCT IN EDIBLE PLANTS

Melatonin at relatively high levels has been detected by radioimmuno assay and high performance liquid chromatography in foodstuffs and plants, such as vegetables, fruits, seeds, rice, wheat, and medical herbs (21). Melatonin is found in leaves and flowers of plants most probably to protect them against an overdose of UV light which may cause an oxidative damage, but, interestingly, it is also identified in seeds of 15 investigated plants. The concentration of melatonin in these seeds was between 2 and 200 ng/g dry weight with the highest concentrations found in seeds of white and black mustard. The levels of melatonin found in seeds are significantly higher compared with those found in human blood under normal conditions, probably due to the vulnerability of germ tissues and their need to be protected against oxidative damage induced by UV irradiation, drought, extreme temperatures, and environmental chemical pollutants (22). It has also been shown that melatonin from plant or plant extract sources is absorbed by the gastrointestinal tract and leads to an increase of melatonin blood levels in humans or rats (23,24). So far, melatonin was shown to be endogenously produced by the pineal gland of vertebrates. Because it is present in food, melatonin is supposed to be also an exogenous antioxidant and, therefore, described as a vitamin because the definition of a vitamin is that of an ingested micronutrient essentially important for life processes being not or insufficiently produced in the animal itself (25,26).

MELATONIN: A FOOD SUPPLEMENT

Melatonin has been shown to reduce the total amount of oxidative damage in many tissues of the rat, such as lung, kidney, and skin (27). Owing to its antioxidant capacities and anti-aging effects concerning the whole organism and in particular the skin, melatonin is taken orally by many people in USA in amounts of 5–20 mg daily. The market share for melatonin at the moment is even more significant than those for vitamins C and E. *In vitro* and *in vivo*, there are many indications that melatonin has immunomodulatory, DNA-protective, and pro-apoptotic properties and, therefore, it may be considered as anticarcinogenic (28). Long-term studies about undesirable side effects were not performed, but so far there are no reports about any toxic or immunosuppressive effects of melatonin. In Europe, melatonin has no registration as a drug nor a food supplement nor a cosmetic substance, as it is regarded as a hormone. By definition, a hormone is a chemical messenger synthesized by an endocrine organ, which is the case with melatonin, and then released into the blood circulation to act in peripheral tissues mediated by a membrane or nuclear receptor. Additionally, a hormone has a feed-back mechanism to its own endogenous synthesis. Melatonin does not fulfill this additional criteria; given in a dosage of 0.5–50 mg per day, melatonin administration in human does not influence significantly the endogenous secretion from the pineal gland in human beings (29,30). Therefore, there is no scientific evidence that melatonin should not be given orally as a food supplement and anti-aging substance.

CONCLUSION

In the last decade, the purpose was to prove the antioxidative properties of melatonin in different organ systems of the human being and, in particular, its protective effect against UV light-induced damage to the skin. In this context, melatonin may be used as a component in topically applied cosmetic anti-aging preparations or as a drug against skin cancer. According to the recent publications, oxidative stress and altered antioxidative response seem to play a role in atopic dermatitis; so, it may be concluded that melatonin may be useful in this condition (31). Melatonin has also been studied and has applications in hair research. Even though the exact mechanism of action is not known, a positive effect of melatonin on hair growth in human beings and fur producing animals has been observed (17,18).

The role of melatonin in clinical and cosmetic use in not fixed so far, and differences exist between USA and Europe. In USA, melatonin is available over the counter as food supplement, whereas in Europe, there is no existing allowance to use melatonin except in clinical studies because of its hormonal profile.

The studies and *in vitro* experiments on melatonin as a sun protector may be promising, but so far it has not been registered as a drug or as a cosmetic product in Europe or in USA. This is a field of future research and development.

REFERENCES

1. Barrett P, Morris M, Choi WS, Ross A, Morgan PJ. Melatonin receptors and signal transduction mechanisms. Biol Signals Recept 1999; 8:6–14.
2. Masana MI, Dubocovich ML. Melatonin receptor signaling: finding the path through the dark. Sci STKE 2000; 107:39.
3. Arendt J. Melatonin. Clin Endocrinol (Oxf) 1988; 29:205–229.
4. Fischer TW, Elsner P. The antioxidative potential of melatonin in the skin. Curr Probl Dermatol 2001; 29:165–174.
5. Halliwell B. Reactive oxygen species and the central nervous system. J Neurochem 1992; 59:1609–1623.
6. Bandyopadhyay D, Biswas K, Bhattacharyya M, Reiter RJ, Banerjee RK. Gastric toxicity and mucosal ulceration induced by oxygen-derived reactive species: protection by melatonin. Curr Mol Med 2001; 1:501–513.
7. Reiter RJ, Tan DX, Sainz RM, Mayo JC, Lopez-Burillo S. Melatonin: reducing the toxicity and increasing the efficacy of drugs. J Pharm Pharmacol 2002; 54:1299–1321.
8. Reiter RJ, Tan DX, Sainz RM, Mayo JC. Melatonin protects the heart against both ischemia/reperfusion injury and chemotherapeutic drugs. Cardiovasc Drug Ther 2002; 16:5–6.
9. Karbownik M, Reiter RJ. Melatonin protects against oxidative stress caused by delta-aminolevulinic acid: implications for cancer reduction. Cancer Invest 2002; 20:276–286.
10. Kim BC, Shon BS, Ryoo YW, Kim SP, Lee KS. Melatonin reduces x-ray irradiation-induced oxidative damages in cultured human skin fibroblasts. J Dermatol Sci 2001; 26:194–200.
11. Ryoo YW, Suh SI, Mun KC, Kim BC, Lee KS. The effects of the melatonin on ultraviolet-B irradiated cultured dermal fibroblasts. J Dermatol Sci 2001; 27:162–169.
12. Fischer T, Scholz G, Knoll B, Hipler UC, Elsner P. Melatonin suppresses reactive oxygen species (ROS) induced by UV-irradiation in leukocytes. J Pineal Res 2004; 37:107–112.
13. Fischer TW, Scholz G, Knoll B, Hipler UC, Elsner P. Melatonin reduces UV-induced reactive oxygen species in a dose-dependent manner in IL-3-stimulated leukocytes. J Pineal Res 2001; 31:39–45.
14. Fischer TW, Scholz G, Knoll B, Hipler UC, Elsner P. Melatonin suppresses reactive oxygen species in UV-irradiated leukocytes more than vitamin C and trolox. Skin Pharmacol Appl Skin Physiol 2002; 15:367–373.

15. Fischer T, Bangha E, Elsner P, Kistler GS. Suppression of UV-induced erythema by topical treatment with melatonin. Influence of the application time point. Biol Signals Recept 1999; 8:132–135.
16. Welch RAS, Gurnsey MP, Betteridge K, Mitchell RJ. Goat fibre response to melatonin given in spring in two consecutive years. Proc N Z Soc Anim Prod 1990; 50:335–338.
17. Nixon AJ, Choy VJ, Parry AL, Pearson AJ. Fiber growth initiation in hair follicles of goats treated with melatonin. J Exp Zool 1993; 267:47–56.
18. Ibraheem M, Galbraith H, Scaife J, Ewen S. Growth of secondary hair follicles of the cashmere goat *in vitro* and their response to prolactin and melatonin. J Anat 1994; 185:135–142.
19. Fischer TW, Fischer A, Knöll B, Hipler UC, Elsner P. Melatonin in low doses enhances *in vitro* human hair follicle proliferation and inhibits hair growth in high doses. Arch Derm Res 2000; 292:147.
20. Fischer TW, Burmeister G, Schmidt HW, Elsner P. Melatonin increases anagen hair rate in women with androgenetic alopecia or diffuse alopecia. Results of a pilot-study. Br J Dermatol 2004; 150:341–345.
21. Hattori A, Migitaka H, Iigo M, Itoh M, Yamamoto K, Ohtani-Kaneko R, Hara M, Suzuki T, Reiter RJ. Identification of melatonin in plants and its effects on plasma melatonin levels and binding to melatonin receptors in vertebrates. Biochem Mol Biol Int 1995; 35:627–634.
22. Manchester LC, Tan DX, Reiter RJ, Park W, Monis K, Qi W. High levels of melatonin in the seeds of edible plants: possible function in germ tissue protection. Life Sci 2000; 67:3023–3029.
23. Reiter RJ, Tan DX, Burkhardt S, Manchester LC. Melatonin in plants. Nutr Rev 2001; 59:286–290.
24. Burkhardt S, Tan DX, Manchester LC, Hardeland R, Reiter RJ. Detection and quantification of the antioxidant melatonin in Montmorency and Balaton tart cherries (*Prunus cerasus*). J Agric Food Chem 2001; 49:4898–4902.
25. Reiter RJ, Tan DX. Melatonin: an antioxidant in edible plants. Ann N Y Acad Sci 2002; 957:341–344.
26. Tan DX, Manchester LC, Hardeland R, Lopez-Burillo S, Mayo JC, Sainz RM, Reiter RJ. Melatonin: a hormone, a tissue factor, an autocoid, a paracoid, and an antioxidant vitamin. J Pineal Res 2003; 34:75–78.
27. Reiter RJ, Tan D, Kim SJ, Manchester LC, Qi W, Garcia JJ, Cabrera JC, El-Sokkary G, Ouvier-Garay V. Augmentation of indices of oxidative damage in life-long melatonin-deficient rats. Mech Ageing Dev 1999; 110:157–173.
28. Pawlikowski M, Winczyk K, Karasek M. Oncostatic action of melatonin: facts and question marks. Neuroendocrinol Lett 2002; 23:24–29.
29. Matsumoto M, Sack RL, Blood ML, Lewy AJ. The amplitude of endogenous melatonin production is not affected by melatonin treatment in humans. J Pineal Res 1997; 22:42–44.
30. Sack RL, Lewy AJ, Blood ML, Stevenson J, Keith LD. Melatonin administration to blind people: phase advances and entrainment. J Biol Rhythms 1991; 6:249–261.
31. Tsukahara H, Shibata R, Ohshima Y, Todoroki Y, Sato S, Ohta N, Hiraoka M, Yoshida A, Nishima S, Mayumi M. Oxidative stress and altered antioxidant defenses in children with acute exacerbation of atopic dermatitis. Life Sci 2003; 72:2509–2516.

24

Topical Niacinamide Provides Skin Aging Appearance Benefits while Enhancing Barrier Function

Donald L. Bissett, John E. Oblong, Abel Saud, Cynthia A. Berge, Amy V. Trejo, and Kimberly A. Biedermann
The Procter & Gamble Company, Miami Valley Laboratories, Cincinnati, Ohio, USA

Introduction	422
Materials and Methods	422
Cell Culture Methods	422
Collagen Synthesis Assay	423
NADPH Level Assay	423
Involucrin Synthesis Assay	424
Filaggrin Synthesis Assay	424
Keratin Synthesis Assay	424
Lipogenesis in Skin Biopsy Samples	425
Clinical Testing	425
Facial Tolerance Testing	425
Facial Benefits Study 1	426
Facial Benefits Study 2	427
Sebum Excretion Measurement Study	427
Pore Size Measurement Study	428
Skin Barrier Evaluation	428
Results	429
NADPH Levels	429

Collagen Synthesis 430
Barrier Layer Components 431
Skin Barrier Function 432
Facial Skin Tolerance of Niacinamide 434
Facial Benefits Study 1 435
Facial Benefits Study 2 435
Reduction in Sebum Excretion and Pore Size 435
Discussion 438
Acknowledgments 439
References 439

INTRODUCTION

The nutritional value of niacinamide is well recognized. However, its use as a topical agent to provide skin care benefits has been less well studied until recently.

There are reports of topical niacinamide providing beneficial effects in prevention of photoimmunosuppression and photocarcinogenesis (1), prevention of the loss of dermal collagen that accompanies photoaging (2), reduction in acne severity (3,4), and improvement in bullous pemphigoid (5). Though effects have been observed in these cases, the likely mechanisms involved have not been clearly defined from these studies.

The physiologic role of niacinamide is as a precursor to important cofactors: nicotinamide adenine dinucleotide (NAD) and its phosphate derivative (NADP). These cofactors and their reduced forms (NADH and NADPH) serve as redox coenzymes in many enzymatic reactions (6). Thus, there is potential for niacinamide to have multiple effects on skin.

In our evaluations of topical niacinamide, we have observed both barrier enhancement properties and several aging skin benefits. We have additionally developed some mechanistic information in regard to these end points. These studies are summarized here.

MATERIALS AND METHODS

Cell Culture Methods

Normal human dermal fibroblasts (ATCC, Rockville, MD) and normal human epidermal keratinocytes (NHEK, Cascade Biologicals, Portland, OR) were grown in standard media as described later. All cells were in passage 1–5 for the experiments described.

Collagen Synthesis Assay

Fibroblasts were plated in DMEM (high glucose) with 10% fetal bovine calf serum at a density of 1×10^5 cells per well. Cells were allowed to attach overnight and media replaced with DMEM containing either 2% or 0.5% fetal bovine serum (FBS) for an additional 24 h. Ten millicuries of ^{14}C-proline (Amersham, UK) was added to each well in addition to ascorbic acid (25 mg/mL). For niacinamide dose responses, a stock solution (10 mM) of niacinamide was prepared in 1X phosphate-buffered saline (PBS) just prior to addition into each culture well. Following a 48 h incubation period, secreted proteins were precipitated with 10% trichloroacetic acid (TCA) on ice for 30 min. Precipitated material was pelleted at 10,000g for 30 min, washed twice with 10% TCA, and resuspeneded in 600 mL of water. Samples were made in 6 N HCl and hydrolyzed overnight at 110°C. The samples were evaporated to dryness, resuspended in 100 mL of water, and filtered through a 0.22 μm filter (Rainin, Woburn, MA). Cells in each well were removed with 0.025% trypsin and cell number determined using a calibrated Coulter counter. ^{14}C-hydroxy protein and ^{14}C-proline in 40 mL from each 100 mL sample were separated using an HPLC equipped with a radiometric detector (β-Ram IN/US Systems, Fairfield, NJ). The stationary phase was a Spheri-5 RP-8 column (220 mm × 4.6 mm) and the mobile phase (0.5 mL/min) was 0.3% sodium lauryl sulfate (SLS) in water–propanol (88:120), pH 2.6 with TCA. The total amount of radioactively labeled hydroxyproline (Hyp) and proline (Pro) in each sample were calculated using a software package provided by the manufacturer (β-Ram IN/US Systems). The amount of total collagen (hydroxyproline), total protein (hydroxyproline + proline), and collagen relative to protein [(hydroxyproline + proline)/hydroxyproline] from each well were normalized to the cell number from the respective well.

NADPH Level Assay

Human dermal fibroblasts (ATCC) were from breast tissue of a 72-year-old female and from the abdomen of a 7-year-old male. They were grown in DMEM containing 10% FBS, with or without 250 μM niacinamide. At 50% confluency, they were spiked with 15–60 μCi of ^{14}C-niacinamide ranging from 15 to 60 μCi, and allowed to grow for an additional 24 h. Cells were then washed with PBS, removed from the culture flasks by scrapping, pelleted by centrifugation, washed with PBS, and resuspended in lysis buffer (50 mM Tris–HCl, 1 mM EDTA, 1% Triton X-100, pH 8.0). Cellular debris was pelleted by centrifugation. The supernatant fraction was assayed for protein and extracted with phenol–CHCl$_3$–IAA (34:24:1). The phenol extracted supernatant solution was then extracted with water-saturated diethyl ether. The aqueous phase of the extraction was then subjected to HPLC analysis for pyridine nucleotides vs. authentic standards on a Supelcosil LC-18-DB column, with profile monitoring at 280 nm and total radioactivity determined with an attached radiometric detector (β-Ram IN/US Systems). The NADPH level was normalized to total protein.

Involucrin Synthesis Assay

Keratinocytes were grown to ~80% confluency prior to addition of niacinamide treatment (250 μM). Following a 24 h incubation period, cells were washed once with sterile PBS and harvested using a plastic scrapper. Cells were pelleted at 1200 rpm and frozen at $-70°C$. The frozen cell pellets were then resuspended in a cell lysis buffer containing 80 mM Tris–HCl, 10% glycerol, 1% SDS, 1 mM EDTA, 50 mM PMSF, 50 mg/mL aprotinin, and 10 mg/mL leupeptin. The suspensions were sonicated and centrifuged at 16,000 rpm. Protein quantitation was performed using a detergent-compatible protein assay kit (DC Protein Assay, Bio-Rad, Hercules, CA). Aliquots of the soluble fraction from cell lysates were used in an involucrin ELISA kit as recommended by the manufacturer (Biomedical Technologies, Stoughton, MA). Quantitation of cell numbers were performed using a Coulter counter.

Filaggrin Synthesis Assay

Keratinocytes were grown to ~80% confluency prior to addition of niacinamide treatment (250 μM). Following a 24 h incubation period, cell culture media was removed and used for quantitation of filaggrin levels. Samples were subjected to SDS–PAGE resolution and resolved proteins were transferred to nitrocellulose. Preblocked blots were then probed initially with rabbit polyclonal anti-filaggrin IgGs at a dilution of 1:2000 in TBST and then with goat anti-rabbit $2°$ conjugated to alkaline phosphatase. Development of alkaline phosphatase reactions followed standard practice. Estimates of changes in filaggrin levels were based on comparisons with vehicle control treatment groups and relative intensity of staining.

Keratin Synthesis Assay

NHEK (Clonetics, Walkersville, MD) were grown in 10 cm Petri dishes in the presence of KBM culture media (Clonetics) supplemented with 0.15 mM calcium. Twenty-four hours after the cells were plated, the growth media was removed and replaced with the either fresh media (control) or media containing 50 μM niacinamide (Sigma, St. Louis, MO). Forty-eight hours after addition of niacinamide to the cultures, the media was removed and the cells were harvested using 200 μL of a lysis buffer containing 2% SDS and 300 mM urea. Forty-five micrograms of each control and niacinamide-treated cell extract were separated using a 4–20% gradient gel (BioRad). The separated proteins were transferred to nitrocellulose using a BioRad Trans-Blot apparatus at 100 W for 90 min. In preparation for Western blot analysis, the nitrocellulose was blocked with a 0.5% milk solution in PBS for 1 h. The nitrocellulose was then incubated overnight at $4°C$ in the presence of a 0.5% milk solution in PBS containing a 1:1000 dilution of an antibody to human keratins 13 and 16 (Sigma clone 8.12). The following day, the nitrocellulose was washed with PBS (three changes for 10 min each) and subsequently incubated at room temperature with 0.5% milk solution in PBS containing a 1:1000 dilution of peroxidase-labeled goat-anti-mouse IgG. Nitrocellulose was washed with PBS as described earlier and was developed using ECL (Amersham). Percent increase in keratin expression was determined via densitometry using BioRad QuantityOne® analysis software.

Lipogenesis in Skin Biopsy Samples

To assess the effect of niacinamide on human sebaceous lipids, a human biopsy culture assay was developed, based on methods from sebaceous gland culture techniques (7,8). Skin biopsies (1–2 mm) obtained from facelift surgery samples were floated in specialized media on sterilized polycarbonate filters and were gently rocked in an incubator at 37°C and 5% CO_2. After 24 h, biopsies were treated with varying concentrations of niacinamide for 4 days. After 4 days treatment, the biopsies were incubated for 6 h with radiolabeled glucose or acetate, and the lipid fraction was isolated and analyzed for incorporation of radioactivity. Individual lipid components were also fractionated using thin layer chromatography. In addition, cell viability (as measured by DNA synthesis and glucose uptake) was assessed over a 4 day period in culture.

Clinical Testing

Before participating in any clinical study, each subject signed a written informed consent that contained all the basic elements outlined in 21 Code of Federal Regulations (CFR) 50.25. It explained the type of study, the procedures to be followed, the general nature of the materials being tested, and any known or anticipated adverse reactions that might result from participation. Owing to the cosmetic nature of these studies, review by an Institutional Review Board (IRB) was usually not required. All studies were monitored for compliance with the protocol.

Facial Tolerance Testing

Forty healthy female Caucasian subjects (age 35–70) were recruited to participate in a double-blind, split-face study with left–right randomization. Each subject received two blind-coded topical test products in 30 g opaque tubes, labeled "left" and "right", one for each side of the face. The pair of test products were identical oil-in-water emulsions except one contained 5% niacinamide. Subjects were instructed to apply a pea-size amount of product (~0.4 g) to each side of the face, twice daily for 6 weeks. Expert redness and dryness grades (0–6 scale, with 0 being normal skin) were taken at baseline and at the end of 4 and 6 weeks of treatment. All 40 subjects completed the study. It was conducted from April to June in Cincinnati, OH.

Facial Benefits Study 1

Healthy Caucasian female subjects (age 35–60; nonpregnant, nonlactating; $n = 40$) were enrolled in a double-blind, split-face study with left–right randomization. All subjects were graded at baseline (0–5 grading scale: 0 being normal skin), and were eligible for study participation with grades of 2.0 or greater in both facial fine lines/wrinkles/texture and facial hyperpigmented spots. Our definition of poor texture encompasses two factors: enlarged pore size and "pebbly, rippled" appearance of older skin in the cheek area.

Prior to study start, there was a 2 week wash-out period in which all subjects used the same facial cleanser commercial product and the same facial moisturizer commercial product twice daily. After 2 week wash-out period, this cleanser product was also used throughout the subsequent 12 week study period, but the moisturizer product was replaced with moisturizer test formulations, which were blind-coded 30 g opaque tubes, labeled "left" and "right". To each side of the face was applied a pea-sized amount ($\sim$0.4 g) of each assigned test formulation, twice daily for 12 weeks, with the evening application occurring at least one hour before bedtime. Subjects were supplied with new containers of test formulations at baseline and at weeks 4 and 8 during the 12 week study.

Subjects were instructed to minimize their UV/sun exposure and to avoid activities that would result in a large amount of such exposure. In addition to the products discussed earlier, subjects also received SPF 15 commercial facial moisturizer sunscreen product to use during outside activities. Other than make-up, subjects were instructed not to use any other skin care products on their faces other than those provided. Subjects washed their faces on the morning of each clinical site visit but did not apply test formulations that day until after the site visit. Subject compliance was checked at a week-one compliance visit and at each subsequent visit to the clinical site (at weeks 4, 8, and 12) by questioning the subjects and weighing test formulation containers to determine usage. Two subjects dropped from the study (5% drop-out rate) for personal reasons unrelated to the test products. This study was conducted from September to December in Cincinnati, OH.

Digital images of each side of the face of all subjects were captured at baseline and at weeks 4, 8, and 12. The facial images were recorded using a wrinkle imaging system (WIS) and color imaging system (CIS). WIS images are captured at high magnification with nonpolarized lighting (incandescent tungsten) that causes a shine that enhances topographical features (fine lines and wrinkles). CIS images are captured at low magnification with direct fluorescent illumination evenly distributed across the face. The fully polarized lighting eliminates all shine allowing for the best assessment of color (spots and redness). All images were taken after the subjects had acclimated their skin in a controlled temperature and humidity room for 30 min. They had their hair and clothing covered with black drapes. The images were taken using the same imaging equipment under the same conditions (lighting, distance, head position, etc.) at all time points.

Test product efficacy was measured by a visual perception study (VPS), wherein expert graders assessed facial image photos for several aging skin attributes. Trained and qualified graders graded the WIS and CIS images. Blind-coded baseline and either 4, 8, or 12 week images were viewed simultaneously on color-calibrated Barco monitors, randomized as to treatment and side of screen. Graders determined which side looked better for a specific skin attribute, then how much better (0–100 scale). Graders had the option of selecting the left-hand image, the right-hand image, or no difference. Three graders independently judged the images. The three grades for each image pair were averaged.

Facial Benefits Study 2

The protocol for this study was as described for Facial Benefits Study 1 with the exceptions as noted in the following description. (1) There were 88 subjects receiving placebo and 5% niacinamide treatments. (2) The study duration was 8 weeks, with skin images captured at 0, 4, and 8 weeks. (3) The only skin measure was texture. (4) The expert grader scoring to determine which image was better for texture was done on a 0–4 grading scale.

During the study, five subjects dropped from the study (6% drop-out rate) for reasons unrelated to test product. The study was conducted from March to May in Cincinnati, OH.

Sebum Excretion Measurement Study

Healthy Caucasian female subjects (age 19–60; $n = 23$ per test formulation) were enrolled in a double-blind, full-face study.

Prior to study start, there was a 2 week wash-out period in which all subjects used the same facial cleanser commercial product and the same facial moisturizer commercial product twice daily. After the 2 week wash-out period, this cleanser product was also used throughout the subsequent 4 week study period, but the moisturizer product was replaced with moisturizer test formulations (2% niacinamide in oil-in-water emulsion or emulsion placebo), which were blind-coded 30 g opaque tubes. To the full face was applied ~ 1.0 g of assigned test formulation, twice daily for 8 weeks, with the evening application occurring at least 1 h before bedtime.

Subjects were instructed to minimize their UV/sun exposure and to avoid activities that would result in a large amount of such exposure. In addition to the products discussed earlier, subjects also received SPF 15 commercial facial moisturizer sunscreen product to use during outside activities. Other than make-up, subjects were instructed not to use any other skin care products on their faces other than those provided. Subjects washed their faces on the morning of each clinical site visit but did not apply test formulations that day until after the site visit. Subject compliance was checked biweekly by questioning the subjects and weighing test formulation containers to determine usage. There were no subject drop-outs in this study. This study was conducted from October to December in Cincinnati, OH.

Sebutape measurements for sebum excretion rates are well documented (9). Briefly, cheek and forehead areas (on both left and right sides of the face) were swabbed with 70% isopropyl alcohol to remove any surface sebum. Sebutapes (CuDerm Corp., Dallas, Texas) were placed on the swabbed areas for 45 min. After removal, the tapes were placed on microscope slides and stored at 5°C until measured by image analysis. The customized image analysis program determined total oil area on the tapes as a measure of sebum content.

Pore Size Measurement Study

Porphyrin fluorescence measurement for pore size determination was done as follows. Healthy Caucasian female subjects (age 19–60; $n = 40$ per test formulation) were enrolled in a double-blind, split-face, left–right randomized study.

Prior to study start, there was a 2 week wash-out period in which all subjects used the same facial cleanser commercial product and the same facial moisturizer commercial product twice daily. After the 2 week wash-out period, this cleanser product was also used throughout the subsequent 4 week study period, but the moisturizer product was replaced with moisturizer test formulations (2% niacinamide in oil-in-water emulsion or emulsion placebo), which were blind-coded 30 g opaque tubes, labeled "left" and "right". To each side of the face was applied a pea-sized amount (~0.4 g) of each assigned test formulation, twice daily for 12 weeks, with the evening application occurring at least 1 h before bedtime.

Subjects were instructed to minimize their UV/sun exposure and to avoid activities that would result in a large amount of such exposure. In addition to the products discussed earlier, subjects also received SPF 15 commercial facial moisturizer sunscreen product to use during outside activities. Other than make-up, subjects were instructed not to use any other skin care products on their faces other than those provided. Subjects washed their faces on the morning of each clinical site visit but did not apply test formulations that day until after the site visit. Subject compliance was checked biweekly by questioning the subjects and weighing test formulation containers to determine usage. There were no subject drop-outs in this study. This study was conducted from April to June in Cincinnati, OH.

For imaging, the face was illuminated with photographic strobes equipped with customized filters that were optimized for the excitation wavelengths (399–407 nm) of the porphyrins in skin pore bacteria. Images under UVA light were then obtained to capture the fluorescence. Pores were evident on the images as fluorescent spots, the diameter of which was determined by a customized image analysis program.

Skin Barrier Evaluation

Healthy Caucasian female subjects (age 30–50; nonpregnant, nonlactating; $n = 41$) were enrolled in a double-blind, dorsal forearm study with left–right randomization. Prior to study start, there was a 1 week wash-out period in which all subjects used the same cleanser commercial product daily. After the 1 week wash-out period, this cleanser product was also used throughout the remainder of the study. One site (5 cm × 13 cm) was marked on each dorsal forearm, and subjects were given treatment formulations (2% niacinamide in oil-in-water emulsion vs. oil-in-water emulsion placebo), which were blind-coded 30 g opaque tubes, labeled "left" and "right". To each forearm site was applied a pea-sized amount (~0.4 g) of each assigned test formulation, twice daily for 24 days, with the evening application occurring at least 1 h before bedtime.

Subjects were instructed to minimize their UV/sun exposure and to avoid activities that would result in a large amount of such exposure. In addition to the products discussed earlier, subjects also received SPF 15 commercial moisturizer sunscreen product to use during outside activities. Subjects were instructed not to use any other skin care products on their arms other than those provided. Subjects washed their arms on the morning of each clinical site visit but did not apply test formulations that day until after the site visit. Subject compliance was checked at a daily compliance visit (5 days per week) by questioning the subjects and weighing test formulation containers to determine usage. The morning application was also done under supervision during those daily visits. There were no subject drop-outs in this study. Redness scoring (0–6 scale) and TEWL measurements (cyberDERM, Dermalab, Media, PA) were taken at baseline and at days 12, 19, and 23.

On day 24, SLS patching and dimethyl sulfoxide (DMSO) chemical probe testing were done to evaluate the resistance of the skin barrier. To an area within the forearm treatment sites, an occlusive 19 mm Hill Top® chamber patch with 150 µL aliquot of a 0.5% aqueous solution of SLS was applied for 24 h. One hour after patch removal, redness scores and TEWL measurements were obtained. These measurements were repeated 24 h later (day 25). Also on day 25, DMSO (at 90%, 95%, and 100%) was applied to the nonpatched area of the treatment sites. Fifteen microliters of each solution was pipetted into 12 mm circles made on the arm with stopcock grease. The amount of time for the whealing response to begin and the amount of erythema produced were scored. Whealing scoring used a 0–4 scale (0 = no response and 4 = elevated tense wheal); erythema used a 0–3 scale (0 = none and 3 = severe confluent redness). Scoring was done on these sites post-DMSO treatment.

No subjects dropped from the study. This study was conducted from September to October in Philadelphia, PA.

RESULTS

NADPH Levels

In cell culture studies, we observed that fibroblasts from old donors had a significantly lower level of NADPH than cells from young donors (Fig. 1). When old

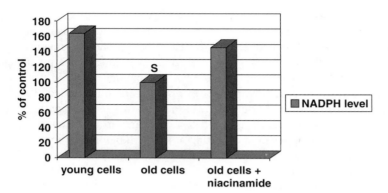

Figure 1 Niacinamide levels in young and old keratinocytes (S indicates significance at $p < 0.05$).

cells were supplemented with niacinamide, the young cell level of NADPH was restored. Thus, old cells have the capacity to synthesize this cofactor if they are provided with sufficiently high levels of the precursor niacinamide, a higher dose than required by young cells. As NADPH is involved in many enzymatic reactions, there is potential for niacinamide to affect many components of skin and thus have multiple effects in improving aging skin.

Collagen Synthesis

Niacinamide was found to increase total protein secreted from quiescent dermal fibroblasts; it also showed selectivity for collagen production over total protein (Table 1). These data suggest that niacinamide will lead to an increase in dermal matrix content via elevated collagen synthesis as well as other secreted proteins. This is above the baseline level attained by low levels of ascorbic acid (25 μg/mL final concentration), an essential component for basal collagen synthesis and that serves as the baseline of collagen synthesis in these experiments.

Table 1 Effect of Niacinamide on Collagen Synthesis from Human Dermal Fibroblasts

	Collagen relative to protein (% of control)	Total collagen (% of control)	Total protein (% of control)	Cell number (% of control)
500 μM Niacinamide	135	154	141	120

Barrier Layer Components

One component that is increased in keratinocyte cultures exposed to niacinamide is skin barrier layer lipids, for example, ceramides (10). In culture studies, we examined the effect of niacinamide on important structural and precursor proteins that are involved in barrier layer development (Fig. 2). There were significant increases in involucrin, filaggrin, and keratin (keratins 13 and 16 which are associated with mature, differentiated corneocytes). Thus, both the intercellular lipids and the protein structural support for those lipids (stratum corneum cell components) are elevated, providing the potential for an enhanced barrier function of niacinamide-treated skin.

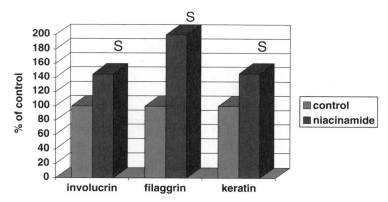

Figure 2 Niacinamide increases barrier layer proteins in keratinocytes (S indicates significance at $p < 0.05$).

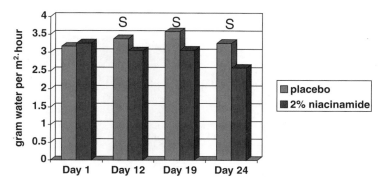

Figure 3 Topical niacinamide treatment reduces forearm TEWL (S indicates significance at $p < 0.002$).

Skin Barrier Function

The dorsal forearms of test subjects were treated topically with placebo vs. 2% niacinamide formulations for 24 days. TEWL was found to decrease significantly in niacinamide-treated skin (Fig. 3) after 12 days, which was the first time point of measurement after initiation of treatment. The TEWL reduction was larger as the study progressed out through the end of the treatment period (day 24). These results indicate barrier enhancement by topical treatment with niacinamide.

After the day 24 TEWL measurements, the treated skin was challenged with either a barrier-damaging level of SLS or a dose of DMSO that will induce a wheal response. SLS treatment dramatically increased TEWL (Fig. 4) and skin redness (Table 2), expected responses of this agent indicative of barrier damage. However, the sites that had been pretreated with niacinamide

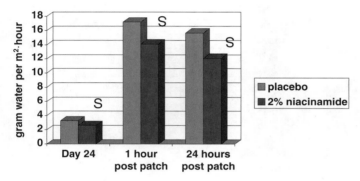

Figure 4 Topical niacinamide treatment reduces the barrier-damaging effect of SLS (S indicates significance at $p < 0.001$).

Table 2 Redness Scores Post-SLS Patching of Placebo or Niacinamide-Treated Forearm Skin

Topical treatment	Redness score (0–6 scale)
Placebo	1.32
2% Niacinamide	0.87 ($p < 0.005$)

Table 3 Whealing Scores Post-100% DMSO Exposure of Placebo or Niacinamide-Treated Forearm Skin

Topical treatment	Whealing score (0–6 scale)
Placebo	3.07
2% Niacinamide	2.61 ($p < 0.05$)

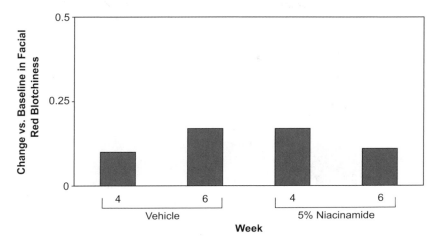

Figure 5 Expert grader assessment of facial skin red blotchiness. The data are presented as change in red blotchiness vs. the baseline (starting) grade.

were significantly more resistant to this barrier destruction both at 1 h and at 24 h post-insult with SLS (Fig. 4). For DMSO-challenged skin, there was significant resistance to DMSO-induced skin whealing in sites pretreated with niacinamide (Table 3). Thus, topical treatment with niacinamide creates a barrier that is more resistant to chemical insults to the skin.

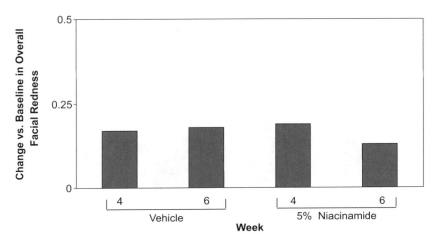

Figure 6 Expert grader assessment of overall facial skin redness. The data are presented as change in redness vs. the baseline (starting) grade.

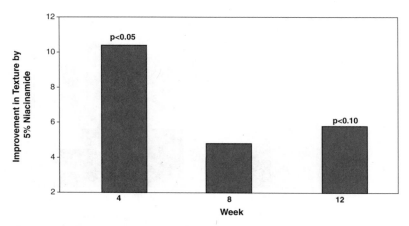

Figure 7 Expert grader assessment of facial skin texture (cheek area). The data are presented as improvement in texture vs. the placebo control.

Facial Skin Tolerance of Niacinamide

To determine how well facial skin can tolerate a moderate dose of niacinamide, test subjects applied placebo and 5% niacinamide formulations twice daily to their faces for 6 weeks (split-face evaluation). The skin was evaluated by expert graders at weeks 4 and 6 for red blotchiness (Fig. 5) and overall facial redness (Fig. 6). There were no significant differences between the two test formulations, indicating lack of significant irritation by 5% niacinamide.

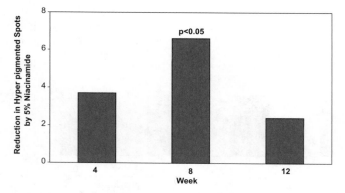

Figure 8 Expert grader assessment of facial skin hyperpigmented spots. The data are presented as reduction in number of spots vs. the placebo control.

Facial Benefits Study 1

The formulations used in the facial tolerance study were evaluated in a 12 week efficacy study for skin benefits (split-face evaluation). One aging skin problem of interest is poor texture, the rippled or pebbly appearance of aged facial skin in the cheek area. Niacinamide improved the appearance of cheek area texture across the study, with significant effects measured at two of the three times points (Fig. 7).

Topical niacinamide also reduced the appearance of hyperpigmented spots in this Caucasian population (Fig. 8). There were improvements across the study, with a statistically significant effect at one of the three time points. This effect is consistent with the spot appearance reduction effect we reported previously for Asian skin in a split-face study using similar clinical methodology (11).

In this study, we also evaluated redness as a measure of irritation. As we saw in the facial tolerance test (Figs. 5 and 6), niacinamide was not irritating to facial skin (Fig. 9). In fact, it reduced the facial skin red blotchiness (e.g., small spider veins or telangiectasia) across the study, with significance at two of the three time points.

Facial Benefits Study 2

A second facial benefit study was conducted to confirm the skin texture benefit of topical niacinamide. In this 8 week study, there was again a significant improvement in skin texture (Fig. 10), confirming the observation from Study 1.

Reduction in Sebum Excretion and Pore Size

A component of poor facial skin texture is enlarged pores. As topical niacinamide improved texture, a possible mechanism could be reduction in sebum excretion,

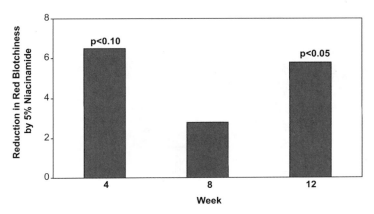

Figure 9 Expert grader assessment of facial skin red blotchiness. The data are presented as reduction in red blotchiness vs. the placebo control.

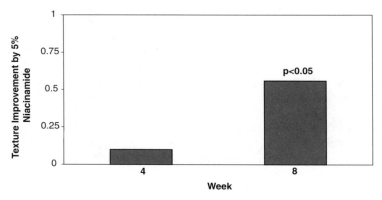

Figure 10 Expert grader assessment of facial skin texture (cheek area). The data are presented as improvement in texture vs. the placebo control.

which may translate into smaller pore size. *In vitro* human skin biopsy samples (1–2 mm) obtained from facelift surgeries can be cultivated in culture media for up to 7 days without significant loss of viability, as measured by both glucose uptake and level of DNA synthesis. Biopsies treated with 25 mM niacinamide for 4 days in the culture media synthesized less total skin lipids, as well as specifically less triglycerides and fatty acids compared with vehicle-treated biopsies (Table 4). In contrast, cholesterol, wax esters, and squalene levels were unaffected by niacinamide treatment.

Clinical testing involving sebutape analysis of treated facial skin was also done. After 4 and 8 weeks of topical treatment, 2% niacinamide reduced the sebum excretion rate, significantly at week 8 (Table 5). In separate testing, after 2 and 4 weeks of treatment, niacinamide was also found to reduce pore diameter, significantly at week 4 (Table 6). Thus, the reduced sebum production appears to lead to a reduced size of the pore.

In a separate human oil control study, sebum compositions were analyzed from the sebutapes of subjects at baseline, and after using the 2% niacinamide or

Table 4 Effect of Niacinamide on Lipid Production in Human Skin Biopsy Samples

Sebum component	% Lipids vs. control[a]
Triglycerides	−60
Fatty acids	−62
Total sebum	−42

[a]After 4 days incubation with 25 mM niacinamide.

Table 5 Sebum Excretion Reduction after Topical Treatment with 2% Niacinamide

Topical treatment	% Change in sebum excretion (8 weeks)
Placebo formulation	−3.5
2% niacinamide formulation	−23.0 ($p < 0.05$)

Table 6 Pore Diameter Reduction after Topical Treatment with 2% Niacinamide

Topical treatment	% Change in pore diameter (4 weeks)
Placebo formulation	−1.3
2% niacinamide formulation	−9.0 ($p < 0.05$)

placebo products for 4 weeks. The average lipid compositions at baseline were as follows: 4.8% diglycerides, 50.7% triglycerides, 16.0% wax esters, 3.3% cholesterol, and 25.2% squalene. At the 4 week time point (Fig. 11), the niacinamide group showed significantly lower total sebum levels, compared with the vehicle group. Specifically di- and triglycerides levels were significantly reduced in the niacinamide group, whereas other lipid fractions were not significantly changed. These clinical results are consistent with the *in vitro* biopsy lipid

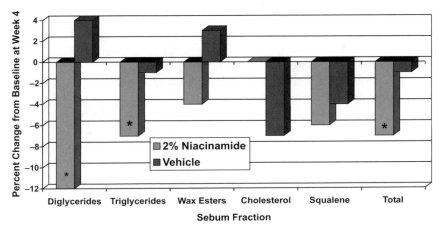

Figure 11 Effect of 4 weeks topical treatment with 2% niacinamide on sebum lipid components. The * indicates significant difference vs. vehicle at $p < 0.05$ (Fisher's *t*-test, 1-tailed analysis).

results and indicate that the oil control activity by niacinamide is due to the specific inhibition of fatty acid or triglyceride synthesis.

DISCUSSION

We have observed a variety of beneficial effects to skin from topical treatment with niacinamide, such as improvement in the appearance of facial skin texture, hyperpigmentation, and red blotchiness. These effects are provided along with enhancement of skin barrier function. This is in contrast to other topical technology such as retinoic acid, which provides appearance improvements but at the expense of barrier, leading to skin sensitivity and redness (12). As niacinamide is nonirritating to facial skin, easily formulated, chemically stable, and compatible with other formulation components, it is an ideal agent for use in cosmetic products.

During the course of the 2–3 month clinical studies reported here, there is variation in the magnitude and level of significance of the observed benefits among time points (4 week intervals). One factor that may contribute to this is the effect of seasonal variations on the skin [e.g., differences in sunlight (UV) levels, differences in humidity and temperature]. Certainly the seasonal change in UV exposure over the course of a 3 month study could impact skin color. Because the underyling cause of facial texture, particularly the rippled appearance aspect of this aging skin problem, is not known with certainty, environmental changes such as humidity and temperature could well contribute to the appearance fluctuations across seasons. Also, the relatively small number of test subjects used in the testing may influence the variability over time.

Though the mechanisms involved in these benefit effects are not specifically defined, there is some information available to suggest associated in-skin effects. On the basis of *in vitro* studies (11), niacinamide has been shown to inhibit melanosome transfer from melanocytes to keratinocytes. This would reduce the total amount of melanin dispersed throughout the epidermis and thus potentially reduce observed skin hyperpigmentation.

Reduction in red blotchiness may be an effect of skin barrier enhancement. Niacinamide increases the stratum corneum barrier layer components, specifically key proteins as we report here and lipids such as ceramides (10). The resulting enhanced barrier is more resistant to damage (e.g., from SLS), which should translate into less irritation and redness when the skin encounters environmental insults, such as surfactants.

For skin texture, a component of this problem is enlarged pore size. Topical niacinamide reduces sebum production and thus reduces pore size. The specific sebum component that is most affected by niacinamide treatment is the fatty acid and triglyceride fraction. Work done with a structurally similar material, the nicotinic acid analog acipimox (13), also indicated inhibition of production of fatty acids and triglycerides. There are likely also other factors involved in skin texture effects because texture as described earlier is more than just a problem of pore size, that is, there is also the rippled appearance component. The underlying problem of this component has yet to be defined.

There is certainly room to explore the specifics of these proffered mechanisms. It is intriguing to speculate that there may be a common underlying mechanism involving the conversion of niacinamide to nicotinamide adenine dinucleotides [e.g., NAD(H) and NADP(H)] (6). As these coenzymes are involved in many cellular processes, there is potential for broad effects as a result. Defining specifically how these dinucleotides fit mechanistically into all the observed skin effects is an opportunity for future studies.

ACKNOWLEDGMENTS

We gratefully acknowledge the technical and administrative assistance of Janet Lynch, Marcia Schnicker, Deanne Lind, Frank Joa, Dan Schaiper, and Cheryl Lepp.

REFERENCES

1. Gensler HL. Prevention of photoimmunesuppression and photocarcinogenesis by topical niacinamide. Nutr Cancer 1997; 29:157-162.
2. Yu J-M, Liu Y, Xie N, Sun W, Wang J-J, Li H-Q. Effects of nicotinamide on levels of dermis hydroxyproline in photoaging skin. Huanjing Yu Jiankang Zazhi 2002; 19:102-104.
3. Shalita AR, Smith JG, Parish LC, Sofman MS, Chalker DK. Topical nicotinamide compared with clindamycin gel in the treatment of inflammatory acne vulgaris. Int J Dermatol 1995; 34:434-437.
4. Girffiths CEM. Nicotinamide 4% gel for the treatment of inflammatory acne vulgaris. J Dermatol Treat 1995; 6:S8–S10.
5. Berk MA, Lorincz AL. The treatment of bullous pemphigoid with tetracycline and niacinamide: a preliminary report. Arch Dermatol 1986; 122:670–674.
6. Matts PJ, Oblong JE, Bissett DL. A review of the range of effects of niacinamide in human skin. Int Fed Soc Cosmet Chem Magazine 2002; 5:285-289.
7. Hall DWR, Van der Hoven WE, Noordzij-Kamermans NJ, Jaitly KD. Hormonal control of hamster ear sebaceous gland lipogenesis. Arch Dermatol Res 1983; 275:1–7.
8. Wheatley VR, Hodgins LT, Coon WM. Cutaneous lipogenesis. I. Evaluation of model systems and the utilization of acetate, citrate, and glucose as compared with other tissues. J Invest Dermatol 1970; 54:288–297.
9. Clarys P, Barel A. Quantitative evaluation of skin surface lipids. Clin Dermatol 1995; 13:307–321.
10. Tanno O, Ota Y, Kitamura N, Katsube T, Inoue S. Nicotinamide increases biosynthesis of ceramides as well as other stratum corneum lipids to improve the epidermal permeability barrier. B J Dermatol 2000; 143:525–531.
11. Hakozaki T, Minwealla L, Zhuang J, Chhoa M, Matsubara A, Miyamoto K, Greatens A, Hillebrand GG, Bissett DL, Boissy RE. The effect of niacinamide on

reducing cutaneous pigmentation and suppression of melanosome transfer. B J Dermatol 2002; 147:22–33.
12. Kang S, Duell EA, Fisher GJ, Datta SC, Wang ZQ, Reddy AP, Tavakkol A, Yi JY, Griffiths CE, Elder JT, Voorhees JJ. Application of retinol to human skin *in vivo* induces epidermal hyperplasia and cellular retinoid binding proteins characteristic of retinoic acid but without measurable retinoic acid levels of irritation. J Invest Dermatol 1995; 105:549–556.
13. Worm D, Vinten J, Vaag A, Henriksen JE, Beck-Nielsen H. The nicotinic acid analogue acipimox increases plasma leptin and decreases free fatty acids in type 2 diabetic patients. Eur J Endocrinol 2000; 143:389–395.

25

Topical Retinyl Propionate Achieves Skin Benefits with Favorable Irritation Profile*

John E. Oblong, Abel Saud, Donald L. Bissett, and Chu Zhu
The Procter & Gamble Company, Miami Valley Laboratories, Cincinnati, Ohio, USA

Introduction	442
Materials and Methods	443
Sources of Materials	443
Stability of Test Materials in Products	443
Human Studies	443
Back Cumulative Irritation Test	443
Facial Irritation Test 1	444
Facial Irritation Test 2	444
Facial Benefits Study 1	445
Facial Benefits Study 2	447
Retinoid Photostability	447
Cell Culture	447
Results	447
Back Cumulative Irritation Test	447
Facial Irritation Test 1	448

*This chapter has been presented in part as posters at the American Academy of Dermatology annual meeting (2002).

Facial Benefits Study 1   450
Retinoid Photostability   455
Facial Irritation Test 2   456
Facial Benefits Study 2   456
Inhibition of Dermal GAG Production   458
Discussion   459
Acknowledgments   461
References   461

INTRODUCTION

Topical *trans*-retinoic acid (*t*-RA) is well known for its activity in improving the appearance of the signs of skin photodamage such as fine lines, wrinkles, and pigmentation problems (1,2). Although *t*-RA provides skin benefits, it can also produce aesthetic negatives such as irritation and dryness (3). To minimize these unwanted side effects and yet still deliver benefits, *t*-RA precursors such as retinol (3) and retinaldehyde (4) and retinyl esters such as retinyl acetate (5) and retinyl palmitate (6) have been used widely in the skin care industry. Although these agents may improve the activity-to-irritation ratio, at least the former three can still have substantial aesthetic issues. The fourth, retinyl palmitate, has an overall weak activity profile (7).

    An additional potential option is retinyl propionate. As with the acetate and palmitate esters of retinol, retinyl propionate must be hydrolyzed to free retinol, a process occurring via a skin esterase (6). Although much of the retinol is then re-esterified via lecithin:retinol acyltransferase (LRAT) to retinyl palmitate for storage, a small percentage is further oxidized to the active acid form (8). The oxidation of free retinol to *t*-RA is the limiting step in the generation of active retinoid metabolites within cells. This process begins when free retinol associates with a specific cytoplasmic retinol-binding protein (cRBP). The retinol–cRBP complex is a substrate for retinol dehydrogenase, a microsomal enzyme uniquely capable of catalyzing the conversion of retinol to retinaldehyde. Retinaldehyde is then rapidly and quantitatively oxidized to *t*-RA by retinaldehyde oxidase (9,10). Once converted, *t*-RA binds to nuclear retinoic acid receptors (RARα, -β and -γ) and regulates gene transcription necessary for skin keratinocyte growth and differentiation (11). This multi-step processing of retinyl esters can serve as a point of regulation to control the level of active retinoid in the skin and may thus contribute to the lower irritation potential of these derivatives.

    Retinyl propionate has been reported to be active in human skin (12) and to have less irritation than other active retinoid options (13). We report here our clinical observations on the reduced irritation of retinyl propionate in comparison with retinol and significant improvements in the appearance of photoaged human skin. We also present clinical data on the efficacy advantage of combining retinyl propionate with niacinamide, an agent that also provides aging skin benefits (14; Chapter 24).

MATERIALS AND METHODS
Sources of Materials

Retinol, retinyl propionate, and retinyl acetate were obtained from BASF (Mount Olive, NJ, USA). All other materials were from standard laboratory suppliers.

Stability of Test Materials in Products

For all studies, retinol and the retinyl esters were prepared in the same oil-in-water emulsion and packaged under nitrogen in aluminum (Glaminate) tubes. Test products were assayed by HPLC to verify retinoid content and stability for the time that products were in the subjects' possession (maximum of 1 month). For studies of greater than 1 month duration, fresh product was supplied to the subjects at monthly intervals.

Human Studies

All studies were conducted double-blind and placebo-controlled. Exclusion criteria included: pregnant or lactating, any chronic disease with skin involvement, history of reactivity to skin care products, and oral Vitamin A $>50,000$ IU/day. The studies were monitored for compliance with the protocol, and test subjects signed a written Informed Consent Statement prior to participation.

For the facial clinical studies, subjects agreed to refrain from the use of oil-based make-up and all skin care products other than that supplied for use during the study. Subjects also agreed to refrain from sun/wind exposure that would result in burning/tanning, and from use of facial scrubbing products and implements, both during the study and for 2 weeks prior to start of the study. In addition, during the conduct of the study and for 4 weeks prior to start of the study, test subjects agreed to refrain from the use of any anti-aging skin care product, anti-acne medication, skin/facial hair lightening or removal products, and topical hormone therapy.

Back Cumulative Irritation Test (15,16)

This study evaluated the irritation potential of test materials, all in the same oil-in-water emulsion base, on the skin of the back. Materials tested were: retinol [0.05% (1.75 mM) and 0.075% (2.62 mM)], retinyl acetate [0.086% (2.62 mM), 0.172% (5.24 mM), and 0.30% (9.15 mM)], retinyl propionate [0.09% (2.63 mM), 0.18% (5.26 mM), 0.30% (8.77 mM)], and emulsion control (in addition to other products which are not relevant to the subject of this report). The study was conducted in December in Scottsdale, Arizona.

An incomplete Latin square design was used for the study in which 16 test materials were evaluated on 10 skin sites per subject located on the back in vertical rows on either side of the spinal area between the scapula and the waistline of 45 healthy subjects (ages 18–65). Treatment assignments were randomized and balanced so that each test material appeared on each skin site an equal number of times.

Blind coded test materials (0.2 mL) were applied to each skin site on a semi-occluded patch (circular non-woven Webril® cotton pad, 2 cm^2) that was covered and held securely to the skin on all sides with a 4.4 × 4.4 cm^2 of porous hypoallergenic Micropore® tape. Adjacent patches were 1 in. apart. Patches remained on the skin for 23 h after which they were removed and after an hour wait, scored for irritation (0–3 scale: 0, no irritation; 3, severe irritation) by a trained and qualified expert grader. Following this daily assessment, patches were re-applied to the same skin sites. This process was repeated on each of 20 consecutive days. In addition to the daily grading, irritation was also assessed with Minolta® Chromameter "a" skin color (red) measurements at baseline and 7, 14, and 21 days. At the conclusion of the study, irritation grades and (separately) chromameter measurements were summed to arrive at cumulative irritation scores for each test material. The use of cumulative irritation scores exaggerates the differences among treatments, and this has been found to be more predictive of subject assessment of relative product irritation on the face than an irritation score from a single time point. Treatment differences were compared using t-tests and were considered statistically significant if $P \leq 0.05$.

Facial Irritation Test 1

Forty healthy female Caucasian subjects (ages 18–65) were recruited to participate in a double-blind, split-face study with left–right randomization. The study was conducted in February–March in Cincinnati, Ohio. Each subject received two topical test products in 30 g opaque Glaminate tubes, labeled "left" and "right", one for each side of the face. The pairs of test products (in identical oil-in-water emulsions) were 0.075% (2.62 mM) retinol vs. vehicle and 0.15% (4.38 mM) retinyl propionate vs. vehicle. Subjects were instructed to apply a pea-size amount of product (∼0.4 g) to each side of the face, twice daily for 3 weeks. An expert skin grader, trained and qualified in the evaluation of skin attributes, assessed redness and dryness (0–6 scales: 0, normal skin) at baseline and at the end of 1, 2, and 3 weeks of treatment. Treatment differences were compared using t-tests and were considered statistically significant if $P \leq 0.05$.

Facial Irritation Test 2

Ninety healthy female Caucasian subjects (ages 18–65) were recruited to participate in a double-blind, split-face study with left–right randomization. The study was conducted in February–March in Cincinnati, Ohio. Each subject received two topical test products in 30 g opaque Glaminate tubes, labeled "left" and "right", one for each side of the face. The pairs of test products (in identical oil-in-water emulsions) were 0.15% (5.24 mM) retinol vs. vehicle and 0.2%

(5.84 mM) retinyl propionate + 3.5% niacinamide vs. 3.5% niacinamide. Subjects were instructed to apply a pea-size amount of product (~0.4 g) to each side of the face, twice daily for 2 weeks. An expert skin grader, trained and qualified in the evaluation of skin attributes, assessed redness and dryness (0–6 scales: 0, normal skin) at baseline and at the end of 1 and 2 weeks of treatment. All other aspects of the study were as described earlier for Facial Irritation Test 1.

Facial Benefits Study 1

Healthy Caucasian female subjects (ages 35–60; non-pregnant, non-lactating; $n = 168$) were enrolled in a double-blind, split-face study with left–right randomization. The study was conducted in June–October in Cincinnati, Ohio. All subjects were graded at baseline (0–5 grading scales: 0, normal skin), and were eligible for study participation with grades of 2.0 or greater in both facial fine lines/wrinkles and facial hyperpigmented spots. Prior to start of the study, there was a 2-week wash-out period in which subjects all used the same cleanser product (Olay Sensitive Skin Foaming Face Wash commercial product) twice daily. This cleanser routine was also used throughout the subsequent 12-week study period. After the 2-week wash-out period, each subject was randomly assigned to one of the three treatment groups, then received topical test products (separate morning and evening products) in 30 g opaque tubes, labeled "left" and "right" (Table 1). A pea-sized amount (~0.4 g) of each assigned test product was applied to each side of the face, once daily for 12 weeks, with the evening application occurring at least 1 h before bedtime.

In addition to the products listed in Table 1, subjects also received Bain de Soleil Extended Protection SPF-30 commercial product and wide-brimmed straw hats to use during outside activities. Subjects kept a daily diary of their product usage and sun exposure during the entire study. Subjects' upper inner arm and facial cheek skin colors were monitored from the skin color images (see later) at weeks 0, 4, 8, and 12 to monitor compliance with minimization of UV/sun exposure. At the same intervals, subjects returned their separate tubes of product (for determination of product usage) and received new tubes of product. Subjects also returned to the clinical site at week 1 for a compliance check (redness scoring, diary review, and product application procedure review).

The degree of irritation was assessed using dermatologist grading at week 1, expert grading (baseline and weeks 4, 8, and 12), and subject self-assessment (weeks 4, 8, and 12). Subject self-assessment was carried out via a questionnaire with a 9-point grading scale. Expert grading (0–6 scale) was carried out using graders trained and qualified in the evaluation of skin attributes.

Product efficacy was determined using a visual perception study (VPS), wherein expert graders assessed facial image photographs for several aging skin attributes. The facial images were recorded using a wrinkle imaging system (WIS) and color imaging system (CIS). WIS images are captured at high magnification with non-polarized lighting (incandescent tungsten) that causes a shine that enhances topographical features (fine lines and wrinkles).

Table 1 Test Materials and Subjects for Facial Benefits Study

Group no.	Treatment	Control	No. of subjects
1	Day-time treatment: oil-in-water emulsion facial moisturizer Night-time treatment: 0.15% all-*trans*-retinol in oil-in-water emulsion	Day-time treatment: oil-in-water emulsion facial moisturizer Night-time treatment: oil-in-water emulsion control	54
2	Day-time treatment: oil-in-water emulsion facial moisturizer with SPF-15 sunscreen[a] Night-time treatment: 0.15% all-*trans*-retinol in oil-in-water emulsion	Day-time treatment: oil-in-water emulsion facial moisturizer with SPF-15 sunscreen Night-time treatment: oil-in-water emulsion control	56
3	Day-time treatment: oil-in-water emulsion facial moisturizer with SPF-15 sunscreen Night-time treatment: 0.30% all-*trans*-retinyl propionate in oil-in-water emulsion	Day-time treatment: oil-in-water emulsion facial moisturizer with SPF-15 sunscreen Night-time treatment: oil-in-water emulsion control	52

[a]SPF-15 sunscreen product contained as actives 7.5% octyl methoxycinnamate and 1% phenylbenzimidazole sulfonic acid.

CIS images are captured at low magnification with direct fluorescent illumination evenly distributed across the face. The fully polarized lighting eliminates all shine allowing for the best assessment of color (spots and redness). Trained and qualified graders graded the WIS and CIS images. Baseline and either 4, 8, or 12 week images were viewed simultaneously on color-calibrated Barco monitors, randomized as to treatment and side of screen. Graders determined which side looked better for a specific skin attribute, then how much better (0–4 scale). Graders had the option of selecting the left-hand image, the right-hand image, or no difference. Three graders judged the 4- and 8-week images, and two graders the 12-week images. The end points evaluated were fine lines/wrinkles, hyperpigmented spots, redness (red blotchiness), and texture. Our definition of poor texture encompasses two factors: enlarged pore size and "pebbly, rippled" appearance of older skin in the cheek area. In addition to VPS grading, efficacy was also assessed by computer image analysis of the captured facial images and by expert grading of the subjects themselves at each time point.

All treatment comparisons were done with t-tests. Levels of significance ($P \leq 0.05, 0.10$) are shown in the figures/tables for comparison.

Facial Benefits Study 2

Healthy Caucasian female subjects (ages 35–60; non-pregnant, non-lactating; $n = 90$) were enrolled in a double-blind, split-face study with left–right randomization. The study was conducted in July–October in Cincinnati, Ohio. All subjects were graded at baseline (0–5 grading scales: 0, normal skin), and were eligible for study participation with grades of 2.0 or greater in both facial fine lines/wrinkles and facial hyperpigmented spots. Prior to start of the study, there was a 2-week wash-out period in which subjects all used the same cleanser product (Olay Sensitive Skin Foaming Face Wash commercial product) twice daily. This cleanser routine was also used throughout the subsequent 12-week study period. After the 2-week wash-out period, each subject was randomly assigned to one of the two treatment groups, then received topical test products in 30 g opaque tubes, labeled "left" and "right". The test products were all prepared in the same oil-in-water formulation base, 45 subjects receiving 0.15% retinol vs. placebo products and 45 subjects receiving 0.2% retinyl propionate and 3.5% niacinamide vs. 3.5% niacinamide products. A pea-sized amount ($\sim$0.4 g) of each assigned test product was applied to each side of the face, twice daily for 12 weeks, with the evening application occurring at least 1 h before bedtime. All other aspects of this study were as described above for Facial Benefits Study 1 earlier.

Retinoid Photostability

Oil-in-water emulsion formulations of 0.26% retinyl propionate and 0.26% retinol were applied (2 mg/cm^2) to triplicate 6 × 6 cm^2 of collagen film (Vitro Skin, IMS Testing, Milford, CT, USA) and exposed to normal room fluorescent light for 4 h. Retinoids were extracted from the films and analyzed by reverse phase HPLC with UV detection at 325 nm. The percentage of the remaining of actives on the film is calculated from the active mass before and after light exposure.

Cell Culture

Normal human fibroblasts (ATCC, Manassa, VA, USA) were neonatal or from a 57-year-old donor (ATCC, Manassas, VA, USA). They were grown in minimal essential medium to near confluency. The supernatant media from duplicate cultures was assayed for hyaluronic acid (HA) as a measure of glycosaminoglycan (GAG) using a commercial HA antibody kit (Corgenic Ltd., Peterborough, UK).

RESULTS

Back Cumulative Irritation Test

To assess the irritation potential of the retinyl esters (acetate and propionate) vs. retinol control, the materials were patched on the backs of subjects for 21 days.

Irritation was measured daily by expert grader scoring (0–3 scale) and is expressed as a cumulative score (Fig. 1). Irritation was also assessed by weekly chromameter a measurements to evaluate skin redness. Cumulative chromameter a scores are shown in Fig. 2. In general, the retinyl esters showed the expected dose–response relationship for both irritation measures. Table 2 shows those dose comparisons that are significantly different from one another. As various groupings of treatments are compared, retinyl propionate was found to cause significantly less irritation than retinyl acetate for both irritation measures. Both esters yielded lower irritation scores than did a comparable amount (mass/volume) of retinol. As the retinyl esters approached 6× the concentration of retinol (0.30% retinyl ester vs. 0.05% retinol) the irritation scores equalized.

Facial Irritation Test 1

Following the back irritation testing, retinyl propionate and retinol were advanced to a split-face irritation test. All 40 subjects completed the study. Both products were well tolerated as assessed by expert graders. No adverse

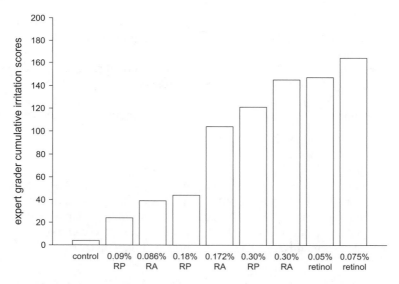

Figure 1 Expert grader scoring of cumulative back irritation following retinoid treatment. Various concentrations of retinyl propionate (RP), retinyl acetate (RA), and retinol, along with vehicle control, were applied to back skin sites via semi-occluded patches. Expert graders assessed irritation daily (0–3 scale); 3-week cumulative irritation scores are shown.

Topical Retinyl Propionate

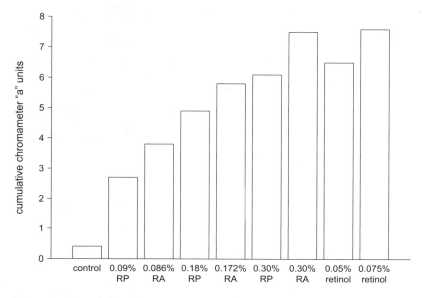

Figure 2 Cumulative chromameter *a* scores following 3 weeks of retinoid treatment. As in Fig. 1, retinoid-induced irritation was assessed each day for 3 weeks by measuring skin redness with a chromameter *a* reading. Cumulative redness scores are shown.

Table 2 Significance of Back Irritation Measures for Retinol and Its Esters

Topical treatment (oil-in-water emulsions)	Expert grader cumulative irritation scores	Significance of expert grader cum scores*	Chromameter *a* measure (day 21)	Significance of chromameter *a* measure*
Emulsion control	3.9	a	0.4	a
0.09% Retinyl propionate	24	b	2.7	b
0.086% Retinyl acetate	39	b	3.8	bc
0.18% Retinyl propionate	44	b	4.9	cd
0.172% Retinyl acetate	104	c	5.8	de
0.30% Retinyl propionate	121	cd	6.1	def
0.30% Retinyl acetate	145	cd	7.5	def
0.05% Retinol	147	d	6.5	def
0.075% Retinol	164	d	7.6	f

*Treatments with the same letter codes are not significantly different from each other ($P < 0.05$).

events were reported. Test product consumption measurements indicated similar usage across the three groups (mean consumption ± SD: retinol = 9.65 ± 3.66 g; retinyl propionate = 11.13 ± 3.00 g; vehicle = 11.51 ± 4.24 g); however, there was a slightly but significantly lower ($P < 0.10$, two-sided test) amount of retinol used as compared with vehicle.

As shown in Figures 3 and 4, the mean scores of expert grading showed that 0.075% retinol led to a pronounced increase in dryness and redness from baseline. The difference from baseline was significantly greater than vehicle control ($P \leq 0.05$) at all time points, except the redness measure at day 7 (data not shown). In contrast, retinyl propionate treated skin was only significantly increased over baseline for day 21 as compared with vehicle control. Comparison between treatments revealed that retinol caused significantly more redness than retinyl propionate at day 14 ($P \leq 0.05$) and day 21 ($P \leq 0.10$). In addition, retinol caused more dryness at day 14 ($P < 0.10$).

Facial Benefits Study 1

After determining that both the retinol and retinyl propionate products had acceptable facial tolerance profiles, the two test products were advanced to a larger study to examine possible facial benefits. Although the percent doses in this study were twice those in the facial irritation study, products in the latter were used twice per day vs. once per day in this study, thus the total daily dosage was the same. Of the 172 subjects recruited for the study, 10 (6%) discontinued

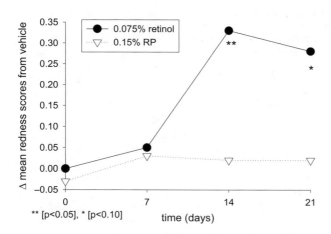

Figure 3 Expert grader scoring of facial redness following retinoid treatment. An expert grader scored facial redness (0–6 scale) at baseline and weekly intervals during 3 weeks of retinoid treatment. Mean redness scores differences from vehicle are shown along with P-values for treatment comparison.

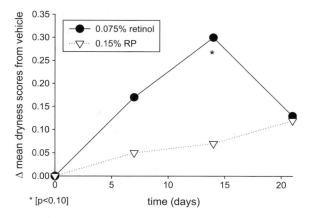

Figure 4 Expert grader scoring of facial dryness following retinoid treatment. As in Fig. 3, an expert grader scored facial dryness at the intervals shown during 3 weeks of retinoid application. Mean dryness differences from vehicle are shown along with P-values for treatment comparison.

prior to completion of the study. All 10 cited various reasons not related to test product effects. Test product usage during the 12-week study was consistent within treatment pairs and across treatment groups (Table 3), except that subjects on retinol treatment and sunscreen tended to use larger amounts of sunscreen moisturizer. The average range of sun exposure per week as recorded in

Table 3 Treatment Product Usage in Facial Benefits Study

Treatment group	Product	Product usage (g)			Average/ 4 weeks
		Week 4	Week 8	Week 12	
1	0.15% Retinol	8.8	9.2	9.6	9.2
1	Vehicle	9.1	9.1	9.9	9.4
1	Moisturizer	24.9	28.0	37.9	30.4
2	0.15% Retinol	10.1	9.6	10.9	10.2
2	Vehicle	9.4	9.2	10.5	9.7
2	Moisturizer + Sunscreen product	38.4	36.5	48.6	41.1
3	0.30% Retinyl propionate	8.6	9.7	10.3	9.5
3	Vehicle	8.8	9.5	10.4	9.5
3	Moisturizer + Sunscreen product	25.5	32.7	38.7	32.2

subject diaries was 1–4 h. Although there were some changes in the CIS readings for overall skin color (darkness, redness) over the course of the study, those changes were all small, indicating good compliance with the instruction to minimize UV/sun exposure.

The relative irritation potential of the test products was assessed by expert grading for dryness and redness (Table 4), subject questionnaire (Table 5), and dermatologist grading at week 1 (Table 6). In general, retinol with and without sunscreen was found to be more irritating than vehicle under these test conditions for all three irritation measures. By expert grader evaluation, the retinol with sunscreen product was more irritating (greater redness, dryness) than vehicle control at all three time points (Table 4). The retinol without sunscreen product was more irritating at week 4. By subject self-assessment, both retinol-containing products were more irritating than vehicle at all time points (Table 5). When subjects were queried about positive attributes indirectly related to irritation (skin looks less dry, skin feels moisturized), the retinol test products were judged more negatively than their vehicles. Similarly, dermatologist assessment (by observation or questioning subjects) deemed both retinol-containing products more irritating (causing erythema, dryness, and burn/itch/tingle) than vehicle controls (Table 6). In contrast, the retinyl propionate product with sunscreen showed parity with its vehicle for irritation. There were no significant differences between retinyl propionate with sunscreen and its vehicle in any of the irritation measures. Finally, the retinyl propionate product showed a significantly lower overall redness attribute as captured by

Table 4 Expert Grader Assessment of Test Product Irritation vs. Vehicle Controls in 12-week Facial Benefits Study

Attribute scored by expert grader	0.30% Retinyl propionate/ sunscreen vs. vehicle/sunscreen control	0.15% Retinol/ moisturizer vs. vehicle/moisturizer control	0.15% Retinol/ sunscreen vs. vehicle/ sunscreen control
Dryness (larger difference = product is more drying)			
4 weeks–baseline	0.13	0.23**	0.32**
8 weeks–baseline	0.09	0.13	0.25**
12 weeks–baseline	0.15	0.08	0.37**
Redness (larger difference = product causes more redness)			
4 weeks–baseline	0.03	0.09*	0.09**
8 weeks–baseline	0.02	0.03	0.08**
12 weeks–baseline	−0.01	0.05	0.19**

*Directionally different ($P < 0.10$) from control.
**Significantly different ($P < 0.05$) from control.

Table 5 Self-Assessment of Test Product Irritation and Related Attributes vs. Vehicle Controls in 12-week Facial Benefits Study

Attribute scored in self-assessment	0.30% Retinyl propionate/ sunscreen vs. vehicle/sunscreen control	0.15% Retinol/ moisturizer vs. vehicle/moisturizer control	0.15% Retinol/ sunscreen vs. vehicle/sunscreen control
Not irritating to skin (larger difference = product is more irritating)			
4 weeks	0.26	0.6**	0.7**
8 weeks	0.14	0.4**	0.7**
12 weeks	0.18	0.4**	0.7**
Skin looks less dry (larger difference = product is more drying)			
4 weeks	0.08	0.31*	0.38**
8 weeks	0.04	0.42**	0.17
12 weeks	0.08	0.41**	0.29
Skin feels moisturized (larger difference = product is less moisturizing)			
4 weeks	0.17	0.50**	0.32*
8 weeks	0.14	0.34**	0.16
12 weeks	0.14	0.30	0.55**

*Directionally different ($P < 0.10$) from control.
**Significantly different ($P < 0.05$) from control.

the CIS system and judged by the expert graders' VPS scores (Fig. 8). This difference was noted by the expert judges at all three timepoints.

When the treatment groups were compared, retinyl propionate with sunscreen was found to be significantly less irritating ($P \leq 0.05$) than retinol with

Table 6 Dermatologist Grading of Reactions to Test Products and Their Vehicles at Week 1

	Dermatologist grading (number of subjects experiencing problem)		
	Erythema	Dryness/peeling	Burn/itch/tingle
0.30% Retinyl propionate/sunscreen	3	5	2
Vehicle/sunscreen control	0	1	1
0.15% Retinol/moisturizer	11**	11**	10**
Vehicle/moisturizer control	2	1	2
0.15% Retinol/sunscreen	13**	19**	11**
Vehicle/sunscreen control	2	1	6

*Directionally different ($P < 0.10$) from control.
**Significantly different ($P < 0.05$) from control.

or without sunscreen as measured by self-assessed irritation at 4 and 8 weeks, and by the dermatologist evaluation of erythema and burn/itch/tingle (data not shown). At 12 weeks, retinyl propionate was also significantly less irritating than retinol with sunscreen as measured by self-assessed irritation and expert grading of dryness and redness. Finally, retinol with sunscreen was significantly more irritating than retinol without sunscreen as measured by self-assessment and expert grading at 12 weeks.

When facial images of the subjects were graded using the VPS system, each of the three treatments delivered an improvement in the appearance of hyperpigmented spots at 4 weeks (Fig. 5). However, retinol with sunscreen no longer delivered a measurable benefit by 8 weeks, whereas retinyl propionate and retinol without sunscreen both yielded measurable benefits at 12 weeks. This result was confirmed by image analysis (data not shown).

VPS analysis of wrinkles yielded a similar result (Fig. 6). Retinyl propionate in sunscreen was significantly better than vehicle control at 4 and 12 weeks, but retinol in sunscreen was not significantly different from it vehicle control at any time point. When the sunscreen was removed from the formulation, retinol was effective at all three time points. This result was confirmed by image analysis (data not shown). Similarly, VPS analysis of texture benefits showed that retinyl propionate delivered a benefit at 4 weeks, retinol without sunscreen did at 12 weeks, but retinol in sunscreen was not significantly improved over its vehicle control at any time point (Fig. 7). This result was confirmed by expert grading (data not shown).

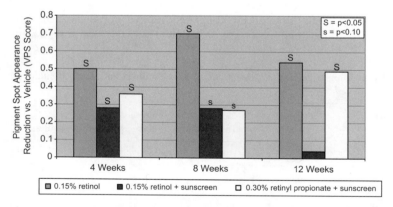

Figure 5 VPS scores of hyperpigmented spots following 12 weeks of retinoid application. Subjects applied retinoid-containing products with and without sunscreen for 12 weeks. Using the CIS images, expert graders completed a visual perception study analysis, comparing facial images at baseline and either 4, 8, or 12 weeks for changes in hyperpigmented spots. The difference in mean score VPS, retinoid vs. vehicle, is shown. Scores significantly different from vehicle are indicated.

Topical Retinyl Propionate

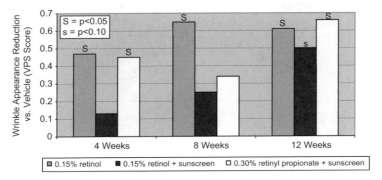

Figure 6 VPS scores of wrinkles following 12 weeks of retinoid application. Subjects applied retinoid-containing products with and without sunscreen for 12 weeks. Using the Wrinkle Imaging System (WIS) images, a visual perception study analysis study was completed, wherein expert graders compared facial images at baseline and either 4, 8, or 12 weeks for changes in wrinkles. As in Fig. 5, these VPS scores are expressed as differences in mean score, retinoid vs. vehicle, with scores significantly different from vehicle indicated.

Retinoid Photostability

In addition to irritation and efficacy evaluations, we also examined photostability of retinyl propionate vs. retinol. On collagen film under fluorescent lighting (4 h), retinyl propionate was found to be substantially more resistant to loss than retinol (Table 7).

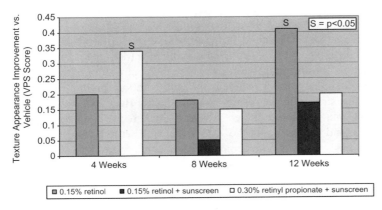

Figure 7 VPS scores of texture following 12 weeks of retinoid application. As in Fig. 6, a VPS analysis was completed using the WIS images. Expert graders compared facial images at baseline and either 4, 8, or 12 weeks for changes in texture. The VPS scores are expressed as differences in mean score, retinoid vs. vehicle, with scores significantly different from vehicle indicated.

Table 7 Photostability of Retinol and Retinyl Propionate After 4 h of Fluorescent Light Exposure

Retinoid	% Remaining after light exposure
Retinol	29.9 ± 1.8
Retinyl propionate	65.7 ± 4.1

Facial Irritation Test 2

In other testing (14; Chapter 24), we have observed good facial tolerance to niacinamide formulations and significant activity of this compound in improving aging facial skin. Therefore, we evaluated the combination of 0.2% retinyl propionate and 3.5% niacinamide to determine if greater benefits could be achieved. In split-face irritation testing of this combination in a test product vs. placebo product control, there was no significant facial redness induced by this combination (data not shown).

Facial Benefits Study 2

Having determined that the test product containing retinyl propionate and niacinamide had acceptable facial tolerance, it and a 0.15% retinol product were advanced to a larger study to examine possible facial benefits. Eight (9%) of the 90 subjects recruited for the study discontinued prior to completion of the study. Six of the eight cited various reasons not related to test product effects. Two subjects (one using the retinol product and one using the retinyl propionate and niacinamide product) withdrew owing to minor irritation that may have been related to test product (specific follow-up not done).

The relative irritation potential of the test products was assessed by VPS analysis of the CIS images for redness (red blotchiness) (data not shown). That analysis revealed no significant differences vs. vehicle control for the retinyl propionate and niacinamide product, whereas the 0.15% retinol product increased facial redness consistent with the results found in Facial Benefits Study 1.

The facial images of the subjects were evaluated for wrinkles, hyperpigmented spots, and texture using the VPS system. In wrinkle assessment, as expected on the basis of the results from Facial Benefits Study 1, both retinoid products provided significant reduction in appearance of wrinkles (data not shown).

In evaluation of hyperpigmented spots, all three products provided significant improvements vs. vehicle control, as shown in Fig. 9. Across all time points, the rank order of effectiveness was 0.2% retinyl propionate and 3.5% niacinamide > 3.5% niacinamide > 0.15% retinol. The magnitude of the spot reduction effect by the combination product was greater than that seen for retinyl propionate alone in Facial Benefits Study 1. This suggests that addition

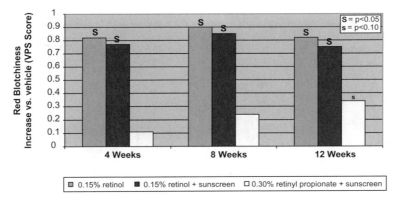

Figure 8 VPS scores of blotchiness following 12 weeks of retinoid application. As in Fig. 5, a VPS analysis was completed using the CIS images. Expert graders compared facial images at baseline and either 4, 8, or 12 weeks for changes in blotchiness. The VPS scores are expressed as differences in mean score, retinoid vs. vehicle, with scores significantly different from vehicle indicated.

of niacinamide resulted in a greater improvement than would be seen with retinyl propionate alone.

In evaluation of skin texture, only the 0.2% retinyl propionate and 3.5% niacinamide and the 3.5% niacinamide products provided significant improvement effects vs. vehicle control, as shown in Fig. 10. Across all time points,

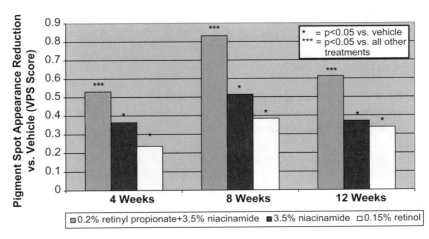

Figure 9 VPS scores of hyperpigmentation spots following 12 weeks of retinyl propionate and niacinamide application. As in Fig. 5, a VPS analysis was completed using the CIS images.

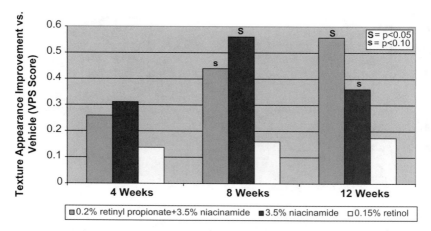

Figure 10 VPS scores of texture following 12 weeks of retinyl propionate and niacinamide application. As in Fig. 7, a VPS analysis was completed using the WIS images.

these two niacinamide-containing products performed similarly, suggesting that all the texture benefit effect was due to niacinamide. This is consistent with other testing we have done showing this benefit for niacinamide (Chapter 24) and the lack of such effect with retinoids in the 3-month time frame of these studies (e.g., Facial Benefits Study 1).

Inhibition of Dermal GAG Production

Elevation in dermal GAG is a characteristic of photodamaged/wrinkled skin (17). In cultures of fibroblasts from young (neonatal) vs. an older donor (57 years old), the older cells produced ~2–3-fold more GAG than young cells, as shown in Table 8.

When cultures of old fibroblasts were exposed to various test agents (at non-cytotoxic doses), a reduction in these excess dermal GAGs was observed, as shown in Table 9. Retinoic acid, as also reported by others (18), reduced dermal fibroblast GAG. Retinyl propionate was also active, although less potent than the benchmark retinoic acid. However, the addition of niacinamide elevated its activity to near that of this benchmark. This GAG reduction activity may contribute to the observed improvement in aging skin (i.e., wrinkle appearance reduction).

Table 8 Ratio of GAG Production by Fibroblasts From Old vs. Young Donors as a Function of Days in Culture.

Days in culture	1	2	3	4	7	11
GAG ratio (old/young)	2.30	2.64	2.68	2.83	3.05	1.98

Table 9 Effect of Niacinamide and Retinoids on Inhibition of GAG Production in Cultured Fibroblasts From Old Donors

Test material	% Reduction in GAG (average of three experiments)
None	0
3 mM niacinamide	29
0.001% retinyl propionate (0.029 mM)	52
0.001% retinyl propionate + 3 mM niacinamide	73
0.001% *trans*-retinoic acid (0.033 mM)	77

DISCUSSION

All *t*-RA, one of the pharmacologically active retinoid forms, is marketed in prescription formulations for treating varying skin conditions such as acne, psoriasis, and photodamage. The latter benefit has driven attempts to identify a cosmetically acceptable retinoid formula that can deliver significant fine lines/wrinkles and color benefits to the consumer. In contrast to the acid form, the alcohol form, retinol, represents a less active retinoid that is still capable of providing significant skin benefits, albeit at much higher concentrations of the molecule due to its required conversion to *t*-RA. Retinyl esters are viewed as still less active forms of retinoids than retinol owing to their prerequisite conversion to retinol by hydrolysis.

A significant side effect of topically applied retinoids is retinoid-induced dermatitis. Retinol is efficacious at levels >0.075%, but also causes significant consumer irritation from normal usage (1–2 applications per day). This study aimed to compare retinol with retinol esters to determine if the esters would have a lower irritation spectrum yet still deliver retinoid-specific benefits.

Our investigations with topical retinyl propionate indicate that it provides skin benefits (e.g., improvement in wrinkles and pigment spots) comparable to those provided by retinol, but with less irritation. A comparison of both products in a sunscreen-containing base showed retinyl propionate to be more efficacious with lower irritation. Preliminary testing of the acetate ester, along with the propionate ester, revealed that retinyl acetate had greater irritation potential than retinyl propionate; thus subsequent studies focused solely on retinyl propionate.

The retinol with sunscreen treatment in our 12-week facial benefit study was significantly irritating at all time points across all measures. Ongoing discussion in the literature regarding potential sensitivity to sunlight of skin treated with retinoids has elucidated the wisdom of adequate sun protection as an adjunct treatment (11,19). The increased skin irritation observed here with retinol and organic sunscreen agents (octyl methoxycinnamate and phenylbenzimidazole sulfonic acid) creates a potential restriction in the choice of aesthetically acceptable skin photoprotection in conjunction with retinol use. However, no such issue was observed with retinyl propionate, thus indicating that it can be used in conjunction with sunscreens without concern for irritation. We hypothesize that the greater irritation caused by retinol with sunscreen is due to retinol enhancing the penetration of the sunscreen components which may themselves have contributed to the irritation responses. Retinol has been reported to decrease the skin's barrier function and sunscreens are reported to be potentially irritating (20,21).

In contrast to our positive results with retinyl propionate, a previous investigation did not detect any benefits (13). Although the two studies involved use of the same total daily dose of retinyl propionate, there were some differences that might account for the divergence in outcome. In the study by Green et al. (13), there was not a positive control, whereas our study involved the use of a high level of retinol for this purpose. (Retinol as a positive control has been effective in several studies we have conducted.) In addition, we monitored chemical stability of the retinoid in product throughout the 3-month duration of the testing. The study by Green et al. (13) did not discuss evaluation of stability. Additionally, Green et al. (13) had only one grader to evaluate the clinical subjects, whereas our work involved evaluations by two–three graders. In addition, the vehicles used were different, which may have affected delivery and thus activity. These differences may have contributed to the different measured clinical outcomes from the two studies.

In addition to a superior efficacy to irritation ratio, retinyl propionate may also have a stability advantage over retinol. A recent study examining the stability of retinyl propionate vs. retinol found that retinyl propionate was about two times more stable than retinol in a simple solution of tetrahydrofuran and water (22). We also have shown here that retinyl propionate has better photostability than retinol after topical application.

We additionally observed that niacinamide in combination with retinyl propionate provided even greater benefits in reduction in hyperpigmented spots and improvement in texture. The texture improvement effect is associated with niacinamide treatment (Chapter 24), and niacinamide alone also has pigment spot reduction activity (14; Chapter 24). Additionally, niacinamide is metabolized to NAD(P)H, and NADP is a required cofactor in the enzymatic conversions of retinol to retinaldehyde and retinaldehyde to retinoic acid, the active retinoid in skin. Thus, once retinyl propionate has been hydrolyzed to retinol in the skin, niacinamide can serve to increase the extent of conversion to retinoic acid leading to greater benefits than with retinyl propionate alone. Our clinical data are consistent with this hypothesized mechanism.

We further hypothesize that at least part of the mechanism by which retinyl propionate (and indeed perhaps other retinoids such as t-RA) provide early skin wrinkle appearance improvement effects is by reducing the elevated dermal content of GAG in older photoaged skin. Elevated GAG is one of the histological observations in photodamaged, wrinkled skin (17). There are other skin disorders in which dermal GAG are excessively elevated, resulting in skin appearance changes, for example, the wrinkled skin of tight-skin mouse (23) and of the Shar Pei dog (24). There are also data illustrating an association between reduction in excess dermal GAG and wrinkle repair. In cell culture (25), excess GAG inhibits collagen bundle assembly and thus would be expected to interfere with dermal repair processes. In addition, reduction in excess dermal GAG with chemical peel (26) and retinoic acid (27) accompanies wrinkle repair.

The combination of the four clinical studies reported herein confirm that retinyl propionate is capable of eliciting positive skin benefits in human skin with reduced overall irritation potential. Given the desirability of a sunscreen component in formulations containing retinoids, the interaction of the retinoid with the sunscreen active ingredients must be considered. Retinol reacted negatively with the sunscreen components, increasing overall irritation. In contrast, retinyl propionate's effects on the skin were not influenced by the presence of sunscreen components. This trait, along with superior stability, are additional advantages to be considered when selecting a retinoid to achieve skin benefits in a cosmetic formulation.

ACKNOWLEDGMENTS

We gratefully acknowledge the technical and administrative assistance of Janet Lynch, Marcia Schnicker, Deanne Lind, Frank Joa, Dan Schaiper, Emilia Mrowczynski, and Sarah Hicks. This work was funded in its entirety by The Procter & Gamble Company.

REFERENCES

1. Kligman AM, Grove GL, Hirose R, Leyden JJ. Topical tretinoin for photoaged skin. J Am Acad Dermatol 1986; 15:836–859.
2. Weiss JS, Ellis CN, Headington JT, Tincoff T, Hamilton TA, Voorhees JJ. J Am Med Assoc 1988; 259:527–532.
3. Kang S, Duell EA, Fisher GJ, Datta SC, Wang ZQ, Reddy AP, Tavakkol A, Yi JT, Griffiths CE, Elder JT, Voorhees JJ. Application of retinol to human skin *in vivo* induces epidermal hyperplasia and cellular retinoid binding proteins characteristic of retinoic acid but without measurable retinoic acid levels of irritation. J Invest Dermatol 1995; 105:549–556.
4. Fluhr JW, Vienne M-P, Lauze C, Dupuy P, Gehring W, Gloor M. Tolerance profile of retinol, retinaldehyde and retinoic acid under maximized and long-term clinical conditions. Dermatol 1999; 199(suppl 1):57–60.
5. Jarrett A, Wrench R, Mahmoud B. The effects of retinyl acetate on epidermal proliferation and differentiation. Induced enzyme reactions in the epidermis. Clin Exp Dermatol 1978; 3:173–188.
6. Boehnlein J, Sakr A, Lichtin JL, Bronaugh RL. Characterization of esterase and alcohol dehydrogenase activity in skin. Metabolism of retinyl palmitate to retinol (vitamin A) during percutaneous absorption. Pharm Res 1994; 11:1155–1159.

7. Counts DF, Skreko F, McBee J, Wich AG. The effect of retinyl palmitate on skin composition and morphometry. J Soc Cosmet Chem 1988; 39:235–240.
8. Kurlandsky SB, Duell EA, Kang S, Voorhees JJ, Fisher GJ. Auto-regulation of retinoic acid biosynthesis through regulation of retinol esterification in human keratinocytes. J Biol Chem 1996; 271:15346–15352.
9. Randolph RK, Simon M. Characterization of retinol metabolism in cultured human epidermal keratinocytes. J Biol Chem 1993; 268:9198–9205.
10. Kurlandsky SB, Xiao J-H, Duell EA, Voorhees JJ, Fisher GJ. Biological activity of all-*trans* retinol requires metabolic conversion to all-*trans* retinoic acid and is mediated through activation of nuclear retinoid receptors in human keratinocytes. J Biol Chem 1994; 269:32821–32827.
11. Davies PJA, Basilion JP, Haake AR. Intrinsic Biology of retinoids in the skin. In: Goldsmith LA, ed. Physiology, Biochemistry, and Molecular Biology of the Skin. Vol 1. New York: Oxford University Press, 1997:385–409.
12. Ridge BD, Batt MD, Palmer HE, Jarrett A. The dansyl chloride technique for stratum corneum renewal as an indicator of changes in epidermal mitotic activity following topical treatment. Brit J Dermatol 1988; 118:167–174.
13. Green C, Orchard G, Cerio R, Hawk JLM. A clinicopathological study of the effects of topical retinyl propionate cream in skin photoaging. Clin Exp Dermatol 1998; 23:162–167.
14. Hakozaki T, Minwalla L, Zhuang J, Chhoa M, Matsubara A, Miyamoto K, Greatens A, Hillebrand GG, Bissett DL, Boissy RE. The effect of niacinamide on reducing cutaneous pigmentation and suppression of melanosome transfer. Brit J Dermatol 2002; 147:20–31.
15. Lanman BM, Elvers WB, Howard CS. The role of patch testing in a product development program. In: Proceedings of the Joint Conference on Cosmetic Sciences, The Toilet Goods. Washington, D.C.: Association, Inc., 1968:135–145.
16. Philips L, Steinberg M, Maibach HI, Akers WA. Comparison of rabbit and human skin response to certain irritants. Toxicol Appl Pharmacol 1972; 21:369–382.
17. Gonzalez S, Moran M, Kochevar IE. Chronic photodamage in skin of mast cell-deficient mice. Photochem Photobiol 1999; 70:248–253.
18. Smith TJ. Retinoic acid inhibition of hyaluronate synthesis in cultured skin fibroblasts. J Clin Endocrinol Metab 1990; 70:655–660.
19. Kligman A. Guidelines for the use of topical tretinoin (Retin-A) for photoaged skin. J Am Acad Dermatol 1989; 21:650–654.
20. Leonardi GR, Gaspar LR, Maia Campos PM. Application of a non-invasive method to study the moisturizing effect of formulations containing vitamins A or E or ceramide on human skin. J Cosmet Sci 2002; 53:263–268.
21. Parrish JA, Pathak MA, Fitzpatrick TB. Letter: facial irritation due to sunscreen products. Arch Dermatol 1975; 111:525.
22. Semenzato A, Bovenga L, Faiferri L, Austria R, Bettero A. Stability of vitamin A propionate in cosmetic formulations. SÖFW-Journal 1997; 123:151–154.
23. Sundberg JP. The tight-skin (Tsk) mutation, chromosome 2. In: Sundberg JP, ed. Handbook of Mouse Mutations with Skin and Hair Abnormalities. Boca Raton, Florida: CRC Press, 1994:463–470.
24. Dunstan RW, Kennis RA. Selected heritable skin diseases of domestic animals. In: Sundberg JP, ed. Handbook of Mouse Mutations with Skin and Hair Abnormalities. Boca Raton, Florida: CRC Press, 1994:524–525.

25. Guidry C, Grinnell F. Heparin modulates the organization of hydrated collagen gels and inhibits gel contraction by fibroblasts. J Cell Biol 1987; 104:1097–1103.
26. Kligman AM, Baker TJ, Gordon HL. Long-term histologic follow-up of phenol face peels. Plast Recontruct Surg 1975; 75:652–659.
27. Schwartz E, Kligman LH. Topical tretinoin increases the tropoelastin and fibronection content of photoaged hairless mouse skin. J Invest Dermatol 1995; 104:518–522.

26

Phyllanthus Tannins

Ratan K. Chaudhuri
EMD Chemicals*, Inc., Hawthorne, New York, USA

Introduction	466
Hydrolyzable Tannins	466
Gallotannins	467
Ellagitannins	467
Gallo-ellagitannins	467
Condensed Tannins (Proanthocyanidins)	467
Phyllanthus Tannins	467
Occurrence of Tannins	469
Tannins of *Phyllanthus emblica*	470
Product Description and Standardization	470
Product Stability	472
Antioxidant Activity	472
Hydroxy Radical Quenching	472
Superoxide Anion Radical Quenching	473
Singlet Oxygen Quenching	474
Nitrogen Radical Quenching	474
Boosting of Antioxidant Defense Enzymes	475
Chelating Activity	476
Chelators as Oxidation Enhancer	476
Antioxidants Act as Pro-Oxidants	476

*An affiliate of Merck KGaA, Darmstadt, Germany.

Chelating Property of *Emblica* Antioxidant	477
Matrix Metalloprotease (MMP) Enzymes	478
Collagenase (MMP-1) Inhibitory Activity of *Emblica* Antioxidant	479
Stromelysin 1 (MMP-3) Inhibitory Activity of *Emblica* Antioxidant	480
Extracellular Matrix (ECM) Proteins	480
Stimulation of Noncollagenic Protein Synthesis	481
Skin Lightening/Skin Even-Toning	481
Emblica Antioxidant Lightens the Normal Skin Color	482
Emblica Antioxidant Reduces Freckle Spots	482
Emblica Antioxidant Reduces UV-Induced Erythema	483
Safety Data	483
Acute Oral Toxicity Study in Rats	483
Primary Eye Irritation Study in Rabbits	483
Evaluation of Phototoxicity Potential by UV-A Irradiation on Human Subjects	483
Repeat Insult Patch Test on Human Subjects/Skin Irritation and Skin Sensitization Evaluation	484
Bacterial Mutagenicity Test	484
Conclusion	484
References	485

INTRODUCTION

Phenolic metabolism in plants is complex, and yields a wide array of compounds ranging from the familiar flower pigments (anthocyanidins) to the complex phenolics of the plant cell wall (lignin). However, the group of phenolic compounds known as tannins is clearly distinguished from other plant secondary phenolics in their structural chemistry and biological activities. The term "tannin" comes from the ancient Celtic word for oak, a typical source of tannins for leather making. Tannins are usually subdivided into two groups: hydrolyzable tannins (HT) and condensed tannins [CT, often-called proanthocyanidins (PA)].

HYDROLYZABLE TANNINS

HTs are molecules with a polyol (generally D-glucose or its derivatives) as a central core. The hydroxyl groups of these carbohydrates are partially or totally esterified with phenolic groups like gallic acid (gallotannins), ellagic acid (ellagitannins), or both (gallo-ellagitannins). HTs are usually present in low amounts in plants. There are some exceptions, namely *Phyllanthus emblica* (syn. *Emblica officinalis*). HT is hydrolyzed by mild acids or mild bases to yield glucose or its derivatives and phenolic acids. Under the same conditions, CT (PA) do not hydrolyze. HTs are also hydrolyzed by hot water or enzymes (i.e., tannase).

Gallotannins

Gallotannins are composed of a core of D-glucose (or its derivatives) and 2–9 galloyl groups. In nature, there is an abundance of mono and di-galloyl esters of glucose (molecular weight ~900 atomic mass unit, amu). They are not considered to be tannins. At least three hydroxyl groups of the glucose must be esterified to exhibit a sufficiently strong binding capacity to be classified as a tannin. The most well-known source of gallotannins is tannic acid obtained from the twig galls of *Rhus semialata*. It has a penta galloyl-D-glucose core and five more units of galloyl linked to one of the galloyl of the core (Fig. 1).

Ellagitannins

Ellagitannins are composed of a core D-glucose (or its derivatives) and the phenolic groups consist of hexahydroxydiphenic acid (dimeric form of gallic acid, or its derivatives), which spontaneously dehydrates to the lactone form, ellagic acid. Molecular weight ranges from ~800 to 5000 (amu).

Gallo-ellagitannins

The phenolic groups in gallo-ellagitannins consist of both gallic and ellagic acid (or its derivatives) as the name implies.

CONDENSED TANNINS (PROANTHOCYANIDINS)

CTs are more widely distributed than HTs. They are oligomers or polymers of flavonoid units (i.e., flavan-3-ol) linked by carbon–carbon bonds not susceptible to cleavage by hydrolysis. CTs are more often called PAs due to their condensed chemical structure. The term, PA, is derived from the acid catalyzed oxidation reaction that produces red anthocyanidins upon heating CTs in acidic alcohol solutions. The most common anthocyanidins produced are cyanidin (flavan-3-ol, from procyanidin) and delphinidin (from prodelphinidin).

CTs may contain from 2 to 50 or greater flavonoid units; CT polymers have complex structures because the flavonoid units can differ for some substituents and because of the variable sites for inter-flavan bonds. Anthocyanidin pigments are responsible for the wide array of pink, scarlet, red, mauve, violet, and blue colors in flowers, leaves, fruits, fruit juices, and wines. They are also responsible for the astringent taste of fruit and wines. CT carbon–carbon bonds are not cleaved by hydrolysis (Fig. 2).

PHYLLANTHUS TANNINS

The plant genus *Phyllanthus* (Euphorbiacea) is a rich source of HT. They are widely distributed in most tropical and subtropical countries. *Phyllanthus* has well over 700 species and subdivided into 10 or 11 sub-genera (1). *Phyllanthus*

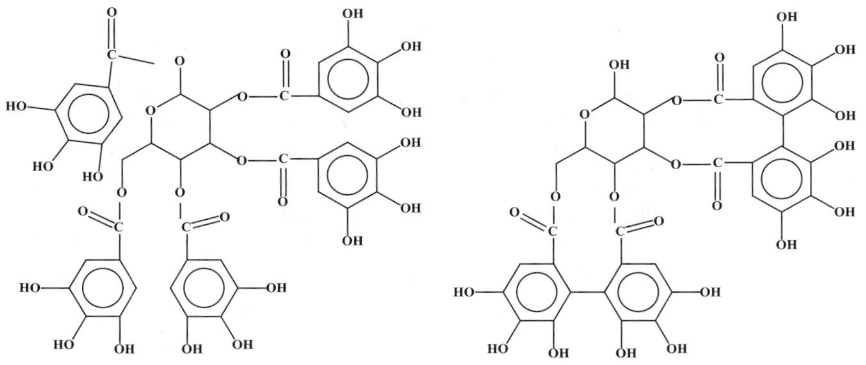

(a) Gallotannin: Pentagalloylglucose   Ellagitannin: Pedunculagin

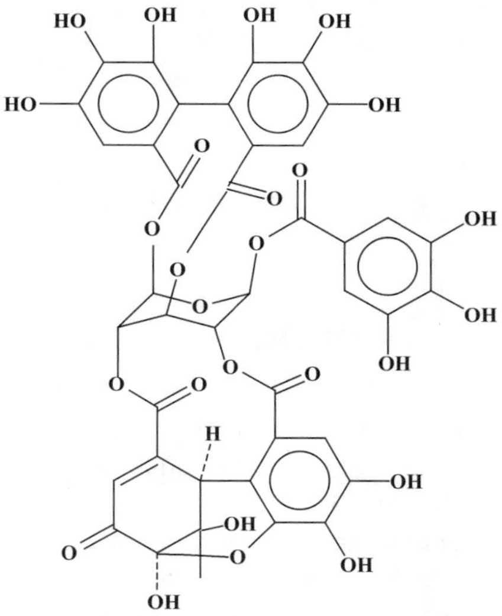

(b) Gallo-ellagitannin: Geraniin

Figure 1 General structure of HT: (a) Examples of gallotannin and ellagitannin; (b) an example of gallo-ellagitannin.

species have long been used in traditional medicine to treat a broad-spectrum of disorders, and there are numerous references. Unander et al. (2–5) published an extensive, four-part survey of the usage of bioassays in the genus *Phyllanthus*. These articles cover published data concerning traditional uses, as well as the results of the laboratory assays. Another recent review (6) on the genus *Phyllanthus* has been published. This review covers the current knowledge of their chemistry, *in vitro* and *in vivo* pharmacological, biochemical, and clinical

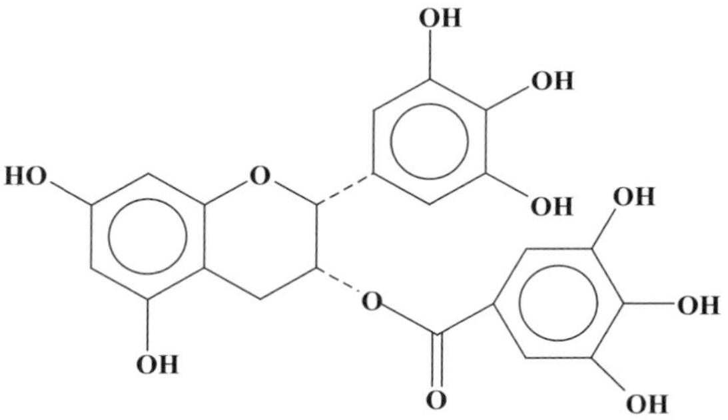

Epigallocatechin 3-Gallate

Figure 2 Example of a condensed tannin.

studies carried out on the extracts, and the main active constituents isolated from different species of plants of the genus *Phyllanthus*.

OCCURRENCE OF TANNINS

A vast amount of literature is available on *Phyllanthus*. On PubMed and Medline, *Phyllanthus* and *Emblica* were used as search criteria to locate literature references on this subject. We included *Emblica* as a search criterion because *Phyllanthus emblica* is synonymous with *Emblica officinalis*. In addition, review articles (6,7) were included for searching relevant information on HT. These publications are mainly related to pharmacological and clinical studies carried out on the extracts. We have found very few literature dealing with the identification and structure determination of tannins of *Phyllanthus*. A list of occurrence of HT in different *Phyllanthus* species with appropriate references is given in Table 1.

In plants, morphological evolution is accompanied by progressive oxidation of secondary metabolites belonging to a particular biosynthetic class (8). This series of oxidative transformations of HT are useful for correlating progressive oxidation with morphological evolution. As HT are generally potent antioxidants whose potency depends on their oxidation stage (9), their correlation with plant evolution may be clearer than with other types of plant metabolites. The evidence presented by Okuda et al. (10) strengthens the basis for this suggestion concerning the evolutionary rationale for the biosynthetic sequence of tannins (11). Examples of each class of the tannins are as follows:

Type 1: Gallotannins (1,2,3,4,6-penta-O-galloyl-β-D-glucose)
Type 2: Ellagitannins (pedunculagin)
Type 3: Dehydroellagitannins (geraniin)
Type 4: Transformed dehydroellagitannins (chebulagic acid)

All these four categories of tannins are present in the *Phyllanthus* genus (10).

Table 1 Occurrence of HT in Different Species of *Phyllanthus*

Species	Tannins	Reference
P. amarus	Amariin, geraniin, corilagin	(56)
(syn. *P. niruri*)	Amariinic acid, amarulone, phyllanthusin D, elaeocarpusin, repandusinic acid A, geraniinic acid B, 1-*O*-galloyl-2, 4-dehydrohexahydrooxydiphenoyl-glucopyranose	(57)
	Niruriside	(58)
P. emblica	Emblicanin A, emblicanin B, pedunculagin, punigluconin	(16)
(syn. *E. officinalis*)	Phyllanemblinins A, B, C, D, E, F 2,3,6-Tetra-*O*-galloylglucose, corilagin chebulanin, chebulagic acid, elaeocarpusin, punicafolin, tercatain, mallonin, putrajivain A	(18)
P. flexuosus	Phyllanthusiins A, B and C	(59)
	Geraniin, geraniinic acid B, corilagin, putranjivain A	
P. virgatus	Virganin	(60)
P. urinaria	Corilagin, geraniin, 1-galloyl-3, 6-hexahydroxydiphenoyl-4-*O*-brevifolincarboxyl-β-D-glucopyranose	(61,62)
P. sellowianus	Geraniin, furosin	(63)
P. myrtifolius	Corilagin, geraniin, chebulagic acid, elaecarpusin, mallotusin, phyllanthusiin C	(62)

TANNINS OF *PHYLLANTHUS EMBLICA*

Documentation of topical application of tannins having well-defined structural information is lacking. The only commercial tannin containing products with well-documented literature known to the author is from *P. emblica* fruits (syn. *E. officinalis*, abbreviated as *Emblica* antioxidant). This review focuses on the currently available knowledge on the HT constituents of *P. emblica* and their effects on skin. Product description, standardization, stability, and toxicity have also been included.

Product Description and Standardization

P. emblica is one of the important ayurvedic (science of life) herbs of India, and has been used for over thousands of years in a wide variety of human ailments (12). Its status ranges from insignificant, in the western world, to highly prized, in tropical Asia. Fruits of *P. emblica* are reputed ayurvedic revitalizers and biological response modifiers and are used for the treatment of a number of diseases and debility states (13). *Emblica* antioxidant is extracted from premium quality fruits using a water-based process (US Patent No. 6,124,268; 6,649,150 and other pending patents). *Emblica* antioxidant is distinctly different from other commercially available extracts of *P. emblica* fruits as it is defined to the extent of well over 50% (typically, 60–75%) in terms of its key bioactive components. Literature reports claiming the presence of vitamin C in *P. emblica* (14,15) are refuted using HPLC and biochemical studies by Ghosal et al. (16) and by Chaudhuri and Schewitz (17). None of the extracts of *P. emblica* in the market compares to *Emblica* antioxidant in terms of composition and consistency of composition, aqueous stability, and color.

The low molecular weight (<1000) HT, namely emblicanin A and emblicanin B, along with pedunculagin and punigluconin are the key ingredients (Fig. 3) in *Emblica* antioxidant. In nature, emblicanin A and emblicanin B have only been found in *P. emblica* plants (16). Interestingly, tannin constituents of *P. emblica* vary due to ecology and process of isolation (18). *Emblica* antioxidant has been standardized (17) using high performance thin layer

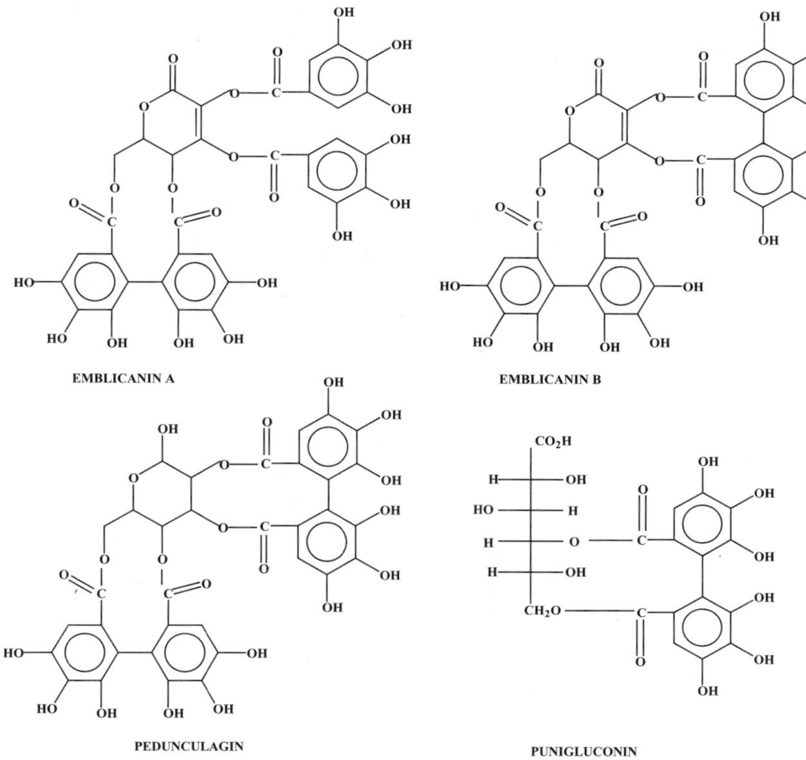

Figure 3 Low molecular-weight HT of *P. emblica*.

chromatography (HPTLC). Alternately, using high performance liquid chromatography (HPLC) the product can also be standardized.

Product Stability

Emblica antioxidant is stable in aqueous as well as in formulated products for well over 2 years (19). *Emblica* antioxidant is very photostable (20), which was determined by irradiating a 1% aqueous solution and a formulated product of *Emblica* to UV-A and UV-B light separately for a period of 4 h (~8 minimum erythemal dose, MED). Photostability of the product was determined from optical density at λ_{max} value at 271 nm and normalized with respect to the time zero. A loss of only 3% activity was observed after irradiating the product for 2 h (4 MED). On the contrary, vitamin E (natural tocopherol, $\lambda_{max} = 263$ nm) in formulated product lost well over 70% in 2 h (4 MED).

The photostability of *Emblica* antioxidant and natural tocopherol in formulations under UV irradiation was tested by ultra-thin film transmission of light. The UV photodegradation of an active is measured from its decrease in the characteristic UV absorption band (optical density), after correction by the light scattering background. Results showed a loss of only 3% of *Emblica* in formulation vs. a loss of 72% of natural tocopherol (20) after irradiating the products for only 2 h (4 MED).

Antioxidant Activity

Over the course of evolution, the skin has developed a complex defense system to protect the organism from oxidative damage. The possible source of oxidative stress to skin is versatile. Ultraviolet light is the primary cause of the oxidative stress. An overload of this system seems to be responsible, at least partially, for the etiology of several skin disorders including skin cancers (21) and photoaging (22). Hence, it seems to be a reasonable strategy to support the natural defense system of the skin by the application of antioxidants.

Tannins are considered superior antioxidants than other polyphenolics as their eventual oxidation lead to oligomerization via phenolic coupling and enlargement of the number of active ROS quenching sites, a reaction which has not been observed with other polyphenolics such as flavonoids. *Emblica* was found to have a very broad antioxidant activity (19,20,23) as it quenches hydroxyl radicals, superoxide anion radical, singlet oxygen, and nitrogen radical. First three ROS are relevant because of exposure of skin to sunlight causes generation of these radicals and nonradical.

Hydroxy Radical Quenching

A comparative (19) study using deoxyribose method (24) showed that *Emblica* is about three- to fourfold more effective in quenching hydroxyl radical than pine antioxidant, grape antioxidant, and Trolox C (vitamin E water-soluble analog).

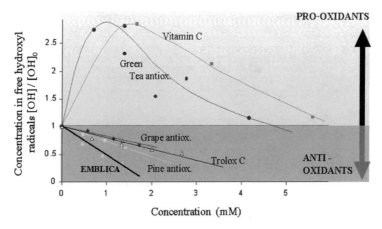

Figure 4 A comparative hydroxyl radical quenching of *Emblica* and other antioxidants.

In this test, green tea antioxidant and vitamin C were found to be pro-oxidant (Fig. 4). A relative efficiency of hydroxyl radical quenching was calculated from the rate constants, which is given in Table 2.

Superoxide Anion Radical Quenching

Chaudhuri et al. (20) have shown that the superoxide radical quenching ability of *Emblica* by two different methods. Both methods use hypoxanthine–xanthine oxidase system to generate superoxide anion radical. The first method is a chemical method, which involves reducing the conversion of nitroblue tetrazolium (NBT) into nitroblue diformazan and determining the reduction in conversion of NBT by measuring the optical density change at 560 nm (25). This study (Fig. 5) showed that *Emblica* antioxidant is several-fold more effective in quenching superoxide radical than Trolox C (vitamin E water-soluble analog) and vitamin C.

Table 2 Relative Hydroxyl Radical Quenching Property of *Emblica* and Other Antioxidants

Antioxidant	Rate constant K (10^9 M^{-1} s^{-1})	Relative % efficiency
Emblica antioxidant	33.9	100
Pine antioxidant	11.0	32.5
Grape antioxidant	7.8	23
Trolox C	8.2	24
Vitamin C	—	Pro-oxidant
Green tea antioxidant	—	Pro-oxidant

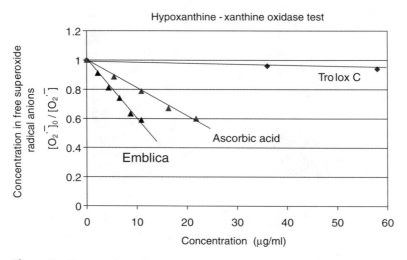

Figure 5 Comparative superoxide anion radical quenching of *Emblica* and other antioxidants.

The second method is a biological method, which involves protecting fibroblast cells from damage caused by superoxide anion radical and determining the cell protection by measuring optical density change at 570 nm (26). This study demonstrated that *Emblica* antioxidant is comparable to vitamin C in protecting fibroblast cells against superoxide damage (20). However, vitamin C is not hydrolytically, thermally, or photochemically stable. Hence, its use in skin care ingredient is limited.

Singlet Oxygen Quenching

The method (27,28) used in generating singlet oxygen involved UV-A irradiation of a sensitizer (methylene blue). Histidine is used as a substrate, which reacts with singlet oxygen to form trans-annular peroxide. The resulting reaction product bleaches *N,N*-dimethyl-*p*-nitrosoaniline (RNO). The bleached form of RNO is then measured spectrally at 440 nm. The singlet oxygen scavenging efficiency of antioxidants will therefore reduce the amount of free singlet oxygen and thus prevent the bleaching of RNO. Results showed (20) that *Emblica* antioxidant (IC_{50} 61 μg/mL) is an excellent singlet oxygen quencher and superior to Trolox C (IC_{50} 84 μg/mL, vitamin E water-soluble analog) (Fig. 6). In this test, vitamin C was found to be a strong singlet oxygen enhancer (pro-oxidant).

Nitrogen Radical Quenching

The method used is a colorimetric method based on the decrease in absorbance at 517 nm of diphenylpicrylhydrazide (DPPH) radical after the addition of an

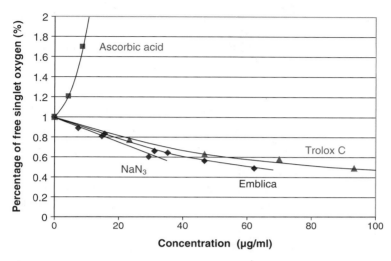

Figure 6 Comparative singlet oxygen quenching ability of *Emblica* and other antioxidants.

antioxidant compound in solution (29). This study showed that *Emblica* is stable in aqueous system for over 1 year at 45°C, whereas all other antioxidants (vitamin E, vitamin C, pine antioxidant, rosemary antioxidant) have lost about or well over 50% activity in 3 months (19). Additionally, a minimum batch to variation in antioxidant activity of *Emblica* antioxidant is seen in this test. Although most antioxidants go from an active to an inactive role, *Emblica* antioxidant utilizes a multilevel cascade of antioxidant compounds resulting in a propagation of its antioxidant capabilities.

Boosting of Antioxidant Defense Enzymes

Superoxide radical is inactivated by superoxide dismutase (SOD) *in vivo*, the only enzyme known to use a free radical as a substrate. However, the free radical scavenging activity of SOD is effective only when it is followed by increases in the activity of catalase (CAT) and/or glutathione peroxidase (GPX). SOD generates hydrogen peroxide as a metabolite, which is also tissue toxic and has to be scavenged by CAT and/or GPX. Thus, a concomitant increase in CAT and/or GPX activity is a prerequisite if a beneficial effect from increase in SOD activity is to be expected. In an animal study, Bhattacharya et al. (30) have shown significant increase in SOD, CAT, and GPX activity in rat brain frontal cortex and striatum when a standardized fruit extract of *E. officinalis* (syn. *P. emblica*) was used. These authors were able to demonstrate a significant reduction in lipid peroxidation in these brain area when rats are administered *Emblica* antioxidant once-a-day for 7 days.

It is quite conceivable that *Emblica* antioxidant would provide a similar boosting of SOD, CAT, and GPX when applied onto skin. This should help to reduce detrimental effects caused by superoxide or its metabolite on the skin.

Chelating Activity

Iron and copper play ambivalent roles in biology because they are required as cofactors for many biological reactions, while at the same time their toxicity threatens cellular integrity. Iron content of human epidermis is greater in sun-exposed than in non-exposed body sites (31). Copper along with iron content in sweat is also increased significantly after exercise (32). It has recently been shown that UV-A and UV-B radiation induce immediate release of iron in skin fibroblasts (33,34). The generation of hydroxyl radicals via Fenton chemistry represents one of the most important mechanisms in various pathological conditions. Therefore, in sun-damaged skin, the significantly increased iron content may drive the production of ROS with subsequent tissue damage and long-term consequences like cancer or premature aging of the skin.

Chelators as Oxidation Enhancer

A wide-range of iron chelators can also stimulate oxidation, especially lipid peroxidation (35). This includes not only Fe^{2+} salts and simple chelates (such as Fe^{2+}-ADP), but also heme, heme proteins and even the iron-containing enzyme phenylalanin hydroxylase (36). Only a few chelators, such as ethylenediamine tetraacetic acid (EDTA) and citric acid are relevant to skin care formulations as they are in wide spread use.

Antioxidants Act as Pro-Oxidants

The chief defense against free radical damage to skin is antioxidants. It is often disregarded that antioxidants not only function as antioxidants, but also intrinsically have pro-oxidant action, in presence of transition metals like iron and copper (37). There is pro-oxidant action even in well-known antioxidants such as vitamin C, vitamin E (tocopherols), glutathione, and plant phenolics (19). Chemistry involved in iron- or copper-induced oxidation is summarized as follows.

Presence of iron (or copper) and H_2O_2

$$Fe^{2+} \text{ (or } Cu^+) + H_2O_2 \longrightarrow \text{Intermediate complex (es)}$$
$$\longrightarrow Fe^{3+} \text{ (or } Cu^{2+}) + OH^{\bullet} + OH^-$$

(very fast reaction)

$$Fe^{3+} \text{ (or } Cu^{2+}) + H_2O_2 \longrightarrow \text{Intermediate complex (es)}$$
$$\longrightarrow Fe^{2+} \text{ (or } Cu^+) + O_2^{\bullet-} + 2H^+ \text{ (slow reaction)}$$

Presence of iron- (or copper-) chelates and H_2O_2

$$Fe^{3+}\text{- (or } Cu^{2+}\text{-) EDTA} + H_2O_2 \longrightarrow Fe^{2+}\text{- (or } Cu^+\text{) EDTA} + O_2^{\cdot -} + 2H^+$$

Presence of Iron (or copper), H_2O_2 & an antioxidant

$$Fe^{3+} + \text{ascorbate} \longrightarrow Fe^{2+} + \text{ascorbate}^{\cdot}$$

$$Fe^{2+} + H_2O_2 \longrightarrow [\text{intermediate complex(es)}] \longrightarrow Fe^{3+} + HO^{\cdot} + HO^-$$

Chelating Property of *Emblica* Antioxidant

An antioxidant can be a true photoprotective agent, provided it chelates all the available coordinate sites in iron and/or copper (38). This is particularly critical as the formation of hydroxyl radicals from superoxide or hydrogen peroxide from iron or copper requires only one coordination site that is open or occupied by water. Water can easily be displaced by a stronger ligand such as the azide anion (N_3^-).

This principle was applied to determine the presence of free coordination site(s) in the iron- (or copper-) *Emblica* and other antioxidant complex by a spectrophotometric method (38). Of all the iron- (or copper-) complex tested (19), only the complex of *Emblica* antioxidant and epigallo catechin-3-gallate (EGCG) and iron (or copper) showed absence of any water coordination. EGCG is the major antioxidant constituent in green tea. This means that the complex is fully and firmly saturated and there is no room for any pro-oxidant activity due to oxo-ferryl or oxo-cuppryl radical formation. All other antioxidants/chelators failed, manifesting pro-oxidant effects, particularly at low concentrations [Tables 3 (iron) and 4 (copper)].

Table 3 Ultraviolet Spectral Data of Fe^{3+}-Chelators

Chelator	Absorption maxima of complex λ_{max} (nm)	
	With Fe^{3+}	N_3-induced shift
EDTA	241, 283	241, 283, 410
Emblica antioxidant	241, 294, 353, 377	241, 294, 353, 377/no shift
Pine antioxidant	241, 294, 353, 384	241, 294, 353, 400, 440
Vitamin C	238, 262	241, 266, 295
Grape antioxidant	247, 295, 353, 396	247, 295, 353, 415, 430
Green tea antioxidant	240, 272, 324, 390	240, 277, 325, 390
Trolox C	240, 284	240, 273, 284, 360
Gallic acid	247, 295, 337	247, 295, 353, 412
EGCG	214, 269, 329, 508	214, 269, 329, 508/no shift

Note: The peak positions are obtained from differential spectroscopic scans of 1.0 mM Fe^{3+} and 5 mM chelator, 1.0 M NaN_3, 50 mM phosphate buffer, pH 7.4, vs. the same solution without sodium azide.

Table 4 Ultraviolet Spectral Data of Cu^{2+}-Chelators

Chelator/Antioxidant	Absorption maxima of complex λ_{max} (nm)	
	With Cu^{2+}	N_3-induced shift
EDTA	240, 278	241, 279, 354
Emblica antioxidant	240, 272, 313	240, 272, 313/no shift
Pine antioxidant	239, 279, 302, 331	239, 280, 307, 430
Vitamin C	239, 263	239, 263, 284, 364
Grape antioxidant	240, 277, 328	240, 277, 328, 359
Green tea antioxidant	241, 276, 327, 403	241, 277, 336, 404
Trolox C	241, 288	241, 261, 352, 440
Gallic acid	240, 258, 321	240, 258, 331, 463

Note: The peak positions are obtained from differential spectroscopic scans of 1.0 mM Cu^{2+} and 5 mM chelator, 1 M NaN_3, 50 mM phosphate buffer, pH 7.4, vs. the same solution without sodium azide.

Matrix Metalloprotease (MMP) Enzymes

MMPs constitute a family of structurally similar zinc-containing metalloproteases, which are involved in the remodeling and degradation of extracellular matrix (ECM) proteins, both as part of normal physiological processes and of pathological conditions. Another important function of certain MMPs is to activate various enzymes, including other MMPs, by cleaving the pro-domains from their protease domains. Thus some MMPs act to regulate the activities of other MMPs, so that over-production of one MMP may lead to excessive proteolysis of ECM by another. At this time more than 20 different MMPs have been identified and classified (39). A few selected MMPs relevant to skin care applications along with their substrates are included in Table 5.

Several studies carried out by Scharffetter-Kochanek's group using dermal fibroblast cells show that both UV-A and UV-B cause four- to fivefold increase in

Table 5 Selected List of MMP Family

Group	Descriptive name	Systematic name	Principal substrate
Collagenase	Interstitial collagenase	MMP-1	Fibrillar collagen types I–III
Gelatinases	Gelatinase A (72 kDa)	MMP-2	Gelatins, nonfibrillar collagen types, IV and V
	Gelatianse B (92 kDa)	MMP-9	Gelatins, nonfibrillar collagen types, IV and V
Stromelysins	Stromelysin-1	MMP-3	Proteoglycans, laminin, fibronectin, nonfibrillar collagens

the production of MMP-1 and MMP-3 (33,40,41). In contrast, the synthesis of tissue inhibitory metalloprotease-1 (TIMP-1), natural inhibitor of MMP, increases only marginally. This imbalance is one of the causes of severe connective tissue damage resulting in photoaging of the skin. A clinical study by Voorhees's group has shown that tretinoin has MMP-1 inhibitory activity and may have a role in preventing some aspect of photoaging attributable to MMP-mediated dermal damage (i.e., wrinkling) (42).

The damage caused by excessive MMP on the ECM proteins does not appear overnight, but is a result of the accumulation of successive molecular damages, especially in the case of overexposure to UV light. The skin repercussion on the degradation of the ECM proteins may then be revealed in many ways depending on age, genetic status, and life-style and of course on the general health status of the individual. Application of MMP inhibitors may be a route to prevent or to minimize damage to ECM proteins (43).

Collagenase (MMP-1) Inhibitory Activity of *Emblica* Antioxidant

A dose-dependant inhibition of gelatinase/collagenase activity by $\sim$55–70% was observed with *Emblica* antioxidant at 150–300 µg/mL (20). Quantification of gelatinase/collagenase inhibitory activity of *Emblica* antioxidant was determined using EnzChek® gelatinase/collagenase kit (E-12055) from Molecular Probe by measuring the substrate fluorescence emission at 515 nm. 1,10-Phenanthroline (Phenan, 10 mM) was used as a positive control and collagenase without inhibitor was used as a negative control. Fluorescence emission was measured at 515 nm. Results of this study are summarized in Fig. 7.

Collagen synthesis in sun-damaged skin appears to remain similar to that of sun-protected sites, although collagen content decreases (44). Thus, evidence suggests that the decrease in collagen content in photoaged skin results from

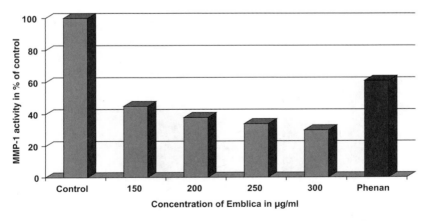

Figure 7 Collagenase (MMP-1) inhibitory activity of *Emblica* antioxidant.

increased collagen degradation without significant changes in production. It seems that the protection of existing collagen is more important than stimulating collagen production.

Stromelysin 1 (MMP-3) Inhibitory Activity of *Emblica* Antioxidant

An inhibition of stromelysin 1 activity by >50% was observed with *Emblica* antioxidant at 100 µg/mL (20). Quantification of MMP-3 inhibitory activity of *Emblica* antioxidant was determined using CHEMICON MMP-3/Stromelysin Activity Assay Kit (ECM 481). The principle of the assay is based upon fluorescence measurement of substrate fragments released upon cleavage of a substrate by MMP-3. Fluorescence intensity of the resulting product is measured and correlated with MMP-3 activity. Result of this study is summarized in Fig. 8.

Extracellular Matrix (ECM) Proteins

The ECM is a complex aggregate of distinct collagenic and noncollagenic protein components, which in physiologic situations are in a dynamic equilibrium. It can include any of several classes of biomolecules, including structural proteins, such as collagens and elastin; adhesion proteins, including fibronectins, laminins, and entactin; proteoglycans; and glycosaminoglycans. Further, the precise composition of the ECM can vary between tissues, and perhaps even in a cell state-specific manner. The ECM not only provides a supportive function for the development and organization of tissues, but also serves as a physical barrier to limit the migration of most normal cells away from their sites of origin.

The optimal quantities of different matrix components and their delicate interactions are clearly necessary to maintain normal physiologic properties of tissues such as skin. In fact, skin is a good example of an organ where the

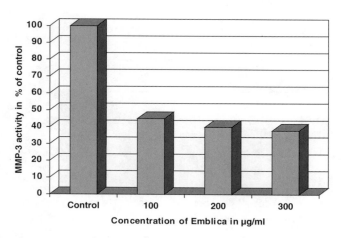

Figure 8 Stromelysin 1 (MMP-3) inhibitory activity of *Emblica* antioxidant.

ECM plays an integral role in providing physiologic properties to the tissue. This point has been well demonstrated by the fact that there are several examples where molecular aberrations in the structure or expression of components of the skin result in a phenotypically recognizable cutaneous disease (45). Most of the dermal ECM is synthesized by fibroblasts. Physical factors such as sunlight play a key role in altering the content and morphology of dermal ECM (44).

Stimulation of Noncollagenic Protein Synthesis

In a *in vitro* study using human skin fibroblast cells, Chaudhuri et al. (20) showed that *Emblica* antioxidant at 50 μg/mL increased the synthesis of noncollagenic proteins by ∼40% over control (without *Emblica*). An immunocolorimetric method (46) was used for quantifying collagenic and noncollagenic proteins. Interestingly, *Emblica* antioxidant had practically no effect on the synthesis of collagenic proteins. Characterization of the individual noncollagenic proteins has not been done.

Recently, Morganti et al. (47) has published a randomized double-blind placebo-controlled clinical study report using *Emblica* as a key component. In this study, Group 1 subjects were given *Emblica*, melatonin, and alpha-lipoic acid topically (twice-a-day) along with a dietary supplement consisting of ascorbic acid, tocopherol, lutein, and alpha-lipoic acid (two capsules a day), whereas the Group 2 subjects received only the carrier topically (placebo, twice-a-day) and the dietary supplement with antioxidants (two capsules a day) and the Group 3 subjects received only the carrier topically (placebo) and orally (placebo, no antioxidants). Results clearly showed statistically significant ($p < 0.005$) increase in skin hydration and skin lipids for both Groups 1 and 2 over a period of 2 months. However, Group 1 showed the highest increase both in skin hydration (55–100%) and skin lipids (55–70%) over placebo control. Moreover, oxidative stress and consequently formation of lipid peroxides in Group 1 subjects were also found to be lower by 30–40% ($p < 0.005$) over placebo control.

Skin Lightening/Skin Even-Toning

Pigmentation of the skin, due to the synthesis and dispersion of melanin in the epidermis, is of great cosmetic and societal significance. An abnormal increase in the amount of melanin in the epidermis can cause excessive pigmentation of the skin, or hyperpigmentation such as melasma and age spots. Pigmentation disorders can be caused by a number of factors—hormonal, inflammation, drugs, UV-radiation, and aging (48). Skin lightening agents have been widely used to either lighten or depigment the skin. Preparations in the European market tend to be used to treat age spots and freckles, whereas the Asian market uses them to change or modify skin color. A wide variety of skin lighteners, namely hydroquinone, kojic acid, and ascorbic acid derivatives such as magnesium ascorbyl phosphate, have been used for these purposes (49–51). A review of the literature showed that many plant extracts with limited standardization have the ability to lighten skin (52).

Chaudhuri et al. (53,54) have demonstrated the ability of *Emblica* antioxidant to lighten and even-tone normal, hyperpigmented and UV-induced pigmented skin color.

Emblica Antioxidant Lightens the Normal Skin Color

Chaudhuri et al. (53,54) performed four clinical studies demonstrating the effect of *Emblica* antioxidant on normal skin. In the first study, 13 Hispanic volunteers were treated for 9 weeks with a cream containing 2% *Emblica* antioxidant vs. 2% hydroquinone in upper arms (left and right). Skin color was determined by measuring individual typology angle (ITA) degree, which was calculated from the mean L^* and b^* Chroma Meter values using the formula:

$$\text{ITA degree} = \left[\frac{\text{Arctangent } (L^* - 50)}{b^*}\right] \frac{180}{3.1416}$$

Skin lightening effects were measured by subtracting the average ITA degree of the treated site from that of the average base line (first day of the study). Results of Δ ITA degree measurement showed that 2% *Emblica* antioxidant had induced a significant (two-tailed $p < 0.001$) lightening effect (Δ ITA = 5.2) at 9 week time-point, which was comparable to 2% hydroquinone (Δ ITA = 5.1). In the second study, 13 Asian volunteers were treated for 9 weeks as described for the first study. Results again showed a significant skin lightening ($p < 0.001$) induced by 2% *Emblica* antioxidant at 9 week time-point, which was comparable to 2% hydroquinone. In the third study, 16 Asian–American subjects were treated separately with 1% *Emblica* antioxidant vs. 3% magnesium ascorbyl phosphate (MAP) for a period of 9 weeks. Results showed a significant skin lightening effect with 1% *Emblica* antioxidant (Δ ITA = 4.5, $p < 0.005$) at 9 week time-point which is much better than 3% MAP (Δ ITA = 3.5, $p < 0.01$). Further scrutiny of the data revealed that the effect of skin lightening is much more pronounced in darker skin subjects (ITA $< +20$) with 1% *Emblica* antioxidant (Δ ITA = 7.0) than with 3% MAP (Δ ITA = 4.0). In the fourth study, 16 African–American subjects were treated separately as described before with 1% *Emblica* antioxidant and 2% kojic acid. Results showed a very significant ($p < 0.001$) skin lightening effect with 1% *Emblica* antioxidant (Δ ITA = 6.7) at 9 week time-point which is comparable to 2% kojic acid (Δ ITA = 7.3). A statistically significant skin lightening was also seen at 6 week time-point for both products.

Emblica Antioxidant Reduces Freckle Spots

Topical application of *Emblica* antioxidant in the form of a 1% lotion has been shown to provide a significant lightening of freckle spots (54,55). After 8 weeks of usage, 84% and 89% of subjects showed a statistically significant

($p < 0.005$) lightening of the freckle spots as determined by Δ ITA value (+6.0) and by L^* value (+1.18), respectively.

Emblica Antioxidant Reduces UV-Induced Erythema

Chaudhuri et al. (20) compared an *Emblica* antioxidant crème to MAP and vitamin E (natural tocopherol) preparations on humans *in vivo*. In this study, 10 subjects were applied topically for 8 days and then exposed to UV-irradiation and assessed the untreated control vs. the site with the product using ITA. Results showed a statistically significant ($p < 0.05$) reduction in erythema with 0.2% *Emblica* antioxidant (Δ ITA = 4.0), and 0.5% vitamin E (Δ ITA = 3.0), but not with 0.5% MAP. In a separate study, erythema was induced by UV-irradiation first and then formulated products were applied topically for 1 week. A statistically significant ($p < 0.05$) reduction in erythema was observed on 5th day with only 0.2% *Emblica* antioxidant. The other two antioxidants failed to show any effect.

Safety Data

Emblica antioxidant is found to be a safe product for cosmetics use as evident from the following studies.

Acute Oral Toxicity Study in Rats

Limit test: an acute oral toxicity test was conducted with rats to determine the potential for *Emblica* antioxidant to produce toxicity from a single dose via the oral route. Under the conditions of this study, the single dose acute oral LD_{50} is >5000 mg/kg of body weight in male and female rats. No animal died at the dose of 5000 mg/kg.

Primary Eye Irritation Study in Rabbits

A primary eye irritation test was conducted with rabbits to determine the potential for *Emblica* antioxidant to produce irritation from a single instillation via the ocular route. Under the conditions of this study, the test substance is classified as minimally irritating to both the un-rinsed and rinsed eyes.

Evaluation of Phototoxicity Potential by UV-A Irradiation on Human Subjects

A phototoxicity test was conducted with 20 human subjects to determine the potential for *Emblica* antioxidant to produce phototoxicity from a single dermal application. Under the conditions of this study, the test substance is classified as nonphototoxic when tested on human subjects at 2% dilution in distilled water. Not a single subject showed any adverse effects.

Repeat Insult Patch Test on Human Subjects/Skin Irritation and Skin Sensitization Evaluation

A repeat insult patch test was conducted with 200 human subjects to determine the potential for *Emblica* antioxidant to produce primary irritation and primary sensitization. Under the conditions of the study, *Emblica* antioxidant (2.0% in water) is considered as a nonprimary irritant and a nonprimary sensitizer to the human skin. Not a single subject showed any adverse effects.

Bacterial Mutagenicity Test

Emblica was examined for mutagenic activity in two series of *in vitro* microbial assays employing *Salmonella typhimurium* (five strains) and *Escheria coli* (one strain) as test organisms. In both series of experiments, each was performed with and without the addition of rat liver S9 mix as the external metabolizing system. Results showed no increase in the number of revertants of any bacterial strain. Under the conditions of the study, *Emblica* antioxidant was found to be not a mutagenic material.

CONCLUSION

Photoaging of skin is a complex biologic process affecting various layers of the skin with major changes seen in the connective tissue of the dermis. The natural shift toward a more pro-oxidant state in intrinsically aged skin can be significantly enhanced by UV-irradiation. *Emblica* antioxidant, has been shown to be a cosmetic ingredient with an extraordinary breadth of cutaneous benefits. It displays distinct advantages over other ingredients with similar benefits such as retinol, vitamin C, in that it is well tolerated, and is easy to formulate with and is not subject to photodegradation.

Melanogenesis is the process of production and subsequent distribution of melanin by melanocytes and is controlled by many factors. Skin lighteners can inhibit tyrosinase activity, or blocking the chain reaction at the various points of the melanogenesis pathway. Tyrosinase inhibition is the key mode of action of most of the commercial skin lighteners. *Emblica* antioxidant, being an excellent chelator for iron and copper, is not a strong tyrosinase inhibitor; instead it reduces melanin synthesis by inhibiting peroxidase-H_2O_2 and non-enzymatic (Fe^{2+}/H_2O_2) pathways (55). *Emblica* antioxidant has been shown to be a safe and effective skin lightener as demonstrated by several clinical studies. It displays distinct advantages over other skin lightening ingredients such as hydroquinone, MAP and kojic acid, in that it is well tolerated, and is easy to formulate with and has no adverse side effects.

A properly constituted *P. emblica* extract (*Emblica* antioxidant), such as the one described here, may provide a great value as a photoprotective agent (in combination with sunscreens and other antiaging ingredients) and skin lightening agent. In short, the multiplicity of effects and formulation benefits seen with *Emblica* antioxidant make it an ideal choice for a variety of cosmetic products targeting young and matured skin alike.

REFERENCES

1. Holm-Nielsen LB. Comments on the distribution and evolution of the genus *Phyllanthus* (Euphorbiacea). In: Larsen K, Holm-Nielsen LB, eds. Tropical Botany. New York: Academic Press, 1979:277–290.
2. Unander DW, Webster GL, Blumberg BS. Records of usage or assays in *Phyllanthus* (Euphorbiaceae). I. Subgenera *Isocladus, Kirganelia, Cicca* and *Emblica*. J Ethnopharmacol 1990; 30:233–264.
3. Unander DW, Webster GL, Blumberg BS. Usage and bioassays in *Phyllanthus* (Euphorbiaceae): a compilation. II. The subgenus *Phyllanthus*. J Ethnopharmacol 1991; 34:97–133.
4. Unander DW, Webster GL, Blumberg BS. Usage and bioassays in *Phyllanthus* (Euphorbiaceae): a compilation. III. The subgenera *Eriococcus, Conami, Gomphidium, Botryanthus, Xylophylla and Phyllanthodendron*, and a complete list of the species cited in the three-part series. J Ethnopharmacol 1992; 36:103–112.
5. Unander DW, Webster GL, Blumberg BS. Usage and bioassays in *Phyllanthus* (Euphorbiaceae). IV. Clustering of antiviral uses and other effects. J Ethnopharmacol 1995; 45:1–18.
6. Calixto JB, Santos ARS, Filho VC, Yunes RA. A review of the genus *Phyllanthus*: their chemistry, pharmacology and therapeutic potential. Med Res Rev 1998. 18:225–258.
7. Okuda T, Yoshida T, Hatano T. Hydrolyzable tannins and related polyphenols. Fort Chem Org Nat 1995; 66:1–117.
8. Gottlieb OR. The role of oxygen in phytochemical evolution towards diversity. Phytochemistry 1989; 28:2545–2558.
9. Hatano T, Edmatsu R, Hiramatsu M, Mori A, Fujita Y, Yashura T, Yoshida T, Okuda T. Effects of the interaction of tannins with co-existing substance. VI. Effects of tannins and related polyphenols on superoxide anion radical. Chem Pharm Bull 1989; 37:2016–2021.
10. Okuda T, Yoshida T, Hatano T. Correlation of oxidative transformations of hydrolyzable tannins and plant evolution. Phytochemistry 2000; 55:513–529.
11. Gardner RO. Systematic distribution and ecological function of the secondary metabolites of the Rosidae–Asteridae. Biochem Sys Ecol 1977; 5:29–35.
12. Chopra RN, Nayar SL, Chopra IC. Glossary of Indian Medicinal Plants. New Delhi: CSIR, 1956.
13. Sharma PV. Dravyaguna Vijnana. Varanasi: Chaukhamba Sanskirt Sansthan, 1978.
14. Naik KG, Shah CC, Pandya HG. Ascorbic acid content of some common fruits and vegetables available in Gujarat. I. Vitamin C content and its stability. J Univ Bombay 1951; 19(Pt. 5 (Science No. 29)):51–58.
15. Nizamuddin M, Hoffman J, Larm O. Fractionation and characterization of carbohydrates from *Emblica officinalis* Gaertn. Fruit. Swedish J Agric Res 1982; 12:3–7.
16. Ghosal S, Triphati VK, Chauhan S. Active constituents of *Emblica officinalis*: Part I—the chemistry and antioxidative effects of two new hydrolyzable tannins, Emblicanin A and B. Indian J Chem 1996; 35B:941–948, and references cited therein.

17. Chaudhuri RK, Schewitz J. Monograph of Emblica. Merck KGaA, Darmstadt: Germany, 2001.
18. Zhang YJ, Abe T, Tanaka T, Yang CR, Kouno I. Phyllanemblinins A-F. New ellagitannins form *Phyllanthus emblica*. J Nat Prod 2001; 64:1527–1532.
19. Chaudhuri RK, Puccetti G. Transition metal-induced oxidation: implications for skin care products. Cosme Toil 2002; 117:43–56.
20. Chaudhuri RK, Puccetti G, Hwang C, Guttierez G, Serrar M. Low molecular-weight tannins of *Phyllanthus emblica* fruits: a new class of anti-aging ingredients. Cosmetics Toiletries, 2003; 119:59–70.
21. Ahmad N, Katiyar SK, Mukhtar H. Antioxidants in chemoprevention. In: Thiele J, Elsner J, eds. Oxidants and Antioxidants in Cutaneous Biology. Current Problems in Dermatology. Basel: Karger, 2001:29, 128–139.
22. Scharffetter-Kochanek K, Brenneisen P, Wenk J, Herrmann G, Ma W, Kuhr L, Meewes C, Wlaschek M. Photoaging of the skin from phenotype to mechanisms. Exp Gerentol 2000; 35:307–316.
23. Chaudhuri RK. Emblica cascading antioxidant: a novel natural skin care ingredient. Skin Pharmacol Appl Skin Physiol 2002a; 15:374–380.
24. Halliwell B, Guttridge JM, Aruoma OI. The deoxyribose method: a simple test tube assay for determination of rate constants for reactions of hydroxyl radicals. Anal Biochem 1987; 165:215–219.
25. Gomes AJ, Lunardi CN, Gonzales S, Tedesco AC. The antioxidant action of *Polypodium leucotomos* extract and kojic acid: reactions with reactive oxygen species. Braz J Med Biol Res 2001; 34:1487–1494.
26. Richard M, Guiraud JP, Monjo AM, Favier A. Development of a simple antioxidant screening system assay using human skin fibroblasts. Free Rad Res Commun 1992; 16:303–314.
27. Kraljic I, El Moshni S. A new method for the detection of singlet oxygen in aqueous solutions. Photochem Photobiol 1978; 28:577–582.
28. Gonzalez S, Pathak MA. Inhibition of ultraviolet-induced formation of reactive oxygen species, lipid peroxidation, erythema and skin photosentization by *Polypodium leucotomos*. Photodermatol Photoimmunol Photomed 1996; 12:45–56.
29. Kato K, Terao N, Shimamoto N, Hirata M. Studies on scavengers of active oxygen species. 1. Synthesis and biological activity of 2-O-alkylascorbic acid. J Med Chem 1988; 31:793–798.
30. Bhattacharya A, Chatterjee A, Ghosal S, Bhattachraya SK. Antioxidant activity of tannoid principles of *Emblica officinalis* (amla). Indian J Exp Biol 1999; 37:676–680.
31. Bissett DL, McBride JF. Iron content of human epidermis from sun-exposed and non-exposed body sites. J Soc Cosmet Chem 1992; 43:215–217.
32. Gutteridge JM, Rowley DA, Halliwell B, Cooper DF, Heeley DM. Copper and iron complexes catalytic for oxygen radical reactions in sweat from human athletes. Clin Chim Acta 1985; 145:267–273.
33. Masaki H, Atsumi T, Sakurai H. Detection of hydrogen peroxide and hydroxyl radicals in murine skin fibroblasts under UVB irradiation. Biochem Biophys Res Commun 1995; 206:474–479.
34. Pourzand C, Watkin RD, Brown JE, Tyrell RM. Ultraviolet A radiation induces immediate release of iron in human primary skin fibroblasts: the role of ferritin. Proc Natl Acad Sci USA 1999; 96:6751-6756.

35. Halliwell B, Gutteridge JM. Role of free radicals and catalytic metal ions in human disease. Meth Enzymol 1990; 186:1–85.
36. Halliwell B, Gutteridge JM. Free radicals in Biology and Medicine, 3rd ed., London: Oxford Science Publications, 1999:298–299.
37. Bast A, Haenen GRM, Doelman CJA. Oxidants and antioxidants: sate of the art. Am J Med 1991; 91(Suppl 3C):2S–8S.
38. Graf E, Mahoney JR, Byrant RG, Eaton JW. Iron catalyzed hydroxyl radical formation, stringent requirement for free iron coordination site. J Biol Chem 1984; 259:3620–3624.
39. Hoekstra R, Eskens FALM, Verweij J. Matrix metalloprotease inhibitors: current developments and future perspectives. Oncologist 2001; 6:415–427.
40. Brenneisen P, Oh J, Wlashek M, Wenk J, Briviba K, Hommel C, Herrmann G, Sies H, Scharffetter-Kochanek K. Ultraviolet B wavelength dependence for the regulation of two major matrix-metalloproteinases and their inhibitor TIMP-1 in human dermal fibroblasts. Photochem Photobiol 1996; 64:877–885.
41. Brenneisen P, Wenk J, Klotz LO, Wlaschek M, Brivia K, Krieg T, Sies H, Scharffetter-Kochanek K. Central role of ferrous–ferric iron in the ultraviolet B irradiation-mediated signaling pathway leading to increased interstitial collagenase (matrix-degrading metalloprotease (MMP)-1) and stromelysin-1 (MMP-3) mRNA levels in cultured human dermal fibroblasts. J Biol Chem 1998; 273:5279–5287.
42. Fisher G, Wang ZQ, Datta SC, Varani J, Kang S, Voorhees J. Pathophysiology of premature skin aging induced by ultraviolet light. New Engl J Med 1997; 337:1419–1429.
43. Thibodeau A. Metalloprotease inhibitors. Cosmet Toiletries 2000; 115:75–82.
44. Bernstein EF, Uitto J. The effect of photodamage on dermal extracellular matrix. Clinics in Dermatology 1996; 14:143–151.
45. Uitto J, Olsen DR, Fazio MJ. Extracellular matrix of the skin: 50 years of progress. J Invest Dermatol, Supplement 1989; 61S–76S.
46. Guerret S, Rojkind M, Druguet M, Chevallier M, Grimaud JA. Collagen Rel Res 1988; 8:249–259.
47. Morganti P, Bruno C, Guarneri F, Cardillo A, Del Ciotto P, Valenzano F. Role of topical and nutritional supplement to modify the oxidative stress. Int J Cosmet Sci 2002; 24:331–339.
48. Perez-Bernal A, Munoz-Perez MA, Camacho F. Management of facial hyperpigmentation. Am J Clin Dermatol 2000; 1:261–268.
49. Morganti P, Fabrizi G, James B. An innovative cosmeceutical with skin whitening activity. J Appl Cosmetol 1999; 18:144–153.
50. Zhai H, Maibach HI. Skin-whitening agents. Cosm Toil 2001; 116:21–25.
51. Zuidhoff HW, van Rijsbergen JM. Whitening efficacy of frequently used whitening ingredients. Cosm Toil 2001; 116:53–59.
52. Gupta S. Formulation of plant-based skin whitening cosmetics. Happi 2001; 38:90–93.
53. Chaudhuri RK. A standardized extract of *Phyllanthus emblica*: A skin lightener with anti-aging benefits. Asia Pacific Personal Care 2005; 6: January issue.
54. Chaudhuri RK, Marchio F. Hydrolyzable tannins from *Phyllanthus emblica*: A new class of safe and effective skin lightening agent, Proceedings of Personal Care Ingredients Asia, Shanghai, 2002:7–15.

55. Chaudhuri RK. 2004, Unpublished work.
56. Foo LY. Amariin, a di-dehydrohexahydroxydiphenoyl hydrolyzable tannin from *Phyllanthus amarus*. Phytochemistry 1993; 33(2):487–491.
57. Foo LY. Amariinic acid and related ellagitannins from *Phyllanthus amarus*. Phytochemistry 1995; 39(1):217–224.
58. Qian-Cutrone J, Huang A, Trimble J, Li H, Lin PF, Alam M, Klohr SE, Kadow KF. Niruriside, a new HIV REV/RRE binding inhibitor from *Phyllanthus niruri*. J Nat Prod 1996; 59:196–199.
59. Yoshida T, Itoh H, Matsunaga S, Tanaka R, Okuda T. Tannins and related polyphenols of euphorbiaceous plants. Part IX: Hydrolyzable tannins with $^1C_4$ glucose core from *Phyllanthus flexuosus* Muell Arg Chem Pharm Bull (Japan) 1992; 40:53–60. Fort Chem Org Nat 1995; 66:1–117.
60. Huang YL, Chen CC, Hsu FL, Chen CF. Tannins, flavonol sulfonates and a norlignann from *Phyllanthus virgatus*. J Nat Prod 1998; 61:1194–1197.
61. Jikai L, Yue H, Henkel T, Weber K. One step purification of corilagin and ellagic acid from *Phyllanthus urinaria* using high-speed countercurrent chromatography. Phytochem Anal 2002; 13:1–3.
62. Liu KCSC, Lin MT, Lee SS, Chiou JF, Ren S, Lien EJ. Antiviral tannins from two *Phyllanthus* species. Planta Med 1999; 65(1):43–46.
63. Miguel OG, Calixto JB, Santos AR, Messana I, Ferrari F, Cechinel FV, Pizzolatti MG, Yunes RA. Chemical and preliminary analgesic evaluation of geraniin and furosin isolated from *Phyllanthus sellowianus*. Planta Med 1996; 62(2):146–149.

27

Management of Unwanted Facial Hair by Topical Application of Eflornithine

Douglas Shander and Gurpreet S. Ahluwalia
Gillette Advanced Technology Center/US, Needham, Massachusetts, USA

Joseph P. Morton
Morton Associates Inc., Silver Spring, Maryland, USA

Management of Unwanted Facial Hair in Women	490
Eflornithine, a Selective Inhibitor of ODC and Hair Growth	491
Eflornithine Delivery to Anagen Hair Follicle	492
Preclinical and Pharmacokinetic Studies with Eflornithine Formulations	494
Percutaneous ADME Studies	494
Clinical Safety of Topical Eflornithine	495
Eflornithine Clinical Studies for Facial Hair Growth Reduction	496
Phase I Clinical Study	496
Phase II and Phase III Clinical Studies (Placebo Controlled)	497
Objective Measures of Facial Hair Growth by Videoimaging in the Phase II and Phase III Studies	500
Phase II Objective Hair Length Reductions	500
Phase II Investigator Perceptions	502
Subject Perception Evaluations	504
Phase III Perception	506
Conclusions	507
References	508

MANAGEMENT OF UNWANTED FACIAL HAIR IN WOMEN

Facial hair is a very disturbing and even psychologically debilitating condition in hirsute women and these women are among the most grateful patients when a treatment is found to lessen the severity of their condition (1). A study from 20 years ago suggested that the level of facial hair, which is regarded as socially unacceptable by the public and distressing to those with the condition, was below that which many physicians would classify as clinical hirsutism (2). Today, the management of unwanted facial hair is not limited to the severe hirsute women, and unwanted facial hair is recognized as a problem confronting a large segment of women. Studies conducted by the NFO Research Group in 1992 and 1999 demonstrated that unwanted facial hair is a chronic problem for $\sim$22 million women in the USA, and of the 13,000 women surveyed, 20% removed facial hair at least weekly and 4% of women found it necessary to remove hair every single day.

A recent web-based survey of 481 women conducted by Yankelovich and Partners found unwanted facial hair to be a pet beauty peeve by >45% of women and 19% of women spend some time every week managing unwanted facial hair, which confirms the NFO research report. These studies indicate that there is a need to improve the effectiveness and convenience of treatments for unwanted facial hair.

A product for facial hair retardation has appeal to a large and heterogeneous audience of women including those with a severe degree of facial hair who would welcome any perceptible improvement in their condition, as well as women bothered by a slight degree of unwanted facial hair who desire smooth hair-free skin without much effort or inconvenience. For clinically hirsute women, pharmaceutical treatments include systemic use of steroidal and nonsteroidal antiandrogens, such as cypoterone acetate, spironolactone, flutamide, finasteride, and cimetidine. However, these agents have serious side effects and have not been approved for treatment of hirsutism in the USA. Although antiandrogens stop the progression of hirsutism, they are not generally very effective in reversing hirsutism and they must be used on a continuous basis to maintain efficacy (3).

An effective management of facial hair requires a combination of approaches and includes such temporary cosmetic measures as plucking, tweezing, waxing, depilatory creams, and shaving. The most effective treatments including laser devices and electrolysis, as both cause damage to the hair follicle and surrounding tissue to provide longer lasting effects of hair inhibition than waxing or tweezing. Electrolysis can provide safe and permanent hair removal when performed by skilled practitioners but may require many treatments over months or years especially for severe conditions or large areas. Each of these systems has certain advantages and disadvantages that range from ease of removal to severe skin irritation and patient awareness of the choices is essential to make informed decisions (4).

FDA approved treatments include laser systems that provide rapid and efficient hair inhibition for larger surfaces but treatments must be performed on a repeated basis to sustain efficacy and it is not known what number of treatments provides maximal benefit and which specific laser treatment regimens are best used for the wide spectrum of consumers with a variety of needs and expectations (5). The treatment outcome varies on the basis of hair color, as patients with blonde, red, or white hair are much less likely to experience the longer lasting reduction than subjects with dark hair and light skin (6). Initially, laser treatments were limited to lighter subjects with lighter skin and dark hair, but diode lasers with long pulse widths (7), as well as long-pulse 1064 nm Nd:YAG lasers (8), appear effective for facial treatments in all skin types. However, additional clinical studies are required to further determine the safe parameters for laser hair removal in skin types IV–VI (9). Unwanted facial hair can also be treated with noncoherent, filtered intense pulsed light source (10). Although light-mediated systems are very effective in hair removal and the relatively minor side effects are transitory, a recent report provides verification of anecdotal accounts indicating that laser treatment of unwanted facial hair can actually stimulate hair growth on the lateral face where new terminal hairs grew at or adjacent to treated sites (11). Facial hair management, therefore, requires special care and a combination of treatment modalities to maximize outcome. Hair retardants that slow hair regrowth offer a safe and effective method to boost efficacy of a variety of epilation, depilation, and hair inhibition regimens and also contribute to increasing safety of other modalities by decreasing their frequency of use. Recently, shave minimizing creams have been offered as over-the-counter treatments for hair reduction; however, there is no convincing clinical evidence that any of these products actually reduce hair growth rate. In fact, these products often claim that repeated use makes hair feel softer, finer, and less noticeable (4). Some products claim that with emergence of softer and finer hairs a reduction in the frequency of shaving occurs and to date there are no placebo-controlled blinded studies using independent investigators to objectively demonstrate facial hair reduction by shave minimizing moisturizers using prospectively defined criteria of efficacy. VANIQA^{TM}, a cream containing 13.9% eflornithine hydrochloride is the only FDA approved topical treatment for unwanted facial hair and it acts to slow the rate of hair growth. It can be used with other hair management procedures such as waxing, tweezing, or shaving to boost their effectiveness in managing the visibility of unwanted hair. Moreover, the treatment increases the ability of facial cosmetics to conceal hair especially in women with heavy facial hair who often suffer from 5 o'clock shadow, which is difficult to hide as lengths of terminal hair approach a readily perceptible threshold in the afternoon.

EFLORNITHINE, A SELECTIVE INHIBITOR OF ODC AND HAIR GROWTH

Ornithine decarboxylase (ODC) catalyzes the metabolism of ornithine to putrescine and subsequently to other polyamines (12). The pattern of increased ODC and DNA synthesis in mouse follicles was found to be congruent with the onset of anagen hair growth cycle of mice (13), and ODC was found to be abundantly expressed in proliferating bulb cells of anagen follicles (14). These reports suggested the involvement of ODC in the regulation of hair growth. It is believed that reduction in cellular polyamine levels results in slowing cellular growth of highly proliferative tissues such as the hair follicle, intestinal epithelium, and neoplastic tissue. Interestingly, inhibition of ODC by eflornithine causes a striking decrease in cell proliferation in skin tumors in mice without any effect on nonneoplastic epidermal keratinocytes (15). On the backs of male Golden Syria hamsters, there are paired oval shaped pigmented spots of $\sim$8 mm diameter called "flank organs" that grow terminal hair, and these structures provide an excellent model to study androgen-dependent hair growth and have been used to screen antiandrogen compounds that reduce hair mass (16). In addition, the follicle growth of flank organs is marked by high levels of ODC and polyamines that are stimulated by androgens and a variety of antiandrogen inhibitors of hair growth affecting ODC activity were screened using the decreases in flank organ ODC as a surrogate endpoint for antiandrogenic activity (17), as well as inhibitors of ODC that act to retard hair growth (18). Among the ODC inhibitors tested, eflornithine was the most effective, and caused a dose-dependent reduction in hair growth as measured by hair mass on the flank organ that was accompanied by a concomitant reduction in hair follicle ODC activity and polyamine levels. The levels of the polyamine putrescine were reduced the greatest and spermidine levels declined moderately, whereas the spermine levels did not change (19). Eflornithine- (DFMO, alpha-difluormethylornithine) is a rationally designed, enzyme activated, irreversible inhibitor of the enzyme ODC (20). Eflornithine was selected as the prime candidate for clinical development in unwanted facial hair as it was the most effective hair growth inhibitor in the model system, and a significant amount of safety data with a substantial toxicological profile had already been generated by the Merrel-Dow company in their efforts to develop this molecule as an anticancer drug. Later, collaborative efforts between Merrell-Dow and the WHO to develop a treatment for trypanosomiasis culminated in the prescription of eflornithine product Ornidyl® for parental use. It has been suggested that eflornithine is a cytostatic rather than a cytotoxic agent (12).

A systematic evaluation of potenial amino acid analog chemotherapuetic agents including eflornithine was conducted in 60 different human-derived cancer cell lines and eflornithine failed to elicit any cytotoxic effects (21). Because of its primarily cytostatic activity the effectiveness of eflornithine in human clinical trials was modest at best and it failed to demonstrate significant efficacy when used as a single treatment.

EFLORNITHINE DELIVERY TO ANAGEN HAIR FOLLICLE

Results from the animal model studies demonstrated specific, potent, and localized effect of eflornithine on hair growth reduction. To translate this efficacy into humans an effective delivery system was needed that could carry this highly hydrophyllic (eflornithine has water solubility of 45%) and charged molecule to a typical 3–5 mm depth of the human facial hair follicle. A hydroalcoholic vehicle containing 68% water, 16% ethanol, 5% propylene glycol, 5% dipropylene glycol, 4% benzyl alcohol, and 2% propylene carbonate was developed to obtain an eflornithine solubility of $\sim$15% (hereafter referred to as the hydroalcoholic vehicle). A 10% eflornithine in this carrier vehicle was stable for over 1 year at room temperature. This combination of ingredients provided the eflornithine penetration enhancement of about two- and four-fold when compared with the simple water–ethanol (80:20) and ethanol–water (70:30) vehicles, respectively.

A single topical application of 10% eflornithine in the hydroalcholic vehicle decreased flank organ follicle levels of ODC two- to threefold between 1 and 24 h after treatment. The putrescine levels were reduced almost twofold within 6 h and threefold within a 24 h period after treatment. The decreases in ODC and putrescine were limited to the treated flank organ (19). These results established that delivery of DFMO in the hydroalcholic vehicle provides a degree of skin penetration that enables rapid inhibition of the target enzyme ODC and the end products, polyamine, in hair follicles without affecting the untreated flank organ. The observed increase in penetration also translated into a corresponding increase in hair growth reduction efficacy. When eflornithine was delivered in simple water–alcohol solutions the effects on hair growth reduction were at best marginal. A significant hair growth reduction was observed, however, with eflornithine delivered in the hydroalcoholic vehicle. Inhibition of hair mass was also dose-dependent, with the 1% and 2% eflornithine doses causing 30% and 50% reduction. Additional studies assessing hair growth rates demonstrated that treatment with 10% eflornithine in the hydroalcholic vehicle caused a 30–40% decrease in hair length within 7 days and a 65–80% decrease after 17 days of treatment. Morphologic studies indicated no adverse effects to the flank organ skin. Most remarkable was the selective effect of eflornithine on the hair follicle as the sebaceous glands and epidermis were unaffected as was the surface diameter of flank organ that contrasts the miniaturization of the follicle and sebaceous glands and the reduction of flank organ diameter by antiandrogens. The DFMO treatment actually caused the follicle to shrink, as the bulb normally embedded in hypodermal fat in the subcutis area retracted back into dermis after treatment. The rapid ODC inhibition and observed follicular shrinkage resulted in hair mass and hair length reductions after topical eflornithine treatment, and strongly support the conclusion that ODC inhibition caused by eflornithine leads to hair growth retardation in which rate of hair growth is slowed without hair cycle changes.

A moisturizing lotion for facial application in women was subsequently developed (22), which showed efficacy in flank organ model comparable to the hydroalcoholic vehicle. The components of this o/w emulsion included water (80.84%), glyceryl stearate (4.24%), PEG-100 stearate (4.09%), cetearyl alcohol (3.05%), ceteareth-20 (2.5%), mineral oil (2.22%), stearyl alcohol

(1.67%), dimethicone (0.56%), and preservative (0.83%) (hereafter referred to as the cream vehicle). A 13.9% eflornithine hydrochloride in this vehicle is now the currently marketed Rx product VANIQA™.

PRECLINICAL AND PHARMACOKINETIC STUDIES WITH EFLORNITHINE FORMULATIONS

Several animal and human pharmacokinetic studies were performed with the hydroalcoholic and the cream eflornithine formulations to assess the extent of dermal penetration into blood and tissues.

The absorption, excretion, and tissue distribution of radioactivity in male and female mice were studied after single dermal application of radiolabeled eflornithine to each mouse. This study was done in three groups of six male and six female mice each. The doses were removed at 4 h after application for group 1, and at 6 h for groups 2 and 3. Mice in groups 1, 2, and 3 were sacrificed at 4, 24, and 96 h after dermal application. The mean dermal absorption of eflornithine (calculated from blood, urine, feces, and tissue activity) was less than 0.84% of the applied dose for all groups and sexes. The mean recovery in urine and feces ranged from 0.11% to 0.44% and <0.005% to 0.39%, respectively. The mean recovery of radioactivity in tissues at the time of sacrifice ranged from <0.005% to 0.04%. The area under the concentration vs. time curve (AUC 0-inf) for total radioactivity in the blood of male and female mice was 2.35 and 2.68 µg equivalent/h per g, respectively. There were no apparent differences in the excretion, absorption, and distribution of radioactivity in male and female mice following single dermal doses of [14C]-eflornithine.

Eflornithine pharmacokinetics, after multiple topical doses, was determined in rats after twice-daily dermal topical treatments with a topical formulation of 15% [14C]-eflornithine (7.5 mg/rat per dose, 30 µCi/dose) delivered in VANIQA™ cream. Rats treated twice daily were sacrificed at 18 h after the second dose on days 1, 3, and 5. On the basis of the recovery of radioactive dose in urine and feces, dermal absorption of eflornithine after twice-daily application ranged from 0.18% to 0.75%. The tissues with the highest concentration of radioactivity were generally the organs associated with elimination, but preferential accumulation did not occur in any tissue.

Percutaneous ADME Studies

Two clinical pharmacology (percutaneous ADME) studies have been conducted in women. The first was an open-label, randomized, parallel-design study with 18 adult women in which the absorption, excretion, and metabolism of topically applied eflornithine were determined. The formulations included 10% eflornithine in the hydroalcoholic vehicle, and 10% and 15% eflornithine in the cream formulation (VANIQA™ base). Single topical doses containing 40 µCi of [U-14C]-eflornithine in each of the three formulations was applied to the chin area (2.0 cm × 2.5 cm area) of three groups of six subjects each. The formulation remained on the site of application for 8 h. Serial blood samples at selected time points and all of the urine and feces were collected over a period of 120 h after dosing. Blood samples from all subjects at all time intervals showed no radioactivity, with the exception of two individuals who showed spurious values at two time intervals that were near the lower limits of radioactivity detection. As a result no pharmacokinetic analysis was possible. The majority of radioactivity excreted in urine was at 12–24 h post-dose time interval for all groups. The average excretion of radioactivity in the cumulative 120 h urine samples accounted for 0.35%, 0.17%, and 0.19% of the applied eflornithine dose in hydroalcoholic (10% eflornithine), 15% eflornithine cream base, and 10% eflornithine cream base, respectively. Because the absorbed eflornithine is rapidly excreted via the renal route, the urinary recovery of radioactivity can be used as a measure of topical absorption. The percutaneous absorption of eflornithine was estimated to be <1% of the applied dose in the two formulations tested.

The topically absorbed eflornithine was recovered predominantly in the urine, unchanged and unmetabolized. Though the molecular mechanism of eflornithine's inhibition of ODC indicates that the molecule is decarboxylated by ODC in the course of its suicidal enzyme inhibition, the metabolite, decarboxylated-eflornithine, was not found in any detectable amounts in the urinary fraction. Essentially, all of the urinary radioactivity co-eluted with the parent molecule on HPLC. This also suggests that only a small fraction of the absorbed eflornithine is involved in enzyme inhibition, and that skin does not appear to play a major role in eflornithine metabolism. This initial percutaneous ADME study was crucial in the development of VANIQA^{TM}, as it provided the first critical safety data on the extent of eflornithine absorption into human skin and the use of eflornithine in the new moisturizer that was later approved as VANIQA^{TM}. This data also supported the Phase II clinical dose–response study using the eflornithine moisturizing formulations.

The effect of multiple dosing on the absorption and excretion profile of eflornithine was determined in a subsequent study that was conducted under the more likely conditions of use (23,24). Plasma levels of eflornithine reached steady state after 4 days of application, and multiple dosing had no apparent effect on the disposition kinetics. Eflornithine was eliminated primarily via renal excretion. The mean percutaneous absorption was determined to be 0.34% of the first single dose and 0.82% of the last dose. Results of this study confirmed the low absorption and rapid excretion of eflornithine found in the first study, with the systemic absorption that remained below the 1% level under conditions of clinical use.

Clinical Safety of Topical Eflornithine

Topical eflornithine is safe and well tolerated, and the most frequent treatment-related adverse events occurred in the skin and were mild. There were no serious treatment-related adverse events in the open-label studies conducted for up to a year (25). The placebo-controlled laboratory tests and physical examinations did not reveal any changes attributable to topical eflornithine and the percentage of subjects reporting adverse events was comparable for both eflornithine and vehicle groups and only transient burning and stinging occurred more frequently in eflornithine-treated subjects than vehicle-treated subjects (26). Eflornithine HCl 13.9% cream does not have contact sensitizing, photocontact allergic or phototoxic properties. It can cause irritation under exaggerated conditions of use. Eflornithine HCl 13.9% cream, therefore, has a favorable dermal safety profile appropriate for a topical treatment to be applied routinely in lifetime use (27).

Presently, eflornithine is also being tested as a systemically administered agent in chemoprevention trials in patient populations that are at elevated risk for the development of specific epithelial cancers, including cutaneous, colon, esophageal, bladder, breast, and prostate malignancies. The side effects of eflornithine at intermediate ($1-3$ g/m^2 per day) doses are few and limited to mild gastrointestinal upset and reversible hearing changes. At the doses (<0.50 g/m^2 per day) of eflornithine being proposed for long-term chemoprevention trials, no systematic side effects (including hearing loss) have been seen (28). Most recently it has been proposed to incorporate eflornithine in sunscreen lotions to improve chemoprevention efficacy and reduce skin cancer incidence, as the Phase II randomized trial of topical eflornithine indicated the treatment reduced AK lesions and suppressed polyamines (29).

EFLORNITHINE CLINICAL STUDIES FOR FACIAL HAIR GROWTH REDUCTION

Phase I Clinical Study

The first clinical test that was sponsored by The Gillette Company included an open-label study in 30 women with mild to moderate degrees of unwanted facial hair who treated areas of their face with unwanted facial hair twice daily with 10% eflornithine HCl in a hydroalcoholic vehicle for 24 weeks. The efficacy measures were based on perceptions of a dermatologist as well as the responses of subjects to questions on the effect of the drug on their unwanted facial hair. A key aspect assessing the perception of efficacy by subjects included their response to the open ended question "Since you started applying the product do you feel the treatment has had a beneficial effect?". Twenty-four of thirty subjects specifically noted a reduction in the rate and/or amount of hair growth in response to the question. The responses were not prompted by any descriptors on hair length or character and illuminated the salient benefits of less visible amounts of hair. Subjects with most severe hair growth as indicated by hair removal frequency on a daily basis also reported a significant reduction in hair removal. These "clearly perceptible" effects of topical eflornithine on growth rate and changes in hair removal frequency were specifically addressed in assessments of perception benefits in Phase II studies in women with pronounced degrees of unwanted facial hair and Phase III studies with women with moderate to excessive degrees of unwanted facial hair. In addition to the subject perception data from the Phase I study, the dermatologist noted that all but two subjects, including those who dropped out of the study prior to the completion of the treatment period, experienced a reduction in the number of hairs in the treated areas. Seven subjects had dramatic reductions and would be considered totally "normal" and completely free of obvious hair growth patterns on their face. In individual interviews after the Phase I, many of the subjects indicated that they felt more comfortable in a variety of social and work-related situations where they previously experienced considerable degrees of self-consciousness and discomfort because to their concern over the visibility of facial hair. The Phase II dose–response and multicenter Pivotal Phase III studies evaluated eflornithine delivered in the more aesthetically appealing cream-based vehicle discussed previously and confirmed and extended the Phase I results that strongly suggested that eflornithine decreased the visibility of facial hair and how the perception of improved appearance had a positive impact on the quality of life in these subjects.

Phase II and Phase III Clinical Studies (Placebo Controlled)

The Phase II dose–response study was sponsored by The Gillette Company (30) and conducted at a single site. At least 30 subjects were initially assigned to each of four groups including vehicle, 5%, 10%, or 15% eflornithine (hydrochloride monohydrate) used in cream base and 106 subjects completed treatments. The subjects were women with more severe degrees of unwanted facial hair as all subjects removed hairs at least three times or more per week and 63% of subjects removed hair daily. The majority of subjects (70%) used shaving as well as tweezing or a combination of both methods to remove hair. Baseline measurements of hair revealed that growth rate of terminal chin hairs in subjects (0.2–0.3 mm/day) was the same as growth rates in adult males. The average density of terminal chin hairs was 27 hairs/cm^2 in the women participants compared with the density of 46 hairs/cm^2 chin hairs in men determined by same method. Subject assignments to groups were stratified by age (18–30 years and 31–46 years) and severity of terminal facial hair area coverage in the chin region. Less severe facial hair was indicated by 50–75% area coverage with terminal hairs of moderate density ($\sim$5–15 hairs/cm^2), and most severe condition of facial hair corresponded to complete chin area coverage with terminal hairs of heavy density ($>$20 hairs/cm^2).

The Phase III multicenter studies jointly sponsored by The Gillette Company and Bristol-Myers-Squibb included 596 subjects divided into two studies, which were randomized double blind vehicle-controlled studies in which subjects applied eflornithine cream or vehicle treatments for 24 weeks followed by 8 week no-treatment period. In Phase III trials women with less severe degrees of unwanted facial hair were eligible for enrollment and inclusion criteria were modified to qualify subjects who removed hairs at least twice weekly with a minimal chin hair density of least 5 terminal hairs/cm^2 in the chin and upper lip regions.

The objectives of the Phase II clinical studies of the cream vehicle were to identify the most effective dose of eflornithine as demonstrated by (1) objective measures of hair length using videoimaging, (2) clinical appraisals of facial hair using a clinical severity scoring system for chin hair length (Table 1), and (3) subject self-perception questionnaires using a visual analog grading scale for perception of decreased hair growth (Fig. 1). The perception questionnaires were designed to determine treatment effectiveness in relation to the subjects perception of decreased facial hair growth.

In Phase III studies, the Physician Global Assessment (Table 2) of the reductions in unwanted facial hair growth was the primary measure of efficacy (26). Subject's perceptions on improvement of their quality of life based on a self-assessment questionnaire evaluating aspects of the subjects' well being and objective reductions in chin hair length were secondary measures of efficacy. Safety assessments were based on the incidence of adverse events, clinical laboratory tests, evaluation of acne and pseudofolliculitis, and physical examinations.

Table 1 Clinical Scoring of Chin Hair Length by Modified Ferriman–Gallwey System

Score (mFG)	Length	Chin length description
0	None	Only vellus hair, no terminal hairs
1	Not visible	Dark areas corresponding to hair tips may be seen at or below epidermal surface and/or terminal hairs are palpable when the skin is brushed lightly with the fingertips
2	Barely visible	Hair tip can definitely be seen above the epidermal surface but the side of the hair is barely visible
2.5		Intermediate between 2.0 and 3.0
3	Definitely visible	Hair unmistakably visible with definite length, and the side as well as the end clearly perceptible
3.5		Intermediate between 3.0 and 4.0
4	Long	Hairs look long in that their side is fully visible. The shape of the hair, for example, straight, curled, and so on is apparent

Effect—Week 9 (Question 8) and Week 25 (Question 9)
Thinking back to before you started treatment what effect do you feel that the treatment has had on your facial hair?

It has made my condition: (Please place a mark along the line indicating how much of a change you feel the treatment has had on your facial hair).

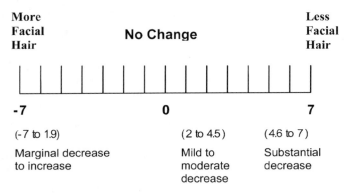

Figure 1 Self-perception question on change in amount of facial hair.

Table 2 Physician's Global Assessment in Phase III Pivotal Study

Grade 3 (clear/almost clear)	There is no or nearly no visible terminal hair on the treated areas of the face; there is no or nearly no darkening on the appearance of the facial skin due to terminal hair
Grade 2 (marked improvement)	There is a considerable decrease in the visibility of terminal hair on the treated areas of the face; there is only minimal darkening in the appearance of facial skin due to terminal hair
Grade 1 (improved)	There is a clinically apparent decrease in visibility of terminal hair on the treated areas of the face; there is noticeable lightening in the appearance due to terminal hair
Grade 0 (no improvement/worse)	There is either no decrease or worsening in visibility of terminal hair on the treated areas of the face; darkening of the terminal hair has not improved or has become worse.

Objective Measures of Facial Hair Growth by Videoimaging in the Phase II and Phase III Studies

For both Phase II and Phase III studies, objective changes in hair length and clinical scoring of hair length changes were focused on the chin as hair is highly visible and more bothersome to the patient in this region. It is also more difficult to conceal and the chin is clearly defined anatomically. Furthermore the density of facial hair and removal methods in the chin are more consistent than other facial regions where there is much greater variability not only in the degree of hair growth but also the removal methods. In Phase III studies, facial hair growth was measured in the chin and upper lip. In both Phase II and Phase III studies, videoimaging was the most objective measure. A specialized video analysis hair measurement system was employed in both Phase II and Phase III studies, which included use of a video fiber microscope with a $15\times$ magnification in Phase II (30) and $50\times$ magnification in Phase III (31). A glass slide was attached to the end of the video-microscope to flatten hairs before imaging. The video images were transferred to a personal computer and digitized for measurements of hair length (length in mm) in Phase II and Phase III as well as spatial mass (area in mm^2) in Phase III by an imaging software program. Digital images of the circumscribed chin regions were obtained 48 h after hair removal by shaving or tweezing in Phase II or shaving in Phase III. In the Phase II study, hairs were identified manually and traced for length measures calculated by imaging program (Fig. 2). In the Phase III studies, hair length and spatial mass in the chin region were measured by an automated image analysis system program.

Phase II Objective Hair Length Reductions

The 15% eflornithine HCl treatment resulted in a decreased growth rate of 47% vs. an 8% in the placebo (control vehicle). The lower 5% and 10% eflornithine doses reduced hair lengths by 26% and 28% but did not differ significantly from the placebo. Statistically repeated measures of analysis of covariance (ANCOVA) showed a significant treatment effect at Wk 25 ($p < 0.009$). Dunnett's method revealed that only the 15% eflornithine HCl group differed significantly ($p = 0.0022$) from controls at Wk 25 (Table 3). Eight weeks after withdrawing treatment, there were no statistical differences between the 15% eflornithine HCl group and the vehicle group ($p > 0.05$) indicating reversibility of the eflornithine effects (Table 3). A 50% reduction in hair growth represents a marked and readily perceptible decrease in hair growth, and 38% of subjects in the 15% eflornithine group had at least a 50% reduction in chin hair length, whereas the percentage of subjects with this magnitude of reduction were only 7% in the control, 11% in the 5% eflornithine group, and 32% in the 10% eflornithine group. The subjects' perceptions of decreased hair growth substantiated that a 50% decrease was viewed as readily perceptible (see perception results) as the subjects in the 15% eflornithine group who demonstrated a 50% reduction

Management of Unwanted Facial Hair

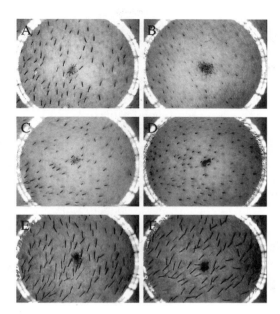

Figure 2 Video images of chin with 48 h hair length. (A) Subject 123 at baseline; (B) subject 123 on 15% eflornithine HCl treatment after 24 weeks, with 71% reduction in hair length and mFG chin decrease of 1.0; (C) subject 57 at baseline; (D) subject 57 on 15% eflornithine HCl treatment after 24 weeks, with 45% reduction and mFG decrease of 1.0 in chin hair length; (E) subject 105 at baseline; (F) subject 105 on placebo after 24 weeks, 7% reduction and mFG change 0 in hair length.

Table 3 Reversible and Dose-Dependent Inhibition of Facial Hair Growth by Eflornithine

	Average hair length on chin (mm)			
Treatment period	15% Treatment group	10% Treatment group	5% Treatment group	Vehicle
Wk 1	0.69	0.53	0.60	0.63
Wk 9	0.39	0.39	0.47	0.56
Wk 25*	0.36	0.40	0.42	0.55
Wk 33	0.52	0.46	0.52	0.58
n	27	18	27	26
	% Change in hair length			
Wk 1 vs. Wk 9	−43	−26	−26	−11
Wk 1 vs. Wk 25**	−48**	−25	−30	−13
Wk 25 vs. Wk 33 (Post-treatment)	+31	+13	+19	+5.2

*Statistically significant overall dose response at $p \leq 0.009$.
**Vehicle vs. 15% statistically significant at $p = 0.0022$ based on two-tail test.

in hair growth were also the most likely to perceive a substantial reduction in facial hair growth. The global scoring (FG Score) on the severity of the condition by the clinical investigator was also consistent with the treatment benefits in the 15% eflornithine group.

In the Phase III study, spatial mass was significantly reduced after 2 weeks ($p < 0.002$) of treatment and this reduction was maintained throughout the entire treatment period and overall there was a 26% reduction in spatial mass at the end of treatment with the 15% eflornithine cream, whereas vehicle treatment had no effect. These benefits were reversed 8 weeks after treatment withdrawal. The 15% eflornithine treatment reduced hair lengths by 23% vs. 4% in placebo ($p < 0.016$), which satisfied the prospectively defined criteria of success for length reduction, requiring a greater proportion of subjects in the eflornithine-treated group exceeding a 50% decrease in hair vs. placebo controls (31).

Phase II Investigator Perceptions

In Phase II, the subjects were evaluated using a modification of the Ferriman–Gallwey method (32), (i.e., mFG scale) at baseline and at 4 week intervals during treatment and 8 weeks post-treatment. The mFG scale was developed by Dr. Geoffrey Redmond (Hormone Help Center of NY, NY) and was designed to more accurately characterize and evaluate changes in growth rate, density, pigmentation, and coarseness corresponding to specific androgen-mediated properties of facial hairs affected by hair growth inhibitors. The clinical scoring for Phase II studies on women with facial hirsutism focused on chin hair length as the chin region is one of the most sensitive and specific indicators of hirsutism (33). The 4 point scale for hair length decreases is described in Table 1 and the magnitude of change is not linear. A score decrease of 1.0 or greater from a baseline of 3.0–4.0 on the mFG scale constitutes a clearly apparent change in hair length in which both the end and side of the hair is changed from being definitely visible (length score ≥ 3.0) to a condition in which only the end of the hair but not the side is barely visible above the epidermal surface (≤ 2.5). The mean chin hair length mFG scores showed a statistically significant ($p = 0.0001$) decrease vs. placebo for subjects treated with the 15% eflornithine HCl formulation after the 24 week treatment interval. The mean value for the 29 subjects completing the trial changed from the baseline of $3.45 \pm (0.39)$ to $2.67 \pm (0.70)$, representing an average change of 0.8 on the mFG scale. This difference was less for the lower concentration formulations (10% and 5%), which did not statistically differ from the placebo. After the 8 week post-treatment period, the difference between baseline and end of treatment scores in the 15% eflornithine group was no longer significant, demonstrating that the effect was reversible after treatment was withdrawn. An mFG chin length score decrease of 1.0 or greater clearly separated the 15% treatment from the other treatment groups (Table 4). Within the 15% eflornithine group, there was a good correlation between decreases in mFG chin length scores and objective

Table 4 Percent Distribution of Changes (delta) in Chin Hair Length Based on Modified Ferriman–Gallwey Scores (Wk 25–Wk 1)

Change in mFG score (delta)	Placebo (vehicle)	Percent of subjects in the group		
		5% Eflornithine treatment group	10% Eflornithine treatment group	15% Eflornithine treatment group
−1 to −1.5 (clearly apparent)	7.4	21.5	22.7	51.7
−0.5 (clinically meaningful)	22.2	32.1	27.3	27.6
0 (no change)	48.1	25.0	36.4	17
≥0.5 (worsened)	22.2	21.5	13.6	3.4
n^a	27	28	22	29

[a]Number of subjects per group.

decreases in hair length. There were 15 of 29 subjects in the 15% eflornithine group who had a clearly apparent chin hair length reductions (mFG reduction 1.0–2.0) after 24 weeks, and 9 of these 15 subjects demonstrated 50% decrease in chin hair length. In the other groups, there was no apparent connection between FG score and hair length reduction and a combined total of 12 subjects out of 72 had FG scores exceeding 1.0 in the placebo, 5% eflornithine, and 10% eflornithine groups and only one subject (5% eflornithine group) had an objective length reduction greater than 50%. These results clearly demonstrate the association between reduction in mFG score for chin hair length and the objective reduction in length as measured by image analysis in the 15% eflornithine group.

Subject Perception Evaluations

In the Phase II dose–response studies, subjects were asked questions about their perception of facial hair growth and responses were recorded on the subject perception form at each monthly visit (Fig. 1). The perceived effectiveness of the treatment by the subjects was measured using a continuous scoring 15 point scale system with -7 representing more facial hair, 0 for no change, and 7 for less facial hair (see Fig. 1). A statistical correlation analysis indicated that higher perception scores, which were indicative of decreased hair visibility, were generated by the higher dosages of eflornithine.

After 8 weeks of treatment 37% of subjects in the 15% eflornithine HCl group observed at least a perceptible reduction by Wk 25 and there was a significant difference ($p < 0.05$) between the percentage of subjects in the 15% eflornithine HCl group scoring at least a perceptible benefit ($y > 3$) at Wk 25 (62%) vs. the percentage of subjects in the placebo group at Wk 25 (29%) as depicted in Table 5.

We were interested in determining an objective reduction in chin hair length (hair decrease >50%) or the perception of the investigator indicating that a clearly apparent reduction in chin hair length (mFG decrease of 1.0–2.0) is associated with a subject's tendency to perceive a substantial reduction in hair as defined by subject self-perception scores exceeding 4.5 in the 15 point scale ranging from -7 (increased facial hair) to 0 (no change) to $+7$ (decreased facial hair). The results are summarized in Table 6. Forty-one percent of the subjects in the 15% eflornithine group (12/29) perceived a substantial reduction of facial hair and 31% had perception scores substantiated by investigator perceptions (mFG change of >1.0). Twenty-four percent of the subjects perceived a substantial reduction in facial hair that was accompanied by investigator scoring of a clearly apparent decrease in chin length as well as a substantial reduction (50% decrease in chin hair length) in objective measures of chin facial hair growth. In contrast, in the control, 5% eflornithine and 10% eflornithine groups the proportion of subjects who perceived either a substantial reduction in hair length accompanied by a substantial objective reduction in hair growth rates (0–5%) or an investigator perceptions of clearly apparent

Table 5 Responses (%) to the Self-Perception Questionnaire of Drug Efficacy

	Number of subjects in response category range* (percentage of subjects)**								
	Placebo (vehicle)		5% Eflornithine treatment group		10% Eflornithine treatment group		15% Eflornithine treatment group	
Score $(y)^*$	Wk 9	Wk 25	Wk 9	Wk 25	Wk 9	Wk 25	Wk 9	Wk 25
$11 < \gamma \leq 15^a$	5*(16.7)**	8 (28.6)	8 (27.6)	11 (39.3)	7 (25)	13 (56.5)	12 (38.7)	18 (62.1)
$8 < \gamma \leq 11^b$	13 (43.3)	11 (39.3)	10 (34.5)	9 (32.1)	18 (64.3)	7 (30.4)	16 (51.6)	7 (24.1)
$\gamma \leq 8^c$	12 (40.0)	9 (32.1)	11 (37.9)	8 (28.6)	3 (10.7)	3 (13.0)	3 (9.7)	4 (13.8)
Sample size (n)	30	28	29	28	28	23	31	29

[a] High to a moderate decrease in facial hair.
[b] Minimal decrease in facial hair.
[c] No change to increase in facial hair.
Statistically significant overall dose response at $p \leq 0.009$.
Vehicle vs. 15% statistically significant at $p = 0.0022$ based on two-tail test.

Table 6 Correlation between Objective Hair Length Reduction, Clinical Scoring, and Subject Perception at the End of Treatment

	Number of subjects in the group (percentage of subjects)			
Efficacy parameter	Placebo (vehicle)	5% Eflornithine treatment group	10% Eflornithine treatment group	15% Eflornithine treatment group
Subjects in perception score range 4.6–7.0 by Wk 25	6 (22)	5 (18)	5 (23)	12 (41)
FG score 1.0–2.0	1 (4)	2 (7)	1 (4)	9 (31)
% Hair inhibition ≥50%	1 (4)	0	1 (5)	7 (28)
FG score 1.0–2.0 and hair inhibition ≥50%	0	0	0	7 (24)
n^a	27	28	22	29

[a]Number of subjects in a group at the end of treatment.

reduction (4–7%) was very low and a subject's perception of substantial decrease in hair growth in these groups was unrelated to their objective length reduction or investigator perception (Table 6). In summary, in the 15% eflornithine group substantial objective reductions in chin hair growth or the perception of the investigator of clearly apparent decreases in chin hair length were associated with the subject's perception of a substantial reduction in facial hair growth and a combination of these two parameters was even more likely to be associated with the subject's perception of substantial efficacy.

Phase III Perception

Each participant in the study completed the self-assessment questionnaire at the start of the study, as well as at intervals during the study and at the end of the study (Table 7). Inclusion in the study required a bother score of 80 on a 100

Table 7 Subject's Self-Assessment of Bother and Discomfort Due to Her Unwanted Facial Hair at Baseline, during Following Treatment Using a 100 Point Analog Scale

How bothered are you by facial hair?
How bothered are you by the time spent removing hair?
How uncomfortable are you when you meet new people?
How uncomfortable are you at work or class?
How uncomfortable are you at social gatherings?
How uncomfortable are you in exchanges of affection?

point scale for all parameters. Bother parameters included how much one was bothered by unwanted facial hair and how much one was bothered by the amount of time spent removing and concealing facial hair. Specific questions on the discomfort experienced in a variety of settings included bother related to (1) intimacy and exchanges of affection; (2) meeting new people; (3) social gatherings with people, dining out or shopping; and (4) the workplace or school. The results of the questionnaire demonstrated a significantly greater decrease in the level of bother and discomfort in women treated with eflornithine (HCl cream) 15% than those on the control.

At the start of the study, the average level of bother and discomfort reported by the 596 participants in Phase III studies was greater than 80 for all situations as results at the end of the study showed that on average women treated with the 15% eflornithine (HCl cream) reported more than a two times greater reduction in their level of bother and discomfort when compared with those in the placebo group (34).

In the eflornithine group those women who demonstrated the most dramatic clinical results by physician assessment had bother index that reduced from a baseline of 85 at the beginning of the study to 30 at the end; those who demonstrated clinical improvements judged as markedly improved had bother indexes reduced from 85 to 50 at the end of study; those showing moderate improvement had bother scores reduced from 85 to 65 and those with no clinical improvement had scores marginally reduced from 85 to 80. The magnitude of clinical score improvements were, therefore, concordant with the subject's perceptions (35).

CONCLUSIONS

The rationale for developing eflornithine to retard the rate of hair regrowth was verified by preclinical research that established that the actions of eflornithine on hair reduction are related to decreased rate of hair growth and the image analysis data on hair length reduction by 15% eflornithine supported these findings. The preclinical biochemical and morphological research in the hamster flank organ as well as the series of penetration studies and pharmacokinetic studies on delivery of eflornithine were critical in developing a consumer acceptable moisturizing formulation that could deliver eflornithine to its follicular target in a safe and effective manner with enough concentration to provide demonstrable clinical benefits. In both Phase II and Phase III studies the 15% eflornithine treatment significantly decreased objective hair length as measured by videoimaging technologies and decreased clinical severity of excessive facial hair measured by the physician's global assessment using the mFG index. The concordance between the investigator's assessment of improvement and the subjects' own perceptions was very compelling in both studies, especially because the methods to assess perceptible benefits by subjects were so different. In Phase II, subject perception research was focused on substantiating that a dose of eflornithine providing objective reductions in hair growth provided visible reduction that was apparent to both the investigator and the subject. More informal information gathered from open ended questionnaires related decreased hair visibility to an increase in self-confidence and less avoidance of uncomfortable situations. The Phase III perception studies were based on specific measures of the emotional outcome and improvements in the quality of life achieved by decreasing the visibility of unwanted facial hair and there was striking correlation between the magnitude of clinical improvement noted by investigators and the magnitude of the overall bother and stress reduction perceived by patient.

Initially eflornithine was used as an adjunct to hair removal by tweezing, waxing, shaving, and chemical depilation. An emerging indication for hair growth retardants such as eflornithine is its use as an adjunct therapy to complement light-mediated hair removal procedures (36).

Overall, the research in eflornithine demonstrates that new product categories including new indications for old drugs and novel treatment synergies can be developed by a strong scientific rationale buttressed with systematic preclinical research coordinated with a series of clinical studies designed to relate biological changes with changes in appearance that deliver meaningful psychosocial benefits.

REFERENCES

1. Rittmaster RS. Medical treatment of androgen dependant hirsutism. J Clin Endocrinol Metab 1995; 80(9):2559–2563.
2. Rabinovitz S, Cohen R, LeRoith, D. Anxiety and hirsutism. Psychol Rep 1983; 53:827–830.
3. Azziz R. The evaluation and management of hirsutism. Obstet Gynecol 2003; 101(5 Pt 1):995–1007.
4. Wooley-Lyoyd H. Hair removal techniques: review. Cosmet Dermatol 2003; 16(6):45–51.
5. Sanchez LA, Perez M, Azziz R. Laser hair reduction in the hirsute patient, a critical assessment. Hum Reprod Update 2002; 8(2):169–181.
6. Dierickx C, Alora MB, Dover JS. A clinical overview of hair removal using light lasers and light sources. Dermatol Clin 1999; 17(2):357–372.
7. Adrian RM, Shay KPJ. 800 nm diode laser hair removal in African American patients: a clinical and histologic study. J Cutan Laser Ther 2000; 2:183–190.
8. Levy JL, Trelles MA, de Ramecourt, A. Epilation with a long-pulse 1064 nm Nd:YAG laser in facial hirsutism. J Cosmet Laser Ther 2001; 3(4):175–179.
9. Nouri K, Rivas MP. Cosemetic dermatology review of laser hair removal in Fitzpatrick skin types IV to VI. Cosmet Dermatol 2003; 16:24–26.
10. Lor P, Lennartz B, Ruedlinger R. Patient satisfaction study of unwanted facial and body hair: 5 years experience with intense pulsed light. J Cosmet Laser Ther 2002; 4:73–79.
11. Hirsch RJ, Farinelli WA, Laughlin SA, Campos V, Dover JS, Pon K, van Labode S, Arndt K, Dierickx C, Anderson RR. Hair growth induced by laser hair removal (Abstract 229). ASLMS/BMLA/ELA Joint International Meeting, Edinburgh, Scotland 2003.

12. Marton LJ, Pegg AE. Polyamines as targets for therapeutic intervention. Annu Rev Pharmacol Toxicol 1995; 35:55–91.
13. Probst E, Krebs A. Ornithine decarboxylase activity in relation to DNA synthesis in mouse interfollicular epidermis and hair follicles. Biochem Biophys Acta 1975; 407:147–157.
14. Nancarrow MJ, Nesci A, Hynd PI, Powell BC. Dynamic expression of ornithine decarboxylase in hair growth. Mech Dev 1999; 84(1–2):161–164.
15. Soler AP, Gilliard G, Megosh L, George K, O'Brien, TG. Polyamines regulate expression of the neoplastic phenotype in mouse skin. Cancer Res 1998; 58:164–169.
16. Kaszynski E. The stimulation of hair growth in the flank organs of female hamsters by subcutaneous testosterone propionate and its inhibition by topical cyproterone acetate: dose–response studies. Br J Dermatol 1983; 109(5):565–569.
17. Shander D, Mudd L, Usdin V. Inhibition of ornithine decarboxylase (ODC) activity in hamster flank organ: a novel assay for topical screening of antiandrogens. (Abstract #655). 65th Annual Meeting Endocrine Society, San Antonio, TX, 1983.
18. Shander D. Hair growth modification with ornithine decarboxylase inhibitors U.S Patent Number 4,720,489. 1988.
19. Shander D, Funkhouser MF, Ahluwalia GS. Pharmacology of hair growth inhibition by topical treatment with eflornithine–HCl monohydrate (DFMO) using flank organ model (Abstract 228). 59th Meeting American Academy Dermatology Washington, DC, 2001.
20. Metcalf BW, Bey P, Danzin C, Hung MJ, Casara JP, Vevert JP. Catalytic irreversible inhibition of mammalian ornithine decarboxylase (E.L. 4.1.1.17) by substrate and product analogues. J Am Chem Soc 1978; 100(8):2251–2253.
21. Ahluwalia GS, Hao Z, Paull K, Stowe E, Cooney D. Control of cancer by amino acid analogs. In: Garth Powis ed. Anticancer Drugs—Antimetabolite Metabolism and Natural Anticancer Agents. New York: Pergamon Press, 1994:1–48.
22. Boxall BA, Amery GW, Ahluwalia GS. Topical Composition for Inhibiting Hair Growth. U.S Patent Number 5, 648,394. 1997.
23. Malhotra B, Palmisano M, Schrode K, Huber F, Altman DJ, Ahluwalia GS, and the eflornithine study group. Percutaneous absorption, pharmacokinetics and dermal safety of eflornithine 15% cream in hirsute women. Abstract Annual Meeting of the American Academy of Dermatology, San Francisco, CA, 1999.
24. Malhotra B, Noveck R, Behr D, Palmisano M. Percutaneous absorption and pharmacokinetics of eflornithine HCl 13.9% cream in women with unwanted facial hair. J Clin Pharmacol 2001; 41:972–978.
25. Schrode KS, Huber F, Staszak H, Altman DJ. Evaluation of the long term safety of eflornithine 15% cream in the treatment of women with excessive facial hair. (Abstract) Annual Meeting of the American Academy of Dermatology, San Francisco, CA, 1999.
26. Schrode KS, Huber F, Staszak H, Altman DJ, Shander D, Ahluwalia GS, Morton J. Randomized, double-blind, vehicle-controlled safety and efficacy evaluation of eflornithine 15% cream in the treatment of women with excessive facial hair. (Abstract) Annual Meeting of the American Academy of Dermatology, San Francisco, CA, 1999.
27. Hickman JG, Huber F, Palmisano M. Human dermal safety studies with eflornithine HCl 13.9% cream (VANIQA), a novel treatment for excessive facial hair. Curr Med Res Opin 2001; 16(4):235–244.

28. Meyskens FL Jr, Gerner EW. Development of difluoromethylornithine (DFMO) as a chemoprevention agent. Clin Cancer Res 1999; 5(5):945–951.
29. Einspahr JG, Bowden GT, Alberts DS. Skin cancer chemoprevention: strategies to save our skin. Recent Results Cancer Res 163:151–164; Discussion 2003; 264–266.
30. Shander D, Funkhouser MF, Ahluwalia GS, Morton J, Harrington FE, Redmond G. Clinical dose range studies with topical application of the ornithine decarboxylase inhibitor eflornithine HCl (DFMO) in women with facial hirsutism. (Abstract 123) 59th Meeting American Academy Dermatology, Washington, DC, 2001.
31. Funkhouser MF, Shander D, Schrode KS, Huber F, Staszak H, Altman DJ. Use of a video-imagining system to obtain hair measurement data in controlled clinical trials evaluating the safety and efficacy of eflornithine 15% cream in the treatment of excessive facial hair in women (Abstract). Annual Meeting of the American Academy of Dermatology, San Francisco, CA, 1999.
32. Ferriman D, Gallwey JD. Clinical assessment of body hair growth in women. J Clin Endocrinal Metab 1961; 24:140–147.
33. Derksen J, Mooleanaar van Seters AP, Kock DFM. Semiquantitative assessment of hirsutism in Dutch women. Br J Dermatol 1993; 128:259–263.
34. Schrode KS, Huber F, Staszak H, Altman DJ, Shander D, Morton J. Outcome of quality of life assessment used in the clinical trials for hirsute women treated with topical eflornithine 15% cream (Abstract) Annual Meeting of the American Academy of Dermatology, San Francisco, CA, 1999.
35. Jackson JD, Shander D, Huber F, Schrode KS, Mathes BM. The evaluation of quality of life in two studies of women treated with topical eflornihtine HCl 13.9% cream for unwanted facial hair. (Abstract), 59th Annual Meeting of American Academy of Dermatology, 259, 2001.
36. Hamzavi I, Tan E, Shapiro J, Lui H. Combined treatment with laser and topical eflornithine is more effective than laser treatment alone for removing unwanted facial hair—a placebo controlled trial (Abstract) 105:32 ASLMS/BMLA/ELA Joint International Meeting, Edinburgh, Scotland, 2003.

28

Ellagic Acid

Koji Takada and Yoshimasa Tanaka
*Biological Science Research Center,
Research & Technololgy Headquarters,
Lion Corporation, Tajima, Odawara, Kanagawa, Japan*

Introduction	511
Skin-Whitening Ingredients	513
General Properties of EA	514
Existence	514
Physicochemical Properties	514
Biochemical Properties	514
Skin-Whitening Activity in Humans	515
Preventing Skin Pigmentation after Sunburn	515
Improving Effect on Skin-Pigmentation Conditions	515
Mode of EA Activity	516
In Vivo Experience	516
In Vitro Experience	517
Summary	520
References	520

INTRODUCTION

Spots and freckles represent general skin-pigmentation conditions that are caused by enhancing and continuous melanogenesis (melanin synthesis). Melanin,

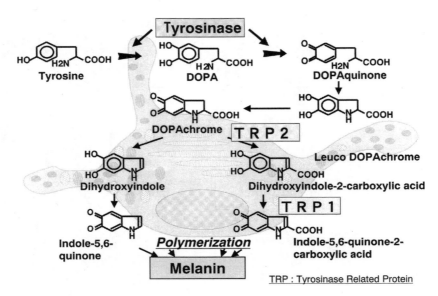

Figure 1 Pathway to melanin from tyrosine. Melanin is synthesized from tyrosine through the action of various enzymes such as tyrosinase (key enzyme in melanin synthesis), TRP1 and TRP2, and nonenzymatic reactions in pigment cells (DOPA: dihydroxy-phenylalanine; TRP: tyrosinase-related protein).

the root factor in such conditions, is synthesized from tyrosine in epidermal melanocytes (pigment cells) via numerous enzymatic and nonenzymatic oxidation and polymerization processes (Fig. 1). Melanin is incorporated into vicinal keratinocytes and determines skin coloration. Keratinocytes containing melanin are discarded through the process of keratinization (Fig. 2). Melanogenesis is enhanced by stimuli such as sunburn [overexposure to ultraviolet (UV) light]. [For the textbook about melanin and its related matters, see Refs. (1) and (2).]

The key enzyme involved in melanogenesis is tyrosinase. Suppression of tyrosinase activity resulting from external stimuli would be the most effective means of preventing or suppressing the formation of spots and freckles. On the basis of this idea, various active substances have been examined. The representative material is ellagic acid (EA), which was approved in 1996 as the active ingredient for a quasidrug* in Japan (3). In this chapter, EA will be introduced after a brief mention of active ingredients (so-called skin-whitening or lightening-active ingredients) that have been approved to inhibit melanogenesis.

---

*This quasidrug will be mentioned in another chapter.

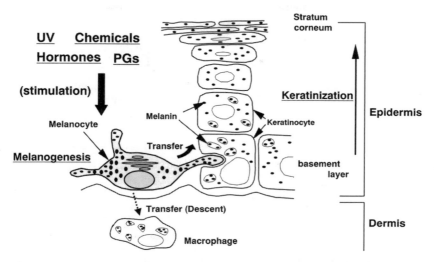

Figure 2 Migration of melanin in the skin. Melanogenesis results from various stimuli. Produced melanin is transferred to vicinal keratinocytes and discarded as dirt followed by keratinization.

SKIN-WHITENING INGREDIENTS

Several ingredients that demonstrate skin-whitening (lightening) effects on topical application have been approved as active ingredients for quasidrugs in Japan. Vitamin C (ascorbic acid) and its derivatives and placenta extract* are well-known ingredients. New ingredients include EA, arbutin, kojic acid[†], butyl resorcin, linoleic acid, chamomile extract, and tranexamic acid. Figure 3 shows representative active ingredients. Although other materials such as azelaic acid, retinoic acid, and numerous plant extracts such as licorice, mulberry, and creeping saxifrage reportedly display skin-whitening effects, they have not been approved as active ingredients for quasidrugs in Japan. Further, innumerable materials have shown *in vitro* inhibition of tyrosinase activity or melanin synthesis, but few have been confirmed to show whitening effects in humans.

Vitamin C, cysteine, and some herb medicines are listed in the Japanese Pharmacopoeia as medicines suitable for internal use.

---

*This usage has been restricted owing to the recent problems with bovine spongiform encephalopathy.
[†]Production of cosmetics containing kojic acid was suspended in 2003 owing to possible carcinogenic effects following ingestion.

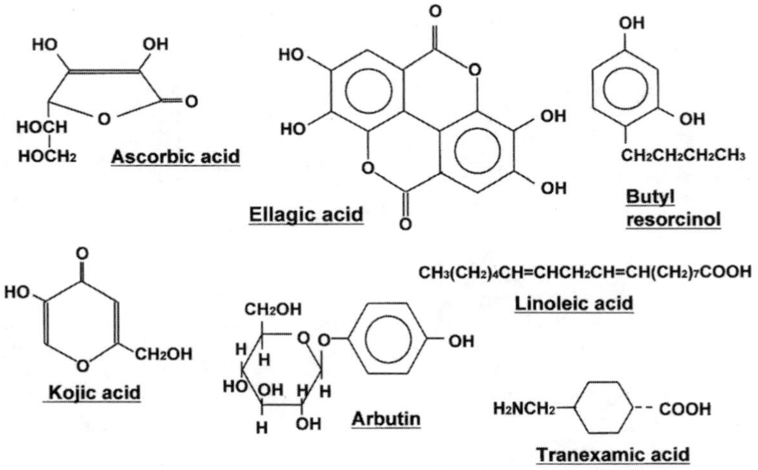

Figure 3 Representative active ingredients that can be used for quasidrugs in Japan. In Japan, nine kinds of active ingredients for quasidrugs have been approved for skin whitening (vitamin C includes some derivatives). Other active ingredients are placenta extract and chamomile extract.

GENERAL PROPERTIES OF EA

Existence

EA is a polyphenol compound, containing two pairs of hydroxyl groups at the ortho position (Fig. 3). EA is present in plants, such as grape, strawberry, raspberry, walnut, green tea, eucalyptus, swertia herb, and tara, existing as substances such as ellagitannin or glycoside (amlitoside) (4–8).

Physicochemical Properties

EA is a white- or cream-colored powder, and is insoluble in water and organic solvents (9–11). Solubility (ppm): water (0.6); ethanol (100); 1,3-butyleneglycol (1000); mono-olein (1000); polyethylene glycol 2000 (4000). EA can chelate to some metals, including copper and iron.

Biochemical Properties

Other than the tyrosinase inhibition described later, EA exhibits anticarcinogenic activity, antioxidative activity (SOD-like activity, suppression of squalene peroxidation, and protection against cell damage caused by hydrogen peroxide) and suppression of nitrogen oxide (NO) production (11–13).

Skin-Whitening Activity in Humans

Preventing Skin Pigmentation after Sunburn

The preventative effects of EA on skin pigmentation (14) after sunburn were evaluated using a model in which bilateral brachia in subjects were irradiated with UV. Figure 4 shows the appearance of pigmentation, which was noticeably reduced on the arm to which EA-containing cream was applied compared with the reference arm to which placebo was applied. The effect of EA appears after 1 week of application and is more pronounced with continued application. Figure 5 shows results from a double-blind trial. Efficacy of EA as determined by dermatologists was verified as "effective or better" by 73% and "moderately effective or better" by 86%. This result was similar to that obtained by image analysis. No adverse effects were observed.

Improving Effect on Skin-Pigmentation Conditions

Table 1 shows the efficacy of EA in treating various skin-pigmentation conditions (15). EA proved particularly effective against postinflammatory pigmentation (95.8% efficacy), chloasma (73.3%), and senile freckles (69.2%).

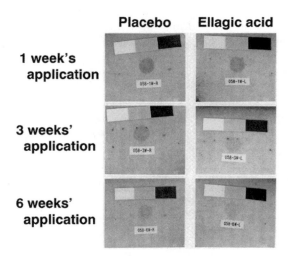

Figure 4 Effect of ellagic acid on reduction of UV-induced human skin pigmentation. Images show the area to which cream containing EA (right) or placebo (left) has been applied. The skin-whitening effect appears after 1 week of application.

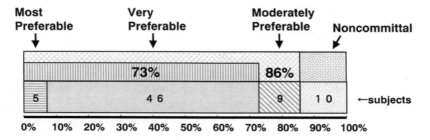

- Volunteer : 70 subjects (20-55 years)
- Investigators : 4 dermatologists
- Method : Double Blind Controlled Test
  UV(A+B) irradiation, 1MED x 3times
- Test period : Application for 6 weeks
- Ingredient : Ellagic acid 0.5%, Placebo

Figure 5 Efficacy for skin-whitening effect of EA on UV-irradiated subjects. The efficacy of EA to pigmentation caused after UV exposure was judged to be 86%.

Mode of EA Activity

In Vivo Experience

Brownish guinea pigs have melanocytes in the skin, as do humans. Figure 6 compares the skin-whitening effect of EA with that of hydroquinone (HQ), a representative depigmenting agent (16). When this animal is UV irradiated, melanogenesis is enhanced and the skin becomes dark brown [Fig. 6(A)]. EA applied to the UV-irradiated area diminishes the coloration, demonstrating suppression of melanogenesis [Fig. 6(B)]. EA, therefore, suppresses melanogenesis and lightens skin color. Furthermore, when the area that had been UV irradiated and treated was irradiated again without treatment, melanogenesis was enhanced on the area originally treated using EA, but not on that using HQ [Fig. 6(C)]. This

Table 1 Efficacy of EA to Some Skin Pigmentation Conditions

	Chloasma (spot) (15 cases)	Postinflammatory pigmentation (24 cases)	Ephelides (freckle) (18 cases)	Senile pigment freckle (13 cases)
Most preferable	2	12	0	0
Very preferable	4	7	1	4
Moderately preferable	5	4	5	5
Noncommittal	4	1	12	4
Effective ratio (%)	73.3	95.8	33.3	69.2

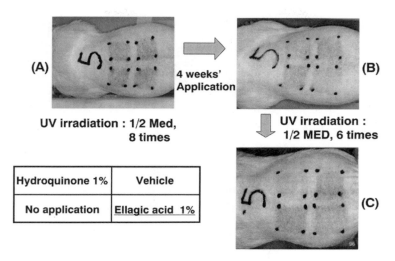

Figure 6 Effect of EA on reduction of UV-induced pigmentation (animal model). When brownish guinea pigs are irradiated with UV, the skin becomes dark brown (A). When EA and HQ are applied to the skin for 4 weeks, coloration at the applied areas becomes fainter than that at non- or vehicle application (B). Furthermore, in cases where UV is irradiated again, the area to which EA was applied becomes dark in the same way as that of non- or vehicle application, whereas the area to which HQ was applied does not.

shows that HQ may damage melanocytes in the skin, whereas EA does not affect the cells and thus does not cause permanent depigmentation (17,18).

Decreases in cutaneous melanin content were ascertained using Fontana–Masson staining (Fig. 7).

In Vitro Experience

Figure 8 shows that melanoma cells cultured with EA (B in Fig. 8) are lighter in color than control cells (A in Fig. 8), indicating inhibition of melanogenesis. If EA is removed from the medium and the culture is continued, the cells regain their original color (C in Fig. 8). This shows that the inhibitory effects of EA on melanogenesis are exhibited only during application, suggesting the safety of EA as a cosmetic agent. Rate of melanogenesis inhibition corresponds to reduction of tyrosinase activity (17,18).

Suppression of tyrosinase activity by EA can be recovered with the addition of copper compounds to the medium (Fig. 9). It is supposed that this is because tyrosinase is a metaloenzyme containing Cu in the active center (19). This was supported by results using tyrosinase derived from mushrooms, as decreased tyrosinase activity coincided with a reduced copper content in the enzyme, and inhibition of enzyme activity was partially recovered on the addition of copper compounds to the tyrosinase treated with EA. Tyrosinase catalyzes the reaction

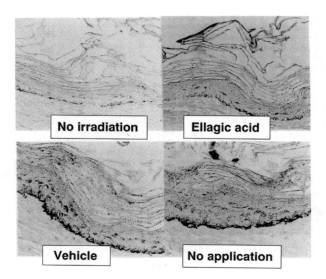

Figure 7 Cross-section features stained using Fontana–Masson method: Black dots show melanin (like materials). The skin to which EA was applied displays less melanin, resembling that of a nonapplication.

from tyrosine to DOPA and DOPAquinone by transferring the electrical charge of Cu between mono- and di-valences (20–22). EA is supposed to chelate with Cu in tyrosinase, suppressing enzymatic activity by shifting Cu from the original active center (Fig. 10).

During melanogenesis, numerous enzymatic and nonenzymatic reactions occur that do not involve tyrosinase. Attention has recently been given to

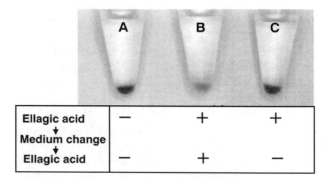

Figure 8 Color of melanoma cells cultured with EA. EA inhibits melanogenesis, but the inhibitory effect appears only under its presence.

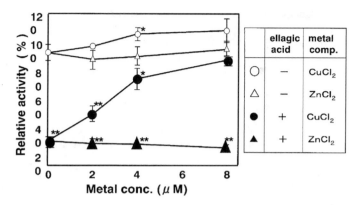

Figure 9 Effect of metal ions on tyrosinase activity of melanoma cells cultured with EA. After B16 melanoma cells were cultured in medium with or without EA, CuCl$_2$, or ZnCl$_2$ was added to the medium and the culture was continued. The inhibitory effect of melanogenesis by EA can be recovered with the addition of CuCl$_2$ to the medium, but CuCl$_2$ itself does not necessarily accelerate melanogenesis.

tyrosinase-related protein (TRP) 1 and 2 (Fig. 1). EA barely affects enzymatic activity, mRNA expression (tested by RT–PCR method), or protein expression (tested by Western blotting) of these enzymes. EA is, therefore, considered to specifically and directly suppress tyrosinase activity.

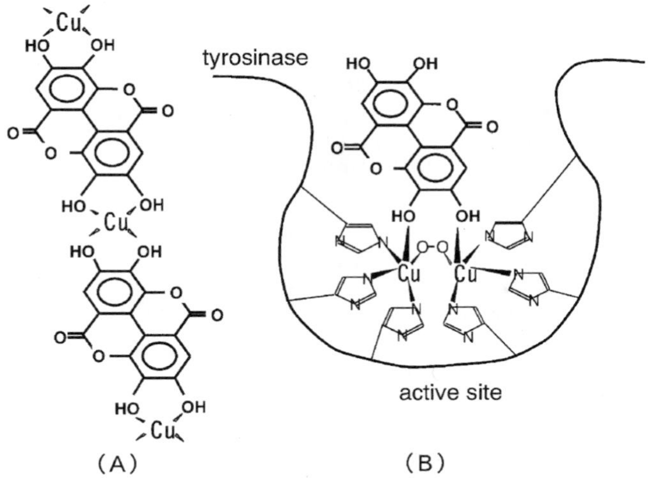

Figure 10 Presumed schema of EA acting on Cu in tyrosinase molecule. EA is assumed to chelate to Cu in the active site of tyrosinase molecule and to inactivate the enzyme activity, followed by the manner of A or B.

SUMMARY

EA suppresses melanogenesis by inhibiting tyrosinase activity, and has been approved as an effective and safe active ingredient. EA is not only useful for cosmetic purposes, but is also expected to be used as a medical adjunct.

REFERENCES

1. Nordlund JJ, Boissy RE, Hearing VJ, King RA, Ortonne J-P, eds. The Pigmentary System (Physiology and Pathophysiology). New York: Oxford University Press, 1998.
2. Levine N, ed. Pigmentation and Pigmentary Disorders. Boca Raton: CRC Press, 1993.
3. Tanaka Y, Masuda M. Trends in skin-whitening agents in Japan. INFORM 1998; 9:306–314.
4. Bate-Smith EC. Chromatography and systematic distribution of ellagic acid. Chem Ind BIF Rev 1956; April:R32.
5. Maas JL, Wang SV, Galletta GJ. Evaluation of strawberry cultivars for ellagic acid content. Hort Sci 1991; 26:66–88.
6. Okuda T, Yoshida T, Nayeshiro H. Gellaniinn, a new ellagitannin from *Gellanium thunbergii*. Tetrahedron Lett 1976; 41:3721–3722.
7. Hills WE, Carle A. The influence of extractives on Eucalyptus pulping and paper making. Appita 1959; 13:74–84.
8. Hatano T, Shida S, Han L, Okuda T. Tannins of Theaceous plants, III, camelliatannins A and B, two new complex tannins from *Camellia japonica* L. Chem Pharm Bull 1991; 39:876–880.
9. Press RE, Hardcastle D. Some physico-chemical properties of ellagic acid. J Appl Chem 1969; 19:247–251.
10. Zhang N-Z, Chen Y-Y. Synthesis of macroporous ellagitannic acid resin and its chelating properties for metal ions. J Macromol Sci, Chem 1988; A25(10 & 11): 1455–1462.
11. Lee C, Briand F, Leaper C. Assessment of copper chelating compounds as tyrosinase inhibitors. IFSCC International Congress, Yokohama, 1992, pp.779–788.
12. Cheng Z, Cheng CC. Ellagic acid. Drugs Future 1986; 11:1029–1033.
13. Osawa T, Ide A, Su J-D, Namiki M. Inhibition of lipid peroxidation by ellagic acid. J Agric Food Chem 1987; 35:808–812.
14. Kamide R, Arase S, Takiwaki H, Watanabe S, Watanabe Y, Kageyama S. Clinical evaluation on the effects of XSC-29 preparation on the pigmentation of the skin by exposure to ultraviolet light. Nishinihon J Dermatol 1995; 57:136–142.
15. Yokoyama M, Ito Y. Clinical evaluation of the use of whitening cream containing ellagic acid for the treatment of skin pigmentation conditions. Skin Res (Hifu) 2001; 43:286–291.
16. Jimbow K, Obata H, Pathak MA, Fitapatrick TB. Mechanism of depigmentation by hydroquinone. J Invest Dermatol 1974; 62:436–449.
17. Shimogaki H, Tanaka Y, Tamai H, Masuda M. *In vitro* and *in vivo* evaluation of ellagic acid on melanogenesis inhibition. Int J Cosmet Sci 2000; 22:291–303.
18. Tanaka Y. Ellagic acid: a new skin-whitening active ingredient. In: Barel AO, Paye M, Maibach HI, eds. Handbook of Cosmetic Science and Technology. New York: Marcel Dekker, 2001:473–478.

19. Nishioka K. Particulate tyrosinase of human malignant melanoma. Solubilization, purification following trypsin treatment, and characterization. Eur J Biochem 1978; 85:137–147.
20. Jackman MP, Huber H, Hajnal A, Lerch K. Stabilization of the oxy form of tyrosinase by a single conservative amino acid substitution. Biochem J 1985; 282:915–918.
21. Maddaluno JE, Faull KF. Inhibition of mushroom tyrosinase by 3-amino-L-tyrosine: molecular probing of the active site of the enzyme. Experientia 1988; 44:885–887.
22. Makino N, McMahill P, Mason HS. The oxidation state of copper in resting tyrosinase. J Biol Chem 1974; 249:6062–6066.

29

Heat Shock Proteins for Cosmeceuticals

Claude Dal Farra, Eric Bauza, and Nouha Domloge
Vincience Research Center, Sophia Antipolis, France

Introduction	523
Hsp: An Overview	524
Hsp70	524
Heat Shock Regulation	525
Medical and Pharmaceutical Interest in Hsp	526
Cosmeceutical Interest in Hsp	527
Inducing Hsp70	527
Supplying Hsp70	527
Effects of Hsp on the Skin: *In Vitro* and *Ex Vivo* Studies	528
Thermal Tolerance	528
Hsp and UV Stress	528
Hsp and Aging	529
Hsp and Retinoids	531
Looking Ahead	532
References	533

INTRODUCTION

Through their long evolution, living cells have developed different mechanisms to counter the increasing stress that they must face. Today, it is well known that stress directly influences our health and well-being, and affects the functioning of most of our organs, including our skin. Stress has different origins including environmental, nutritional, and psychological causes. In recent years, interest in environmental stresses has increased and has become especially focused on UV stress, as UV plays a central role in photoaging and skin cancer. Other important causes of stress in living cells include thermal shock, oxygen free radicals, chemical substances, as well as inflammatory and infectious states, among other causes.

When cells are exposed to stress, depending on the degree, damage can vary from huge energy consumption (to protect their constituents and to repair damaged structures and proteins) to cell death. As a result, living cells have developed different ways to respond to stress and this defense against stress is one of the most preserved mechanisms shared between species.

Among these defense processes, the family of "heat shock proteins" (Hsp) represents one of the principal mechanisms of cell defense and protection from different kinds of aggression and stress. This chapter reviews many studies that reveal the cosmeceutical interest of both "stress-free induction and administration" of Hsp70 in the field of skin care.

Hsp: AN OVERVIEW

The first data about stress response was published by Ritossa in 1962 (1). Since then, many studies have followed and have progressively demonstrated that Hsp, or "molecular chaperones", play an important role in protecting the cell from different types of stress. Hsp represent a family of widely expressed chaperone proteins implicated in maintaining cell integrity after an exposure to a stress stimulus. This protein family is found expressed not only in mammalian organisms but also in bacteria, yeast, and so on.

Under nonstressful conditions, Hsp are important for cell development and differentiation. Hsp also survey and aid new protein folding and assembly. In mammalian cells, Hsp synthesis is induced by hyperthermia and can be triggered by a broad range of stressors that lead to the accumulation of nonnative proteins. These stressors include exposure to UV, heavy metals, amino acid analogs, cytotoxic drugs, hypoxia, glucose deprivation, and virus infection (2,3).

Hsp70

Hsp are divided into many families depending on their molecular weights: Hsp110 kDa, Hsp90, 70, 60, 47, and small Hsp18-30 including Hsp27 (Table 1).

Among these different Hsp families, Hsp70 is the most abundant Hsp in eukaryotes and includes two types: constitutive (Hsc) (c for cognate) and stress-inducible Hsp70 (also known as Hsp72). Both types are very similar in amino acid sequence. Moreover, earlier data have provided evidence that heat-induced Hsp70 cells were protected from lethal stimuli (4–7). Although some

Table 1 Hsp Families and Their Main Effects

Principal families of Hsp	Main effects
Small weight Hsp (10–27)	Tolerance of ischemia; resistance of tumors cells
Hsp47	Interaction with collagen
Hsp60	Wound healing; tumor regression; actin dynamics
Hsp70	Thermal protection: tolerance of hyperthermia and hypothermia; role in wound healing and photoaging; resistance to apoptosis; tolerance of ischemia, endoxin, UV
Hsp90	Resistance to apoptosis, tolerance of ischemia, and role with steroid receptors
Hsp110	Tolerance of hyperthermia and ischemia

Hsp are localized into endoplasmic reticulum (8) or cell mitochondria, both Hsp70 types are localized in the nucleus and in the cytoplasmic cytosol (9).

Under normal conditions, Hsp70 function as molecular chaperones by assisting in the folding of newly synthesized polypeptides, the assembly of multiprotein complexes, and the transport of proteins across cellular membranes. When under stress, Hsp70 can also effectively inhibit aggregation and assist in the refolding of denatured proteins. In addition, Hsp70 can reduce cellular damage by retaining the damaged proteins in soluble form, as well as by binding to unfolded or misfolded proteins to assist in their proper refolding.

Heat Shock Regulation

In eukaryotic cells, regulation of heat shock gene expression requires the activation and translocation to the nucleus of transregulatory proteins, heat shock factors (HSF), which recognize and bind to specific sequences in the promoter region of heat shock genes called heat shock element (HSE) (10,11). Although a single type of HSF has been described in yeast, an HSF multigene family has been identified in plants and vertebrates. At least four HSF have been isolated in humans (2).

With the discovery of different classes of HSF, their relevant functions are becoming progressively revealed. It is now known that HSF1 is responsible for heat-induced Hsp, HSF2 is rebellious to classical stress, and HSF4 is expressed in a tissue-specific manner (12). Moreover, the role of the HSF family has gained more attention as it was discovered that the function of HSF may include regulation of other target genes in response to diverse stimuli. It has also been proposed that different members of the HSF family cooperate in order to regulate the expression of their target genes (12–24). Under nonstressful conditions, activation of the transcription of Hsp genes is modulated during cell cycle, development, and differentiation, and following exposure to molecules that regulate cell proliferation (2,3,25).

MEDICAL AND PHARMACEUTICAL INTEREST IN Hsp

It has become evident and well-established that Hsp are utilized by cells during the repair process, following different types of injury, to prevent damage resulting from the accumulation and aggregation of nonnative proteins (2,3,26). These studies suggest that induction of Hsp70 by pharmaceutical or genetic means may prove useful in surgery, transplantation, and treatment of sepsis and ischemic conditions of the heart, brain, and other organs. Consequently, the use of Hsp70 to improve grafted skin tolerance against ischemic and oxidative stress (8), and its potential protective role in heart and liver transplantation were both seriously considered (27,28). Moreover, the importance of Hsp in pathogenesis, and as diagnostic markers and prognostic indicators, is beginning to be appreciated. The potential of these molecules (and corresponding genes) both as targets for treatment and as therapeutic tools has emerged and is being explored (9).

Data have shown that Hsp also play an accompanying role in the repair process involved in wound healing. Recent data indicates that Hsp70 is expressed in wound healing and that the Hsp70 protein is prominent in the epithelium and in the inflammatory cells migrating into the granulation tissue matrix. RT-PCR demonstrates upregulation of Hsp70 within 12 h after wounding, lasting until day 3, and decreasing thereafter (29).

In animal models, including studies on mice with Cushing-like syndrome, for instance, there is evidence that both diabetes and the hypercortisolemic state that is associated with delay in wound healing are also associated with reduction in Hsp70 (30). In these studies, Hsp70 expression in the wound bed peaked at 24 h in the nondiabetic mice. In contrast, the expression of Hsp70 was delayed for 3 days in the diabetic mice, which corresponded with the clinical delay in healing.

Moreover, stress-induced protein glycosylation (in parallel with Hsp synthesis) is a component of cellular stress response. Protein glycosylation is known to occur when proteins are unfolded and potential glycosylation sites are exposed (31). This finding has considerably increased the interest of protecting the skin from stress in order to limit the glycosylation process.

As Hsp are induced by stress, their protective biological role has been subject to various studies and controversies. Some researchers have wondered whether Hsp serve more as therapeutic targets. However, a recent review has confirmed the protective role of Hsp and gives evidence that there is a potential role for Hsp as therapeutic agents rather than as therapeutic targets (32). Recently, it has been shown that Hsp–peptide complexes serve as successful vaccines, producing antitumor immune responses in animals and humans, and their role in cancer immunotherapy is also gaining increased interest (33).

COSMECEUTICAL INTEREST IN Hsp

Throughout this long history of study, Hsps, in particular Hsp70, have demonstrated numerous beneficial properties and have been shown to exhibit multiple protective effects on human cells and organ functions. These results have inevitably attracted the interest of skin biologists and dermatologists, and it has become increasingly evident that the scientific background behind the Hsp concept is of great cosmeceutical interest. As a result of this interest, two possible approaches to the skin have been revealed: inducing Hsp70 in the cells or providing skin cells with ready-made Hsp70 from another source.

Inducing Hsp70

Studies of the mRNA and Hsp70 protein level provide evidence that Hsp70 is induced by skin cells. These studies can be performed on cultured human keratinocytes and fibroblasts, as well as by immunostaining on human skin biopsies (34–36). As it is already known that stress is not conducive to Hsp synthesis, and in order to offer solely the beneficial protective effect of Hsp, it is essential to induce Hsp in a stress-free manner. A panel of tests are necessary in order to ensure that the induction of Hsp by an active ingredient or a molecule does not involve cell stress (34,35). Such tests may include cell viability using MTT colometric (tetrazolium) assay, or neutral red test, to verify that there is no loss or change in cell viability.

Likewise, studies of cell metabolism and protein synthesis after Hsp70 induction, as well as studies of cytokine synthesis by epidermal keratinocytes and fibroblasts (by ELISA), such as IL-1 and IL-8 synthesis, can indicate the absence of cellular stress. These studies must be associated with the routine toxicology tests for the proposed molecule or active ingredient that is used to induce Hsp. The tests must show that there is no toxicity in the cells or organs after the administration of the molecule or active ingredient in the recommended dose for Hsp induction.

Supplying Hsp70

Another approach to increase cell content of Hsp without stress is to provide the skin cells with ready-made Hsp70. This approach evokes Hsp synthetic preparation or Hsp70 induction in living organisms, as in yeasts by biotechnology (37). Interestingly, studies have shown that yeast and human Hsp70 are both recognized by anti-human Hsp70 antibody, which confirms the great sequence homology of 70% to 85% between yeast and human Hsp.

The stress-free administration of Hsp to the cells is an important aim. The panel of tests proposed earlier is of great interest to ensure a stress-free state. Studies have confirmed that administration is stress-free in the case of the use of yeast Hsp70 (35,37). In addition, immunostaining and immunoblotting studies have shown that after administration of yeast Hsp70 to human skin cells, the cells exhibit a very rapid increase (within 30 min) in their Hsp70 content. This increase is at its maximum 6 h after yeast extract administration and lasts up to 24 h. These findings confirm the rapid uptake of the administered Hsp70 by human cells, thanks both to the great homology between yeast and human Hsp, and the importance of the molecule to the cells.

EFFECTS OF Hsp ON THE SKIN: *IN VITRO* AND *EX VIVO* STUDIES

In recent years, scientists have concentrated strongly on the study of the harmful effects of environmental stress on the human body and, especially on the largest human organ, the skin. For a long time now, studies on UV damage to the skin have been at the center of pharmaceutical and cosmetic skin care research. Based on both the aggressive results of environmental stress on the skin and the known role of Hsp70 in the defense against stress, different studies have focused on investigating the effects of Hsp70 in increasing the skin cell defense against some common environmental stresses, such as "thermal" and "UV" stresses.

Thermal Tolerance

These studies were performed on cultured human fibroblasts that were either Hsp70-treated or Hsp70-induced. After treatment or induction, the cells were exposed to heat stress. Viability test showed that the cells prepared by Hsp resisted better to heat stress than the control cells, and their viability was well-preserved (34,37).

Similar results were obtained on *ex vivo* skin. Human skin samples that were either treated with Hsp70 or were Hsp70-induced prior to heat stress, showed significantly less stress and signs of tissue damage than the control skin. Skin samples where Hsp70 level was increased also presented a well-preserved structure and minimal signs of heat-injury when compared with the control skin (34,37).

Hsp and UV Stress

It is now known that protection of epidermal cells from UV-induced damage is mediated by diverse mechanisms including Hsp70 expression. *In vitro* studies using UVB rays have demonstrated that UVB irradiation activates HSF1 in human keratinocytes, as evidenced by HSF phosphorylation and binding of this transcription factor to the HSE in the Hsp70 gene promoter region (38,39).

Studies on both cultured human epidermal cells and *ex vivo* skin showed that induction or administration of Hsp70 prior to stress significantly diminished UV-related morphological changes and sunburn cell number (34,36,37). Moreover, further studies demonstrated that Hsp70 induction modulated inflammatory cytokine synthesis in human skin cells (40), which is of special interest in diminishing sun damage and inflammatory symptoms.

Furthermore, using comet assay, studies on UV-induced DNA degradation revealed an interesting finding that the induction of Hsp70 prior to UV stress was accompanied by a decrease in DNA fragmentation and cell death (41). Moreover, studies on apoptosis showed that heat-induced apoptosis was blocked in Hsp70-expressing cells. Heat-induced cell death was associated with the activation of the stress-activated protein kinase SAPK/JNK, whose activation was strongly inhibited in cells where Hsp70 was induced, suggesting that Hsp70 is able to block apoptosis by inhibiting signaling events upstream of SAPK/JNK activation (42,43).

In addition, further results have shown that overexpression of Hsp70 in cells make them resist apoptosis induced by ceramides, lipid signaling molecules that are linked to SAPK/JNK activation and are generated by apoptosis-inducing conditions. Likewise, it has been demonstrated that Hsp is able to inhibit apoptosis at some point downstream of SAPK/JNK activation (42). Recent studies have shown that Hsp70 inhibits apoptosis by preventing recruitment of procaspase-9, the Apaf-1 apoptosome. More recent studies have also revealed that Hsp70 antagonizes apoptosis-inducing-factor (44,45).

Furthermore, earlier data have suggested that Hsp may protect cells from energy deprivation (46,47) and that Hsp may prevent ATP depletion associated with cell death (48), as other data have suggested that Hsp protect mitochondrial ATP synthesis from damage (49). Indeed, recent data strongly suggest that Hsp exhibit a regulative effect on cellular balance, which determines whether cells go into apoptosis. These studies reveal an important link between Hsp and apoptotic mechanisms, and show that Hsp play a pivotal role in maintaining this delicate balance (50).

Hsp and Aging

Earlier studies on the cultured cells of rodents have shown that aging alters the ability of their tissues to express Hsp70 in response to stress (43,51–55). Moreover, in cultured cells reaching the end of their replicative life span, a biological step known as "cellular senescence", the induction of Hsp70 has been reported to decline (51). Today, aging is thought to be associated with a reduced response to environmental stress (56). Through aging, skin becomes fragile towards different stresses, UV stress in particular. Protein damage progressively accumulates and both stress tolerance and the ability to express Hsp deteriorate (9,51,56,57).

A prior *in vivo* study on 30 individuals has shown that although the time course of the heat-induced Hsp70 expression was similar in young and aged groups, a lower level of induction of Hsp70 was observed in the latter group (56). Additional results have shown that under normal conditions, aged skin may exhibit a normal constitutive level of Hsp70, but the binding activity of the "heat shock transcription factor" decreases with aging.

Recent studies compared the Hsp70 level in aged and younger skin under normal conditions and after a stress, such as UV stress. They also investigated the modulation of Hsp70 level in these skin samples after Hsp70 induction in relation to UV stress (58). These studies were carried out on 10 volunteers between the ages of 50 and 70, and five younger volunteers between the ages of 30 and 40. Three punch biopsies from each volunteer were kept in culture, for 48 h, following organ culture methods. The first biopsy was the control skin, which was kept in culture for 48 h. The second biopsy was irradiated, after 24 h of culture, with UVB ($100 \, \text{mJ/cm}^2$), then kept in culture for another 24 h. For the third biopsy, Hsp70 was induced in a stress-free manner, 24 h prior to its irradiation with UVB, and then was kept in culture for another 24 h. After the 48 h of skin culture protocol, all skin samples were stained by H&E for morphological studies. This was followed by immunostaining studies of Hsp70 expression in the skin biopsies.

The results demonstrated that in stress-free conditions, both aged and younger skin exhibited a similar level of constitutive Hsp70 in the epidermis and superficial dermis, thus confirming earlier data. After UV stress, aged skin failed to produce a significant increase in Hsp70 and exhibited a remarkable decrease in Hsp70 staining intensity. In contrast, the Hsp70 level of younger skin increased significantly after UV stress in all samples, as expected.

Interestingly, when Hsp70 was induced in aged skin, prior to UV stress, samples exhibited a higher level of Hsp70 than in Hsp-uninduced skin, and this increase in Hsp lasted after UV irradiation, similar to younger skin (Figs. 1 and 2).

Accordingly, H&E staining of skin biopsies showed usual UV-morphological changes in the irradiated skin, such as apoptotic sunburn cells (SBC) and some edema. Aged skin suffered more and showed a higher number of SBC when compared with younger skin. When aged skin samples were Hsp-induced, prior to UV irradiation, a significant decrease in sun damage was seen. The samples showed milder signs of UV-aggression, similar to younger skin (Fig. 3).

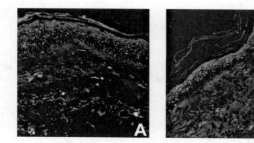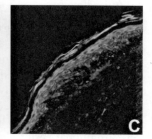

Figure 1 Immunofluorescence of Hsp70 in the skin from a 50-year-old woman: (A) Control skin; (B) irradiated skin; and (C) irradiated and Hsp-induced skin.

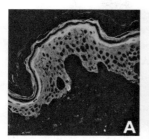 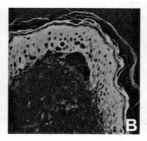 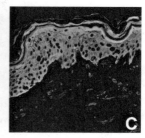

Figure 2 Immunofluorescence of Hsp70 in the skin from a 31-year-old woman: (A) Control skin; (B) irradiated skin; and (C) irradiated and Hsp-induced skin.

These studies show that although aged skin may exhibit a "normal" level of Hsp70 under nonstressful conditions, it fails to produce the typical protective increase of Hsp70 when faced with UV stress when compared with the Hsp increase in younger skin. These results also demonstrate that stress-free induction of Hsp70 in aged skin compensates for the decrease in stress-induced Hsp70 in aged skin, and improves its defense against UV stress.

Hsp and Retinoids

Another very interesting application for Hsp in the field of skin treatment is "retinoids". In the pharmaceutical and cosmeceutical field of skin care products, the use of retinoids in the treatment of some skin pathologies and the treatment of skin aging has taken a central role for many years. Retinoic acid and its derivatives have been widely used in topical skin care products for both short- and long-term applications.

As retinoid-treated skin is known to be fragile toward stress, in particular UV stress, and as Hsp70 is known to be important for skin protection from different types of stress, different studies have focused on investigating Hsp level after retinoids administration to the skin (59–62). This data has shown that long-term

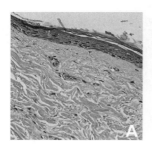 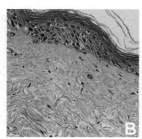 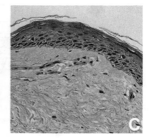

Figure 3 H&E staining of the skin from a 55-year-old woman: (A) Control skin; (B) irradiated skin; and (C) irradiated and Hsp-induced skin.

treatment with retinoids induces a post-transcriptional decrease in constitutive Hsp70 level. In a study on HL-60 cells (60), after 8 days of exposure to "all-*trans* retinoic acid" (ATRA) and "9-*cis* retinoic acid", Hsp70 was reduced by 40% in ATRA-treated cells and by 28% in 9-*cis* retinoic acid-treated cells, compared with untreated cells.

Other studies showed that in human fibroblasts, ATRA administration at the dose of 10^{-7} M decreased Hsp70 protein level in these cells. This effect was seen within the first week of ATRA administration, and became increasingly clear with time (3–7 weeks). Interestingly, these studies also showed that Hsp70 induction significantly restored Hsp70 in these aged ATRA-treated cells to a level which approached the control constitutive level (61).

Recent studies (62) have investigated the effect of stress-free induction of Hsp70 in UVB-irradiated and ATRA-treated cells, in both short- and long-term studies. These studies demonstrate that in cells treated for a short time with ATRA, UV irradiation induces an increase in total IL-1 level, whereas stress-free induction of Hsp70 down-regulated IL-1 level in ATRA-treated cells. IL-1 assessment by ELISA in long-term studies (up to 2 months), on cultured human fibroblasts treated with ATRA for long periods of time with and without UV irradiation with 100 mJ/cm^2, revealed that cells treated with ATRA and irradiated with UV exhibited a consistently higher level of IL-1 than control cells. Interestingly, stress-free induction of Hsp70 in ATRA-treated cells significantly decreased the level of UV-induced IL-1 in these cells (62) (Fig. 4).

LOOKING AHEAD

Taken together, the above studies provide support to the idea that Hsp are of considerable cosmeceutical interest to sun and after-sun care products. Moreover, today we have a relevant amount of studies and data that show the potential

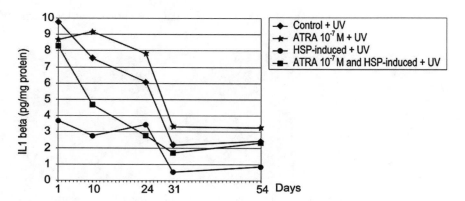

Figure 4 Effect of Hsp70 induction on IL-1 level in ATRA-treated and irradiated cells.

cosmeceutical application of Hsp70. The use of Hsp70 in skin-aging therapy and in association with retinoids skin therapy seems to be increasingly essential, in order to compensate for loss in skin defense and increase skin comfort toward environmental stress, especially UV stress.

REFERENCES

1. Ritossa F. A new puffing pattern induced by temperature shock and DNP in *Drosophila*. Experimentia 1962; 18:571–573.
2. Santoro MG. Heat shock factors and the control of the stress response. Biochem Pharmacol 2000; 59:55–63.
3. Feige U, Morimoto RI, Yahara I, Polla BS, eds. Stress-Inducible Cellular Responses. Basel-Boston-Berlin: Birkhäuser-Verlag, 1996.
4. Jäättelä M, Saksela K, Saksela E. Heat shock protects WEHI-164 target cells from the cytolysis by tumor necrosis factors alpha and beta. Eur J Immunol 1989; 19:1413–1417.
5. Jäättelä M. Effects of heat shock on cytolysis mediated by NK cells, LAK cells, activated monocytes and TNFs alpha and beta. Scand J Immunol 1990; 31:175–182.
6. Maytin EV, Murphy LA, Merrill MA. Hyperthermia induces resistance to ultraviolet light B in primary and immortalized epidermal keratinocytes. Cancer Res 1993; 53:4952–4959.
7. Bellmann K, Wenz A, Radons J, Burkart V, Kleemann R, Kolb H. Heat shock induces resistance in rat pancreatic islet cells against nitric oxide, oxygen radicals and streptozotocin toxicity *in vitro*. J Clin Invest 1995; 95:2840–2845.
8. Jäättelä M. Heat shock proteins as cellular lifeguards. Ann Med 1999; 31:261–271.
9. Macario AJ. Heat-shock proteins and molecular chaperones: implications for pathogenesis, diagnostics, and therapeutics. Int J Clin Lab Res 1995; 25:59–70.
10. Wu C. Heat shock transcription factors: structure and regulation. Annu Rev Cell Dev Biol 1995; 11:441–469.
11. Morimoto RI, Kroeger PE, Cotto JJ. The transcriptional regulation of heat shock genes: a plethora of heat shock factors and regulatory conditions. In: Feige U, Morimoto RI, Yahara I, Polla BS, eds. Stress-Inducible Cellular Responses. Basel-Boston-Berlin: Birkhäuser-Verlag, 1996:139–163.
12. Pirkkala L, Nykänen P, Sistonen L. Roles of the heat shock transcription factors in regulation of the heat shock response and beyond. FASEB J 2001; 15:1118–1131.
13. Tanabe M, Sasai N, Nagata K, Liu XD, Liu PC, Thiele DJ, Nakai A. The mammalian HSF4 gene generates both an activator and a repressor of heat shock genes by alternative splicing. J Biol Chem 1999; 274:27845–27856.
14. Scharf KD, Rose S, Zott W, Schöffl F, Nover L. Three tomato genes code for heat stress transcription factors with a region of remarkable homology to the DNA-binding domain of the yeast HSF. EMBO J 1990; 9:4495–4501.
15. Nakai A, Morimoto RI. Characterization of a novel chicken heat shock transcription factor, heat shock factor 3, suggests a new regulatory pathway. Mol Cell Biol 1993; 13:1983–1997.
16. Råbergh CM, Airaksinen S, Soitamo A, Bjorklund HV, Johansson T, Nikinmaa M, Sistonen L. Tissue-specific expression of zebrafish (*Danio rerio*) heat shock factor 1 mRNA in response to heat stress. J Exp Biol 2000; 203:1817–1824.

17. Stump DG, Landsberger N, Wolffe AP. The cDNA encoding *Xenopus laevis* heat-shock factor 1 (XHSF1): nucleotide and deduced amino-acid sequences, and properties of the encoded protein. Gene 1995; 160:207–211.
18. Nover L, Scharf KD, Gagliardi D, Vergne P, Czarnecka-Verner E, Gurley WB. The Hsf world: classification and properties of plant heat stress transcription factors. Cell Stress Chaperones 1996; 1:215–223.
19. Nakai A. New aspects in the vertebrate heat shock factor system: Hsf3 and Hsf4. Cell Stress Chaperones 1999; 4:86–93.
20. Leppä S, Sistonen L. Heat shock response—pathophysiological implications. Ann Med 1997; 29:73–78.
21. McMillan DR, Xiao X, Shao L, Graves K, Benjamin IJ. Targeted disruption of heat shock transcription factor 1 abolishes thermotolerance and protection against heat-inducible apoptosis. J Biol Chem 1998; 273:7523–7528.
22. Xiao X, Zuo X, Davis AA, McMillan DR, Curry BB, Richardson JA, Benjamin IJ. HSF1 is required for extra-embryonic development, postnatal growth and protection during inflammatory responses in mice. EMBO J 1999; 18:5943–5952.
23. Pirkkala L, Alastalo TP, Zuo X, Benjamin IJ, Sistonen L. Disruption of heat shock factor 1 reveals an essential role in the ubiquitin proteolytic pathway. Mol Cell Biol 2000; 20:2670–2675.
24. Liu XD, Liu PC, Santoro N, Thiele DJ. Conservation of a stress response: human heat shock transcription factors functionally substitute for yeast HSF. EMBO J 1997; 16:6466–6477.
25. Sistonen L, Sarge KD, Phillips B, Abravaya K, Morimoto RI. Activation of heat shock factor 2 during hemin-induced differentiation of human erythroleukemia cells. Mol Cell Biol 1992; 12:4104–4111.
26. Morimoto RI, Santoro MG. Stress-inducible responses and heat shock proteins: new pharmacologic targets for cytoprotection. Nat Biotechnol 1998; 16:833–838.
27. Baba HA, Schmid KW, Schmid C, Blasius S, Heinecke A, Kerber S, Scheld HH, Bocker W, Deng MC. Possible relationship between heat shock protein 70, cardiac hemodynamics, and survival in the early period after heart transplantation. Transplantation 1998; 65:799–804.
28. Flohe S, Speidel N, Flach R, Lange R, Erhard J, Schade FU. Expression of Hsp70 as a potential prognostic marker for acute rejection in human liver transplantation. Transpl Int 1998; 11:89–94.
29. McMurtry AL, Cho K, Young LJ, Nelson CF, Greenhalgh DG. Expression of Hsp70 in healing wounds of diabetic and nondiabetic mice. J Surg Res 1999; 86:36–41.
30. Bitar MS, Farook T, John B, Francis IM. Heat-shock protein 72/73 and impaired wound healing in diabetic and hypercortisolemic states. Surgery 1999; 125:594–601.
31. Henle KJ, Jethmalani SM, Li L, Li GC. Protein glycosylation in a heat-resistant rat fibroblast cell model expressing human Hsp70. Biochem Biophys Res Commun 1997; 232:26–32.
32. Pockley AG. Heat shock proteins in health and disease: therapeutic targets or therapeutic agents? Expert Rev Mol Med 2001; 1–21.
33. Manjili MH, Wang XY, Park J, Facciponte JG, Repasky EA, Subjeck JR. Immunotherapy of cancer using heat shock proteins. Front Biosci 2002; 7:D43–D52.
34. Cucumel K, Botto JM, Bauza E, Dal Farra C, Roetto R, Domloge N. Artemia extract induces Hsp70 in human cells and enhances cell protection from stress. J Invest Dermatol 2001; 117(2): 454.

35. Dal Farra C, Domloge N. Stressing out. Soap Perfumery Cosmetics 2002; 75:83–86.
36. Domloge N, Bauza E, Cucumel K, Peyronel D, Dal Farra C. Artemia extract toward more extensive sun protection. Cosmet Toiletries 2002; 117:69–78.
37. Botto JM, Cucumel K, Dal Farra C, Domloge N. Treatment of human cells with Hsp70-rich yeast extract enhances cell thermotolerance and resistance to stress. J Invest Dermatol 2001; 117(2):452.
38. Zhou X, Tron VA, Li G, Trotter MJ. Heat shock transcription factor-1 regulates heat shock protein-72 expression in human keratinocytes exposed to ultraviolet B light. J Invest Dermatol 1998; 111:194–198.
39. Trautinger F, Kokesch C, Klosner G, Knobler RM, Kindas-Mügge I. Expression of the 72-kD heat shock protein is induced by ultraviolet A radiation in a human fibrosarcoma cell line. Exp Dermatol 1999; 8:187–192.
40. Bauza E, Dal Farra C, Domloge N. Hsp70 induction by Artemia extract exhibits an anti-inflammatory effect and down-regulates IL-1 and IL-8 synthesis in human HaCaT cells. J Invest Dermatol 2001; 117(2):415.
41. Cucumel K, Dal Farra C, Bauza E, Domloge N. Stress-free Hsp70 induction by Artemia extract modulates p53 and p21 expression and enhances human cell protection from UVB. J Invest Dermatol 2001; 117(2):497.
42. Mosser DD, Caron AW, Bourget L, Denis-Larose C, Massie B. Role of the human heat shock protein hsp70 in protection against stress-induced apoptosis. Mol Cell Biol 1997; 17:5317–5327.
43. Gabai VL, Meriin A, Mosser DD, Caron AW, Rits S, Shifrin VI, Sherman MY. Hsp70 prevents activation of stress kinases. A novel pathway of cellular thermotolerance. J Biol Chem 1997; 272:18033–18037.
44. Beere HM, Wolf BB, Cain K, Mosser DD, Mahboubi A, Kuwana T, Tailor P, Morimoto RI, Cohen GM, Green DR. Heat-shock protein 70 inhibits apoptosis by preventing recruitment of procaspase-9 to the Apaf-1 apoptosome. Nat Cell Biol 2000; 2:469–475.
45. Ravagnan L, Gurbuxani S, Susin SA, Maisse C, Daugas E, Zamzami N, Mak T, Jäättelä M, Penninger JM, Garrido C, Kroemer G. Heat-shock protein 70 antagonizes apoptosis-inducing factor. Nat Cell Biol 2001; 3:839–843.
46. Kabakov AE, Gabai VL. Heat shock proteins and cytoprotection: ATP-deprived mammalian cells (Molecular Biology Intelligence Unit series). Austin, TX: R.G. Landes Company, 1997.
47. Gabai VL, Kabakov AE. Rise in heat-shock protein level confers tolerance to energy deprivation. FEBS Lett 1993; 327:247–250.
48. Wong HR, Menendez IY, Ryan MA, Denenberg AG, Wispe JR. Increased expression of heat shock protein-70 protects A549 cells against hyperoxia. Am J Physiol 1998; 275:836–841.
49. Polla BS, Kantengwa S, François D, Salvioli S, Franceschi C, Marsac C, Cossarizza A. Mitochondria are selective targets for the protective effects of heat shock against oxidative injury. Proc Natl Acad Sci USA 1996; 93:6458–6463.
50. Xanthoudakis S, Nicholson DW. Heat-shock proteins as death determinants. Nat Cell Biol 2000; 2:E163–E165.
51. Gutsmann-Conrad A, Heydari AR, You S, Richardson A. The expression of heat shock protein 70 decreases with cellular senescence *in vitro* and in cells derived from young and old human subjects. Exp Cell Res 1998; 241:404–413.

52. Wu B, Gu MJ, Heydari AR, Richardson A. The effect of age on the synthesis of two heat shock proteins in the hsp70 family. J Gerontol 1993; 48:B50–B56.
53. Blake MJ, Fargnoli J, Gershon D, Holbrook NJ. Concomitant decline in heat-induced hyperthermia and Hsp70 mRNA expression in aged rats. Am J Physiol 1991; 260:663–667.
54. Pardue S, Groshan K, Raese JD, Morrison-Bogorad M. Hsp70 mRNA induction is reduced in neurons of aged rat hippocampus after thermal stress. Neurobiol Aging 1992; 13:661–672.
55. Fargnoli J, Kunisada T, Fornace AJ, Schneider EL, Holbrook NJ. Decreased expression of heat shock protein 70 mRNA and protein after heat treatment in cells of aged rats. Proc Natl Acad Sci USA 1990; 87:846–850.
56. Muramatsu T, Hatoko M, Tada H, Shirai T, Ohnishi T. Age-related decrease in the inductability of heat shock protein 72 in normal human skin. Br J Dermatol 1996; 134:1035–1038.
57. Feder ME, Hofmann GE. Heat-shock proteins, molecular chaperones, and the stress response: evolutionary and ecological physiology. Annu Rev Physiol 1999; 61:243–282.
58. Cucumel K, Dal Farra C, Domloge N. Artemia extract "compensates" for age-related decrease of Hsp70 in skin. J Invest Dermatol 2002; 119(1):257.
59. Santin AD, Hermonat PL, Ravaggi A, Chiriva-Internati M, Pecorelli S, Parham GP. Effects of retinoic acid on the expression of a tumor rejection antigen (heat shock protein gp96) in human cervical cancer. Eur J Gynaecol Oncol 1998; 19:229–233.
60. Tosi P, Visani G, Ottaviani E, Gibellini D, Pellacani A, Tura S. Reduction of heat-shock protein-70 after prolonged treatment with retinoids: biological and clinical implications. Am J Hematol 1997; 56:143–150.
61. Cucumel K, Bauza E, Dal Farra C, Domloge N. Treatment of human cells with Artemia extract helps to restore the decrease in hsp70 level caused by cell treatment with "all *trans* retinoic acid". J Invest Dermatol 2002; 119(1):257.
62. Bauza E, Cucumel K, Roux E, Dal Farra C, Domloge N. Artemia extract significantly down-regulates ATRA-induced IL-1 after UV-exposure in human fibroblasts. J Invest Dermatol 2003; 1082(1):500.

30

Evelle® Supplementation

Dörte Segger
Skin Investigation and Technology, Hamburg, Germany

Frank Schönlau
University of Münster, Münster, Germany

Introduction	537
Clinical Study with Evelle®	538
Results	540
Discussion	541
References	543

INTRODUCTION

The skin protects our body from environmental harm, plays an important role in controlling water retention and body temperature, and is an essential part of the immune system. Further to the vital biological functions, the skin plays a pivotal role in the feeling of well being and physical attractiveness, determined by color, surface texture, and physiological properties such as elasticity, sweat, scent, and sebum production (1). With increasing age, skin appearance gradually declines, ultimately leading to reduction and coarsening of collagen, elastosis, wrinkling, laxity, atrophy, irregular pigmentation, and dryness (2). Various environmental factors are understood to accelerate this process: UV radiation, free radicals, toxic and allergic compounds, immune and hormonal status, mechanical strain, cigaret smoking, and stress.

Skin functioning and attractiveness rely on specific nutritional needs, as evidenced by the development of skin disorders in response to various nutritional deficiencies (3). Supplementation with deficient vitamins, minerals, and other dietary constituents were shown to improve skin conditions (4). Vitamin C is essential as a cofactor of prolyl 4-hydroxylase (5). Dietary supplementation with vitamins C and E as well as carotenoids provides significant antioxidant activity in human skin with demonstrated UV-protection and enhancement of cutaneous immune response (1). Selenium as component of antioxidant selenoproteins was shown to protect skin cells from UV-induced damage, DNA oxidation, and lipid peroxidation (6). Zinc is an essential element of more than 200 metalloenzymes, such as superoxide dismutase, and enzymes required for DNA replication, gene transcription, and RNA and protein synthesis. Roughened skin and impaired wound healing have been reported in association with mild zinc deficiency, implicating changes in skin (7). Biotin is an essential cofactor for several carboxylases that catalyze vital steps in intermediary metabolism in skin. Deficiency of biotin is known to manifest in various skin disorders, including dermatitis, scaling, and alopecia (8).

An approach to retard progression of skin aging has been proposed to rest on the requirement of antioxidant defense and sufficient density and geometry of collagen and elastic fibers (9). Although the earlier-mentioned vitamins and minerals fulfill the basic needs for healthy skin tissue, another micronutrient has been suggested to support collagen skin density. An extract of French maritime pine bark (*Pinus pinaster*), Pycnogenol®, a mixture of procyanidins and phenolic acids, display pronounced selective affinity to collagen and elastin. Moreover, Pycnogenol as well as its two major human metabolites δ-(3,4-dihydroxyphenyl)-γ-valerolactone and δ-(3-methoxy-4-hydroxylphenyl)-γ-valerolactone strongly inhibit matrix-metalloproteinases MMP-1, MMP-2, and MMP-9 (10). On a weight per volume basis, the metabolites appeared to be more effective than Pycnogenol. It was concluded that Pycnogenol might favorably act on an imbalance between MMPs and their natural inhibitors, tissue inhibitors of metalloproteinases (TIMPs). This assumption is supported by pharmacological studies showing statistical significant acceleration of wound healing by administration of Pycnogenol (11).

Clinical Study with Evelle®

We carried out a clinical study to evaluate whether a proprietary formulation "Evelle" (registered trademark of Pharmanord, Denmark) with Pycnogenol in combination with vitamins, antioxidants, minerals, and other micronutrients may favorably alter skin roughness and elasticity in women aged 45 years or older (12).

A total of 62 women, aged 45–75 years with phototypes I–IV, were recruited for this study. The inner side of the left forearm was chosen as investigation site because it is more homogeneous and covered from environmental factors such as sunlight and to refrain from using cosmetic products is more feasible than for example in the face. The investigation site had to be free of acute skin diseases, such as warts, scabs, with little or no hair, and no tattoo. Exclusion criteria were chronic diseases, pregnancy or breastfeeding, as well as other studies on the forearms during the past 2 weeks. Subjects were advised to refrain from sauna and swimming, and discontinue the use of skin care products, shower oils, and dermatological therapeutics on the tested area of the arm during the trial period. Written informed consent was obtained from all subjects.

The study design was double-blinded and placebo-controlled. After a run-in period of 7 days for conditioning subjects, they were assigned to either verum or placebo group according to their initial skin roughness value to ensure equal distribution. One group of 31 women was advised to take two Evelle tablets twice a day, a trademarked proprietary blend of ingredients geared to support optimal nutrition of the skin as well as hair and nails (Pharmanord, Denmark). One Evelle tablet provides the following micronutrients: Pycnogenol (10 mg), vitamin C (30 mg), vitamin E (D-α-tocopherylacetate) (5 mg), biotin (75 μg), selenium (25 μg), zinc as gluconate (7.5 mg), Bio-Marine Complex (hydrolyzed collagen and glycosaminoglycans from salmon) (50 mg), Horsetail herb extract (natural source of silicate) (40 mg), blueberry extract (15 mg), tomato extract (dietary carotenoids, $\beta + \gamma$-carotene, lycopene, and lutein) (34 mg). The control group received identically looking tablets containing none of the above-mentioned ingredients.

Skin elasticity was recorded using the instrument "Cutometer SEM 575" (Courage & Khazaka Electronics, Cologne, Germany) 1 day before start of supplementation and then again after 6 weeks. Measurements of viscoelastic properties were performed according to the manufacturer's instructions (available on website www.courage-khazaka.de) with the following parameter settings: 350 mbar, on-time 5 s, and off-time 5 s followed by computer-aided evaluation using parameter R5 ($=Ur/Ue$). Measurements were always repeated twice.

Skin roughness was evaluated using a three-dimensional microtopography imaging system "PRIMOS" (GF Messtechnik, Teltow, Germany; www.gfmesstechnik.com). The scanned skin area size was 13×18 mm^2, with three separate sites of the investigation site being measured. Calculation of skin roughness was carried out using the PRIMOS computer program using the parameter star roughness (polynom level 5) according to the manufacturer's instructions. Each line of the star had a length of 12.8 mm, with 16 lines being analyzed. The result was recorded as skin roughness in micrometers. Evaluation of skin roughness was carried out 1 day before start of supplementation and a second time after 12 weeks.

Skin parameters were measured in a climate controlled room at 21.5°C (± 1°C) and 50% (± 5%) relative humidity. Subjects were conditioned to this indoor climate 20 min before performing measurements.

Statistical analysis was carried out using computer programs Excel (Microsoft) and STATISTICA. Excel was used for calculation of relative data, the means and standard deviation. STATISTICA was applied to test significance of differences between verum and placebo. The distribution of original and relative data was checked using the Kolmogorov–Smirnov test. In the case of normal distribution of data, the test of significance of differences between verum and placebo was performed with the t-test for independent samples. Differences between treatment situations with a p-value of ≤ 0.05 were accepted as statistically significant.

RESULTS

A total of 58 women completed the trial, 29 each in placebo and verum groups. Two subjects in the placebo group and another two in the verum group discontinued the study. All four subjects described symptoms of gastric discomfort which resolved after termination of tablet intake.

The initial skin elasticity of both groups was comparable and not statistically significantly different. The mean skin elasticity in the verum and placebo groups was 0.638 ± 0.119 and 0.677 ± 0.104, respectively. After 6 weeks, the mean elasticity in the placebo group decreased to 0.675 ± 0.117, whereas the mean elasticity in the Evelle group rose to 0.681 ± 0.085. The results are presented relative to t_0 in Fig. 1, with verum relative elasticity being statistically significantly higher by 9% than placebo.

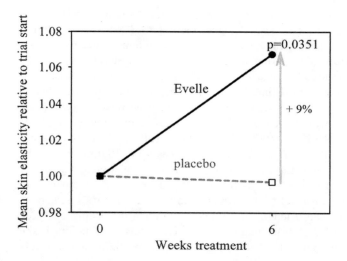

Figure 1 Mean skin elasticities of both treatment groups are presented relative to the initial value ($=1$) measured at t_0. Skin elasticity was measured prior to start of supplementation and again after 6 weeks of supplementation with either verum or placebo. Presented are mean values of 29 subjects in each group and SD. Statistical significance of difference between treatment groups was obtained by the t-test after normal distribution of data was found according to the Kolmogorov–Smirnov test. [From Segger and Schönlau (12).]

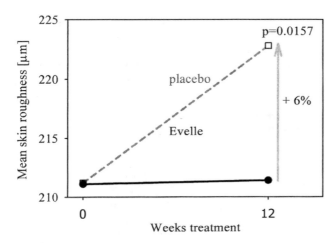

Figure 2 Mean of subject's skin roughness values in both treatment groups are presented. Skin roughness was measured by three-dimensional microtopography imaging at trial start and after 12 weeks of supplementation with either verum or placebo. Presented are mean values of 29 subjects in each group and SD. Statistical significance of difference between treatment groups was obtained by the t-test after normal distribution of data was found according to the Kolmogorov–Smirnov test. [From Segger and Schönlau (12).]

At trial start, the skin roughness of investigated sites in both the groups was statistically significantly indistinguishable from another. The starting level was 211.1 ± 21.6 μm in the verum group and 211.2 ± 29.5 μm in the placebo group. After 12 weeks of oral treatment, there was an increase of skin roughness in the placebo group, whereas the verum group did not encounter increase of skin roughness. As shown in Fig. 2, the mean skin roughness of the placebo-treated group was statistically significantly higher by 6% than in the verum-treated group.

DISCUSSION

In our study objective parameters, skin elasticity and roughness, were favorably altered by oral treatment with a supplement created for improved skin nutrition. Placebo treatment had no measurable effect on skin elasticity. In our study, we chose to first study an effect of the nutritional supplement on skin elasticity, as we expected this parameter to be affected first. Only when the result were promising, the study was planned to be continued for further 6 weeks to measure a possible effect on skin roughness. Unexpectedly, the skin roughness in the placebo group rose considerably, whereas this was not the case in the verum group. We suspect that outdoor climate might have contributed to this finding as the study was carried out in the course from winter to summer. At trial start, the outdoor climate represented mild winter weather conditions with temperatures ~6°C and moderate humidity. After 6 weeks when the effect on skin elasticity was measured, a moderately warm spring weather prevailed (~ 22°C and low relative humidity). At the end of the study, when skin roughness was measured, hot spring weather with ~22°C and low relative humidity predominated.

Despite the unexpected increase of skin roughness in the placebo group, skin roughness in the verum group was statistically significantly lower. This finding together with the improved elasticity suggests that Evelle bears nutritional benefits for the skin.

As reviewed by Boelsma et al. (1) vitamins C and E and carotenoids have been extensively researched for skin nutrition, showing protection against photoaging, antioxidant protection, and improved cutaneous immune responses. Because studies have suggested that broad mixtures of carotenoids are more effective than isolated species, a tomato extract was chosen as carotenoid source in Evelle as it provides lycopene and lutein and further carotenoids species in addition to β- and γ-carotene (13). In addition to providing the minerals selenium and zinc, which are essential cofactors of various enzymes, blueberry extract was added because of the ascribed potent antioxidant activity (14).

In order to warrant abundant supply with amino acids necessary for collagen production, a standardized fish extract (Bio-Marine Complex), consisting of hydrolyzed collagen and glycosaminoglycans, was incorporated into Evelle. Glycosaminoglycans represent modified carbohydrates such as hyaluronic acid, which play an important role in skin hydration. A need for supplementation appears reasonable in light of the documented age-related decreased content of glycosaminoglycans in aged skin (15).

A pivotal ingredient of Evelle is Pycnogenol®, a standardized extract of *Pinus pinaster* bark. Pycnogenol is a powerful antioxidant which can recycle oxidized ascorbate and protect vitamin E from oxidation, thus prolonging the activity of these vitamins (16). Furthermore, Pycnogenol was found to inhibit collagenase from degrading collagen (10). Interestingly, the two major metabolites formed in humans after consumption of Pycnogenol, δ-(3,4-dihydroxyphenyl)-γ-valerolactone and δ-(3-methoxy-4-hydroxylphenyl)-γ-valerolactone (17), were found to be more potent MMP inhibitors than the parent molecules (10). The 50% inhibitory concentration of the metabolites on MMP-1, MMP-2, and MMP-9 was 20 μM or lower. An imbalance between MMPs and their natural inhibitors, TIMPs, occurs in aging skin and prevails during UV-exposure and cigarette smoking. Indeed, the common perception that smokers and sun-lovers look older is believed to be the consequence of increased dermal collagen degradation (18). Pharmacological studies have demonstrated that Pycnogenol accelerates wound healing, suggesting increased collagen matrix remodeling (11). MMPs are up-regulated during inflammatory conditions, causing proteolytic tissue damage. It was shown that MMP-9 secretion by stimulated human monocytes was strongly inhibited by Pycnogenol metabolites with IC50 value of 0.5 μM. The metabolites were shown in this experiment to be more effective than the endogenous glucocorticoid hydrocortisone (10).

Oral consumption of Pycnogenol was shown to increase UV-light-induced minimal erythema dosage in humans in dose-dependent manner (19). Pycnogenol's antioxidant activity prevents redox regulated activation of gene transcription factor NF-κB, thus preventing expression of pro-inflammatory adhesion molecules and cytokines. In pharmacological studies, Pycnogenol was shown to reduce incidence of skin tumors during chronic exposure of skin to UV-light, indicating potent photoaging protection (20). Oral Pycnogenol administration was found to be helpful for women with hyper-pigmentation (chloasma). Size of affected skin area as well as pigmentation intensity was significantly reduced, most likely because of an tyrosinase inhibitory effect (21). Furthermore, in pharmacological and clinical studies, Pycnogenol was found to increase microcirculation by enhancing production of endothelial nitric oxide (22). The improved microcirculation has been proposed to support better oxygen and nutrient supply as well as better waste removal in the skin (23).

In conclusion, our clinical studies suggests that the chosen combination of micro-nutrients in Evelle can potentially alleviate visible signs of skin aging.

REFERENCES

1. Boelsma E, Hendriks HFJ, Roza L. Nutritional skin care: health effects of micronutrients and fatty acids. Am J Clin Nutr 2001; 73:853–864.
2. Kurban RS, Bhawan J. Histologic changes in skin associated with aging. J Dermatol Surg Oncol 1990; 16:908–914.
3. Miller SJ. Nutritional deficiency and the skin. J Am Acad Dermatol 1989; 21:1–30.
4. Roe DA. Current etiologies and cutaneous signs of vitamin deficiencies. In: Roe DA, ed. Nutrition and the Skin. Contemporary Issues in Clinical Nutrition. New York: Alan R Liss Inc., 1986:81–98.
5. Davidson JM, LuValle PA, Zoia O, Quaglino D, Giro MG. Ascorbate differentially regulates elastin and collagen biosynthesis in vascular smooth muscle cells and skin fibroblasts by pre-translational mechanisms. J Biol Chem 1997; 372:345–352.
6. McKenzie RC. Selenium, ultraviolet radiation and the skin. Clin Exp Dermatol 2000; 25:631–636.
7. Rostan EF, DeBuys HV, Madey DL, Pinnel SR. Evidence supporting zinc as an important antioxidant for skin. Int J Dermatol 2002; 41:606–611.
8. Mock DM. Skin manifestations of biotin deficiency. Semin Dermatol 1991; 10:296–302.
9. Murad H, Tabibian MP. The effect of an oral supplement containing glucosamine, amino acids, minerals, and antioxidants on cutaneous aging: a preliminary study. J Dermatol Treat 2001; 2:47–51.
10. Grimm T, Schäfer A, Högger P. Antioxidant activity and inhibition of matrix metalloproteinases by metabolites of maritime pine bark extract (Pycnogenol®). Free Radic Biol Med 2004; 36:811–822.
11. Blazsó G, Gábor M, Schönlau F, Rohdewald P. Pycnogenol® accelerates wound healing and reduces scar formation. Phytother Res 2004; 18:579–581.

12. Segger D, Schönlau F. Supplementation with Evelle® improves skin smoothness and elasticity in a double-blind placebo controlled study with 62 women. J Dermatol Treat 2004; 15:222–226.
13. Khachik F, Carvalho L, Bernstein PS, Muir GJ, Zhao DY, Katz NB. Chemistry, distribution, and metabolism of tomato carotenoids and their impact on human health. Exp Biol Med 2002; 227:845–851.
14. Prior RL, Cao G, Martin A, Sofic E, McEwan J, O'Brien C, Lischner N, Ehrenfeldt M, Kalt W, Krewer G, Mainland M. Antioxidant capacity is influenced by total phenolic and anthocyanin content, maturity, and variety of *Vaccinium* species. J Agric Food Chem 1998; 46:2686–2693.
15. Ghersetich I, Lotti T, Campanile G, Grappone C, Dini G. Hyaluronic acid in cutaneous intrinsic aging. Int J Dermatol 1994; 33:119–122.
16. Packer L, Rimbach G, Virgili F. Antioxidant activity and biologic properties of a procyanidin-rich extract from pine (*Pinus maritima*) bark, Pycnogenol®. Free Radic Biol Med 1999; 27:704–724.
17. Grosse Düweler K, Rohdewald P. Urinary metabolites of French maritime pine bark extract in humans. Pharmazie 2000; 55:364–368.
18. Lahmann C, Bergemann J, Harrison G, Young AR. Matrix metalloproteinase-1 and skin ageing in smokers. Lancet 2001; 357:935–936.
19. Saliou C, Rimbach G, Moini H, McLaughlin L, Hosseini S, Lee J, Watson RR, Packer L. Solar ultraviolet-induced erythema in human skin and nuclear factor-kappa-B-dependent gene expression in keratinocytes are modulated by a French maritime pine bark extract. Free Radic Biol Med 2001; 30:154–160.
20. Sime S, Reeve VE. Protection from inflammation, immunosuppression and carcinogenesis induced by UV radiation in mice by topical Pycnogenol. Photochem Photobiol 2004; 79:193–198.
21. Ni Z, Mu Y, Gulati O. Treatment of melasma with Pycnogenol®. Phytother Res 2002; 16:567–571.
22. Rohdewald P. A review of the French maritime pine bark extract (Pycnogenol®), a herbal medication with a diverse pharmacology. Int J Clin Pharmacol Ther 2002; 40:158–168.
23. Schönlau F. The cosmeceutical Pycnogenol®. J Appl Cosmetol 2002; 20:241–246.

31

Retinaldehyde: A New Compound in Topical Retinoids

F. Verrière
Pierre Fabre Dermo-Cosmétique, Lavaur, France

Regulatory Environment 545
References 546

REGULATORY ENVIRONMENT

All-*trans* retinal or retinaldehyde (RAL) belongs to the group of natural retinoids issued from vitamin A metabolism. Next to retinol, RAL is the key metabolite as the immediate precursor of retinoic acid (RA) and can be physiologically stored in the keratinocytes of the skin. With a similar activity (1) and a better tolerability than RA, RAL is used as cosmetic mainly in skin aging (2).

In the epidermis, RAL increases cells differentiation and keratinocytes turnover (3) with induction of synthesis of low-molecular-weight keratins that are characteristic of young skin. In parallel, RAL reduces the thickness of epidermis and decreases stratum corneum thickness and cell cohesion (4). These pharmacological effects justify the use of RAL in skin aging.

The pharmacological effect of RAL is dose dependent up to concentrations of 0.1% with a convenient tolerability (5), and the efficacy tolerance ratio of 0.05% concentration used for skin aging during several months is supported by a significant clinical experience.

The clinical effect of RAL 0.05% in skin aging has been assessed under profilometric evaluation using skin silicon replicas. In a comparative study (6) vs. vehicle, 18 weeks of RAL treatment can significantly reduce wrinkles and skin rugosity in patients with photodamaged skin of the face. Another study conducted on a large number of patients confirms the clinical efficacy of RAL to reduce wrinkles, lines, pigmentary spots, and complexion of the face (7). Both studies confirm the high tolerability of RAL 0.05% used once a day in the evening. RAL is a convenient ingredient for cosmetic formulations in skin aging.

In the dermis, by decreasing the vascular endothelial growth factor of keratinocytes (8) involved in the neoangiogenesis, topical RAL has a clinically confirmed interest in rosacea and in general in red skin conditions (9). RAL also has a repairing action of different proteins of the dermis, including elastic fibers (10), and a potential interesting hypopigmentation effect.

Involved in other skin functions, RAL decreases the number and diameters of comedones (11). The aldehyde chemical radical contributes to the microcidal effect of RAL (12) against *Propionibacterium acnes*. This supports the interest of RAL in acne skin conditions.

With a clinical background of now 10 years in skin aging, RAL proposes other potential therapeutic outcomes in skin conditions such as rosacea and acne.

REFERENCES

1. Didierjean L, Carraux P, Grand D, Sass JO, Nau H, Saurat JH. Topical retinaldehyde increases skin content of retinoic acid and exerts biologic activity in mouse skin. J Invest Dermatol 1996; 107:714–719.
2. Edwards H. Topical retinol and retinaldehyde in cosmetics as alternative to retinoic acid: evidence of efficacy. Retinoids Lipid-Soluble Vitam Clin Practice 2001; 17(4):98–102.
3. Didierjean L, Tran C, Sorg O, Saurat JH. Biological activities of topical retinaldehyde. Dermatology 1999; 199:19–24.
4. Diridollou S, Vienne MP, Alibert M, Aquilina C, Briant A, Dahan S. Efficacy of topical 0.05% retinaldehyde in skin aging by ultrasound an rheological techniques. Dermatology 1999; 1899:37–41.
5. Saurat JH, Didierjean L, Masgrau E, Piletta PA. Topical retinaldehyde on human skin: biologic effect and tolerance. J Invest Dermatol 1994; 103(6):354–356.
6. Creidi P, Vienne MP, Ochonovski S, Lauze C, Turlier V, Lagarde JM, Dupuy P. Profilometric evaluation of photodamage after topical retinaldehyde and retinoic acid treatment. J Am Acad Dermatol 1998; 39:960–965.
7. Verrière F, Nocera T, Segard S, Guerrero D. Efficacy of the retinaldehyde 0.05% and pretocopheryl 0.05% association: I. The correction of skin aging. Nouv Dermatol 2002; 21:295–298.
8. Lachgar S, Chharveron M, Gall Y, Bonafe JL. Inhibitory effects of retinoids on VEGF production by cultured huma skin keratinocytes. Dermatology 1999; 199:25–27.
9. Vienne MP, Ochando N, Borrel MT, Gall Y, Lauze C, Dupuy P. Retinaldahyde alleviates rosacea. Dermatology 1999; 199:53–56.

10. Boisnic S, Branchet MC, Le Charpentier Y, Segard C. Repair of UVA inducing elastic fiber and collagen damage by 0.05% retinaldehyde creal in an *ex vivo* human skin model. Dermatology 1999; 199:43–48.
11. Fort-Lacoste L, Verscheure Y, Tisne Versailles J, Navarro R. Comedolytic effect of topical retinaldehyde in the rhino mouse model. Dermatology 1999; 199:33–35.
12. Pechère M, Pechère JC, Siegenthaler G, Germanier L, Saurat JH. Antibacterial activity of retinaldehyde against *Propionibacterium acnès*. Dermatology 1999; 199:29–31.

32

Copper Peptide and Skin

Mary Beth Finkey and Yohini Appa
Neurogena Corporation, Los Angeles, California, USA

Sulochana Bhandarkar
University of California at San Francisco, San Francisco, California, USA

Introduction	550
Molecular Biology	550
Absorption and Transport	550
Metabolism and Excretion	550
Molecular Pharmacology	551
Copperceuticals and Skin: The GHK–Cu Tripeptide	552
GHK–Cu Analogs	552
The Importance of the Copper Peptide Complex	554
Skin Penetration Study of GHK–Cu	554
Immunohistological Assessment	555
Controlled Usage Study in Photodamaged Skin	555
Methods	556
Clinical Results	557
Viscoelastic Properties	558
Ultrasound Measurements	559
Digital Images	559
Safety of GHK–Cu Complex	559
Conclusions	561
References	561

INTRODUCTION

Copper peptide, a recent addition to the cosmeceutical pantheon, has an extensive scientific background. This chapter focuses on cutaneous implications.

Molecular Biology

The average diet of adult humans in western countries contains from 0.6 to 1.6 mg Cu/day (1–3). Foods rather than water contribute to virtually all of the copper consumed, and the copper content of different foods varies considerably. Shellfish and organ meats are the richest sources of copper, whereas muscle meats contain much less. Among plant foods, seeds (including nuts and grains) have a high abundance of copper; fruits and vegetables have less (1,4).

Absorption and Transport

Absorption of copper occurs primarily in the small intestine, after digestion of food in the stomach and duodenum. Absorption of the metal ion is high; values for apparent absorption by adult humans average between 55% and 75% (1,3,5). The recommended dietary allowance for copper has been designated as 1.5–3.0 mg/day (1,6). Absorption of copper across the brush border into the cells of intestinal mucosa, and its subsequent transfer across the basolateral membrane into interstitial fluid and blood, occur by different mechanisms. Transfer across the mucosal barrier occurs by non-energy-dependent diffusion, whereas transfer of copper across the basolateral membrane is mediated by a saturable, energy-dependent mechanism (1).

Transport of copper in the blood plasma and interstitial fluid is through albumin and transcuprein in the protein bound state (1,7). Most of this bound copper is then rapidly deposited in the liver and lesser amounts to the kidney (1,2,8,9). Ceruloplasmin binds the majority of copper ($\sim$65%), and it is this form that is available for uptake by other tissues (1).

Metabolism and Excretion

On entering cells, copper finds its way readily to the different sites where it is needed. It plays a role as a cofactor for specific enzymes and electron transport proteins involved in energy or antioxidant metabolism. Besides its incorporation into ceruloplasmin, it is also a part of cytochrome oxidase, superoxide dismutase (SOD), and metallothionein. Various other intracellular and extracellular enzymes depend on copper for their activity (1).

The excretion of copper, though not fully understood, is mainly through bile. The minimal loss of copper through the urine is consistent with the low levels of free copper in blood plasma, suggesting that any low-molecular-weight copper complexes that might be filtered by the glomeruli are specifically reabsorbed. The sloughing of epithelial cells also does not appear to be a major excretory route for copper, and although hair and nails have high concentrations of copper, average daily losses from cutting hair and nails do not account for much (1).

Molecular Pharmacology

Copper is required for several intracellular and extracellular enzymes. Cytochrome c oxidase, the terminal enzyme of the electron transport chain in mitochondria, is required for oxygen utilization. Cytochrome c is mediated by two heme moieties and two copper atoms. Copper deficiency results in a reduction of cytochrome c oxidase activity and the respiratory capacity of mitochondria, particularly in liver, heart, and brain (1,2,10).

Superoxidase dismutase (SOD), a copper-containing enzyme is critical to the antioxidant defense system (1,11). The peroxide produced by SOD is disposed of by other enzymes, notably heme-dependent catalase and selenium-dependent glutathione peroxidase (1,12). Without these enzymes, there would be formation of destructive hydroxyl radicals which are implicated in damage to unsaturated lipids in cell membranes (2).

Metallothioneins are small polypeptides which contain copper and are sites for storage and detoxification of this ion which otherwise can interfere with reactions of metabolism. Owing to this detoxification property, they play a role in resistance to metal toxicity. Deletion of the metallothionein genes renders cells hypersensitive to copper poisoning (1,2). These also have a role in antioxidant defense, and may explain why metallothionein expression is up-regulated in inflammation (1,13–15).

Ceruloplasmin is among those copper enzymes involved in the acute-phase reaction of inflammation, in the scavenging of oxygen radicals to protect cells against oxidative damage and to aid the release of stored iron to transferrin (1,16,17). Ceruloplasmin has ferroxidase activity and its deficiency is accompanied by accumulation of iron in liver, brain, and a few other organs (1).

Blood clotting factors (V and VIII), copper containing proteins, are produced by endothelial cells such as those lining blood vessels (1,2). Chondrocytes, involved in the production of cartilage, have a copper containing glycoprotein referred to as cartilage matrix glycoprotein (1,18,19).

Lysyl oxidase is another extracellular copper enzyme critical to the formation and function of connective tissue throughout the body (1,2). Its function is to catalyze cross-linking of newly formed collagen and tropoelastin fibers through the oxidative deamination of lysine side chains on these proteins. Lack of collagen maturation and defective sheathing of blood vessels by elastic fibers is thus seen as a result of copper deficiency (1).

Tyrosinase, the Cu-containing enzyme responsible for synthesis of melanin pigment, is required for protection against excess ultraviolet exposure and for hair, skin, and eye color (1,2).

Dopamine-β-monoxygenase is a key enzyme in the production of catecholamines, which are involved in nerve transmission in the adrenergic nerve system (1,2). Production of brain norepinephrine is impaired in severe copper deficiency in various regions of the brain (20,21).

Another copper-dependent enzyme in the brain catalyzes the α-amidation of neuropeptides and is found particularly in hypothalamic granules (1,2). Studies indicate that brain dopamine synthesis as well as myelination during development are copper dependent (1).

Copper additionally has inhibitory effects on interleukin 1β (22). IL-1β mediates an acute inflammatory response, which increases free radical formation leading to prolonged activation of the scavenger enzyme, Cu, Zn-SOD (22–24). This leads to depletion of Cu (II) stores and impairs function of Cu (II)-depending enzyme, cytochrome c oxidase (22). IL-1β thus impairs mitochondrial functions (22,25). Addition of Cu (II)–GHK (glycyl-L-histidyl-L-lysine) may prevent the IL-1β induced inhibition of mitochondrial glucose oxidation (22).

Copperceuticals and Skin: The GHK–Cu Tripeptide

The natural tripeptide glycyl-L-histidyl-L-lysine (Gly-His-Lys, GHK) was first isolated by Pickart et al. (26,27) from human plasma. GHK acts synergistically with copper and plays a role in copper ion uptake into cells (26,28–32). It has also been recognized as a metal ion carrier in biological fluids (30). A GHK structure–activity study led to the hypothesis that the His-Lys sequence and Lys side chain are essential for its biological activity (26,33). The mechanism of action is through the first two residues of the tripeptide binding to the copper ion forming a 1:1 complex while the Lys side chain is involved in the recognition of the hypothetical receptor on the cell surface. This forms the basis for the copper uptake into cells and most of GHK's biological activities (29) (Table 1).

GHK–Cu Analogs

SPARC, secreted protein that is acidic and rich in cysteine is a metalloprotein that binds to Cu^{2+} and Ca^{2+} (34). It is produced at high levels by cells in tissues undergoing remodeling as a consequence of injury, disease, or development (34,35). SPARC inhibits endothelial cell proliferation, but proteolysis of this metalloprotein leads to the source of circulating GHK which has angiogenic and proliferative activities (34). The three stages of progression are: (1) proliferation, stimulated by cytokines is necessary for the provision of cells for incorporation into neovessels (36); (2) cord formation and elongation, facilitated by release of (K) GHK from SPARC by plasmin (34,37,38); and (3) inhibition of proliferation and subsequent lumen formation, the former mediated by intact SPARC, which inhibits endothelial cell proliferation (34,39). In this way, SPARC functions at several levels to control the progression of neovessels (34).

Table 1 Biological Activity of GHK–Cu

Compound	Endpoint	Results	Comments	References
GHK–Cu^{2+}	Lipid peroxidation	Inhibition of ferritin iron release	Ferritin dependent lipid peroxidation and iron release in damaged tissues is inhibited preventing inflammation and microbial infections	Miller et al., 1990 (40)
GHK–Cu^{2+}	Wound healing	Increased wound strength	Enhanced synthesis of glycosaminoglycans from fibroblasts	Wegrowski et al. (41)
GHK–Cu^{2+}	Tissue remodeling	Increased matrix metalloproteinase-2	Modulates MMP-2 mRNA, TIMP-1, and TIMP-2 expression and release by fibroblasts	Siméon et al., 2000 (42)
GHK–Cu^{2+}	Wound healing	Increased wound strength	Increased decorin expression, increased collagen deposition in GHK–Cu injected wounds	Siméon et al., 2000 (43)
GHK–Cu^{2+}	Scar formation	Decreased secretion of TGF-beta1	Modulation of TGF-b1, possible role in decreasing excessive scar and keloid formation	McCormack et al., 2001 (44)

The Importance of the Copper Peptide Complex

To better understand the mechanism of action of GHK–Cu, GHK and Cu on adult skin, the effect of the complex and its components on the collagen synthesis in normal human dermal fibroblast culture established from adult donors was studied (45). Collagen synthesis rate was assessed by measuring the level of proline incorporation into newly synthesized collagen molecules after collagenase extraction of the protein in the culture supernatant. Under the conditions of the experiment, GHK–Cu was able to significantly stimulate collagen synthesis. This stimulation was ~50% of the effect observed with 1 ng/mL of TGFβ used as a positive control, indicating a significant stimulating activity on collagen formation by the GHK–Cu. In order to investigate whether this activity could be attributed to copper or to the tripeptide, each of the components was evaluated separately. The peptide GHK did not exhibit any stimulating effect on collagen synthesis. For copper evaluation, one inorganic salt, copper chloride, and one organic salt, copper gluconate, were tested. Both copper salts also failed to stimulate collagen synthesis. Treatment of the cell with GHK peptide and copper chloride added separately to the culture at the same ratio compared with the copper peptide complex also failed to stimulate the collagen synthesis.

These results demonstrate that the complex formation of the copper with GHK is the decisive factor in the stimulating activity of GHK–Cu on collagen synthesis as the *in situ* association of copper and the tripeptide was not efficient in generating GHK–Cu (Table 2).

Skin Penetration Study of GHK–Cu

To determine the skin penetration of the copper tripeptide complex, GHK–Cu on the skin, Cao et al. followed a published skin persistence method. A cosmetic cream formulation containing GHK–Cu was applied in 2.5 cm diameter test sites on the cheek of four subjects aged 24–55. The sites were sampled at 0, 2, 4, and 6 h post-application. Samples for assay were obtained by swabbing three times with cotton-tipped swabs moistened in ethanol and put into the test

Table 2 Stimulation of Extracellular Collagen Synthesis Rate vs. Untreated Control

Dose (µg/mL of raw material)	1	10	100
Copper peptide	−1.5%	+9%	+66%*
Dose (µg/mL of raw material)	0.6	6	60
Peptide GHK	−34%	−40%*	−46%**
Dose (µg/mL of raw material)	0.17	1.7	17
Copper chloride	+3%	+7%	−24%*
Dose (µg/mL of raw material)	0.17 + 0.6	1.7 + 6	17 + 60
Copper chloride + peptide GHK	−32%	−12%	−27%*

*$p \leq 0.05$.
**$p \leq 0.01$.

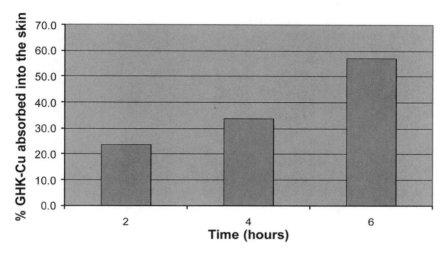

Figure 1 GHK–Cu adherence to skin.

tube. A 1 mL solution of 0.25% EDTA was pipetted and vortexed for 1 min. The concentration of GHK–Cu was determined by high performance liquid chromatograpy (HPLC) and gas chromatography (GC) analyses. The data showed that 24% of the GHK–Cu containing cream adhered to the skin after 2 h, 34% after 4 h, and 57% after 6 h (Fig. 1). To conclude, the study indicated that GHK is delivered and readily absorbed on the skin in the given formulation (46).

Immunohistological Assessment

The copper-binding tripeptide complex has been shown to be effective in the induction of procollagen synthesis *in vitro*, in synthesis of glycosamingolycans and in extracellular matrix accumulation *in vivo* (41,47–49). Five women ages 50-plus with moderate to advanced photodamage participated in a 12-week study using a cream containing the GHK–Cu tripeptide complex. Histological assessment of forearm skin biopsies showed a remarkable increase in keratinocyte proliferation (49) (see Figs. 2 and 3).

CONTROLLED USAGE STUDY IN PHOTODAMAGED SKIN

To quantify the benefits of a facial product containing GHK–Cu for firming and ameliorating the appearance of photodamaged skin, a 12-week controlled usage study was conducted.

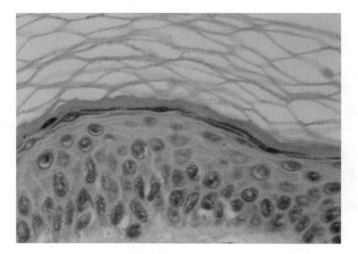

Figure 2 A 52-year-old subject before treatment (40×).

Methods

Sixty-seven women with mild to advanced photodamage (Fitzpatrick and Glogau type I–III) participated in this randomized, two-celled, placebo-controlled full-face, double blind study. During the study period subjects applied the face cream or placebo twice daily.

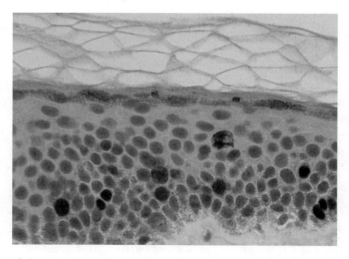

Figure 3 The darkly stained (Ki67 stain) keratinocyte nuclei indicate immunoreactivity for cell proliferation-associated antigens expressed in all active stages of cell division (40×).

A trained clinician conducted evaluations at baseline, 2, 4, 8, and 12 weeks. Skin attributes evaluated were fine lines, wrinkles, laxity (via physical pinch recoil in crows feet area), clarity, roughness, mottled pigmentation, and overall skin appearance. A 10 cm analog scale was used to grade the attributes, where 0 indicated absence of the condition and 10 indicated severity.

Subjects were graded globally on the face for objective irritation (erythema, edema, and scaling) and subjective irritation (burning, stinging, itching, tightness, and tingling) using a three-point scale in which 0 indicated none and 3 indicated severe (50). Digital photographs were taken of the left and right sides of subjects' faces at baseline and week 12.

Firmness of the skin was measured using a hand-held ballistometer. Triplicate measurements were taken in the temple area on the right side of the face (51). Prior to instrumentation measurements, subjects rested quietly for 30 min in a room with controlled temperature and humidity. The room's temperature was maintained between 66°F and 72°F, and the humidity ranged from 29% to 61%.

Ultrasound measurements to evaluated skin density were performed on the temple area. A DUBplus (Taberna, Pro Medicum, AG) system consisting of a hand-held probe containing an ultrasonic transducer interfaced to a specially configured computer was employed. A standard 50 MHz transducer with a focal distance of 12 mm, 40 dB resolution, and gain setting of 28 dB was used (52).

Clinical Results

Results indicated that the GHK–Cu cream delivered statistically significant improvements in skin benefits when compared with placebo (Table 3 and Fig. 4). By week 4, clinical grading indicated statistically significant improvements for all attributes for the GHK–Cu cream (Fig. 5) vs. baseline.

In the clinical testing described, minimal irritation was noted in safety assessments, subjects reported good tolerability, and there were no subject discontinuations for treatment-related events.

Table 3 Skin Benefits

Attribute	Baseline	Week 1	Week 2	Week 4	Week 8	Week 12
Overall appearance	5.50	4.99*	4.52*	3.95*	3.48*	3.14*
Laxity	4.52	4.41*	4.13*	3.65*	3.08*	2.74*
Clarity	3.85	7.95*	8.86*	9.20*	9.29*	9.35**
Fine lines	4.30	4.19	3.85*	3.11*	2.35*	2.01*
Mottled hyperpigmentation	4.57	4.49	4.45	4.19	3.90*	3.60*
Coarse wrinkles	1.21	1.20	1.17	1.02	0.69*	0.54**

*Statistically significant improvement vs. placebo paired t-test ($p \leq 0.05$).
**Statistically significant improvement vs. placebo paired t-test ($p \leq 0.10$).

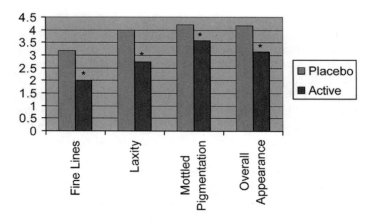

Figure 4 Clinical efficacy week 12. *Indicates a significantly greater decrease (improvement) for the active cream (ANOVA Fisher's LSD, $p \leq 0.05$). 0 indicates absence of the condition and 10 indicates severity.

Viscoelastic Properties

Pinch recoil times with the GHK–Cu cream improved significantly compared with placebo beginning at week 2, supporting a rapid onset of enhanced skin resiliency.

Ballistometer measurements (indentation and area parameters), decreased significantly compared with baseline by week 1 and after, an indication of skin firming.

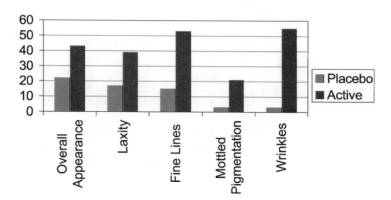

Figure 5 Percent change in average clinical scores, indicating improvement in skin condition, week 12 when compared with baseline.

Ultrasound Measurements

Ultrasound density measurements significantly increased at weeks 4, 8, and 12, when compared with baseline. Thick, uniform entry echoes and intense echo reflexes are shown in post-treatment images (Figs. 6 and 7). The average percent increase in skin thickness over the duration of the study was 17.8%.

Digital Images

Before (left) and after (right) digital images (Fig. 8) illustrate typical improvements after 12 weeks of treatment. Note the improvement in skin firmness, peroicular fine lines, crow's feet wrinkles, and nasolabial fine lines (51-year-old subject).

SAFETY OF GHK–Cu COMPLEX

Human Repeated Insult Patch Testing of the GHK–Cu complex at 20× use levels did not indicate potential to induce allergic contact dermatitis. In humans studies, the GHK–Cu-containing creams were classified as minimally irritating in cumulative irritation studies and were determined to be noncomedogenic. Acute eye installation determined an eye cream to have little or no potential for ocular irritation.

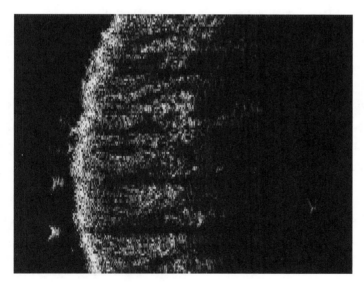

Figure 6 Baseline: ultrasound scan of a 50-year-old woman. The image shows a faint echolucent band with serrated ridges or pockets of translucency extending into the subepidermal area. Translucent banding and ridging in ultrasound images are characteristic of photodamaged (45) skin.

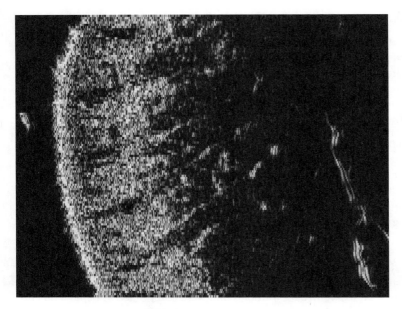

Figure 7 Post-treatment: ultra sound image shows a dense, entry echo that is typical of subjects using the test material. This may reflect deposition of the copper peptide complex into the stratum corneum layer and upper epidermis. The echolucent bands observed in baseline images are markedly diminished and replaced with echo-rich material.

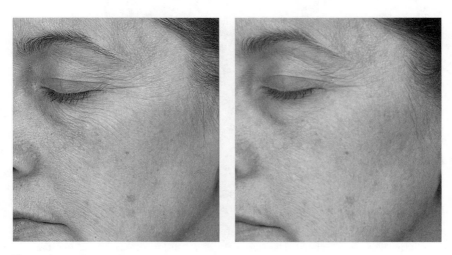

Figure 8 Before (left) and after (right) digital images illustrate typical improvements after 12 weeks of treatment.

CONCLUSIONS

Copper peptide is a new weapon in the anti-aging arsenal. *In vitro* work established that this molecule enhances the rate of collagen synthesis in dermal fibroblasts and skin penetration studies confirmed bioavailability. Histological assessment of skin treated with a personal care cream containing GHK–Cu indicated that it enhanced procollagen synthesis. On the basis of clinical evidence, this cream demonstrated the advantages of being extremely mild, providing both rapid and sustained skin care benefits. Viscoelastic and ultrasound measurements are consistent with the *in vivo* findings that the GHK–Cu cream provided increased skin density and firmness. Results from a series of studies have been presented that confirm the ability of GHK–Cu-containing creams to deliver skin benefits similar to those described here (45,53,54).

REFERENCES

1. Maria C Linder, Maryam Hazegh-Azam. Copper biochemistry and molecular biology. Am J Clin Nutr 1996; 63:797S–811S.
2. Linder MC. The Biochemistry of Copper. New York: Plenum, 1991.
3. Johnson PE, Milne DB, Lykkken GI. Effect of age and sex on copper absorption, biological half-life, and status in humans. J Clin Nutr 1992; 56:917–925.
4. Dunham R, Smith HE. Lead and copper—a model home approach. Proc Water Qual Technol Conf 1992; 1991:341–352.
5. Turnlund JR, Keyes WR, Anderson HL, Acord LL. Copper absorption and retention in young men at three levels of dietary copper using the stable isotope, 65Cu. Am J Clin Nutr 1989; 49:870–878.
6. National Research Council. Recommended Dietary Allowances. 10th ed. Washington, DC: National Academy Press, 1989.
7. Linder MC, Weiss KC, Vu HM, Rucker RB. Structure and function of transcuprein in transport of copper by mammalian blood plasma. In: Hurley LC, Lonnerdal B, Keen C, eds. Trace Elements in Man and Animals (TEMA-6). New York: Plenum, 1987:141–144.
8. Owen CA Jr. Biochemical Aspects of Copper. Copper Deficiency and Toxicity. Physiological Aspects of Copper. Park Ridge, NJ: Noyes, 1982.
9. Weiss KC, Linder MC. Copper transport in rats involving a new plasma protein. Am J Physiol 1985; 249:E77–E88
10. Tavassoli M, Kishimoto T, Kataoka M. Liver endothelium mediates the hepatocyte's uptake of ceruloplasmin. J Cell Biol 1986; 102:1298–1303.
11. Bode AM, Miller LA, Faber J, Saari JT. Mitochondrial respiration in heart, liver and kidney of copper deficient rats. J Nutr Biochem 1992; 3:668–672.
12. Linder MC. Nutrition and metabolism of trace elements. In: Linder MC, ed. Nutritional Biochemistry and Metabolism. 2nd ed. New York: Elsevier, 1991:215–276.
13. Felix K, Lengfelder, Hartmann H-J, Weser U. A pulse radiolytic study on the reaction of hydroxyl and superoxide radicals with yeast Cu (I) thionein. Biochim Biophys Acta 1993; 1203:104–108.
14. Satoh M, Naganuma A, Imura N. Effect of preinduction of metallothionein on paraquat toxicity in mice. Arch Toxicol 1992; 66:145–148.

15. Miesel R, Hartmann H-J, Weser U. Antiinflammatory reactivity of copper (I)-thionein. Inflammation 1990; 14:471–483.
16. Miura T, Muraoka S, Ogiso T. Adriamycin-induced lipid peroxidation of erythrocyte membranes in the presence of ferritin and the inhibitory effect of ceruloplasmin. Biol Pharm Bull 1993; 16:664–667.
17. Linder MC. Interactions between copper and iron in mammalian metabolism. In: Elsenhans BE, Forth W, Schumann K, eds. Metal–Metal Interactions. Gutersloh, Germany: Bertelsheim Foundation, 1994:11–41.
18. Fife RS, Kluve-Beckerman B, Houser DS et al. Evidence that a 550,000 dalton cartilage matrix glycoprotein is a chondrocyte membrane associated protein closely related to ceruloplasmin. J Biol Chem 1993; 268:4407–4411.
19. Fife RS, Moody S, Houser D, Proctor C. Studies of copper transport in cultured bovine chondrocytes. Biochim Biophys Acta 1994; 1201:19–22.
20. Prohaska JR, Bailey WR. Persistent regional changes in brain copper, cuproenzymes and catecholamines following perinatal copper deficiency in mice. J Nutr 1993; 123:1226–1234.
21. Prohaska JR, Bailey WR. Regional specificity in alterations of rat brain copper and catecholamines following perinatal copper deficiency. J Neruochem 1994; 63:1551–1557.
22. Vinci C et al. Copper and IL-1b effects on islets. Diabetolgia 1995; 38:39–45.
23. Sorenson JRJ. In: Sigel H, ed. Metal Ions in Biological Systems. New York: RRR. Dekker, 1982.
24. Klevay LM. In: Sorensen JRJ, ed. Inflammatory Diseases and Copper. Clifton, NJ: RRR. Humana, 1982.
25. Sandler S, Andersson A, Hellerstrom C. Inhibitory effects of interleukin 1 on insulin secretion, insulin biosynthesis and oxidative metabolism of isolated rat pancreatic islets. Endocrinology 1987; 121:1424–1431.
26. Conato et al. Copper complexes of glycyl-histidyl-lysine and two of its synthetic analogues: chemical behaviour and biological activity. Biochim Biophys Acta 1526 2001; 199–210
27. Pickart L, Thaler MM. Tripeptide in human serum which prolongs survival of normal liver cells and stimulates growth in neoplastic liver. Nat New Biol 1973; 234:85–87.
28. Pickart L, Thaler MM, Millard M. Effect of transition-metals on recovery from plasma of the growth-modulating tripeptide glycylhistidyllysine. J Chromatogr 1979; 175:65–73.
29. Pickart L, Freedman JH, Loker WJ, Peisach J, Perkins CM, Stenkamp RE, Weinstein B. Growth-modulating plasma tripeptide may function by facilitating copper uptake into cells. Nature 1980; 288:715–717.
30. Darwish HM, Cheney JC, Schmitt RC, Ettinger MJ. Mobilization of copper(II) from plasma components and mechanism of hepatic copper transport. Am J Physiol 1984; 246:G72–G79.
31. Hartter DE, Barnea A. Brain-tissue accumulates copper-67 by 2 ligand-dependent saturable processes—A high-affinity, low capacity and a low affinity, high-capacity process. J Biol Chem 1988; 263:799–805.
32. Antholine WE, Petering DH, Pickart L. ESR studies of the interaction of copper(II) GHK, histidine, and ehrlich cells. J Inorg Biochem 1989; 35:215–224.
33. Pickart L, Thaler MM. Growth-modulating human-plasma tripeptide—relationship between molecular-structure and DNA-synthesis in hepatoma-cells. FEBS Lett 1979; 104:119–122.

34. Sage EH, Vernon RB. Regulation of angiogenesis. J Hypertens 1994; 12: S145–S152.
35. Lane TF, Sage EH: The biology of SPARC, a protein that modulates cell–matrix interactions. FASEB J 1994; (8):163–173.
36. D'amore PA. Mechanisms of endothelial growth control. Am J Respir Cell Mol Biol 1992; 6(1):1–8.
37. Iruale-Arispe ML, Sage EH. Endothelial cells exhibiting angiogenesis in vitro proliferate in response to TGF-beta-1. J Cell Biochem 1993; 52(4):414–430.
38. Pepper MS, Vassalli J-D, Orci L, Montesano R: Biphasic effect of transforming growth factor-b1 on in vitro angiogenesis. Exp Cell Res 1993; 204(2):356–363.
39. Montesanto R. Regulation of angiogenesis in vitro. Eur J Clin Invest 1992; 22(8):504–515.
40. Miller D, DeSilva D, Pickart L, Aust S. Effects of glycyl-histidyl-lysyl chelated Cu(II) on feritin dependent lipid peroxidation. In: Emerit I et al., eds. Antioxidants in Therapy and Preventive Medicine. New York: Plenum Press, 1990:79–84.
41. Wegrowski Y, Maquart FX, Borel JP. Stimulation of sulfated glycosaminoglycan synthesis by the tripeptide copper complex glycyl-L-histidyl-L-lysine-Cu^{2+}. Life Sci 1992; 51:1049–1056.
42. Simeon A, Emonard H, Hornebeck W, Marquart FX. The tri-peptide-copper complex glycyl-L-histidyl-L-lysine-Cu^{2+} stimulates matrix metalloproteinase-2 expression by fibroblast cultures. Life Sci 2000; 67:2257–2265.
43. Simeon A, Wegrowski Y, Bontemps Y, Marquat FX. Expression of Glycosaminoglycans and small proteoglycans in wounds: modulaton by the tripeptide-copper complex glycyl-L-histidyl-L-lysine-Cu^{2+}. J Investigative Derm 2000; 115(6):962–968.
44. McCormack M, Nowack K, Koch RJ. The effect of copper tripeptide and tretinoin on growth factor production in a serum-free fibroblast model. Arch Facial Plast Surg 2001; 3:28–32.
45. Leyden JJ, Grove G, Stephens TJ, Finkey MB, Barkovic S, Appa Y. Skin benefits of copper peptide containing face cream. Presented at the 60th Annual American Academy of Dermatology Meeting, New Orleans, LA, 2002.
46. Orth DS, Widjaja J, LY L, Cao N, Shapiro WB. Stability of Skin Persistence of Topical Products. Cosmet Toiletries Oct 1119; V. 113:51–63.
47. Maquart FX, Pickart L, Laurent M, Gillery P, Moboisse JC, Borel JP. Stimulation of collagen synthesis in fibroblast cultures by the tri-peptide-copper complex glycycl-L-histidyl-L-lysine–Cu^{2+}. FEBS Lett 1988; 238:343–346.
48. Buffoni F, Pino R, Dal Pozzo A. Effect of tripeptide-copper complexes on the process of skin wound healing and on cultured fibroblasts. Arch Int Pharmacodyn Ther 1995; 330:345–360.
49. Abdulghani AA, Sherr A, Shirin S, Solodkina G, Morales Tapia E, Wolf B, Gottlieb AB. Effects of creams on skin ultrastructure. DMCO 1998; 1(4):136–141.
50. Lammintausta K, Maibach HI, Wilson D. Irritant reactivity in males and females. Contact Dermat 1987; 17(5):276–280.
51. Jemec GB, Selvaag E, Agren M, Wulf HC. Measurements of the mechanical properties of skin with ballistometer and suction cup. Skin Res Technol 2001; 7(2):122–126.
52. Pellacani G, Seidenari S. Variations in facial skin thickness and echogenicity with site and age. Acta Dermatol Venereol 1999 Sep; 79(5):366–369.

53. Sigler ML, Stephens TJ, Barkovic S, Finkey MB, Appa Y. A clinical evaluation of a copper-peptide-containing liquid foundation and cream concealer designed for improving skin condition. Presented at the 60th Annual American Academy of Dermatology Meeting, New Orleans, LA, 2002.
54. Stephens TJ, Sigler M, Finkey MB, Appa Y. Skin benefits of an SPF 20 copper peptide containing face cream. Presented at the 61st Annual American Academy of Dermatology Meeting, San Francisco, CA, 2003.

Toxicology

33

Dermatotoxicology Overview

Philip G. Hewitt
Merck kGaA, Darmstadt, Germany
Howard I. Maibach
University of California, San Francisco, California, USA

Introduction	568
Dermatopharmacokinetics: Relation to Predictive Assays	568
In Vivo Percutaneous Absorption Assays	569
In Vitro Percutaneous Penetration Assays	570
Allergic Contact Dermatitis	570
Quantitative Structure Activity Relationships	571
Guinea Pig Sensitization Tests	571
Draize Test	571
Open Epicutaneous Test	572
Buehler Test	573
Freund's Complete Adjuvant Test	573
Optimization Test	573
Split Adjuvant Test	574
Guinea Pig Maximization Test	574
Human Sensitization Assays	575
Repeat Insult Patch Tests	575
Modified Draize Human Sensitization Test	577

Irritant Dermatitis	577
In Vitro Assays	577
Irritation Tests in Animals	578
Draize-Type Tests	578
Non-Draize Animal Studies	578
Human Irritation Tests	578
Contact Urticaria Syndrome	579
Nonimmunological Contact Urticaria	580
Immunological Contact Urticaria	580
Guinea Pig Ear Swelling Test	581
Trimellitic Anhydride-Sensitive Mouse Assay	581
Subjective Irritation and Paresthesia	581
Human Assay	582
References	582

INTRODUCTION

Cosmeceuticals are presumably relatively "safe". Adverse skin responses associated with repetitive, low-dose exposure to consumer products are all too often not accurately predicted by the required assays. The need to market products with low risk of producing dermal and systemic injury to increase consumer satisfaction has led to the development of numerous assays to rank chemicals for their ability to injure the skin. Although these assays are not routinely mandated by regulatory agencies for cosmetics and skin care, the frequency with which they are conducted and their utility warrant attention.

The field of dermatotoxicology includes measurement of absorption of materials as well as assays that evaluate the ability of topically applied chemicals to induce or promote the development of neoplasia, trigger an immune response in the skin, directly destroy the skin (corrosion), irritate the skin, produce urticaria (hives), and produce noninflammatory painful sensations. The inflammatory responses of skin are the most common chemically induced dermatoses in humans.

DERMATOPHARMACOKINETICS: RELATION TO PREDICTIVE ASSAYS

Although the skin's barrier properties are impressive, it has been shown to be a major route of entry under some exposure situations. Interest in dermatopharmacokinetics has increased as the skin has been reconsidered to be a route for systemic administration of drugs and chemicals, as well as a route of entry for toxins. A variety of assays, both *in vivo* and *in vitro*, for measuring absorption through the skin, have been developed (1,2) and many factors that govern absorption through the skin have been determined.

A major diffusion barrier of the skin is considered to be the stratum corneum. Absorption of chemicals through shunts, openings of skin appendages, and gaps in the stratum corneum associated with these structures has been considered (3). Absorption can be described as passive diffusion across this membrane by the equation, $J = (K_m C_v D_m)/\delta$, where J is the rate of absorption, K_m is the vehicle/stratum corneum partition coefficient, C_v is the skin surface concentration, D_m is the diffusion constant of penetrant in stratum corneum, and δ is the thickness of stratum corneum (4). Other factors that affect thermodynamic activity of the solution at the skin surface (e.g., pH and temperature) may vary flux (5,6). Vehicle influence cannot be overstated; for a specific concentration of chemical, thermodynamic activity may vary by 1000-fold from one vehicle to another (6). Other factors that affect percutaneous absorption include condition of the skin (7), age, surface area to which the material is applied (8), penetrant volatility, temperature and humidity (9), substantivity, and wash-and-rub resistance to removal from the skin and binding to the skin (10).

Once a chemical has gained access to the viable epidermis, it may initiate a local effect, be absorbed into the circulation and produce an effect, or produce no local or systemic effects. The viable epidermis contains enzymes capable of metabolizing exogenous chemicals (11), including a substantial cytochrome P450 system, esterases, mixed-function oxidases, and glucuronyltransferases. Early studies conducted *in vitro* using whole skin indicated that enzymatic activity in skin was only a fraction of the activity of the liver. However, when the surface area of the epidermis is taken into account, the enzymatic activities of the epidermis can range from 80% to 240% of those in liver (12).

IN VIVO PERCUTANEOUS ABSORPTION ASSAYS

Percutaneous absorption can be determined by applying a known amount of chemical to a specified surface area and then measuring levels of the chemical in the urine and/or feces. Because the analytical techniques to measure the chemical are not always available and because some chemicals may be metabolized, radiolabeled chemicals, ^{14}C or ^{3}H, are often used.

In vivo studies have been conducted in humans and other species (12). Comparison of absorption rates of a number of compounds showed that absorption rates in the rat and rabbit tend to be higher than humans and that the skin permeability of monkeys and swine more closely resembles that of humans. No significant mouse–human skin comparisons exist. Guinea pig–human comparisons offer some promise for refinement of guinea pig–human irritation and sensitization extrapolations (13). Although these differences are not predicted by any single factor, they are not unexpected in light of differences in metabolism and in routes of excretion. Therefore, the metabolic capabilities of the species should be considered when selecting an animal model and designing the experiment. Although there is no question that pharmacokinetic studies of this type in humans or animals provide the best estimate of percutaneous absorption, the cost and difficulty in conducting well-controlled studies have led to the use of other *in vivo* assays that are poorer predictive tools and to the development of *in vitro* models.

IN VITRO PERCUTANEOUS PENETRATION ASSAYS

The excised skin of humans or animals can be used to measure penetration of chemicals. *In vitro* assays using excised skin utilize specially designed diffusion cells (1,14,15). The skin is stretched over the opening of a collecting receptacle, epidermal side up. The chemical is applied to the epidermis, and fluid from the receptacle is assayed to measure the penetration of the chemical. This type of *in vitro* assay offers some advantages over *in vivo* assays: highly toxic compounds can be studied in human skin, large numbers of cells can be run simultaneously, diffusion through the membrane (eliminating other pharmacokinetic factors) can be studied, and these assays may be easier to conduct.

Comparison of penetration rates obtained from *in vitro* and *in vivo* assays has been made (1), often with a good correlation; however, with some, correlation was poor. Differences in the methods for some compounds could be explained on the basis of solubilities in the receptacle fluid and blood; others could not be explained. Skin of the weanling pig and miniature swine appear to be good *in vitro* models for most compounds (2). Although a limited number of studies have been reported, the skin of monkeys also appears to be a good model (8). Rat skin appears to be a good model for some compounds; however, when differences have been noted, they have been large.

ALLERGIC CONTACT DERMATITIS

Jadassohn (16) demonstrated that in some patients dermatitis was due to increased sensitivity following repeated contact with a substance and not the irritant properties of the material. By 1930, a procedure for producing this hypersensitivity to chemicals in guinea pigs had been developed (17). Landsteiner and associates (18) demonstrated that low-molecular-weight chemicals conjugate with proteins to form an antigen that stimulates the immune system to form a hyperreactive state. Immunogenicity is related to chemical structure (19), and two types of immunological response exist, one transferable by serum and the other transferable by suspensions of white blood cells (20). These mechanisms are succinctly provided by von Blomberg (21).

Appropriate planning and execution of predictive sensitization assays is critical. The first priority is to choose an appropriate experimental design. A common error in choosing an animal assay is using Freund's complete adjuvant

(FCA) when setting dose–response relationships. The adjuvant provides such sensitivity that dose–effect relationships are muted. Choice of dose and vehicle appropriate to the assay and the study question is the second priority. Although dose must be high enough to ensure penetration, it must be below the threshold at challenge to avoid misinterpretation of irritant inflammation as allergic. Knowing the irritation potential of compounds will allow the investigator to design and execute these studies appropriately. Vehicle choice determines in part the absorption of the test material and can influence sensitization rate, ability to elicit response at challenge, and the irritation threshold.

QUANTITATIVE STRUCTURE ACTIVITY RELATIONSHIPS

Quantitative structure activity relationships describe a relationship of chemical structure to biological activity—in this case allergic contact dermatitis. A computer-assisted database describing the chemical structure and physicochemical parameters of an array of chemicals provides a facile approach to designing appropriate *in vitro*, animal, and human sensitization studies (22). In essence, searching the prior experimental data not only permits determination of relationship between structures and allergenicity, but also provides insight into planning a given experiment. For example, if a closely related structure to the chemical of interest has been shown to be a potent allergen, the new chemical may be examined with a more quantitative assay.

GUINEA PIG SENSITIZATION TESTS

Predictive animal tests to determine the potential of substances to induce delayed hypersensitivity in humans are conducted most often in guinea pigs. Several tests have been described. All utilize young (1–3 months), randomly bred, albino guinea pigs. Most visually evaluate the responses using descriptive scales for erythema and edema. The tests differ significantly in route of exposure, use of adjuvants, induction interval, and number of exposures. The principal features of the most commonly used assays and assays acceptable to regulatory agencies to predict sensitization are summarized in Table 1 (23–25).

DRAIZE TEST

The Draize sensitization test (DT) (26,27) was the first predictive sensitization test accepted by regulatory agencies. One flank of 20 guinea pigs is shaved and 0.05 mL of a 0.1% solution of test material in saline, paraffin oil, or polyethylene glycol is injected into the anterior flank on day 0. Every other day through day 20, 0.1 mL of the test solution is injected into a new site on the same flank. After a 2 week rest period, the opposite untreated flank is shaved and 0.05 mL of test solution is injected into each animal (challenge). Twenty previously untreated controls are injected at the same time. The test site is visually evaluated

Table 1 Features of Most Commonly Used Assays to Predict Sensitization

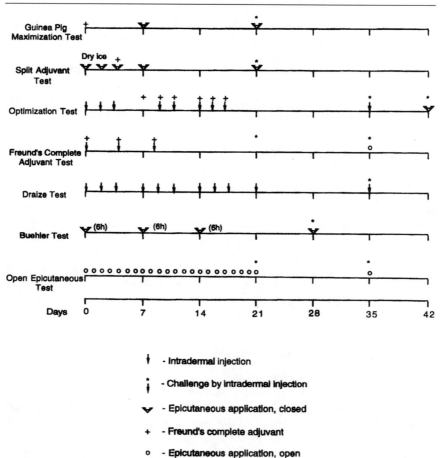

24 and 48 h after injection. A larger or more intensely erythematous response than that of controls is considered a positive response.

OPEN EPICUTANEOUS TEST

The open epicutaneous test (OET) (28) simulates the conditions of human use by utilizing topical application of the test material. The procedure determines the doses required to induce sensitization and to elicit a response in sensitized animals. The irritancy profile is determined by applying 0.025 mL of varying concentrations to a 2 cm^2 area of the shaved flanks of six to eight guinea pigs.

Test sites are visually evaluated 24 h after application of test solutions to erythema. The dose not causing a reaction in any animals (maximal nonirritant concentration) and the dose causing a reaction in 25% of the animals (minimal irritant concentration) are determined. During induction, test solution is applied to flank skin of six to eight guinea pigs for 3 weeks, or five times a week for 4 weeks. A control group is treated with vehicle only. The highest dose tested is usually the minimal irritant concentration and lower doses are based on usage concentration or a stepwise reduction. Each animal is challenged on the untreated flank 24–72 h after the last induction treatment. The minimal irritant concentration, the maximum nonirritant concentration, and five solutions of lower concentrations are applied. Skin reactions are read on an all-or-none basis at 24, 48, and 72 h after application. The maximum nonirritating concentration in the vehicle-treated group is calculated. Animals in test groups that develop inflammatory responses to lower concentrations are considered sensitized.

BUEHLER TEST

The Buehler test (occlusion only) (29) also employs topical application. An absorbent patch, or vehicle alone, is placed on the shaved flanks of 10–20 guinea pigs. Test concentration varies from undiluted to usage levels. A concentration that produces slight erythema is optimum and is selected on the basis of an irritancy screen conducted in other animals. This procedure is repeated 7 and 14 days after the initial exposure. Animals are challenged with patches saturated with a nonirritating concentration of test material and with the vehicle, 2 weeks after the last induction patch. After 6 h, the patch is removed and the area depilated. Test sites are visually evaluated 24 and 48 h after patch removal. Animals developing erythematous responses are considered sensitized (if irritant control animals do not respond).

FREUND'S COMPLETE ADJUVANT TEST

Freund's complete adjuvant test (FCAT) is an intradermal technique incorporating test material in a 50/50 mixture of FCA and distilled water. The description is summarized by Klecak (30).

OPTIMIZATION TEST

The optimization test resembles the DT, but incorporates the use of adjuvant for some induction injections and both intradermal and topical challenges (27). On day 1, one injection into the shaved flank and one into a shaved area of dorsal skin are given. One injection into a new dorsal site is given 2 and 4 days later. The test material is administered in saline during the first week. During the second and third weeks, test material is administered in FCA/saline every other day to a shaved area over the shoulders; 20 test animals are treated and

20 controls are injected with vehicle alone. Thickness of a skinfold over the injection site is measured with a caliper. Any animal developing a reaction volume at challenge greater than the mean plus 1 standard deviation during induction is considered sensitized. A second challenge is conducted 45 days after the first injection. A nonirritating concentration of the test material in a suitable vehicle is applied to the flank skin, away from injection sites. Reactions are visually evaluated after 24 h using the four-point erythema scale of the Draize primary irritancy scale. To classify materials as strong/moderate/weak/nonsensitizer, a classification scheme has been devised using results of exact Fisher test and number of positives detected.

SPLIT ADJUVANT TEST

The split adjuvant test (30) utilizes skin damage and FCA as adjuvants. An area of back skin of 10–20 guinea pigs is shaved to glistening, then treated with dry ice for 5–10 s. A layer of loose mesh gauze and stretch adhesive with a 2×2 cm^2 opening over the shaved area is placed around the animal. Approximately 0.2 mL of creams or solid test material, 0.1 mL if liquid, is spread over the test site and occluded. The concentration tested varies by irritancy potential, use conditions, and so on. After 2 days, the occlusive filter paper is removed, the test material reapplied, and the covering replaced. On day 4, the filter paper cover is removed, two injections of 0.075 mL FCA are given into the edges of the test site, the test material reapplied, and the site resealed. On day 7, the test material is reapplied and on 9 the dressing is removed. Animals are challenged by topical application of 0.5 mL of test material to a 2×2 cm^2 area of the shaved midback 22 days after the initial treatment. A group of native controls, 10–20 animals, is treated by the same procedure at challenge. The dressing is removed and the test site is visually evaluated using a descriptive visual scale 24, 48, and 72 h after application. Sensitization of individual animals is indicated by significantly stronger reactions than those of controls.

GUINEA PIG MAXIMIZATION TEST

The guinea pig maximization test (GPMT) (27,30) combines FCA, irritancy, intradermal injection, and occlusive topical application during the induction period. Two identical sets of 0.1 mL intradermal injections of 50/50 FCA/water, test material in water, paraffin oil, or propylene glycol, and the same dose of test material in FCA/vehicle are placed on a filter paper, placed over the shaved injection site, covered with $\sim 4 \times 8$ cm^2 occlusive surgical tape, and secured in place. If the test material is nonirritating, the test site is pretreated with 10% sodium lauryl sulfate (SLS) in petrolatum on day 6 to provoke an irritant reaction. After 48 h, test and control (vehicle alone) animals are challenged on the shaved flank with the highest nonirritating concentration and with the vehicle. Solutions are applied to filter paper secured in place and patches removed 24 h later. Reactions are visually evaluated 24 and 48 h after patch removal. Reactions are considered positive when they are more intense than the response to vehicle and the responses to the test materials in controls. The test material is rated as a weak-to-extreme sensitizer, on the basis of the incidence of positives in the test group (Table 2).

HUMAN SENSITIZATION ASSAYS

Chemicals can be tested for their ability to induce contact hypersensitivity in panels of human volunteers from whom informed consent is obtained. Allergic contact dermatitis to materials already in commercial use is sometimes detected by early induction patches. This does not reflect the particular test material's ability to induce sensitization. It merely indicates that under patch conditions, the material may elicit a response in presensitized individuals.

There are four basic predictive human sensitization tests in current use: (i) a single inducion/single challenge patch test; (ii) repeated insult patch test (RIPT); (iii) RIPT with continuous exposure (modified Draize); and (iv) the maximization test, all of which use similar customized patches (31,32). Principal features of human sensitization assays are summarized in Table 3. For assays other than maximization, 150–200 subjects are usually tested. Henderson and Riley (33) statistically showed that if no positive reactions are observed in 200 randomly selected subjects, as many as 15/1000 of the general population may react (95% confidence). As sample size is reduced, the likelihood of unpredicted adverse reactions in the general population increases.

REPEAT INSULT PATCH TESTS

In the Draize humun sensitization test (34), an occlusive patch containing the test material is applied to the upper arm or upper back of 200 volunteers for 48 h. The test site is evaluated at patch removal for erythema and edema. This process is repeated until a total of 9–10 patches have been applied. Subjects are challenged via a patch applied to a new site for 48 h, 10–14 days after application of the last induction patches. Sites are visually evaluated at removal

Table 2 GPMT Rating of Weak-to-Extreme Sensitizers

Sensitization rate (%)	Grade	Class
0–8	I	Weak
9–28	II	Mild
29–64	III	Moderate
65–80	IV	Strong
81–100	V	Extreme

Table 3 Principal Features of Human Sensitization Assays

Test	No. of subjects	Concentration/amount of test material	Vehicle	Skin site	Patch type	Induction No. of patches	Duration	Rest	Challenge
Schwartz	200	Fabric			Fabric	1	5 days	10 days	48 h patch; observe 10 days
Schwartz	200	1 in. fabric, liquid or powder		Arm, thigh, or back	Cellophane covered with 2×2 in.^{2} Elastoplast	1	72 h	7–10 days	72 h; same site; observe 3 days
"Prophetic," Schwartz–Peck	200	1/4 in.^{2} 4-ply gauze, liquid saturated[a]	Petrolatum or corn oil	Arm or back	1 in.^{2} nonwaterproof cellophane covered with 2 in.^{2} adhesive plaster	1	24, 72, or 96 h	10–14 days	48 h; observe 3 days: compare new and old formulas
"Repeated insult" Shelanski	200	Proportional to area of ultimate use	Mineral oil		Occlusion: follows Schwartz test	10–15	24 h every other day: same site	2–3 weeks	48 h patch
"Repeated insult" Draize	100 males 100 females	0.5 mL or 0.5 g		Arm or back	1 in.^{2}	10	24 h alternate days	10–14 days	Repeat patch on new site
Modified Draize	200	0.5 mL or 0.5 g high concentration	Petrolatum	Arm	Square BandAid, no perforations	10	48 h	2 weeks	Patch on new site 72 h with nonirritant concentration
"Maximization" (Kligman)	25	1 mL 5% SLS[b], followed by 1 mL 25% test material	Petrolatum	Forearm or calf	1.5 in.^{2} Webril occluded with Blenderm held with perforated plastic tape	5 (same site)	24 h SLS followed by 48 h test material for each of 5 inducing applications	10 days	1 in.^{2} patch on lower back or forearm: 0.4 mL of 10% SLS for 1 h followed by 0.4 mL of 10% test material for 48 h
Modified "maximization"	25	Same as maximization	Petrolatum	Forearm or calf	Same as maximization	7	24 h SLS followed by 48 h test material for each of 7 inducing applications	10 days	2% SLS for 0.5 h followed by 48 h patch with test material

[a]Modified for solids, powders, ointment, and cosmetics. Concentration, amount, area, and site of application are considered important in evaluating results. Authors recommended that cosmetics be tested uncovered.
[b]SLS pretreatment is used to produce moderate inflammation. SLS is mixed with test material when compatible. SLS is eliminated when the test material is a strong irritant.
Source: Modified from Patrick E, Maibach HI. Predictive skin irritation tests in animals and humans. In: Marzulli FN, Maibach HI, eds. Dermatotoxicology, 3rd ed. New York: Hemisphere Publishing, 1991:201–222.

of the patch and the response at challenge is compared with the response to patches applied early in induction.

MODIFIED DRAIZE HUMAN SENSITIZATION TEST

The RIPT procedure was modified to provide continuous patch exposure to the test material during a 3 week induction period (35,36). Patches are applied to the outer upper arm each Monday, Wednesday, and Friday, until a total of 9–10 patches have been applied. Fresh patches are applied to the same site unless moderate inflammation has developed when the patches should be placed on adjacent noninflamed skin. This produces a continuous exposure of 504–552 h compared with a total exposure period of 216–240 h for RIPT of comparable induction periods. In addition, induction concentrations are increased to levels above usage exposure. Subjects are challenged by exposure of a new site to a patch for 48–72 h at a nonirritating concentration, 2 weeks after induction. Test sites are evaluated at 0 and 24 h after removal.

IRRITANT DERMATITIS

Historically, skin irritation has been described by exclusion as localized inflammation not mediated by either sensitized lymphocytes or antibodies (i.e., nonimmunogenic). Application of some chemicals directly destroys tissue, producing skin necrosis at the site of application (i.e., corrosive chemicals). Chemicals may disrupt cell functions and/or trigger the release, formation, or activation of autocoids that produce local increases in blood flow, increase vascular permeability, attract white blood cells in the area, or directly damage cells. The additive effects of these mediators result in local skin inflammation (i.e., acute irritants). A number of as-yet poorly defined pathways involving different processes of mediator generation appear to exist. Although no agent has yet met all the criteria to establish it as a mediator of skin irritation, histamine, 5-hydroxytryptamine, prostaglandins, leukotrienes, kinins, complement, reactive oxygen species, and products of white blood cells have been strongly implicated as mediators of some irritant reactions (37).

Some chemicals do not produce acute irritation from a single exposure but may produce inflammation following repeated application to the same area of skin [cumulative irritation (38)]. Studies on skin corrosion are conducted in animals, using standardized protocols as it is not appropriate to conduct screening studies in humans. But acute irritation is sometimes evaluated in humans after animal studies have been completed. Tests for cumulative irritation in both animals and humans have been reported.

IN VITRO ASSAYS

Numerous *in vitro* assays for irritation exist. Rougier et al. (39) summarize these assays and offer guidelines as to their potential validation.

IRRITATION TESTS IN ANIMALS

Draize-Type Tests

Primary irritation and corrosion are most often evaluated by modifications of the method described by Draize (24). The Federal Hazardous Substance Act (FHSA) adopted one modification as a standard procedure (22). The backs of six albino rabbits are clipped free of hair. Each undiluted material is tested on two 1 in.^{2} sites on the same animal (one site is intact and the other is abraded in such a way that the stratum corneum is opened but no bleeding produced). Each test site is covered with two layers of 1 in.^{2} surgical gauze and secured in place. The entire trunk of the animal is then wrapped with rubberized cloth or other occlusive impervious material to retard evaporation of the substances and hold the patches in position. The wrappings are removed and the test sites evaluated for erythema and edema, using a prescribed scale, 24 and 48 h after application. Modifications of the Draize procedure that have been proposed include changing the species tested (40), reduction of exposure period, use of fewer animals, and testing on intact skin only (41). Several governmental bodies utilized their own modification of the Draize procedure for regulatory decisions. The FHSA, DOT, Environmental Protection Agency (EPA), Federal Insecticide, Fungicide, Rodenticide Act (FIFRA), and OECD guidelines are contrasted to the original Draize methods. All Draize-type tests are used to evaluate corrosion as well as irritation. When severe reactions that may not be reversible are noted, test sites are observed for a longer period. Delayed evaluations are usually made on days 7 and 14, but maybe as late as 35 days.

Non-Draize Animal Studies

Animal assays to evaluate the ability of chemicals to produce cumulative irritation have been developed (42). Those assays used often are not as well standardized as Draize-type tests, and many variables have been introduced by multiple investigators.

Repeat application patch tests in which diluted materials are applied to the same site each day for 15–21 days have been reported using several species (the guinea pig or rabbit being most commonly used) (42). Because the degree of occlusion is an important determinant of percutaneous penetration, the choice of covering materials may determine the sensitivity of a given test (43). A reference material of similar use or one that produces a known effect in humans is included in almost all repeat application procedures. Test sites are evaluated for erythema and edema, either using the scales of the Draize-type tests or more descriptive scales developed by the investigator.

Human Irritation Tests

Because only a small area of skin need be tested, it is possible to conduct predictive irritation assays in humans, provided systemic toxicity (from absorption) is low. Human tests are preferred to animal tests in some cases because of the uncertainties of interspecies extrapolation. Many forms of a single application patch test have been published. Custom-made apparatus to hold the test material have been designed (29,43). Duration of patch exposure has varied between 1 and 72 h. The single application patch procedure outlined by the National Academy of Sciences (NAS) Publication 1138 (44) incorporates important aspects of assays. For new materials or volatiles, a relatively nonocclusive tape (e.g., Micropore, Dermical, or Scanpore) should be used. Increasing the degree of occlusion with occlusive tapes (e.g., Blenderm) or chamber devices generally increases the severity of responses. A 4 h exposure period was suggested by the NAS panel. However, it is desirable to test new materials and volatiles for shorter periods (30–60 min) and many investigators apply materials intended for skin contact between 24 and 48 h periods. After the period of exposure, the patches should be removed and the area cleaned with water to remove any residue. Responses are evaluated 30 min to 1 h and 24 h (to allow hydration and pressure effects to subside) after patch removal. Persistent reactions may be evaluated for 3–4 days. The Draize scales for erythema and edema have no provision for scoring papular, vesicular, or bullous responses. Therefore, integrated scales ranging 4–16 points have been published and are generally preferred to the Draize scales.

Most multiple application patch tests were patterned after human sensitization studies with 24 h exposures, with or without a rest period between patches. The early work of Kligman and Wooding (45) forms the basis for the irritant dose 50 (ID_{50}) comparative system.

The cumulative irritation assay (46) was used to compare antiperspirants, deodorants, and bath oils to provide guidance for product development. A 1 in.^{2} patch of Webril was saturated with test compound and applied to the skin of the upper back. After 24 h, the patch was removed, the area evaluated, and a fresh patch applied. The procedure was repeated daily for up to 21 days. The IT_{50} [as described by Kligman and Wooding (45)] was used to evaluate and compare test materials. Modifications of the cumlative irritation assay have been reported (44,47) and newer chamber devices have replaced Webril with occlusive tape by some. Many variables of the chosen test procedure (e.g., vehicle, type of patch, concentration tested) may modify the intensity of the response (48,49). Differences in intensity of responses have also been linked to differences in age (50), sex (50), and race (51).

CONTACT URTICARIA SYNDROME

Contact urticaria syndrome (CUS) has been defined as a wheal-and-flare response that develops within 30–60 min after exposure of the skin to certain agents (52,53). Symptoms of immediate contact reactions can be classified according to their morphology and severity:

> Itching, tingling, and burning with erythema is the weakest type of immediate contact reaction.

Local wheal-and-flare with tingling and itching represents the prototype reaction of contact urticaria.
Generalized urticaria after local contact is rare, but can occur from strong urticaria.
Symptoms in other organs can appear with the skin symptoms in cases of immunological CUS.

The strength of the reactions may vary greatly and often the whole range of local symptoms can be seen from the same substance if different concentrations are used (54). In addition, a certain concentration of contact urticant may produce strong edema and erythema reactions on the skin of the upper back and face but only erythema on the volar surfaces of the lower arms or legs. In some cases, contact urticaria can be demonstrated only on damaged or previously eczematous skin and it can be part of the mechanism responsible for maintenance of chronic eczemas (25). Because of the risk of systemic reactions (e.g., anaphylaxis), human diagnostic tests should be performed only by experienced personnel with facilities for resuscitation on hand. Contact urticaria has been divided into two main types on the basis of proposed pathophysiological mechanisms, namely, nonimmunological and immunological (55).

NONIMMUNOLOGICAL CONTACT URTICARIA

Nonimmunological contact urticaria (NICU) is the most common form and occurs without previous exposure in most individuals. The reaction remains localized and does not cause systemic symptoms to spread to become generalized urticaria. Typically, the strength of this type of contact urticaria reaction varies from erythema to a generalized urticarial response, depending on the concentration, skin site, and substance. The mechanism of NICU has not been delineated, but a direct influence on dermal vessel walls or a nonantibody-mediated release of histamine, prostaglandins, leukotrienes, substance P, other inflammatory mediators, or different combinations of these mediators represents possible mechanisms (56). The most potent and best studied substances producing NICU are benzoic acid, cinnamic acid, cinnamic aldehyde, and nicotinic esters. Under optimal conditions, more than half of a random sample of individuals show local edema and erythema reactions within 45 min of application of these substances if the concentration is high enough.

IMMUNOLOGICAL CONTACT URTICARIA

Immunological contact urticaria (ICU) is an immediate type 1 allergic reaction (52). The molecules of a contact urticant react with specific IgE molecules attached to mast-cell membranes. The cutaneous symptoms are elicited by vasoactive substances, mainly histamine, released from mast cells. Other mediators of inflammation may influence the degree of response. ICU reaction can extend beyond the contact site and generalized urticaria may be accompanied by other symptoms, such as rhinitis, conjunctivitis, asthma, and even anaphylactic shock. The term "contact urticaria syndrome" was therefore suggested by Maibach and Johnson (55). Fortunately, the appearance of systemic symptoms is rare, but it may be seen in cases of strong hypersensitivity or in a widespread exposure and abundant percutaneous absorption of an allergen.

GUINEA PIG EAR SWELLING TEST

Predictive assays for evaluating the ability of materials to produce NICU have been developed. Lahti and Maibach (57) developed an assay in guinea pigs using materials known to produce urticaria in humans. One-tenth of a milliliter of the material (or control solvent) is applied to one ear of the animal. Ear thickness is measured before application and then every 15 min for 1 or 2 h after application. The maximum response is a 100% increase in ear thickness (within 50 min after application).

Materials can also be screened for NICU in humans. A small amount of the test material is applied to a marked site on the forehead and the vehicle is applied to a parallel site. The areas are evaluated at $\sim 20-39$ min after application for erythema and/or edema (52).

Differentiation between nonspecific irritant reactions and contact urticaria may be difficult. Strong irritants (e.g., hydrochloric acid, lactic acid, and phenol), can cause clear-cut immediate wheals if the concentration is high enough, but the reactions do not usually fade away quickly. Instead, they are followed by signs of irritation (erythema, scaling, or crusting) 24 h later. Some substances have only irritant properties (e.g., benzoic acid and nicotinic acid esters), some are pure irritants (e.g., SLS), and some have both these features [e.g., dimethyl sulfoxide (DMSO) and formaldehyde].

TRIMELLITIC ANHYDRIDE-SENSITIVE MOUSE ASSAY

The respiratory allergen, trimellitic anhydride (TMA), has been shown to induce IgE production and immediate ear swelling in mice sensitized to it (58). Lauerma et al. showed that TMA-sensitized mice have a biphasic ear-swelling response with early (30–120 min) and late (24–48 h) phases after topical application of TMA. It was concluded that the first swelling was due to either immediate-type immunological processes or NICU, and the second swelling was due to contact hypersensitivity (i.e., allergic contact dermatitis). This relatively simple method could possibly be a useful tool to study the pharmacology of contact urticaria. However, further validation of this model is still required.

SUBJECTIVE IRRITATION AND PARESTHESIA

Cutaneous application of some chemicals elicits sensory discomfort—tingling and burning without visible inflammation. This noninflammatory painful response has been termed subjective irritation (59). Materials reported to produce subjective irritation include DMSO, salicylic acid, amyl-dimethyl-*p*-amino benzoic acid, and 2-ethoxy ethyl-*p*-methoxy cinnamate, which are ingredients of cosmetics and over-the-counter drugs. Pyrethroids, a group of broad-spectrum insecticides, produce a similar condition that may lead to temporary numbness, which has been called paresthesia (60). Only a portion of the human population seems to develop nonpyrethroid subjective irritation. For example, only 20% of subjects exposed to 5% aqueous lactic acid in a hot, humid environment developed stinging response (59). Prior skin damage (e.g., sunburn, pretreatment with surfactants, and tape stripping) increases the intensity of responses in stingers. Recent data show that stingers develop stronger reactions to materials causing NICU. The mechanisms by which materials produce subjective irritation have not been extensively investigated. Pyrethroids directly act on the axon, interfering with the channel-gating mechanism and impulse firing (61). It has been suggested that agents causing subjective irritation act via a similar mechanism because no visible inflammation is present.

An animal model was developed to rate paresthesia to pyrethroids and may be useful for other agents (60). Both flanks of 300–450 g guinea pigs are shaved and 100 μL of the test material (or vehicle) is spread over ~ 30 mm^2 on separate flanks. The animal's behavior is monitored by an unmanned video camera for 5 min at 0.5, 1, 2, 4, and 6 h after application. Subsequently, the film is analyzed for the number of full turns of the head made, usually accompanied by attempted licking and biting of the application sites. Using this technique, it was possible to rank pyrethroids for their ability to produce paresthesia; it corresponded to the ranking available from human exposure.

HUMAN ASSAY

As originally published, the human subjective irritation assay required the use of a 110°F environmental chamber with 80% relative humidity (59). Sweat was removed from the nasolabial fold and cheek, then a 5% aqueous solution of lactic acid was briskly rubbed over the area. Those who reported stinging for 3–5 min within the first 15 min were designated as stingers and were used for subsequent tests. Subjects were asked to evaluate the degree of stinging as 0, 1, 2, and 3 for no stinging, slight stinging, moderate stinging, and severe stinging, respectively.

REFERENCES

1. Bartek MJ, LaBudde JA. Percutaneous absorption *in vitro*. In: Maibach HI, ed. Animal Models in Dermatology. New York: Churchill-Livingstone, 1975:103–120.
2. Bartek MJ, Labudde JA, Maibach HI. Skin permeability *in vivo*: comparison in rat, rabbit, pig and man. J Invest Dermatol 1972; 58:114–123.

3. Simpson WL, Cramer W. Fluorescence studies: carcinogens in skin. Cancer Res 1943; 3:362–369.
4. Dugard PJ. Skin permeability theory in relation to measurements of percutaneous absorption in toxicology. In: Marzulli FN, Maibach HI, eds. Dermatotoxicology, 2d ed. New York: Hemisphere, 1983:91–116.
5. Scheuplein RJ. Permeability of skin: a review of major concepts. Curr Probl Dermatol 1978; 7:58–68.
6. Scheuplein RJ, Bronough RL. Percutaneous absorption. In: Goldsmith LA, ed. Biochemistry and Physiology of the Skin. New York: Oxford Press, 1983:1255–1295.
7. Feldmann RJ, Maibach HI. Regional variation in percutaneous penetration of [^{14}C]cortisone in man. J Invest Dermatol 1967; 48:181–183.
8. Wester RC, Maibach HI. Cutaneous pharmacokinetics: 10 steps to percutaneous absorption. Drug Metab Rev 1983; 14:169–205.
9. Frosch PJ. Irritancy of soap and detergent bars. In: Frost P, Horwitz SN, eds. Principles of Cosmetics for the Dermatologist. St. Louis: CV Mosby, 1982:5–12.
10. Ostrenga J, Steinmetz C, Poulsen B, Yett S. Significance of vehicle composition. II. Prediction of optimal vehicle composition. J Pharm Sci 1971; 60:1180–1183.
11. Noonan PK, Wester RC. Cutaneous biotransformations and some pharmacological and toxicological implications. In: Marzulli FN, Maibach HI, eds. Dermatotoxicology, 2nd ed. New York: Hemisphere, 1983:71–90.
12. Hotchkiss SAM. Skin as a xenobiotic metabolising organ. In: Gibson GG, ed. Progress in Drug Metabolism. Vol. 13. London: Taylor and Francis, 1992:217–262.
13. Anderson C, Sundberg K, Groth O. Animal model for assessment of skin irritancy. Contact Derm 1986; 15:143–151.
14. Franz TJ. Percutaneous absorption. On the relevance of *in vitro* data. J Invest Dermatol 1975; 64:190–195.
15. Bronaugh, Maibach HI. *In Vitro* Percutaneous Absorption. Boca Raton: CRC Press, 1992.
16. Jadassohn J. Zur Kenntniss der medicamentosen Dermatosen. Verh Dtch Dermatol Ges 5 Congress 1896:103–129.
17. Bloch B, Steiner–Wourlisch A. Die Sensibilisierung des Meerschweinchens gegen Primeln. Arch Dermatol Syph 1930; 162:349–378.
18. Landsteiner K, Jacobs J. Studies on the sensitization of animals with simple chemical compounds. II. J Exp Med 1936; 64:625–629.
19. Landsteiner K, Jacobs J. Studies on the sensitization of animals with simple chemical compounds. J Exp Med 1935; 61:643–648.
20. Landsteiner K, Chase MW. Studies on the sensitization of animals with simple chemical compounds. IV. Anaphylaxis induced by picryl chloride and 2:4-dinitrochlorobenzene. J Exp Med 1937; 66:337–351.
21. von Blomberg BME, Bruynzeel DP, Scheper RJ. Advances in mechanisms of allergic contact dermatitis: *in vitro* and *in vivo* research. In: Marzulli FN, Maibach HI, eds. Dermatotoxicology, 4th ed. New York: Hemisphere, 1991:255–362.
22. Magee PS, Hostynek JJ, Maibach HI. A classification model for allergic contact dermatitis. Quant Struct Act Relat 1994; 13:22–33.
23. Code of Federal Regulations. Office of the Federal Registrar, National Archives of Records Service. General Services Administration 1985: Title 16, parts 1500.40–1500.41.
24. Environmental Protection Agency. Pesticides registrations: proposed data requirements. Sec. 158, 135: toxicology data requirements. Fed Reg 1982; 47:53192.

25. Andersen KE, Maibach HI. Multiple-application delayed-onset contact urticaria: possible relation to certain unusual formalin and textile reactions. Contact Derm 1983; 10:227–234.
26. Draize JH, Woodard G, Calvery HO. Methods for the study of irritation and toxicity of substances applied topically to the skin and mucous membrane. J Phamacol Exp Ther 1944; 82:377–390.
27. Klecak G. Identification of contact allergens: predictive tests in animals. In: Marzulli FN, Maibach HI, eds. Dermatotoxicology, 2d ed. New York: Hemisphere, 1983: 193–236.
28. Kero M, Hannuksela M. Guinea pig maximization test, open epicutaneous test and chamber test in induction of delayed contact hypersensitivity. Contact Derm 1980; 6:341–344.
29. Buehler EV. A new method for detecting potential sensitizers using the guinea pig. Toxicol Appl Pharmacol 1964; 6:341.
30. Klecak G. The Freund's Complete Adjuvant test and the open epicutaneous test. In: Maibach HI, Anderson KE, eds. Contact Allergy, Predictive Tests in Guinea Pigs. Basel: Karger, 1985:152–171.
31. Kaminsky M, Szivos MM, Brown KR. Application of the Hill Top Patch Test Chamber to dermal irritancy testing in the albino rabbit. J Toxicol Cutaneous Ocul Toxicol 1986; 5(2):81–87.
32. Frosch PJ, Kligman AM. The Duhring chamber: an improved technique for epicutaneous testing of irritant and allergic reactions. Contact Derm 1979; 5:73.
33. Henderson CR, Riley EC. Certain statistical considerations in patch testing. Invest Dermatol 1945; 6:227–230.
34. Draize JH. Procedures for the appraisal of the toxicity of chemicals in foods, drugs, and cosmetics. VIII. Dermal toxicity. Food Drug Cosmet Law J 1955; 10:722–731.
35. Marzulli FN, Maibach HI. Antimicrobials: experimental contact sensitization in man. J Soc Cosmet Chem 1973; 24:399–421.
36. Marzulli FN, Maibach HI. Use of graded concentrations in studying skin sensitizers: experimental contact sensitization in man. Food Cosmet Toxicol 1974; 12:219–227.
37. Prottey C. The molecular basis of skin irritation. In: Breuer MM, ed. Cosmetic Science, Vol. 1. London: Academic Press, 1978:275–349.
38. Shelanski HA. Experience with and considerations of the human patch test method. J Soc Cosmet Chem 1951; 2:324–331.
39. Irritation: *in vitro* approaches. In: Rouger A, Goldberg L, Maibach H, eds. *In Vitro* Toxicology. London: Academic Press, 1994:23–185.
40. Motoyoshi K, Toyoshima Y, Sato M, Yoshimura M. Comparative studies on the irritancy of oils and synthetic perfumes to the skin of rabbit, guinea pig, rat, miniature swine, and man. Cosmet Toilet 1979; 94:41–42.
41. Guillot JP, Gopnnet JF, Clement C, Caillard L, Truhauf R. Evaluation of the cutaneous-irritation potential of compounds. Food Chem Toxicol 1982; 20:563–572.
42. Phillips L, Steinberg M, Maibach HI, Akers WA. A comparison of rabbit and human skin response to certain irritants. Toxicol Appl Pharmacol 1972; 21:369–382.
43. Magnusson B, Hersle K. Patch test methods. I. A comparative study of six different types of patch tests. Acta Dermatol 1965; 45:123–128.
44. Mathias CGT, Maibach HI. Dermatoxicology monographs. I. Cutaneous irritation: factors influencing the response to irritants. Clin Toxicol 1978; 13:333–346.

45. Kligman AM, Wooding WM. A method for the measurement and evaluation of irritants on human skin. J Invest Dermatol 1967; 49:78–94.
46. Lanman BM, Elvers WB, Howard CS. The role of human patch testing in a product development program. In: Proceedings of the Joint Conference on Cosmetic Sciences. The Toilet Goods Association. Washington DC, 1968:135–145.
47. Rapaport M, Anderson D, Pierce U. Performance of the 21 day patch test in civilian populations. J Toxicol Cutaneous Ocul Toxicol 1978; 1:109–115.
48. Emery BE, Edwards LD. The pharmacology of soaps. II. The irritant action of soaps on human skin. J Am Pharm Assoc 1940; 29:251–254.
49. Maurer T, Thomann P, Weirich EG, Hess R. The optimization test in the guinea pig. A method for the predictive evaluation of the contact allergenicity of chemicals. Agents Actions 1975; 5:174–179.
50. Kligman AM. A biological brief on percutaneous absorption. Drug Dev Ind Pharm 1983; 19:521–560.
51. Weigand DA, Gaylor JR. Irritant reaction in negro and caucasian skin. South Med J 1976; 67:548–551.
52. von Krogh C, Maibach HI. The contact urticaria syndrome. Semin Dermatol 1982; 1:59–66.
53. Lahti A. Nonimmunologic contact urticaria. Acta Derm Venereol (Stockh) 1980; 60(Suppl):1–49.
54. Maibach HI, Johnson HL. Contact urticaria syndrome. Contact urticaria to diethyltoluamide (immediate-type hypersensitivity). Arch Dermatol 1975; 111:726–730.
55. Lahti A, Maibach HI. Species specificity of non-immunologic contact urticaria: guinea pig, rat and mouse. J Am Acad Dermatol 1985; 13:66–69.
56. Lahti A, Maibach HI. An animal model for non-immunologic contact urticaria. Toxicol Appl Pharmacol 1984; 76:219–224.
57. Frosch PJ, Kligman AM. A method for appraising the stinging capacity of topically applied substances. J Soc Cosmet Chem 1977; 28:197–207.
58. Lauerma AI, Fenn B, Maibach HI. Trimellitic anhydride-sensitive mouse as an animal model for contact urticaria. J Appl Toxicol 1997; 17(6):357–360.
59. Cagen SZ, Malloy LA, Parker CM, Gardiner TH, van Gelder CA, Jud VA. Pyrethroid mediated skin sensory stimulation characterized by a new behavioral paradigm. Toxicol Appl Pharmacol 1984; 76:270–279.
60. Vijverberg HP, VandenBercken J. Frequency dependent effects of the pyrethroid insecticide decamethrin in frog myelinated nerve fibers. Eur J Pharmacol 1979; 58:501–504.
61. Vijverberg HP, VandenBercken J. Neurotoxicological effects and the mode of action of pyrethroid insecticides. Crit Rev Toxicol 1990; 21(2):105–126.

34

Contact Urticaria Syndrome and Claims Support

Saqib J. Bashir and Howard I. Maibach
University of California, San Francisco, California, USA

Introduction	588
Symptoms and Signs	588
Epidemiology	588
Mechanisms of Contact Urticaria	589
Nonimmunological Contact Urticaria	589
Immunological Contact Urticaria	590
Site Specificity of Contact Urticaria Reactions	591
Human Experimental Protocols	591
Subject Selection	591
Site Selection	592
Paired Comparison Studies	592
Serial Doses	592
Application Techniques	593
CUS Inhibition	593
Clinical Assessment and Quantitative Methods	594
Visual Scoring of Contact Urticaria	594
Measurement of Erythema	594
Measuring Color	595
Laser-Doppler Blood Flowmetry	595
Measurement of Edema	596

Animal Experimental Protocols   596
   NICU   596
   ICU   596
Conclusion   597
References   597

INTRODUCTION

Contact urticaria syndrome (CUS) was first defined by Maibach and Johnson (1) and, since then, numerous reports of contact urticaria to a variety of compounds, such as foods, preservatives, fragrances, plant and animal products, metals, and other things, continue to be reported. Therefore, it is important to determine, in a scientific manner, whether and in what dose a particular substance causes contact urticaria. Accurate experimental models are required to document urticaria-inducing properties of a substance; protocols to quantify efficacy of formulations that putatively inhibit CUS are also proposed. This chapter outlines current scientific knowledge and approaches to experimental methodology.

SYMPTOMS AND SIGNS

Immediate contact reactions, such as contact urticaria, appear within minutes to ~1 h after exposure of the urticariant to the skin. The patient may complain of local burning, tingling, or itching, and swelling and redness may be seen (wheal and flare). Symptoms may extend extracutaneously, inducing, for example, bronchial asthma. In the most severe cases, anaphylactoid reactions may occur. A staging system of CUS has been described (Table 1).

EPIDEMIOLOGY

Kanerva and colleagues (2,3) gathered statistical data on occupational contact urticaria in Finland. The incidence more than doubled from 89 reported cases in 1989 to 194 cases in 1994. From 1990 to 1994, a total of 815 cases were reported. The most common causes were, in decreasing order, cow dander, natural rubber latex (NRL), and flour/grains/feed. These three groups comprised 79% of all cases. Reflecting this, the most affected occupations (per 100,000 workers) were bakers, processed food preparers, and dental assistants, in decreasing order. Contact urticaria is, therefore, a common problem that may affect many people in the course of their daily lives.

Table 1 Staging of Contact Urticaria

Cutaneous reactions only	
Stage 1	Localized urticaria (redness and swelling)
	Dermatitis (eczema)
	Nonspecific symptoms (itching, tingling, burning)
Stage 2	Generalized urticaria
Extracutaneous reactions	
Stage 3	Bronchial asthma (wheezing)
	Rhinitis, conjunctivitis (runny nose, watery eyes)
	Orolaryngeal symptoms (lip swelling, hoarseness, difficulty swallowing)
	Gastrointestinal symptoms (nausea, vomiting, diarrhea, cramps)
Stage 4	Anaphylactiod reactions (shock)

Source: Ref. (11).

MECHANISMS OF CONTACT URTICARIA

CUS can be described in two broad categories: nonimmunological contact urticaria (NICU) and immunological contact urticaria (ICU). The former does not require presensitization of the patient's immune system to an allergen, whereas the latter does. However, there are contact urticaria reactions of unknown mechanism, and these are unclassified.

Nonimmunological Contact Urticaria

NICU is the most frequent immediate contact reaction (4) and occurs, without prior sensitization, in most exposed individuals. The symptoms may vary according to the site of exposure, the concentration, the vehicle, the mode of exposure, and the substance itself (5).

The mechanism of NICU is not well understood. It was previously assumed that histamine was released from mast cells in response to exposure to an eliciting substance. However, the H_1 antihistamines, hydroxyzine and terfenadine, do not inhibit NICU to benzoic acid, cinnamic acid, cinnamic aldehyde, or methyl nicotinate in prick tests, but they do inhibit reactions to histamine itself (5,6). Therefore, mechanisms that do not involve histamine may mediate NICU for these substances.

Evidence suggests that prostaglandins may mediate NICU. Oral and topical nonsteroidal anti-inflammatory drugs (NSAIDs) inhibit nonimmunological reactions (7). Lahti (6) used laser-Doppler flowmetry (LDF) to demonstrate a reduction in NICU-induced erythema in subjects pretreated with NSAIDs. This group believed that inhibition of prostaglandin metabolism may explain this effect.

Supporting this, Morrow et al. (8) demonstrated an increase in plasma PGD_2 following the topical application of 1% sorbic acid to the human forearm. The time course of PGD_2 peaks correlated temporally with the observed intensity of cutaneous vasodilatation. Notably, histamine and PGE_2 levels at peak erythema were not significantly higher than pretreatment levels. This suggests that the release of vasodilatory prostaglandins induced by sorbic acid was selective for PGD_2, and that histamine is not involved in sorbic acid contact urticarial reactions. The release of PGD_2 was a dose-dependent effect, increasing with greater concentrations of sorbic acid, until reaching a plateau between 1% to 3%. Pretreating the subjects with oral aspirin (325 mg b.i.d. for 3 days) attenuated the observed cutaneous vasodilatation and inhibit release of PGD_2. In later studies, on the basis of the same model, this group demonstrated similar results with benzoic acid- and nicotinic acid-induced contact urticaria (9,10).

These studies add evidence to the argument that prostaglandin metabolism is significant in the pathophysiology of CUS. In addition, they not only suggest that NSAIDs are useful as a treatment, but also suggest that experimental subjects should avoid these drugs when participating in a contact urticaria study.

Ultraviolet A and ultraviolet B light also inhibits immediate nonimmunological contact reactions. Notably this effect can last for 2 weeks after irradiation and inhibits skin sites that were not directly irradiated (7). The authors suggest that there may be a systemic effect rather than simply a local one; however, the mechanism by which ultraviolet light inhibits NICU is not known.

Immunological Contact Urticaria

ICU is less frequent in clinical practice than the NICU form. It is a type-1 hypersensitivity reaction mediated by IgE antibodies, specific to the eliciting substance (11). Therefore, prior immune (IgE) sensitization is required for this type of contact urticaria.

This sensitization can be at the cutaneous level, but also via mucous membranes, for example, in the respiratory or gastrointestinal tracts. Notably, ICU reactions may spread beyond the site of contact and progress to generalized urticaria and, in the most severe case, to anaphylactic shock.

People with an atopic background (personal or family background of eczema, hayfever, or asthma) are predisposed toward the ICR.

A well-studied example of ICU is allergy to NRL, which is found in a wide variety of products such as balloons, condoms, and, importantly, surgical or protective gloves. ICU to NRL is a major occupational hazard in occupations that utilize such gloves (e.g., the health-care profession).

Typically, latex gloves cause a wheal-and-flare reaction at the site of contact. This can affect either the person wearing the gloves or the person being touched by the wearer. In a study of 70 German patients with contact urticaria, 51% suffered rhinitis, 44% conjunctivitis, 31% dyspnea, 24% systemic symptoms, and 6% severe systemic reactions during surgery (12). In addition to direct skin contact, allergy may be caused by airborne NRL (13). Clearly, sensitized, yet undiagnosed, individuals are at risk when contacting ICU allergens.

Cross allergy can also induce ICU reactions: the patient may be sensitized to one protein but reacts to other proteins that contain the same (or similar) allergenic molecule. In the example of latex allergy, patients may also experience symptoms from banana, chestnut, and avocado (14). This phenomenon places ICU patients at further risk.

SITE SPECIFICITY OF CONTACT URTICARIA REACTIONS

Characteristics of the skin and also of its sensitivity to urticariants vary from site to site. This is an important consideration in experimental design, discussed in what follows, and in diagnosis. Schriner and Maibach (15) used LDF to map the regions of the human face most sensitive to NICU induced by benzoic acid: the neck was the most sensitive area, followed by the perioral and nasolabial folds. The least sensitive area was the volar forearm. The authors conclude that the neck, nasolabial, and perioral areas are most sensitive to test for potential NICU to this agent. In his study of benzoic acid sensitivity at various body sites, Lahti (5) found that the back was more sensitive than the hands, ventral forearms, or the soles of the feet.

HUMAN EXPERIMENTAL PROTOCOLS

Human subjects may be used to determine the potential for a product to cause CUS in the human population. The protocols for ICU and NICU are the same, although ICU requires volunteers who are presensitized to the product. Subject selection, dosing, test site, application methods, and analysis are discussed in this section.

Subject Selection

To test a product for use in the general population, it is desirable to recruit a random pool of volunteers. However, this may introduce several confounding factors such as age, skin disease, atopic tendency, and medication (such as NSAIDs) that may alter the results. Therefore, subjects must be chosen with particular regard to the aim of the study and screened carefully for inclusion and exclusion criteria and for possible confounding factors.

Spriet et al. (16) suggest that subjects can be classified into three categories: serious sufferers, symptomatic volunteers, and healthy volunteers. It is likely that the latter are most suitable for testing new products, whereas the former two groups may be better suited to ICU studies or investigating claims that a product already in use causes CUS. Ideally, subjects should be the representative of the population at which the product is aimed.

Site Selection

In the diagnostic investigation of a patient, the site affected in the patient's history may be tested. However, in a new product test trial, it is preferable to test the site at which the product is to be used. However, this may not be convenient for volunteers, and therefore concealed sites such as the volar aspect of the forearm or the upper back may be chosen. Importantly, the site selected should be consistent in patients and controls, as different areas of the skin may demonstrate different sensitivities to the urticariant, thereby distorting comparability of the data. As mentioned earlier, different areas of the skin have varying capacity to induce urticaria, which should be considered when a site is chosen. Even in ICU, different skin sites may vary in their ability to elicit contact urticaria (17).

A history of skin disease may also affect the result. A test that is negative in nondiseased skin may in fact be positive in previously diseased or currently affected skin (18a). If the initial studies are negative, it may be desirable to select subjects who are symptomatic and use the affected sites to test the substance.

Paired Comparison Studies

Paired comparison studies allow rapid comparison between treated and untreated groups. Randomized matched pairs can be grouped for treatment and control, or the subjects can be used as their own controls by applying the test substance and controls on separate sites. The latter is preferred, because each subject may have several doses applied to their skin, providing more data from a smaller pool of subjects. Furthermore, this decreases intersubject variation and confounding, thus providing better control.

Serial Doses

Performing studies at different doses of the product will allow the investigator to build a dose–response profile. This may indicate a minimum dose that causes a threshold response in the study group and also the dose at which a maximum response is seen. Extrapolating these data to the general population may give manufacturers an indication of a safe concentration for an ingredient to be included in a product. Dose–response analysis may also demonstrate that there is no safe concentration for that ingredient, or, indeed, that there is relatively little risk.

Examples of concentrations that have been used in dilution series in alcohol vehicles are 250, 125, 62, 31 mM for benzoic acid and 50, 10, 2, 0.5 mM for methyl nicotinate (7).

Application Techniques

Commonly used topical application techniques in both ICU and NICU are the *open test* and the *chamber test*. A *use test* can be employed in known sufferers. A positive reaction comprises a wheal-and-flare reaction and sometimes an eruption of vesicles.

1. In the *open test*, 0.1 mL of the test substance is spread over a 3×3 cm^2 area on the desired site. Lahti (7) suggests that using alcohol vehicles, with the addition of propylene glycol, enhances the sensitivity of this test compared with previously used petrolatum and water vehicles. The test is usually read at 20, 40, and 60 min in order to see the maximal response. ICR reactions appear within 15–20 min and nonimmunological ones appear within 45–60 min after application (11).
2. The *chamber test* is an occlusive method of applying the substance to be tested. These are applied in small aluminum containers (Finn Chamber, Epitest Ltd., Hyrylä, Finland) and attached to the skin via porous tape. The chambers are applied for 15 min, and the results are read at 20, 40, and 60 min. The advantages of this method are that occlusion enhances percutaneous penetration, and therefore possibly the sensitivity of the test; in addition, a smaller area of skin is required than in an open test. For unexplained reasons, this occlusion may provide less responsivity than in the open test.
3. The *use test* is a method in which a subject known to be affected uses the substance in the same way as when the symptoms appeared (e.g., putting surgical gloves on wet hands provokes latex ICU).

Other techniques used in the assessment of ICU are the prick test, the scratch test, and the chamber prick test. RAST can be used to determine cross-reactivity (11,13).

CUS Inhibition

The earlier-mentioned models can be employed to test the capability of a substance to inhibit CUS. This may be by topical application or by systemic means. Topical putative inhibitors can be studied by the paired comparison method, using multiple test sites and a control on the same subject. This allows serial dosing, with either the urticariant or the inhibitor, to identify its protective potential against a known urticariant. In systemic studies of an oral putative CUS inhibitor, for example, subjects can be randomized into matched pairs for treatment and control. Following systemic administration, a known urticariant can be applied topically in various doses, as mentioned earlier, and the response assessed.

CLINICAL ASSESSMENT AND QUANTITATIVE METHODS

Previously, dermatological studies of the skin have scored the degree of urticaria by means of visual assessment by an experienced observer, usually a dermatologist. There are several advantages and disadvantages to this technique. Advantages are that it is inexpensive, visual scoring is rapid, subjects are regularly assessed so that the study can be curtailed if adverse reactions are severe, and unexpected findings can be handled by the investigator. However, simple observation may introduce error, inter- and intra-observer variations. This is especially important in larger studies, which may involve a team of investigators.

Visual observations are also often graded on an ordinal (nonlinear) scale (e.g., rating reactions as weak, moderate, or severe). As these data are not in linear numerical form, statistical analysis is not as powerful as for quantitative data. In many studies, subjects report symptoms, also on an ordinal scale; this, again, is a subjective analysis prone to variation error.

In contrast, a quantitative analysis may provide linear numerical data that are easily reproducible and accurate in standardized conditions. Rather than providing a score, measured data allow for statistical comparisons such as mean values and standard deviations. This adds to our understanding of the properties of the test substance. Thus, objective measurements can clearly benefit dermatology studies.

Visual Scoring of Contact Urticaria

Contact urticaria can be graded visually by marking the degree of erythema and edema on an ordinal scale. Examples are given in Tables 2 and 3.

Measurement of Erythema

Erythema, redness of the skin, is a part of the skin inflammatory response that reflects localized increase in capillary blood flow elicited. Therefore, erythema can be measured by both the redness and the blood flow in the inflamed area.

Table 2 Scale to Score Erythema

Score	Description
1+	Slight erythema, either spotty or diffuse
2+	Moderate uniform erythema
3+	Intense redness
4+	Fiery redness with edema

Source: Ref. (18b).

Table 3 Scale to Score Edema

Score	Description
1	Slight edema, barely visible or palpable
2	Unmistakable wheal, easily palpable
3	Solid, tense wheal
4	Tense wheal, extending beyond test area

Source: Ref. (18c).

Measuring Color

Two techniques have been used to measure color: remittance spectroscopy and tristimulus chromametry. Elsner gave detailed descriptions of the two techniques (19,20). Essentially, both methods detect light remitted from illuminated skin. Remittance spectroscopy employs multiple sensors to "scan" the light over the whole visible spectrum, producing a spectrogram. This differs from a tristimulus chromameter, in which the remitted light is transmitted to three photodiodes, each with a color filter with a specific spectral sensitivity: 450 nm (blue), 550 nm (green), 610 nm (red). The data from a colorimeter are expressed as a color value.

Remittance spectroscopy has been used to measure erythema in contact urticaria (21,22). This group evaluated remittance spectroscopy compared with visual scoring in the assessment of urticarial prick test reactions. They found that there was a significant difference between negative and positive reactions, and between positive and strong positive reactions $(+/++)$. Baseline skin had an erythema index of 36, compared with 72 for a positive reaction. Negative skin sites had a slightly, but not significantly, raised erythema index, resulting from a dermographic reaction related to the procedure of the test itself. Notably, remittance spectroscopy was not as effective in discerning between the stronger reactions $(++/+++)$, possibly because of the reduction of blood flow and hemoglobin content associated with the whitening of the center of the lesion and also because the blood flow may already have been maximized.

Laser-Doppler Blood Flowmetry

Several studies have identified a reliable correlation between skin blood flow measured by LDF and cutaneous inflammation (23–27). Bircher (28) reviews the use of LDF to study the role of various mediators in altering cutaneous blood flow.

The LDF technique measures the Doppler frequency shift in monochromatic laser light backscattered from moving red blood cells. This shift is proportional to the number of erythrocytes times their velocity in the cutaneous microcirculation. This noninvasive technique measures a surface are of 1 mm^2 and a depth of 1–1.5 mm. The 1 mm depth will therefore measure the upper horizontal plexus, consisting of arterioles, capillaries, and postcapillary venules. LDF does not measure the deep horizontal plexus that lies at the subcutaneous dermal junction. Detailed review of the principles, techniques, and methodology can be found by Berardesca (22).

The changes in blood flow can be expressed in two ways. Either as the net change in cutaneous blood flow over the time of the experiment, which is given by the area under the curve, or as the maximal increase in flow over the baseline value (PEAK). Following a measurement of baseline blood flow, the product can be applied and post-treatment flow can be measured. The change in blood flow provides an indication of the degree of inflammation caused.

Measurement of Edema

Ultrasound has been used to quantify the edema component of urticaria. Agner and Serup (29) demonstrated a significant difference in skin thickness compared with controls in irritant reactions to sodium lauryl sulfate, nonanoic acid, and hydrochloric acid. Serup et al. (30) used ultrasound to measure edema in patch tests, expressed in millimeters. Agner (31) suggests that A-mode ultrasound scanning is a simple, reproducible method of measuring skin thickness. However, one disadvantage is that the technique is dependent on an experienced operator, which can potentially introduce observer error.

ANIMAL EXPERIMENTAL PROTOCOLS

Animal models are potentially useful to identify putative contact urticariants.

NICU

The guinea pig ear lobe resembles human skin in its reaction to contact urticariants (7,32), and is an established model for NICU. A positive reaction is seen as erythema and swelling of the ear, which can be quantified by measuring the thickness of the ear.

ICU

Lauerma and Maibach (33) considered a possible animal model for ICU, topically presensitizing mice to trimellitic anhydride (TMA), which is known to cause IgE-mediated reactions. Topical TMA was applied to the dorsum of mice ears 6 days after they had been sensitized, eliciting a biphasic ear-swelling response. However, further studies are required to validate this model.

CONCLUSION

In conclusion, study of contact urticaria is possible with both human and animal subjects in whom a combination of subjective and objective analysis can identify potential ICU and NICUs.

REFERENCES

1. Maibach HI, Johnson HL. Contact urticaria syndrome: contact urticaria to diethyltoluamide (immediate type hypersensitivity). Arch Dermatol 1975; 111:726–730.
2. Kanerva L, Susitaival P. Cow dander—the most common cause of occupational contact urticaria in Finland. Contact Derm 1996; 35:309–310.
3. Kanerva L, Jolanki R, Toikkanen J, Estlander T. Statistics on occupational contact urticaria. In: Amin S, Lahti A, Maibach HI, eds. Contact Urticaria Syndrome. Boca Raton: CRC Press, 1997:55–70.
4. Lahti A. Immediate contact reactions. In: Rycroft RJG, Menné T, Frosch PJ, Benezra C, eds. Textbook of Contact Dermatitis. Berlin: Springer-Verlag, 1992:62–74.
5. Lahti A. Nonimmunologic contact urticaria. Acta Dermatol Venereol (Stockh) 1980; 60:1.
6. Lahti A. Terfrenadine (H_1-antagonist) does not inhibit nonimmunological contact urticaria. Contact Derm 1987; 16:220.
7. Lahti A. Nonimmunologic contact urticaria. In: Amin S, Lahti A, Maibach HI, eds. Contact Urticaria Syndrome. Boca Raton: CRC Press, 1977 (Chapter 3).
8. Morrow JD, Minon TA, Awad JA, Roberts LJ II. Release of markedly increased quantities of prostaglandin D_2 from the skin *in vivo* in humans following the application of sorbic acid. Arch Dermatol 1994; 130:1408.
9. Morrow JD. Prostaglandin D_2 and contact urticaria. In: Berardesca E, Elsner P, Maibach HI, eds. Bioengineering of the Skin: Cutaneous Blood Flow and Erythema. Boca Raton: CRC Press, 1995 (Chapter 8).
10. Jackson Roberts L II, Morrow JD. Prostaglandin D_2 mediates contact urticaria caused by sorbic acid, benzoic acid, and esters of nicotinic acid. In: Amin S, Lahti A, Maibach HI, eds. Contact Urticaria Syndrome. Boca Raton: CRC Press, 1997 (Chapter 8).
11. Amin S, Maibach HI. Immunologic contact urticaria definition. In: Amin S, Lahti A, Maibach HI, eds. Contact Urticaria Syndrome. Boca Raton: CRC Press, 1997 (Chapter 2).
12. Jaeger D, Kleinhans D, Czuppon AB, Baur X. Latex specific proteins causing immediate type cutaneous, nasal, bronchial and systemic reactions. J Allergy Clin Immunol 1992; 89:759.
13. Turjanmaa K, Mäkinen-Kiljunen S, Ruenala T, Alenius H, Palosuo T. Natural rubber latex allergy: the European experience. Immunol Allergy Clin Am 1995; 15(1):71–88.
14. Hannuksela M. Mechanisms in contact urticaria. Clin Dermatol 1997; 15:619–922.

15. Schriner DL, Maibach HI. Regional variation of nonimmunologic contact urticaria Functional map of the human face. Skin Pharmacol 1996; 9:312–321.
16. Spriet A, Dupin-Spriet T, Simon P. Selection of subject. In: Methodology of Clinical Drug Trials. Basel: Karger, 1994 (Chapter 3).
17. Maibach HI. Regional variation in elicitation of contact urticaria syndrome (immediate hypersensitivity syndrome): shrimp. Contact Derm 1986; 15:100.
18. (a) Lahti A, Maibach HI. Immediate contact reactions (contact urticaria syndrome). In: Maibach HI, ed. Occupational and Industrial Dermatology, 2d ed. Chicago: Year Book Medical, 1986:32–44; (b) Frosch PJ, Kligman AM. The soap chamber test. J Am Acad Dermatol 1979; 1:35; (c) Gollhausen R, Kligman AM. Human assay for identifying substances which induce non-allergic contact urticaria: the NICU test. Contact Derm 1985; 13:98–105.
19. Elsner P. Chromametry: hardware, measuring principles, and standardisation of measurements. In: Berardesca E, Elsner P, Maibach HI, eds. Bioengineering of the Skin: Cutaneous Blood Flow and Erythema. Boca Raton: CRC, 1995 (Chapter 19).
20. Andersen PH, Bjerring P. Remittance spectroscopy: hardware and measuring principles. In: Berardesca E, Elsner P, Maibach HI, eds. Bioengineering of the Skin: Cutaneous Blood Flow and Erythema. Boca Raton: CRC, 1995 (Chapter 17).
21. Berardesca E, Gabba P, Nume A, Rabbiosi G, Maibach HI. Objective prick test evaluation: non-invasive techniques. Acta Dermatol Venereol 1992; 72:261.
22. Berardesca E. Erythema measurements in diseased skin. In: Berardesca E, Elsner P, Maibach HI, eds. Bioengineering of the Skin: Cutaneous Blood Flow and Erythema. Boca Raon: CRC, 1995 (Chapter 20).
23. Bircher AJ, Guy RH, Maibach HI. Skin pharmacology and dermatology. In: Shepherd AP, Oberg PS, eds. Laser-Doppler Blood Flowmetry. Boston: Kluwer Academic Publishers, 1990:141–174.
24. Blanken R, van der Valk PGM, Nater JP. Laser-Doppler flowmetry in the investigation of irritant compounds on the human skin. Dermaotsen Beruf Umwelt 1986; 34:5–9.
25. Pershing LK, Heuther S, Conklin RL, Krueger GG. Cutaneous blood flow and percutaneous absorption: a quantitative analysis using a laser Doppler flow meter and a blood flow meter. J Invest Dermatol 1989; 92:355–359.
26. Li Q, Aoyama K, Matsushita T. Evaluation of contact allergy to chemicals using a laser Doppler flowmetery (LDF) technique. Contact Derm 1992; 26:27–33.
27. Wilhelm KP, Surber C, Maibach HI. Quantification of sodium lauryl sulfate irritant dermatitis in man: comparison of four techniques: skin colour reflectance, transepidermal water loss, laser Doppler flow measurement and visual scores. Arch Dermatol Res 1989; 281:293–295.
28. Bircher AJ. Skin pharmacology. In: Berardesca E, Elsner P, Maibach HI, eds. Bioengineering of the Skin: Cutaneous Blood Flow and Erythema. Boca Raton: CRC Press, 1995:73–84.
29. Agner T, Serup J. Skin reactions to irritants assessed by non-invasive bioengineering methods. Contact Derm 1989; 20:352–359.
30. Serup J, Staberg B, Klemp P. Quantification of cutaneous edema in patch test reaction by measurement of skin thickness with high frequency pulsed ultrasound. Contact Derm 1984; 10:88–93.

31. Agner T. Ultrasound: a mode measurement of skin thickness. In: Serup J, Jemel GBE, eds. Handbook of Non-invasive Methods and the Skin. Boca Raton: CRC Press, 1995 (Chapter 12.5).
32. Lahti A, Maibach HI. An animal model for nonimmunologic contact urticaria. Toxicol Appl Pharmacol 1984; 76:219–224.
33. Lauerma AI, Maibach HI. Model for immunologic contact urticaria. In: Amin S, Lahti A, Maibach HI, eds. Contact Urticaria Syndrome. Boca Raton: CRC, 1997:27–32.

Product Development

35

Process Engineering in Cosmetics to Utilize Active Ingredients

Kazuyuki Takagi
Mizuho Industrial Co., Ltd., Osaka, Japan

Introduction	603
Application for Decreasing the Amount of Emulsifier	604
Application Correspondence in Order to Decrease Preservatives	607
Application to Solubility and Dispersion	608
Application for Improvement in Usability and Feeling	610
Scale-up	610
Conclusion	611
References	612

INTRODUCTION

Many cosmetics are manufactured according to the process classified in chemical engineering as emulsification or distribution. Various emulsification and distribution technologies have been developed in recent years. Regarding formulation emulsification technology, the phase inversion emulsifying method, the gel emulsifying method, and the D phase emulsifying method are used. As a form of mechanical emulsification technology, there is also the emulsifying method in which mechanical power (mainly shear, impact, and cavitation is applied).

In the interest of increasing the use of natural cosmetics and using properties of natural active ingredients that are mild to the skin (in accordance with recent conceptions of "mild"), application of materials and additives with skin stimulatives, such as emulsifiers, perfumes, and preservatives, is lessening and many of these products are no longer included.

In emulsification, an emulsifier of natural origin is used or a formulation where the emulsifier is reduced or not used at all is constructed, using high molecule materials. Powerful machinery is needed for manufacturing a product when the amount of an emulsifier is decreased or it is not used at all. Although many cosmetics that use natural emulsifiers, such as a lecithin, have already been manufactured, a high-pressure homogenizer and an ultra high-speed rotating design for applying powerful mechanical forces are necessary for dispersion of the extremely stable hydrogenated lecithin (1).

In recent times, the use of preservatives by which a skin stimulus is strengthened more than by an emulsifier is decreasing. Additionally, the demand for manufacturing a product that does not contain preservatives is increasing.

Use of mechanical emulsification as the manufacturing technology helps in such a formulation. The search for a harmonization of formulation, materials, manufacturing process, and production equipment for new product development is increasingly important. Moreover, as the manufacturing process becomes more complicated, the problem of scaling-up also becomes more significant.

Efficient use of new equipment and mechanical emulsification may be applied to manufacturing cosmetics, utilizing the properties of the active ingredients.

APPLICATION FOR DECREASING THE AMOUNT OF EMULSIFIER

The skin stimulative of an emulsifier varies with molecular weight or structure, and although all emulsifiers are not bad, the demand for generally decreasing levels of an emulsifier has been strong. In order to decrease the level of emulsifier, the microfluidizer method is used, (Fig. 1), which uses mechanical power.

In the following, the relation between mechanical force and the quantity of an emulsifier is investigated.

Basic formulation: 71% water, 25% liquid paraffin, and 4% (Tween/Span HLB $= 10$) emulsifiers (an emulsifier reduced ratio; 4% vs. $1/4, 1/8, 1/20, 1/22$).

Processing conditions: Total quantity, 500 mL; temperature, 70°C. The formulation is applied as a pre-emulsification for 30 min using the rotating homogenizing mixer at 5000 rpm. After pre-emulsification, a microfluidizer is used for

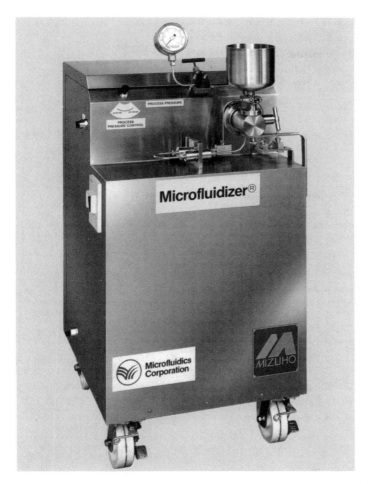

Figure 1 Schematic diagram of microfluidizer.

high-pressure processing at 172 Mpa; one pass is performed. The result is shown in Fig. 2.

When only a rotating homogenizing mixer is used, as this graph shows, the diameter of a particle when the amount of relative particles is 50% becomes ~5 μm. Using the same formulation, but using a microfluidizer, a 0.1 μm particulate is obtained. In fact, using the microfluidizer, a particle diameter of ~5 μm is obtained when the amount of emulsifier is managed at 0.18%.

It is shown that an emulsifier can be decreased from 4% to 0.18% when using a microfluidizer, compared with using only a rotating homogenizer, and still retain the same particle diameter. Separation will be caused when 0.18% of this emulsifier is required to make the emulsification system stable, and it

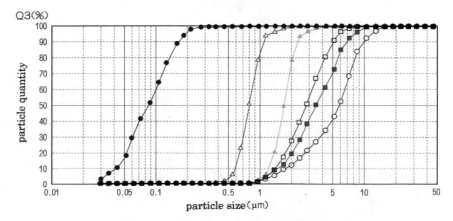

Figure 2 Graphical representation of high-pressure processing.

has been removed until now. However, an emulsifier will become completely unnecessary if an emulsification system can be made stable by other factors. Factors for making the emulsification system stable include the following:

1. the specific gravity difference is made small and the onset of surfacing and separation rates is delayed;
2. strong formation and electric restitution of an interface film protect the union of an emulsification particle; and
3. by increasing viscosity of a product, control of the particle movement is increased or the onset of surfacing and separation rates is delayed, and union of an emulsification particle is prevented. Increasing product viscosity can be easily attained by using high molecule materials.

If a particulate is distributed by mechanical force and viscosity is raised using high molecule materials, a product that does not use an emulsifier may be made. However, the selection of high molecule materials suitable for formulation or a manufacturing process becomes important. This is because shearing forces may result in the chain of a high molecule being turned off, depending on the kind of high molecule materials, or a liquid phase component may ooze. Instead of high molecule materials, a method is available that uses clay (bentonite, silica), protein, and ester oil.

When raising the viscosity of a product and making an emulsification system stable, it also becomes possible to use the rotating homogenizing mixer. A base with sufficiently high viscosity maintaining stability is made to distribute water droplets using the ultra-mixer, which combines the high viscosity at 100 Pa or the Nerimaze-type kneader (Fig. 3) with the ultra-mixer. By this method, vaseline ointment containing a water-soluble agent is manufactured, without using an emulsifier.

APPLICATION CORRESPONDENCE IN ORDER TO DECREASE PRESERVATIVES

For decreasing the level of preservatives, large mechanical forces (shearing, impact, and cavitation), such as those provided by microfluidizers, are used. Originally, such high-pressure homogenizer equipment was developed for the purpose of cell rupture. As shown in Fig. 4, such force crushes cells; consequently numbers bacteria in materials can be sharply decreased. Therefore, if such mechanical power is used in the current application, the type and quantity of preservatives may be decreased.

In cosmetics, countermeasures for bacterial contamination at filling and secondary pollution are also needed. Regarding the filling environment, if the

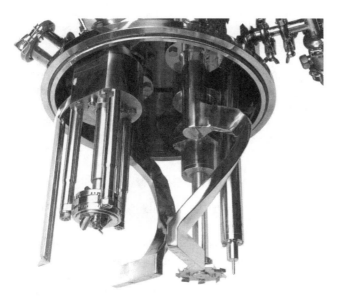

Figure 3 Schematic diagram of Nerimaze-type kneader.

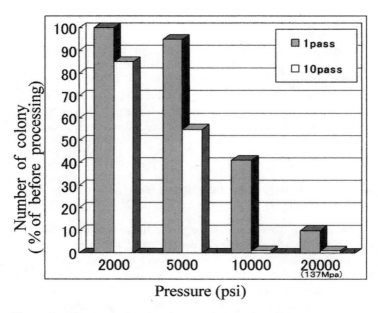

Figure 4 Histogram showing decrease in bacteria number at pressures.

filling is on a small scale, and the place has a high degree of cleanliness, a small filling machine may be installed onto a clean bench (Fig. 5) or an isolator (Fig. 6). Regarding the container, cosmetics (Fig. 7) produced by the Blow Fill Seal filling equipment are presently available, and the containers are currently used for eyewash medicine.

When a product is used over a long period of time, for example, a cream, countermeasures against bacteria are needed. Use of an airless pump container is increasing for this purpose. This is a sealing type of container, and since fingers do not contact the product in the container at the time of use, secondary contamination by the bacteria can be prevented.

APPLICATION TO SOLUBILITY AND DISPERSION

Mechanical force is used also for providing functionally to cosmetics by dispersing efficiently low-solubility ingredients.

1. Products that have the effects of whitening or anti-aging are increasing. Using a microfluidizer, the amount of oil-phase dissolving and dispersing ceramides, which are an active ingredient, is increased. It is said that osmosis of such an ingredient in a keratin layer becomes easy.

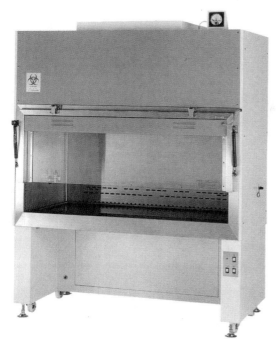

Figure 5 Schematic diagram of bench used for installing filling machine (2).

2. Dissolving and dispersing low-solubility materials alternatively to the inside or outside of emulsion can increase the effect of an active ingredient. Furthermore, regarding improvement of osmosis to a keratin layer, it can be attained by fine particle emulsification with powerful mechanical force such as those provided by a microfludizer.
3. By distributing a lecithin with the microfluidizer, liposomes are made, thereby controlling the release speed of the active ingredients.
4. A microfluidizer is used also for dispersion of a kind of cellulose as a base material (3).
5. In order to heighten the ultaviolet ray prevention effect, the microfluidizer is used to enable distribution and stabilization of ultra-fine particles of titanium oxide.
6. A microfluidizer is used also for manufacturing organic solvent-free consmetics such as makeup cosmetics.

It is expected that the use of new materials and the effective use of active ingredients will increase with increased application of mechanical forces.

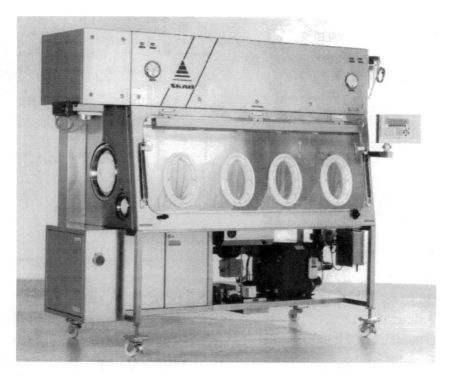

Figure 6 Schematic diagram of isolator used for installing filling machine (4).

APPLICATION FOR IMPROVEMENT IN USABILITY AND FEELING

Although a product present inside will not come out even if a container is toppled, it can be arranged that a milky lotion may come out when the container is shaken.

Products whose qualities are completely different, using the same formulation, can also be manufactured by changing the equipment and process used. For example, a milky lotion can be manufactured using the formulation of a cream by cutting out the high molecule materials using powerful mechanical forces or by destroying structural viscosity.

SCALE-UP

When the amount of emulsifier is decreased or materials of weak emulsification power are used more often in formulation, and because the manufacturing process is becoming more complicated, scale-up is difficult. It is not for the equipment maker to decide the scale-up in terms of motor horsepower and

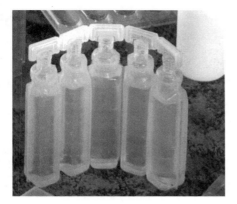

Figure 7 Schematic diagram of blow fill seal filling equipment.

the size of agitator, but rather for the user to scale up the equipment to make the quality of the sample at the laboratory and the factory product similar, by deciding upon the operating conditions of the equipment. The tendency to decrease the amount of an emulsifier is strong and mechanical force is important in scale-up. Moreover, it is important to decide the evaluation method for the effects of a scale-up and the desired value, especially in the validation of medical supplies.

The important points for scale-up are as follows:

1. formulation power cannot be changed in a scale-up,
2. depending on the purpose, selection of the optimal mechanical force is the most important point,
3. emulsion has thixotropy property, a non-Newtonian viscosity property. Then, it becomes important that path clearance is small; if path clearance of a test machine and a production machine is made the same, in order to acquire the same shearing force, it will be effective to make the tip-speeds of the agitator equal,
4. by using particle diameter and particle size distribution, it is easy to evaluate scale-up.

CONCLUSION

It is expected that development of manufacturing technology that considers the balance of formulation force and mechanical force will become the main development method for new products. Moreover, the importance of searching for the harmonization of formulation, materials, manufacturing process, and production equipment is also increasing.

REFERENCES

1. Maeyama K, Tsujide M, Ueda S, Kato T. Characterization of cosmetic colloidal dispersion of plate-shaped inorganic compounds prepared by the use of an ultahigh-pressure homogenizer. J Soc Cosmet Chem Jpn 1995; 29(3):234–241.
2. The clean bench catalog of Yuyama Company.
3. Ono H. New cellulose material; structure and properties of transparent cellulose gel (TCG). Cellulose 1999; 6(2):101–105.
4. The isolator catalog of Bosch Company.

The Industry View

36

Cosmeceuticals or Not? The Industry View: Europe

C. Bouillon
R&D, Cosmetic Scientist and Senior R&D Consultant, Soisy-sous-Montmorency, France

European Union	617
USA	618
Advances in the Science of Skin and Cosmetic Care	619
References	622

Before discussing the need for creating or managing a room for a category of in-between products which cannot enter either within cosmetics or within the scope of drugs, it seems reasonable as a first approach to give consideration to the present frame and scope of cosmetics vs. drugs.

We cannot but acknowledge that opposing cosmetics and drugs is quite a common attitude in most countries for various reasons: cultural, regulatory, scientific, or on the basis of background, lobby groups, or time serving. Most of the time, the prevailing attitude, even if discreet or unexpressed, is to distinguish between what is, in short, viewed as frivolous, superfluous, inactive and even artificial and what is brought forward as essential, scientifically formulated, medically tested, effective, and highly beneficial to health.

The aesthetics of appearance as opposed to the science of medical care. Beauty aids as opposed to health concern.

However, surprisingly enough, when the question of controlling or registering cosmetic products is at stake, the trend is generally to apply or rely on rules and procedures inspired by the drug approach. Experts in charge of drug control mostly are not trained to grasp the very nature of a cosmetic product. Drug is the reference despite irrelevance.

Cosmetics have indeed nothing to do with drugs. By their nature, composition, related specifications, and concept, cosmetics are clearly distinct from drugs.

A drug is identified by its *active ingredient*, potential side effects of which have been cataloged and for which a risk/benefit ratio has been established, which means that a certain number of untoward effects which might even be severe and a certain number of toxic effects which might have negative repercussions on the body's organs and on the individual's health in general are considered an acceptable risk in view of the potential therapeutic benefits of alleviating the disorder for which the drug is indicated.

All medicines present a risk, which has to be outweighed by the potential benefit. In contrast, cosmetics must present a minimal risk.

A drug implies a number of questions to be addressed and satisfied:

- dosage regimen
- usage restrictions and cautions
- warnings on contraindications
- supervision exercised by the dispensing pharmacist
- quite often the requirement for medical prescription.

A drug is generally designed for a target population in which a certain level of associated risk is acceptable as long as the therapeutic effects are substantial. In contrast, a cosmetic product is mostly designed for a very large, diverse population of users and it should present optimal skin compatibility.

By concept and composition, the cosmetic and drug are characterized by rather opposite designs.

A drug product is an active ingredient in a usually simple vehicle. Everything is directed, concentrated, and focused on the active ingredient (toxicity, dosage, purity, quality control, hygiene inspections, drug monitoring, etc.).

Cosmetics have no relationship with the concept of a drug. Unlike a drug, a cosmetic product is not a simple active ingredient in an inert vehicle. It is a multifunctional complex formulation involving numerous ingredients that contribute toward the overall effect which encompasses a comfortable feel, pleasure upon use, high compatibility with the skin or mucous membrane to which it is applied, delightful texture, gentle perfume, and so on.

With ingredients which contribute to stability, preservation from microbial contamination, and maintenance of the characteristics of the composition over time, it is not uncommon to find 20–30 constituents, or more, in the formulation of a cosmetic product.

Whereas pharmacy is the science of the active ingredient, cosmetology is the complex science of combinations.

As a consequence, cosmetic products and claims should not be viewed with the rationale, the concept, the approach, and the rules and assessment procedures which are applied to drugs. They need *specific consideration, specific evaluation, and specific education and expertise.*

The efficacy of a cosmetic product is not dictated or conferred by a single active ingredient. It is the combined result of a variety of ingredients selected for the contribution they can provide to overall quality and their compatibility with all the other ingredients, which, together, build up to make a product appreciated for its sensory attributes and for its ability to withstand impairment or contamination upon use.

Unlike the case of drugs, it makes no sense to seek to define very precisely what is due to one particular ingredient or another, one concentration or another, given the actual construction of a cosmetic product. It is worked out for optimal synergy to provide at the same time, both pleasure and beneficial effects.

These considerations are also of prime importance in the management of "clinical" studies to evaluate the effects of a cosmetic product. By its very nature, it does not lend itself to the procedures for evaluation of a drug, and such procedures would not yield the information sought.

However, it has to be kept in mind that testing procedures for drugs were developed with the aim of proving the absolute efficacy of the active ingredient, while eliminating all the other factors which could contribute to the overall efficacy. For a dermatological product, the contribution of an adequate vehicle is well known. The trial is carried out on patients selected based on criteria characterizing the targeted disorder or disease, hence very far from a normal condition. In other words, the goal is to test an active ingredient, specifically targeting a disease in patients specifically affected by the disease, that is, those most likely to exhibit a positive response. Despite such ideal conditions, the vehicle effect in dermatology is usually at least 60% and sometimes as high as 80%. Therefore, it is necessary to test under double-blind conditions against the vehicle to demonstrate the efficacy of the active ingredient itself.

However, it is evident that applying the same testing procedure to a cosmetic, for which any ingredient is part of the perceived activity, is absurd. For a cosmetic product, a placebo does not exist. The efficacy of a cosmetic product can only be viably tested in comparison to nothing or to a benchmark cosmetic product with similar claims. Now the issue is "Do regulations adequately recognize that drug and cosmetics are poles apart and need a different evaluation process"?

EUROPEAN UNION

It has to be emphasized that EU cosmetics regulation (1) recognized at an early stage that the peculiar role and composition of cosmetic products needed a unique status and specific, proper provisions.

First and paramount is the definition of a cosmetic product as stated in Article 1 of related regulation, which is appended with an open representative list of products. Merely representative, because there are no limits to the creativity of cosmeticians. The future cannot be restricted to today's vision and scope.

The European definition firstly indicates the targets of cosmetic products. They are exclusively applied to skin and its appendages, which include hair, nails, eyebrows, teeth, and so on. It clearly restricts the route and the scope when compared with a drug. Administration, inhalation, injection, and so on are clearly excluded, as opposed to drugs. Moreover, cosmetics do not address diseases or pathological conditions, which are the territory and targets of drugs. The EU drug definition unambiguously, makes the distinction.

A major provision of EU definition of cosmetics is the functions ascribed to it, which has to be continuously emphasized and reminded. Apart from cleansing, perfuming, and correcting body odors, pivotal functions are "change the appearance" and "protect and keep in good condition", which implies that skin should also be given appropriate care to recover when its condition is impaired albeit nonpathological.

Second, Article 2 clearly establishes the responsibility of the manufacturer and/or marketer, while further differentiating from drugs, on the basis of the absence of potential harmfulness for human health under normal and foreseeable conditions of use.

Another crucial aspect of EU regulation is the Committee for Adaptation to Technical Progress (CATP) procedure which ensures permanent consideration is given to scientific and technological advances and account taken of them in updating provisions (7 amendments and 30 adaptations to technical progress since 1976). This process is illustrative of a regulation that is not stuck to outdated knowledge in contrast to some countries like USA whose regulation for cosmetics is still anchored to the situation in 1938.

USA

As a first and major feature, it should be reminded that US regulation (1) does not specifically address cosmetic products. By long-standing statute, the world of topicals is divided into two distinct groups: drugs and cosmetics. Stated simply, a topical product is a drug when it is used to prevent or to treat a disease. On the other hand, cosmetics are used for beautification and enhancement of appearance. The separation seems to be neat and simple. However, in contrast with EU regulation, not only does the FDA definition ignore the major role of "protection" and "keeping in good condition" of cosmetic products, but it also provides for a legal structure which thoroughly confounds the issue, namely that a cosmetic must "not affect the structure and function of skin", which is "the territory of a drug". As a consequence, cosmetics should never be applied or spread using a finger; skin care products should be applied at a distance in order to avoid any risk of affecting the cutaneous structure and functions even by ultra-mild massage. All scientists dealing with the skin know that lightly touching the skin instantly induce a physiological response including messages sent to the brain and systemic effects or reactions as a result, which are hardly comparable with local effects of cosmetics.

Another point of US regulation turns anyone from confused to disconcerted or taken aback, when reading the statement that the same product may be either a cosmetic or a drug or both. The deciding factor is the claim or the interpretation of the claim. In other words, it is not the ingredients in a product but the claims in labeling or advertising that determine whether the product will be classified as a cosmetic or a drug.

As an example, a new UV filter may be used in a cosmetic product as long as no claims are made about its protective effects as a sunscreen even if substantiated. Such claims are deemed to be drug claims and require to go through a highly unpredictable process of application to get the filter approved (only one approved in 25 years).

The inadequacy of such a regulation frame is that it dates back to 1938. In addition, it is still running as if nothing had happened in science and technology since that time. Albert Kligman, a worldwide reputed, prominent American professor of dermatology, has repeatedly denounced the inadequacy of a regulation that denied a cosmetic skin care product might have any effect on the physiology of the skin (2). All scientists in the field of dermatology, skin physiology, and cosmetology know that it is impossible to think of a single substance that when applied to the skin does not, under some circumstances, alter the structure and function of the skin. No topical is completely inert, including water.

The science of normal skin and its care was primitive in 1938. Cosmetic science was simply non-existent. Even the biology of diseased skin was ignored. Skin diseases were known only by the clinical description of symptoms associated with. Most knowledge in skin biology has been acquired in the last 30 years. It has been progressing at an ever growing speed in recent years, as has cosmetic technology.

ADVANCES IN THE SCIENCE OF SKIN AND COSMETIC CARE

What have we learnt about normal skin since 1938? A two-day course would be hardly enough to overview the diversity of advances in the biology of the skin since that time. One of the most significant breakthroughs for cosmeticians and for skin care has been the progressive awareness of the very role of the horny layer or stratum corneum (3). The outermost compartment of the epidermis has long been thought of as a dead, desquamating part of the skin. We all know nowadays that the so-called horny layer whose thickness averages not more than one hundredth of a millimeter (except on the palms) plays a paramount role both as a barrier to potentially harmful exogenous, environmental factors and in the control of homeostasis, of which timely renewal of epidermis is an essential part.

The skin is a dynamic organ, continuously renewed to cope with exposure to the various stimuli of daily life and to adapt to any change in its environment (cold, warmth, dryness, etc.). The uppermost layers communicate down to basal layer. The basal epidermis is stimulated for renewal and interacts with the dermis for proactive co-operation by feedback mechanisms.

These findings have stimulated basic research and raised enormous interest among cosmetic scientists who consider the stratum corneum as the familiar, prevailing site of action of their products. These findings have thoroughly demonstrated the reality of the benefits provided by cosmetic products to achieve healthy renewal and cohesiveness.

A major factor learnt from skin science is that maintaining the stratum corneum in an optimal condition is pivotal in the prevention of the premature aging imprinted on exposed areas of the skin.

The primary requisite to retard or prevent or minimize the appearance of symptoms of aging is to provide appropriate daily care and protection. The primary need for the skin to fight against aging or wrinkling is to have available all the equipment, nutrients, and potential to face daily environmental factors that may weaken it and contribute to premature aging.

Moreover, when skin is wrinkled or shows symptoms of aging, it means it is weakened and woundable, more prone to impairment and disorganization, more prone to deeper, and irreversible weakening with less potential to face, resist, or scavenge the factors which induce aging.

Numerous basic studies have taught us that skin must be protected from oxidative stress triggered daily by UVA, from acute, deleterious effects of UVB photons at peak sunshine hours, from pollution, dry air, and so on. In addition, the stratum corneum has to provide an optimally effective barrier function which requires an optimal architecture of bound water, lipid organization, and protein network.

There are different ways to help restore skin functions, optimal moisturization, and normal condition; to promote strength, tonicity, and cohesiveness; to assure the healthy renewal of the epidermis and active monitoring of environmental changes. This is usually the role of cosmetics. They are cosmetics, which means they comply with the requirements of not being potentially harmful to human health in normal or reasonably foreseeable conditions of use, of containing no ingredients forbidden in cosmetic products or ingredients failing to meet the conditions laid down for safe use in cosmetic products.

However, there is also the well-known example of a drug which is used for cosmetic purposes (retinoic acid) whose efficacy in reducing wrinkles has been demonstrated but whose side effects are also well-known and justify drug status [>90% of more or less severe reactions reported in a peer-reviewed study (4)].

This incidental example raised the opportunity to create an additional category designed to embrace so-called "active cosmetics" (which would suggest that other cosmetics should fall within the register of inactive consumer products).

Japanese regulation (1) has established a subtle discrimination of cosmetics into two categories which segregates a major part of cosmetics as so-called "quasi-drugs" based on obscure, odd-sounded reasons. Thus, the "quasi-drug" category jumbles a variety of types of product including hair coloring products, hair perming and relaxing, bath preparations, depilatories, products for combating dandruff, itching, hair loss, body odors, products for smoothing the roughness of the skin, for keeping the skin healthy, preventing dry skin, providing sun protection, and most innovative skin care preparations among others. The rationale of such a classification looks groundless and lacks consistency.

As in other countries enacting similar approach, it reflects an ancient view on skin biology and cosmetics, out of touch with the physiological reality. We now know from a Japanese paper (5) and from increasing reports that even applying make-up products results in biological benefits that may be profound and well beyond what might be expected. They may influence immune, nerve, and endocrine functions all at once just by improving self-esteem and reducing stress.

Because we know more about the effects of cosmetics, the question is whether they should be parceled out into cosmeceuticals or quasi-drugs or some other coinage. However, the issue is to get regulations that address the whole reality of cosmetics appropriately.

In the context of the American regulations, whereby a cosmetic is still supposed to not affect skin physiology and solely inactively improve its appearance; this proposal was spread by Albert Kligman (2), who is worldwide known for his pugnacity in the face of obscurantism. It was spread as a way to compensate for obsolete regulation. In the context of the European regulations and ongoing harmonization process in most countries of the world where cosmetics are assumed, expected, demanded, and used to maintain the skin in good condition and to have no toxic effects, such a proposal would only create a category of products for which a certain degree of toxicity could be acceptable in view of some cosmetic benefits expected. It seems there is a general agreement for rejecting such a speculative, disturbing, gray area.

In conclusion, I would place the emphasis again on what we have learnt from science and expertise as guidance for our way forward in the third millennium.

Progress in science never stops: as in other fields of science, cosmetology is continuously advancing and discovering new technologies and new benefits of cosmetic products for skin and consumers. Boundaries between cosmetics and drugs are prone to evolve unpredictably as our understanding is enlarged. However, the safety in use is the definitive threshold.

Such a context makes the idea of a third category groundless, raising many questions and providing nothing but confusion and muddle.

Cosmetic products address superficial but essential functions with deep echoes and active signaling that may stimulate the skin at all levels to regain its optimal qualities. Any cosmetic ingredient has an effect on the biology of the skin. Any embellishing product may significantly influence the functions of the body by the positive image reflected which makes feel and experience the life differently.

Stating that a cosmetic product should not elicit any physiological effect is denying basic evidence in the same way as Galileo was forced, by the obscurantism of his time, to admit that the Earth did not revolve around the Sun. It is like ignoring the Internet.

The toxic potential makes the drug: as stated by EU Cosmetic Regulations, a cosmetic product should not be harmful to human health under normal conditions of use.

Unlike drugs, cosmetics are not concerned with fine-tuning a benefit/risk ratio and defining the category(ies) of individuals at potential risk.

Aging is the problem of exposed areas of the skin, such as the face, aging far earlier than never exposed sites of the body. Environmental factors are determinants. As a consequence, the fight against the effects of aging is a major everyday role and function ascribed to cosmetics.

Maintaining skin and hair in good condition is a key task for and a prime requisite from cosmetics. It is the prime requisite for beauty, combating aging, facing daily environmental stress, maintaining the skin (and hair) at its best, affording the potential for optimal defense, and promoting homeostasis (adaptability). These are not the business of a drug.

Cosmetics have much to offer the future. Through the pleasure, comfort, and care they provide, cosmetics make a very real contribution to the quality of life, self-image, social integration, and definitely contribute to health as defined by WHO: "physical, mental, and social well-being". It is to the merit of research in cosmetology that the true effects of cosmetics have been measured and substantiated, although their record of safety today far exceeds that of food products and continues to do so.

REFERENCES

1. Pierrard-Meillon D. Regulation of cosmetic products. In: Bouillon C, Wilkinson JD, eds. The Science of Hair Care. New York: Marcel Dekker, 2005 (Chapter 13).
2. Kligman AM, Maibach HI. Why Cosmeceuticals? A dermatological view. Cosmet Toiletries 1993; 108(8):37.
3. Jass AE, Elias JP. The living Stratum Corneum: implications for cosmetic formulation. Cosmet Toiletries 1991; 106:47.
4. Weiss JS, Ellis CN, Headington JH, Tincoff T, Hamilton TA, Voorhees JJ. Topical tretinoin improves photoaged skin. JAMA 1986; 259:529–532.
5. Kan C, Kumura S. Psychoneuroimmunological benefits of cosmetics. Proceedings IFSCC Congress, Venezia, 1994.

Regulatory

37

Legal Distinction in USA between Cosmetic and Drug

Peter Barton Hutt
Covington & Burling, Washington, DC, USA

Historical Overview	626
Legislative History of the Cosmetic and Drug Provisions of the 1938 Act	627
Implementation of the FD&C Act	629
Initial FDA Action under the FD&C Act	630
Wrinkle Remover Cases of the 1960s	631
OTC Drug Review	632
Warning Letters of the Late 1980s	633
The Alpha-Hydroxy Acid (AHA) Products of the 1990s	635
Use of Foreign Marketing Experience	635
Rationale of the Tobacco Initiative	637
Labeling and Manufacturing Difficulties for Cosmetic Drugs	638
Budgetary Impact on the FDA	638
Potential Future Approaches	639
Conclusion	640
References	640

The Federal Food, Drug, and Cosmetic Act (FD&C Act) establishes substantially different regulatory requirements in USA for cosmetics and drugs. This chapter traces the history of US regulatory policy for these two categories of products, discusses the application of US law to products that fall within both categories at the same time (i.e., cosmetic drugs*), and considers potential strategies for resolving the long-standing concern that the drug provisions of the Act impose overly stringent requirements on cosmetic drugs.

HISTORICAL OVERVIEW

Cosmetic products have been used by humans since before recorded history. Archeologists date the earliest discovered cosmetics to about 10,000 BC (1). By the height of the ancient Roman civilization, virtually all types of cosmetics that are available today were in widespread use. In his landmark *Natural History*, Pliny, the Elder (23–79 AD), described such cosmetic products as hair dye, eyelash dye, eyebrow dye, freckle removers, rouge, deodorants and antiperspirants, depilatories, wrinkle removers, hair preservatives and restorers, bust firmers, sunburn products, complexion aids, moisturizers, mouthwashes and breath fresheners, toothpaste, face powder, and perfume (2). Cosmetics have continued to be widely used from these ancient times to the present.

During the 19th century, virtually all government regulation of private enterprise in USA was conducted at the city, county, and state levels. Because of the Supreme Court's narrow interpretation of the power of the federal government to regulate interstate commerce, federal laws regulating consumer products did not emerge until the decade of the 20th century. Thus, the first laws explicitly regulating cosmetics were enacted by the states. The earliest known state regulatory law explicitly mentioning cosmetics was enacted by Massachusetts in 1886. This law included all cosmetics within the statutory definition of a drug, thus imposing the same regulatory requirements on both cosmetics and drugs (3).

From 1879 through 1906, Congress held hearings and debated the enactment of a federal food and drug law (4). Although bills introduced in Congress during 1898–1900 explicitly defined the term "drug" to include all cosmetics (5), the inclusion of cosmetics was deleted from the drug definition in 1900 as part of a legislative compromise (6). As a result, cosmetics were not included when the legislation was finally enacted as the Federal Food and Drugs Act of 1906 (7).

Implementation of the 1906 Act was delegated by Congress to the US Department of Agriculture (USDA). Subsequently, it was redelegated to the Federal Security Agency (FSA), then to the Department of Health, Education, and Welfare (DHEW), and now to the Department of Health and Human Services (DHHS). Since 1930, the specific agency responsible for the 1906 Act and its successor statute, the Federal Food, Drug, and Cosmetic Act (FD&C Act) of

---

*The term "cosmeceutical" has no legal or regulatory meaning and no other accepted definition, and is therefore not used in this chapter.

1938 (8) has been the Food and Drug Administration (FDA) (9). For editorial purposes, throughout this chapter, all references to the agencies and departments responsible for implementing federal food and drug laws shall be to the FDA.

Not long after enactment of the 1906 Act, FDA concluded that its jurisdiction should be expanded to include both cosmetics and medical devices (10). When the Roosevelt Administration introduced a bill to replace the 1906 Act (11), cosmetics were included (12) through a separate definition and separate regulatory requirements. Although the provisions relating to cosmetics were revised periodically during the 5 years of congressional consideration, the separate definition and separate regulatory requirements were retained in the final FD&C Act when it was enacted 1938 (9). In the intervening 66 years, these provisions have not been amended.

LEGISLATIVE HISTORY OF THE COSMETIC AND DRUG PROVISIONS OF THE 1938 ACT

The 1906 Act (13) had defined a drug to include:

> ... all medicine and preparations recognized in United States Pharmacopoeia or National Formulary for internal or external use, and any substance or mixture of substances intended to be used for the cure, mitigation, or prevention of disease of either man or other animals.
>
> Stat. (1906)

From the time that the legislation that ultimately became the FD&C Act was initially introduced until it was finally enacted, substantial attention was focused on the specific definitions of food, drug, and cosmetic, and the interaction among these three definitions. Out of these deliberations, the following important principles and policies emerged.

First, the 1938 Act, like the 1906 Act, classified products according to their intended use. In a paragraph from the 1935 Senate Report (14) on the legislation, Congress established the policy that the representations of the sellers with respect to a product would determine its classification:

> The use to which the product is to be put will determine the category into which it will fall. If it is to be used only as food it will come within the definition of food and none other. If it contains nutritive ingredients but is sold for drug use only, as clearly shown by the labeling and advertising, it will come within the definition of drug, but not that of food. If it is sold to be used both as a food and for the prevention or treatment of disease it would satisfy both definitions and be subject to the substantive requirements for both. The manufacturer of the article, through his representations in connection with its sale, can determine the use to which the article is to be put. For example, the manufacturer of a laxative which is a medicated candy or chewing gum can bring his product

within the definition of drug and escape that of food by representing the article fairly and unequivocally as a drug product.

S. Rep. No. 361 (1935)

This principle remains the touchstone for product classification under the 1938 Act.

Second, from the outset, the FDA sought to expand the definition of a drug from the narrow definition included in the 1906 Act. The 1906 Act limited the drug definition to products intended to prevent or treat disease. The FDA was concerned that, although it was able to regulate food products represented for use in weight reduction, it could not exert jurisdiction over nonfood chemicals represented for the same purpose because obesity was not regarded as a disease. Accordingly, from the initial bill to the final law, the drug definition was expanded to include articles "intended to affect the structure or any function of the body of man or other animals" (15).

Third, Congress determined that the definitions of food, drug, and cosmetic should not be mutually exclusive. Because the representations made for the product would determine the proper classification of the product, and thus classification was within the sole control of the seller, Congress concluded that the product should be subject to whatever statutory requirements are established for whatever product classifications applied, on the basis of those representations (14):

> It has not been considered necessary to specify that the definitions of food, drug, and cosmetic shall not be construed, other than to the extent expressly provided, as mutually exclusive. The present law does not have such a clause relating to the definitions of food and drug and there has never been a court decision to the effect that these definitions are mutually exclusive, despite the fact that repeated actions have been brought, for example, against filthy foods bearing unwarranted therapeutic claims, alleging these products to be adulterated as food because of their filth, and misbranded as drugs because of their false and fraudulent therapeutic claims.
>
> S. Rep. No. 361 (1935)

Thus, dual and even triple classifications of a product as a food, drug, and cosmetic was contemplated by Congress under the 1938 Act.

Congress realized that there must be one exception to the general rule of nonexclusive definitions. All food is intended to affect the structure or function of the human body. Accordingly, Congress explicitly excluded food from the structure/function prong of the drug definition, but not from the disease prong.

In the Senate debate on the legislation in April 1935, the exclusion of food from the structure/function prong of the drug definition was expanded, without discussion, to include cosmetics (16). However, that bill was not passed by the House of Representatives, and no subsequent legislation retained the cosmetic

Legal Distinction between Cosmetic and Drug

exclusion. Accordingly, any cosmetic represented to affect the structure or function of the human body is classified as a drug as well as a cosmetic and must meet the statutory requirements for both categories of products.

Finally, Congress also included in the 1938 Act, as it had in the 1906 Act, a third prong of the drug definition to include articles recognized in specified pharmacopeias. However, this was intended to include pharmacopeial articles only when they are in fact represented for disease or structure/function purposes (17). Accordingly, this prong of the definition may be excluded from further consideration in this chapter.

With these principles and policies established, Congress enacted the FD&C Act in 1938 with the following two pertinent definitions. A drug was defined in section 201(g) to mean:

> ... (1) articles recognized in the official United States Pharmacopeia, official Homeopathic Pharmacopeia of the United States, or official National Formulary, or any supplement to any of them; (2) articles intended for use in the diagnosis, cure, mitigation, treatment, or prevention of disease in man or other animals; and (3) articles (other than food) intended to affect the structure or any function of the body of man or other animals ...

A cosmetic was defined in section 201(i) to mean:

> ... articles intended to be rubbed, poured, sprinkled, or sprayed on, introduced into, or otherwise applied to the human body or any part thereof for cleansing, beautifying, promoting attractiveness, or altering the appearance ...

Parts of the drug definition not pertinent here have been revised since 1938, but the central core of the definition has not been altered. No part of the cosmetic definition has been changed. Thus, the controlling definitions have remained in place for the entire 66 year history of the FD&C Act.

IMPLEMENTATION OF THE FD&C ACT

The regulatory consequences of classifying a product as a drug rather than as a cosmetic are substantial. A drug will almost invariably be determined by the FDA to be a "new drug" that requires substantial preclinical toxicological testing, clinical testing under an investigational new drug (IND) application, submission of a new drug application (NDA) requesting FDA approval, and ultimately marketing under substantial FDA postapproval requirements, including drug good manufacturing practices (GMP) regulations (18). New drugs typically require a decade or more for research and development prior to FDA approval and require the investment of hundreds of millions of dollars. In short, it is only the very rare cosmetic product that could justify this level of investment.

It is therefore essential that cosmetic products be formulated and labeled in such a way as to avoid the drug definition.

Initial FDA Action under the FD&C Act

FDA scientists recognized very early that all cosmetics penetrate the skin and thus inherently affect the structure or function of the body (19):

> ... there are few if any substances which are not absorbed through the intact skin, even though the idea is prevalent that the skin is a relatively effective barrier to its environment.
>
> Calvery (1944)

Nonetheless, the FDA recognized that Congress fully intended a separate category of cosmetic products regardless of their inherent effect on the structure or function of the body, as long as no structure/function or disease claims were made for them.

The FDA sought to establish policy on the distinction between a cosmetic and a drug in three ways. First, FDA issued formal trade correspondence that set forth advisory opinions on the classification of products. Second, the agency published pamphlets and other educational materials with examples of product classification. Third, it brought court action to contest the legality of cosmetic products with labeling that contained what the agency concluded to be drug claims. From this body of literature and precedent have emerged, over six decades, a number of well-developed examples:

> A suntan product is a cosmetic, but a sunscreen product is a drug.
> A deodorant is a cosmetic, but an antiperspirant is a drug.
> A shampoo is a cosmetic, but an antidandruff shampoo is a drug.
> A toothpaste is a cosmetic, but an anticaries toothpaste is a drug.
> A skin exfoliant is a cosmetic, but a skin peel is a drug.
> A mouthwash is a cosmetic, but an antigingivitis mouthwash is a drug.
> A hair bulking product is a cosmetic, but a hair growth product is a drug.
> A skin product to hide acne is a cosmetic, but an antiacne product is a drug.
> An antibacterial deodorant soap is a cosmetic, but an antibacterial anti-infective soap is a drug.
> A skin moisturizer is a cosmetic, but a wrinkle remover is a drug.
> A lip softener is a cosmetic, but a product for chapped lips is a drug.

This list is illustrative and not exhaustive.

Products that are represented only to change the structure or function of the hair or nails are regarded as cosmetics and not drugs. For example, permanent waves and cuticle removers are cosmetics and not drugs (20). On the other hand, products that are represented to affect the hair or nails systemically are regarded as drugs.

Legal Distinction between Cosmetic and Drug

Cosmetic products represented as "hypoallergenic", and thus with reduced allergic potential, remain classified as cosmetics and not as drugs (21). If these products are represented to treat specific reactions or diseases, they would be classified as drugs.

Inclusion of an active ingredient in a cosmetic does not automatically classify it as a drug, unless the active ingredient is so closely identified with therapeutic properties that the mere use of the term would connote a drug claim. For example, use of the term "penicillin" or "AZT" would preclude classification of the product solely as a cosmetic because of their well-recognized therapeutic purposes (22). However, in many instances, ingredients can be used in both cosmetic and drug products. When the FDA banned all topical nonprescription drug products containing hormones, the agency stated that cosmetics could continue to contain hormones without becoming drugs if the chemical name of the specific hormone was included in the ingredient statement and the word "hormone" was not used in the labeling or advertising (23).

In many instances, the context of a word or phrase must be considered before a determination can be made about proper classification of the product as a drug or cosmetic. A product represented as a treatment for disease is a drug, but a product represented as a beauty treatment is a cosmetic. A product represented to kill germs that cause infection is a drug, but a product represented to kill germs that cause odor is a cosmetic.

These examples illustrate the difficulty in drawing a clear and definitive distinction between these two categories of products. Nonetheless, these distinctions have come to be understood by both FDA and industry, and serve the extremely useful purpose of guiding decisions in this area.

Wrinkle Remover Cases of the 1960s

In the early 1960s, the cosmetic industry developed a line of products, broadly characterized as "wrinkle remover" products, containing ingredients intended to smooth, firm, and tighten the skin temporarily and thus to make wrinkles less obvious. In 1964, the FDA seized several of these products, alleging that they were drugs under the FD&C Act. The resulting litigation produced three decisions by US District Courts and two decisions by US Courts of Appeals involving three products: Line Away, Sudden Change, and Magic Secret.

The District Court in the Line Away case took the position that, by intending to smooth and tighten the skin, Line Away had as its objective affecting the structure of the skin and thus was a drug (24). The Court of Appeals agreed, citing the "strong therapeutic implications" of the promotional material (25).

The District Court in the Sudden Change case concluded that the product was represented merely to alter the appearance of the skin and thus was a cosmetic (26). However, The Court of Appeals reversed the District Court in a split decision. The majority held that the claims that the Sudden Change product would give a "face lift without surgery" and would "lift out puffs" had "physiological connotations" (27). However, the majority went out of its way to state that all of the traditional cosmetic claims (e.g., that a product will soften or moisturize the skin) remain within the cosmetic category. One judge dissented on the ground that the two claims cited by the majority as drug claims were indistinguishable from such cosmetic claims as smooths, firms, tones, and moisturizes the skin.

Finally, the District Court in the Magic Secret case determined that the product was a cosmetic, not a drug, on the basis of the conclusion that the claims were less exaggerated than in the other two cases. The court held that the claim that the product caused an "astringent sensation" would not be regarded by consumers as doing anything other than altering their appearance (28).

By this time, it was apparent to both the FDA and the regulated industry that further litigation would be unproductive. Industry sought to modify its claims in order to bring them within the cosmetic boundaries established by the FDA administrative precedent and the judicial decisions. The FDA concluded to provide any further guidance with respect to the distinction between a drug and a cosmetic through the OTC Drug Review, which was initiated in the early 1970s.

OTC Drug Review

Under the Drug Amendments of 1962 (29), which were enacted following the thalidomide disaster in order to strengthen drug regulation in USA, the FDA was required to review every new drug application (NDA) that had become effective on the basis of an agency safety review between 1938 and 1962 in order to determine whether the drug was effective as well as safe. For prescription drugs, FDA submitted the pre-1962 NDAs for review by the National Academy of Sciences, under the Drug Efficacy Study Implementation (DESI) program. For nonprescription drugs (also called over-the-counter or OTC drugs), the FDA chose a different approach. Under procedures promulgated in 1972 (30), the FDA established advisory committees to review all of the pharmacological categories of OTC drugs and to prepare reports on the safety, effectiveness, and labeling for all existing OTC drugs. The advisory committee reports, together with a proposed monograph, were published in the Federal Register for public comment. After reviewing the public comment, the FDA published its own conclusions together with a tentative final monograph for further public comment. Following its consideration of the second round of public comments, the FDA promulgated a final monograph establishing the conditions for safe and effective use, including required and permitted labeling of the OTC drugs that fall within that drug category. An OTC drug ingredient that was not included in a final monograph could no longer be used as an active ingredient in an OTC drug following the effective date of the final monograph, but could be used as an inactive ingredient or as a cosmetic ingredient.

Legal Distinction between Cosmetic and Drug

The OTC Drug Review inherently raised issues relating to the distinction between a cosmetic and a drug. All of the traditional cosmetic drug products—sunscreens, antiperspirants, antidandruff shampoos, anticaries toothpaste, skin protectants, hormone creams, acne products, and so forth—were reviewed under the OTC Drug Review. The FDA made clear that only the drug and not the cosmetic aspects of cosmetic drugs were subject to review and evaluation, and ultimately a final monograph, under this program. Thus, in many of the advisory committee meetings and subsequent reports (31), as well as in the preambles to the tentative final (32) and final (33) monographs, there has been substantial discussion about the dividing line between a drug claim and a cosmetic claim for a cosmetic drug. In several instances, the FDA has explicitly stated that a final monograph covered only products making drug claims and did not cover cosmetic claims for the product or products making only cosmetic claims.

The distinction between a cosmetic and a drug became important early in the OTC Drug Review process. On the basis of an advisory committee recommendation, FDA published regulations banning three substances as unsafe for use: hexachlorophene (34), TBS (35), and zirconium (36). Recognizing that these substances could properly be used in both drugs and cosmetics, the FDH published parallel regulations to assure that both types of uses would be banned.

For the most part, the OTC Drug Review has proceeded without major controversy with respect to the classification of cosmetic and drug claims. In general, the FDA has followed the traditional cosmetic/drug distinctions described earlier in this chapter. In a few remaining monographs, however, the FDA has proposed to change its policy with respect to important products. It has proposed to reclassify "kills germs that cause odor" from the cosmetic category to drug status (37). It initially proposed to set a limit on cosmetic use of hormone ingredients, above which they would automatically become drugs (38), and then withdrew the proposal on the ground that substantial time had passed since it was proposed and it was no longer a priority (39). Although the FDA had previously stated that suntan products are cosmetics (40), it proposed to reclassify them as drugs, but then retained them as cosmetics (with a required sunburn warning) in the final regulations (41). Industry, in turn, has asked the FDA to classify sunscreen ingredients when used in nonbeach traditional cosmetic formulations as cosmetic ingredients rather than as drugs, in order to encourage the cosmetic industry to include sunscreen ingredients in skin-care products for public health protection wherever feasible, but the FDA rejected this approach.

Warning Letters of the Late 1980s

For a period of 15 years following the conclusion of the wrinkle remover cases, the FDA pursued cosmetic/drug issues largely through the OTC Drug Review and seldom, if ever, through Regulatory or Warning Letters or direct court action. On the basis of new product technology and the conclusion that the consuming public was becoming increasingly sophisticated about skin-care products and their claims, the cosmetic industry gradually became more aggressive with cell rejuvenation and other antiaging promotional claims. As a result of research and development in the intervening years, new and more effective products were now on the market.

Two defining events served to initiate a new round of FDA enforcement activities against skin-care claims in the late 1980s (42). First, in 1986 the well-known South African heart surgeon, Christiaan Barnard, made a tour of USA on behalf of a cosmetic company to promote its skin-care product, Glycel. Barnard made extravagant claims for Glycel on the television program, Nightline, with FDA Commissioner Frank Young participating on the same program. Second, an attorney for a major cosmetic company wrote Dr. Young to protest the claims being made for Glycel. As a result, the FDA began to issue Regulatory Letters not only to the manufacturer of Glycel, but also to other leading members of the industry (43). More than 20 Regulatory Letters were sent in the first wave, and when the FDA concluded that the response was unsatisfactory the agency sent another 20. Complex negotiations ensued among the FDA, individual companies, and a consortium of companies. The FDA established the agency position on the matter with a letter from the FDA Associate Commissioner for Regulatory Affairs, John Taylor (44):

> We consider a claim that a product will affect the body in some physiological way to be a drug claim, even if the claim is that the effect is only temporary. Such a claim constitutes a representation that the product is intended to affect the structure or function of the body and thus makes the product a drug under 21 U.S.C. 321(g)(1)(C). Therefore, we consider most of the anti-aging and skin physiology claims that you outline in your letter to be drug claims. For example, claims that a product "counteracts", "retards", or "controls" aging or the aging process, as well as claims that a product will "rejuvenate", "repair", or "renew" the skin, are drug claims because they can be fairly understood as claims that a function of the body, or that the structure of the body, will be affected by the product. For this reason also, all of the examples that you use to allege an effect within the epidermis as the basis for a temporary beneficial effect on wrinkles, lines, or fine lines are unacceptable A claim such as "molecules absorb" ... and expand, exerting upward pressure to "lift" wrinkles "upward" is a claim for an inner, structural change.
>
> John M. Taylor (1987)

The Associate Commissioner did offer some guidelines for cosmetic claims:

> While we agree with your statements that wrinkles will not be reversed or removed by these products ... we would not object to claims that products will temporarily improve the appearance of such outward signs of aging. The label of such products should state that the product is intended to cover up the signs of aging, to improve the appearance by

Legal Distinction between Cosmetic and Drug

adding color or a luster to skin, or otherwise to affect the appearance through physical means . . .

However, we would consider a product that claims to improve or to maintain temporarily the appearance or the feel of the skin to be a cosmetic. For example, a product that claims to moisturize or soften the skin is a cosmetic.

Following the FDA letter, one company brought court action to obtain a declaratory judgment that its product was a cosmetic rather than a drug, but the court ruled that a Regulatory Letter could not be contested in this way, and the issue remained unresolved (45). Individual companies eventually worked out their issues with the FDA and thus the agency was not required to bring formal court action against even one product.

The Alpha-Hydroxy Acid (AHA) Products of the 1990s

In the early 1990s, the cosmetic industry developed and marketed a line of products containing alpha-hydroxy acids such as glycolic, lactic, and citric acid that occurred in natural food products to cleanse dead cells from the surface of the skin and assist moisturization. The AHAs have been used in consumer products at relatively modest levels, usually at $\leq 10\%$, in contrast with very high levels used in professional skin peeling products (46). It is universally accepted that the AHA products are the most effective skin-care beauty products that the industry has ever developed. As a result, they have become extremely popular with consumers and gained substantial media and regulatory attention.

The FDA has raised two questions about the AHA products. First, the agency has questioned the claims being made. The FDA has sought to adhere to the guidelines established in the November 1987 letter on the antiaging and cell rejuvenation products. Second, the FDA has also questioned the safety of these products, not on the ground that there are known toxicological concerns but rather on the ground that their safety is unproven. However, in contrast with the cell rejuvenation claims of the 1980s, the FDA has not launched another wave of Warning Letters. A company that had obtained FDA approval of NDAs for antiaging drugs, frustrated by this lack of FDA action, brought a private false advertising case under section 43(a) of the Lanham Act (47) against a competitor making aggressive claims for a cosmetic product, but lost in both the District Court (48) and the Court of Appeals (49).

Use of Foreign Marketing Experience

As mentioned earlier, the cosmetic industry has been forced to stay within the confines of traditional cosmetic claims for skin-care products, which could potentially justify stronger promotion, because the only other alternative is the bottomless pit of the IND/NDA process for drugs. To create a more realistic alternative, the FDA has sought to modify its position on OTC drugs.

When the OTC Drug Review was initiated in 1972, the FDA announced two policies that were designed to confine the scope of the Review. First, the Review included only those products on the market prior to the final procedural regulations, published in June 1972. This date was later extended to December 1975. Second, the Review included only products marketed in USA and excluded those marketed abroad. As a result, it was impossible to market in USA any nonprescription drug that had been sold abroad before the cutoff date or that was developed at any time, anywhere in the world, after the cutoff date.

These two policies were adopted for management, not legal, reasons. The OTC Drug Review was an enormous undertaking, and the FDA concluded that it was essential to establish limitations in order to avoid a perpetual process. Nonetheless, these two policies had a major adverse impact. Some products marketed abroad have important public health benefits. For example, sunscreen products providing protection against both ultraviolet A (UVA) radiation and ultraviolet B (UVB) radiation were available in Europe for at least 15 years before they became available in USA. The FDA refused to bring these products within the OTC Drug Review until it finally relented in 1997 (50). In the interim, US residents were denied important public health protection solely because of this policy.

Recognizing the adverse public health consequence of its policy and in light of a court decision invalidating a parallel policy for food ingredients (51), the FDA has now opened up the OTC Drug Review to include new conditions under the OTC drug monograph system based upon foreign marketing experience (52). The FDA has promulgated a final regulation establishing this policy, but is so narrowly circumscribed that it has only very limited utility.

In the interim, additional pressure is being placed on the FDA to change its policy in order to achieve international harmonization in the regulation of cosmetics and nonprescription drugs. It is difficult, if not impossible, to reconcile the FDA policy that excludes foreign marketing experience with the requirements of the General Agreement of Tariffs and Trade (GATT) (53). The recently enacted Food and Drug Administration Modernization Act of 1997 also requires the FDA to work toward international harmonization and mutual recognition agreements relating to drugs between the European Union and USA (54). The combination of all of these efforts may well produce a more flexible approach toward FDA approval of nonprescription cosmetic drugs.

If the FDA were to recognize foreign marketing experience and engage in international harmonization, the distinction between a cosmetic and a drug in USA could become less crucial. A number of products that are marketed as cosmetic drugs in USA are classified solely as cosmetics in Europe. Cosmetic drugs can also be marketed in Europe with less restrictions than apply in USA. Once a cosmetic drug is on the market in Europe, entry into USA could become easier on the basis of international harmonization and mutual recognition principles.

Rationale of the Tobacco Initiative

In August 1995, the FDA published two notices in the Federal Register relating to the proposed regulation of tobacco (55). The first notice set forth the proposed regulation governing cigarettes. The second notice consisted of an analysis supporting the agency's decision on the matter. Normally, regulation of cigarettes would have little or nothing to do with regulation of cosmetics. However, the rationale provided by the FDA for asserting its jurisdiction over cigarettes, as well as some of the specific discussion in the Federal Register preambles, is of substantial importance to the cosmetic/drug distinction.

As discussed earlier, the FD&C Act provides that a drug includes articles "intended to affect the structure or any function of the body". In its analysis relating to cigarettes, the FDA took the position that the "intent" required under this definition means the "objective" intent of the manufacturer, not the "subjective" intent (i.e., the manufacturer's representation for the product). The FDA contended that "objective" intent requires a "reasonable person" test, and that a manufacturer is charged with the reasonable foreseeability—the natural and foreseeable consequences—of its action. Thus, the FDA asserted that it has authority under the FD&C Act to classify products as drugs, where they inherently result in nontherapeutic but pharmacological effects even though no pharmacological or therapeutic claims are made for the products. The following examples were given by the FDA: topical hormones and sunscreens. However, the FDA analysis stated that courts have distinguished between "remote physical effects" that would not make a product inherently a drug and "significant effects on structure or function" which the agency concluded clearly fall within the drug definition (56).

In its final regulation published in August 1996 (57), the FDA adhered to this position. The FDA categorically rejected the contention that the intended use of a product must be derived solely from the manufacturer's subjective intent (i.e., promotional claims for the product). However, the FDA did reiterate that the structure/function provision would not extend to products that have a "remote physical effect on the body" (58).

The US District Court that reviewed this matter upheld the FDA position on "intended use" (59). However, on appeal, the US Court of Appeals overturned the District Court and declared the FDA regulations unlawful (60). In a divided decision, the majority of the Court of Appeals agreed with the District Court that "no court has ever found that a product is 'intended for use' or 'intended to affect' within the meaning of the [Act] absent manufacturer claims as to that product's use", but then went on to decide the case on completely different grounds. The majority concluded, as a matter of statutory construction, that the FDA has no jurisdiction over tobacco products under the FD&C Act, and thus it was unnecessary to determine the scope of the "intended use" provision in the structure/function prong of the drug definition. The dissenting judge agreed with the FDA interpretation of intended use. The US Supreme Court upheld the Court of Appeals in a 5-4 divided decision (61). The majority did not address the "intended use" issue and the minority agreed with the FDA interpretation.

As a result, we are left with an FDA interpretation, a District Court agreement with that interpretation, two judges on the Court of Appeals who questioned the FDA interpretation but determined it was irrelevant, one judge on the Court of Appeals who also agreed with the FDA interpretation, four Supreme Court justices who agreed with the FDA interpretation, and five Supreme Court justices who determined it was irrelevant. In short, the state of the law remains quite uncertain in this area. However, even if the FDA interpretation were upheld, it would still exclude all cosmetics with structure/function effects that are remote or insignificant.

Since the Supreme Court's decision, FDA has repudiated the extreme interpretation the agency advanced in the Federal Register notices announcing the tobacco initiative. The FDA Chief Counsel has written an opinion stating that the "intended use" of a product is determined by the claims made for the product, not by the foreseeable effects of the product (62). Based on this opinion, FDA reclassified decorative contact lens as cosmetics rather than as medical devices, because they are presented solely for cosmetic purposes (63).

Labeling and Manufacturing Difficulties for Cosmetic Drugs

Compliance with the combined cosmetic and drug provisions of the FD&C Act can be difficult and aggravating. However, FDA regulations have in the past sought to accommodate cosmetic drug labeling requirements (64), and the FDA Modernization Act specifically reconciled the two different approaches to ingredient labeling (65). To the extent that FDA continues to ignore the labeling complexities of cosmetic drugs—as it did, for example, in promulgating the final regulations for nonprescription sunscreen drugs (66) and for the new labeling requirements for all nonprescription drugs (67)—concerns about the dividing line between a cosmetic and a drug will be greatly aggravated. Although the FDA has declined formally to acknowledge different good manufacturing practice standards for cosmetic drugs (68), in practice cosmetic drugs are usually not held to the identical requirements.

Budgetary Impact on the FDA

The ability of the FDA to monitor and bring regulatory action with respect to claims for cosmetic products must take into account the resources available to the agency for this purpose. During the past several years, the FDA has experienced a flat budget. Because of the inexorable impact of inflation, this has been tantamount to a substantial reduction in available resources. At the same time, the FDA has been pursuing its tobacco initiative and a presidential initiative on food safety. As a result of all of these budgetary factors, the FDA announced in 1998 that it was reducing the staff of the Office of Cosmetics and Colors by 50%

Legal Distinction between Cosmetic and Drug 639

and cutting back or eliminating many cosmetic regulatory programs (69). This reduction is so substantial that it propelled the cosmetic industry to request and obtain restoration by Congress of adequate funds to assure that the FDA has a credible cosmetic regulatory program. FDA cosmetic officials are also reaching out to FDA drug officials for co-operation and assistance in discharging their duties.

POTENTIAL FUTURE APPROACHES

For more than 40 years, there has been widespread debate about whether, and how, the current statutory definitions of cosmetic and drug should be changed. Virtually, every option has been considered, from making no change at all to modest or even substantial legislative changes.

Advocates of leaving the statute unchanged contend that, in general, there is already sufficient flexibility in the law to permit valid cosmetic claims and that any attempt to change the legislation might well result in a worse situation rather than a better one. Even the November 1987 FDA guidelines provide industry with a great deal of flexibility. Creative marketing has found a way to convey the benefit of innovative new cosmetic products to consumers, as shown by experience with the AHA products. Thus, there is a little to be gained, and potentially a great deal to be lost, by Congress considering changes in the cosmetic provisions of the FD&C Act that have stood the test of 66 years of experience without a single amendment.

Advocates of moderate change contend that all that would be needed is to insert the two words "and cosmetics" in the parenthetical exclusion that currently exists in the structure/function prong of the drug definition—the approach taken by the Senate in April 1935 (16)—with the result that both food and cosmetics would be excluded from this portion of the definition. This would allow cosmetics to make structure/function claims comparable with the structure/function claims available to dietary supplements and conventional food (70). It would be necessary to obtain clear legislative history that a structure/function claim is not an implied disease claim, as the FDA once contended for food products (15). However, advocates of this minimalist legislative approach acknowledge that they can offer no assurance that Congress would not re-examine other portions of the cosmetic provisions of the FD&C Act and perhaps make additional changes.

Advocates for a more extensive legislative approach offer a wide variety of potential statutory changes. Some advocate creating an entire new category of cosmetic drugs that would have its own separate regulatory requirements and prohibitions, halfway between those for drugs and those for cosmetics. Others argue for imposing the same premarket safety requirements for cosmetic drugs as for other drugs, but excluding claims from premarket review or approval. Once again, these advocates acknowledge that Congress could, in the process of establishing any such new statutory scheme, also review and change the existing cosmetic provisions of the FD&C Act.

In the more than 40 years that this subject has been debated, no new legislation has been proposed to address the matter. Over the same period of time, industry has found ways to accommodate the existing FDA requirements and to reconcile advances in technology with current regulatory policy.

CONCLUSION

The history set forth in this chapter reflects the inherent uncertainty in attempting to formulate any bright line between a cosmetic and a drug. Even with the legislation, whatever new statutory definitions or standards that might be enacted would inevitably raise close questions of judgment that would continue to evolve over time. Accordingly, the legislation will not eliminate the uncertainty inherent in the cosmetic/drug distinction and thus is not the only or even the preferred solution to this matter.

The FDA has substantial administrative discretion to determine the line between a cosmetic and a drug. By assuring the safety of cosmetic ingredients through the Cosmetic Ingredient Review program (71), the cosmetic industry has substantially reduced concern about the safety of marketed cosmetic products. International harmonization activities have already led the FDA to explore opening US requirements to include foreign marketing experience, and the FDA Modernization Act requirements with respect to international harmonization and mutual recognition will accelerate this approach. Thus, it is more likely that a reasonable approach to the cosmetic/drug distinction will be found through administrative and international action rather than through legislation.

REFERENCES

1. Corson R. *Fashions in Makeup from Ancient to Modern Times* 8 (1972).
2. Pliny, *Natural History*, Vols I–X. (H. Rackham & W. H. S. Jones eds. 1938–1962).
3. L. Mass 1886, c. 171 (April 29, 1886).
4. Hutt PB, Hutt PB II. *A history of government regulation of adulteration and misbranding of food.* 39 Food Drug Cosmet L J 2, 47–53 (1984).
5. H.R. 9154, 55th Cong., 2d Sess. (1898); S. 4144, 55th Cong., 2d Sess. (1898).
6. Anderson OE. *Pioneer statute: The Pure Food and Drugs Act of 1906.* 13 J Publ Law 189–195 (1964).
7. 34 Stat. 768 (1906).
8. 52 Stat. 1040 (1938), 21 U.S.C. 301 et seq.
9. Hutt PB. *A historical introduction.* 45 Food Drug Cosmetic L J 17 (1990).
10. *1917 Report of Bureau of Chemistry* 15–16, in Food Law Institute, *Federal Food, Drug, and Cosmetic Law Administrative Reports: 1907–1949*, 355, 369–370 (1951).
11. S. 1944, 73d Cong., 1st Sess. (1933).

12. *1933 Report of Food & Drug Administration* 13, in Food Law Institute, S. 1944, 73d Cong., 1st Sess. (1933) at 787–799.
13. Section 6, 34 Stat. 768, 769 (1906).
14. S. Rep. No. 361, 74th Cong., 1st Sess. 4 (1935).
15. The legislative history of this prong of the drug definition is reviewed exhaustively in *American Health Products Co., Inc. v. Hayes*, 574 F. Supp 1498 (S.D.N.Y. 1983), affirmed on other grounds, *American Health Products Co. v. Hayes*, 744 F.2d 912 (2d Cir. 1984) (per curiam).
16. 79 Cong. Rec. 4845 (April 2, 1935).
17. *United States v. An Article of Drug ... Ova II*, 414 F. Supp. 660 (D.N.J. 1975), affirmed without opinion, 535 F.2d 12448 (1975).
18. Peter Barton Hutt, Richard A. Merrill, *Food and Drug Law Cases and Materials* Chapter III (1991).
19. Calvery HO. *Safeguarding foods and drugs in wartime*. 32 Am Sci, No. 2, at 103, 119 (1944).
20. FDA, *Facts for Consumers—Cosmetics*, Pub. No. 26 at 6 (1965); FDA Trade Correspondence No. 245 (April 25, 1940).
21. *Almay, Inc. v. Califano*, 569 F.2d 674 (D.C. Cir. 1977).
22. Cf. *United States v. Articles of Food and Drug*, 444 F. Supp. 266, 271 (E.D. Wisc. 1978).
23. 54 Fed. Reg. 40618, 40619–40620 (October 2, 1989); 21 C.F.R. 310.530(a).
24. *United States v. An Article ... "Line Away"*, 284 F. Supp. 107 (D. Del. 1968).
25. *United States v. An Article ... "Line Away"*, 415 F.2d 369 (3rd Cir. 1969).
26. *United States v. An Article ... Sudden Change*, 288 F. Supp. 29 (E.D.N.Y. 1968).
27. *United States v. An Article ... Sudden Change*, 409 F.2d 734 (2d Cir. 1969).
28. *United States v. An Article ... "Helene Curtis Magic Secret*," 331 F. Supp. 912 (D. Md. 1971).
29. 76 Stat. 780 (1962).
30. 37 Fed. Reg. 85 (Jan. 5, 1972); 37 Fed. Reg. 9464 (May 11, 1972); 21 C.F.R. Part 330.
31. 48 Fed. Reg. 46694, 46701–46702 (October 13, 1983) (vaginal douche products).
32. 54 Fed. Reg. 13490, 13491 (April 3, 1989) (astringent products).
33. 56 Fed. Reg. 63554, 63555 (December 4, 1991) (dandruff products).
34. 37 Fed. Reg. 219 (January 7, 1972); 37 Fed. Reg. 20160 (September 27, 1972).
35. 39 Fed. Reg. 33102 (September 13, 1974); 40 Fed. Reg. 50527 (October 30, 1975).
36. 40 Fed. Reg. 24328 (June 5, 1975); 42 Fed. Reg. 41374 (August 16, 1977).
37. 59 Fed. Reg. 31402, 31440 (June 17, 1994). Cf. *United States v. Undetermined Quantities ... "Pets Smellfree" or "Fresh Pet"*, 22 F.3d 235 (10th Cir. 1994).
38. 58 Fed. Reg. 47611 (September 9, 1993).
39. 68 Fed. Reg. 19766, 19769 (April 22, 2003); 69 Fed. Reg. 68831 (November 26, 2004).
40. FDA Trade Correspondence No. 61 (February 15, 1940).
41. 58 Fed. Reg. 28194, 28203–28206 (May 12, 1993); 64 Fed. Reg. 27666 (May 21, 1999).
42. Egli RJ. The cosmeceutic-drug regulatory distinction. In: Hori W, ed. Drug Discovery Approaches for Developing Cosmeceuticals 1.2.1 (1997).
43. " 'Antiaging' Creams Challenged," FDA Talk Paper No. T87-24 (May 14, 1987).

44. Letter from FDA Associate Commissioner for Regulatory Affairs John M. Taylor (November 19, 1987).
45. *Estee Lauder, Inc.* v. *FDA*, 727 F. Supp. 1 (D.D.C. 1989).
46. FDA issued a strong public warning about "chemical skin peeling products" in FDA Press Release No. P92-13 (May 21, 1992).
47. 15 U.S.C. 1125(a).
48. *Ortho Pharmaceutical Corp.* v. *Cosprophar, Inc.*, 828 F. Supp. 1114 (S.D.N.Y. 1993).
49. *Ortho Pharmaceutical Corp.* v. *Cosprophar, Inc.*, 32, F.3d 690 (2d Cir. 1994).
50. 62 Fed. Reg. 23350 (April 30, 1997).
51. *Fmali Herb, Inc.* v. *Heckler*, 715 Fed. 1385 (9th Cir. 1985).
52. 61 Fed. Reg. 51625 October 3, 1996; 64 Fed. Reg. 71062 (December 20, 1999); 67 Fed. Reg. 3060 (January 23, 2002); 21 C.F.R. 330.14.
53. 108 Stat. 4809 (1994).
54. 21 U.S.C. 383(c), added by 111 Stat. 2296, 2373 (1997).
55. 60 Fed. Reg. 41314 & 41453 (August 11, 1995).
56. 60 Fed. Reg. at 41467–41470.
57. 61 Fed. Reg. 44396 (August 28, 1996).
58. 61 Fed. Reg. at 44667.
59. *Coyne Beahm* v. *FDA*, 966 F. Supp. 1374 (M.D.N.C. 1997).
60. *Brown & Williamson Tobacco Corp.* v. *FDA*, 153 F.3d 155 (4th Cir. 1998).
61. *Food and Drug Administration* v. *Brown & Williamson Tobacco Corp.*, 529 U.S. 120 (2000).
62. Letter from Daniel E. Troy to Jeffrey N. Gibbs (October 17, 2002).
63. 68 Fed. Reg. 16520 (April 4, 2003).
64. 21 C.F.R. 701.3(d).
65. 21 U.S.C. 352(e)(1)(A)(iii), added by 111 Stat. 2296, 2357 (1997).
66. 58 Fed. Reg. 28194 (May 12, 1993); 64 Fed. Reg. 27666 (May 21, 1999).
67. 62 Fed. Reg. 9024 (February 27, 1997); 64 Fed. Reg. 13254 (March 17, 1999).
68. 43 Fed. Reg. 45014, 45027–45028 (September 29, 1978).
69. Letter from FDA Director of the Center for Food Safety and Applied Nutrition Joseph A. Levitt to CTFA President E. Edward Kavanaugh (March 30, 1998).
70. 63 Fed. Reg. 23624 (April 29, 1998).
71. "Potential Health Hazards of Cosmetic Products" *Hearings before the Subcommittee on Regulation and Business Opportunities of the Committee on Small Business, House of Representatives*, 100th Cong., 2d Sess. 89 (1988).

38

Drugs versus Cosmetics: Cosmeceuticals?

Kenkichi Oba and Mitsuteru Masuda
Lion Corporation, Tokyo, Japan

Regulatory Environment	643
Cosmeceuticals in Japan	650
Cosmeceuticals in the Future	651
References	652

REGULATORY ENVIRONMENT

The legal classification of topical products in Japan is different from that in the USA and Europe, where they are classified into only two categories—drugs and cosmetics. In Japan, there are also regulations covering cosmetic products with pharmacological action, called quasidrugs, which are ranked between cosmetics and drugs (1). Each definition of drugs, cosmetics, and quasidrugs in the regulations of The Pharmaceutical Affairs Law (2,3) reads as follows.

Drugs are articles that are defined as follows

1. Articles recognized in the official Japanese Pharmacopoeia.
2. Articles (other than quasidrugs) that are intended for use in the diagnosis, cure, or prevention of disease in humans or animals, and that are

not equipment or instruments (including dental materials, medical supplies, and sanitary materials).
3. Articles (other than quasidrugs and cosmetics) that are intended to affect the structure or any function of the body of humans or animals, and that are not equipment or instruments (paragraph 1, Article 2 of the law).

Quasidrugs are articles that have the following purposes and exert mild actions on the human body, or similar articles designated by the Minister of Health, Labor, and Welfare (Tables 1–3). They exclude not only equipment and instruments but also any article intended, in addition to the following purposes, for the use of drugs described earlier in categories 2 and 3.

Quasidrugs prescribed by the law

1. Prevention of nausea or other discomfort, or prevention of foul breath or body odor;
2. Prevention of prickly heat, sores, and the like;
3. Prevention of falling hair, or hair restoration or depilation;
4. Killing or prevention of rats, flies, mosquitoes, fleas, and so on, for maintaining the health of humans or animals.

Quasidrugs designated by the Minister of Health, Labor, and Welfare (MHLW notification no. 14, 1961, MHLW notification no. 202, 1995, and MHLW notification no. 31, 1999)

1. Cotton products intended for sanitary purpose (including paper cotton);
2. The following products with a mild action on the human body:
    i. Disinfecting solutions for soft contact lenses;
    ii. Products used to disinfect or protect abrasions, cuts, puncture wounds, scratches, and wound surfaces;
    iii. Products that combine the purposes of use as stipulated in paragraph 3, Article 2 of the law (on cosmetics), with the purpose of prevention of acne, chapping, itchy skin rash, chilblain, and so on, as well as disinfection of the skin and mouth;
    iv. Products used to improve such symptoms as chapped skin, prickly heat, sores, corns, calluses, and dry skin;
    v. Hair dyes;
    vi. Agents for permanent waving;
    vii. Bath preparations;
    viii. Products used to alleviate discomfort of the throat;
    ix. Products used to alleviate discomfort of the stomach;
    x. Products intended to supply vitamins or calcium to the fatigued or middle-aged body;
    xi. Products used to nourish the body or improve a weak body (diet supplements).

Table 1 Types, Purposes of Use, Indications, and Effects of Quasidrugs

Type of quasidrugs	Purpose of use	Principal product form	Indications and effects
1. Mouth refreshers	Oral preps for prevention of nausea or other indisposition	Pill, plate, troche, liquid	Heartburn, nausea and vomiting, motion sickness, hangover, dizziness, foul breath, choking, indisposition, sunstroke
2. Body deodorants	External agents to prevent body odor	Liquid, ointment, aerosol, powder, stick	Body odor, perspiration odor, suppression of perspiration
3. Talcum powders	Agents to prevent prickly heat, sore, etc.	Powder for external application	Prickly heat, diaper rash, sore, thigh sores, razor burn
4. Hair growers (hair nutrients)	External agents to prevent loss of hair and to grow hair	Liquid, aerosol	Hair growth, prevention of thinning hair, itching and falling hair, promotion of hair growth, dandruff, loss of hair after illness or childbirth, hair nutrition
5. Depilatories	External agents for hair removal	Ointment, aerosol	Hair removal
6. Hair dyes (including color and dye removers)	External agents for dying hair, removing hair or dye colors. Excluding agents for physical hair dying	Powder, tablet, liquid, cream, aerosol	Hair dying, hair decoloring, removal of hair color dye
7. Permanent waving agents	External agents for waves in the hair etc.	Liquid, cream, powder, paste, aerosol, tablet	Creation and retention of waves in the hair, straightening the frizzy, curly or wavy hairs, and retaining that condition
8. Sanitary cotton products	Cotton (including paper cotton) used for sanitation	Cotton products, gauze	Sanitary napkins: for absorbing and managing menses; cotton for cleaning: for wiping clean the skin and cavities of babies, for wiping clean the breasts and nipples when nursing, for wiping clean the eyes, genitals, and anus

(*continued*)

Table 1 *Continued*

Type of quasidrugs	Purpose of use	Principal product form	Indications and effects
9. Bath preparations	External agents to be dissolved, as a rule, in the bath (excluding bath soaps)	Powder, granule, tablet, soft capsule, liquid, etc.	Prickly heat, roughness, ringworm, bruises, stiff shoulder, sprains, neuralgia, eczema, frostbite, hemorrhoids, tinea, chills, athlete's foot, scabies, itch, lumbago, rheumatism, fatigue recovery, chaps, cracks, chills before and after childbirth, acnes
10. Medicated cosmetics (including medicated soaps)	External agents combining cosmetic purposes and resembling cosmetics in forms	Liquid, cream, jelly, solid, aerosol	See table 2.
11. Medicated dentifrices	External agents combining cosmetic purposes and resembling ordinary dentifrices in forms	Paste, liquid, powder, solid, tooth wet-powder	Making the teeth white, cleaning and refreshing the mouth, prevention of pyorrhea, prevention of gingivitis, prevention of tartar, prevention of dental caries, prevention of occurrence and progress of dental caries, prevention of foul breath, removal of tobacco stains
12. Repellents	Agents for repelling insects such as flies, mosquitoes, fleas, etc.	Liquid, stick, cream, aerosol	Repelling mosquitoes, gnats, stinging flies, fleas, house ticks and bedbug, etc.
13. Insecticides	Agents for killing and eliminating insects such as flies, mosquitoes, fleas, etc.	Mat, stick-incense, powder, liquid, aerosol, paste	Killing of insects; exterminating and preventing sanitary insects pest such as flies, mosquitoes, fleas, etc.
14. Rodenticides	Agents for killing and eliminating rats and mice		Killing of rats and mice; expelling, exterminating or preventing rats and mice
15. Soft contact lens disinfectants	Agents to disinfect soft contact lens		Disinfectant for soft contact lens

Source: Modified from Refs. (2,3,10).

Table 2 Types of Medicated Cosmetics

Type	Indications and effects
1. Shampoos	Prevention of dandruff and itching
	Prevention of perspiration odors in the hair and on the scalp
	Cleaning of the hair and scalp
	a. Keeping the hair and scalp healthy
	b. Making the hair supple (choose either a or b)
2. Rinses	Prevention of dandruff and itching
	Prevention of perspiration odors in the hair and on the scalp
	Supplementing and maintaining moisture and fat of the hair
	Prevention of split, broken, or branched hairs
	a. Keeping the hair and scalp healthy
	b. Making the hair supple (choose either a or b)
3. Skin lotions	Chapping and roughness of the skin
	Prevention of prickly heat, frostbite, chaps, cracks, acnes
	Oily skin
	Prevention of razor burn
	Prevention of spots and freckles due to sunburn
	Burning sensation after sunburn or snow burn
	Bracing, cleaning, and conditioning the skin
	Keeping the skin healthy; supplying the skin with moisture
4. Creams, milky lotions, hand creams, cosmetic oils	Chapping and roughness of the skin
	Prevention of prickly heat, frostbite, chaps, cracks, acnes
	Oily skin
	Prevention of razor burn
	Prevention of spots and freckles due to sunburn
	Burning sensation after sunburn or snow burn
	Bracing, cleaning, and conditioning the skin
	Keeping the skin healthy; supplying the skin with moisture
	Protection of the skin; prevention of dry skin
5. Shaving agents	Prevention of razor burn
	Protection of the skin for smoother shave
6. Sunburn prevention agents	Prevention of chapping due to sunburn and snow burn
	Prevention of sunburn and snow burn
	Prevention of spots and freckles due to sunburn
	Protection of the skin
7. Packs	Chapping and roughness of the skin
	Prevention of acnes
	Oily skin
	Prevention of spots and freckles due to sunburn
	Burning sensation after sunburn or snow burn
	Making the skin smooth
	Cleaning the skin
8. Medicated soaps (including face cleaning agents)	⟨Soaps which are mainly bactericides⟩
	Cleaning, sterilizing and disinfecting the skin
	Prevention of body odor, perspiration odor, and the acnes
	⟨Soaps mainly containing antiinflammatory agents⟩
	Cleaning of the skin; prevention of acnes, razor burn, and chapping

Source: Refs. (2,3,10).

Table 3 Newly Designated Quasidrugs

Category	Dose form	Efficacies/indications
1. Products such as throat candies (to be melted in the mouth) that contain mild natural drugs such as senega	Troche, drop	Sputum; hoarse voice, rough throat, throat inflammation, discomfort in the throat, sore throat, and swollen throat associated with throat inflammation
2. Digestive aids containing natural stomachic remedies as their main active ingredients	Tablet, pill, capsule, granule, powder, oral liquid	Discomfort in the stomach due to overeating and overdrinking; nausea (retching, stomach nausea, retching due to hangover/overdrinking, vomiting)
3. Disinfectants/bactericides containing ethanol, iodine tincture, benzalkonium chloride, benzethonium chloride, chlorhexidine gluconate, etc. as their main active ingredients (for external use only)	Topical liquid, ointment	Cleansing and disinfecting abrasions, cuts, stabs, scratches, shoe sores, and wounds; cleansing and disinfecting fingers and skin
4. Adhesive plasters containing disinfectants/bactericides for treating cuts and wounds	Plaster, water plaster, gauze	Disinfecting and protecting abrasions, cuts, stabs, scratches, shoe sores, and wounds
5. Chlorhexidine (ointment for external application)	Ointment	Chaps, crack, abrasions; shoe sores
6. Products for external application containing metholated camphor as the main active ingredient	Ointment	Chaps, frostbites, and skin cracks
7. Products for external application with zinc oxides as the main active ingredient	Ointment	Mitigation of chaps, frostbites, skin cracks, and roughness of hands and legs
8. Adhesive plasters containing salicylic acid (for external use only)	Ointment, topical liquid	Mitigation and prevention of heat rashes and erosion
9. Ointments containing urea (for external use only)	Plaster	Corns and callus
10. Ointments containing vitamins A and E (for external use only)	Ointment	Mitigation of dried and rough hand and legs

(*continued*)

Table 3 *Continued*

Category	Dose form	Efficacies/indications
11. Vitamin C preparations (for oral administration)	Tablet, capsule, pill, granule, powder, jelly, drop, oral liquid	Supplement of vitamin C for physical fatigue, pregnant and nursing period, during and after illnesses, and those in middle-to-advanced ages
12. Vitamin E preparations (for oral administration)	Tablet, capsule, pill, granule, powder, jelly, drop, oral liquid	Supplement of vitamin E for those in middle-to-advanced ages
13. Vitamins E and C preparations (for oral administration)	Tablet, capsule, pill, granule, powder, jelly, drop, oral liquid	Supplement of vitamins C and E for physical fatigue, weakness during and after illnesses, and those in middle-to-advanced ages
14. Vitamins B1, B2, and B6 preparations (for oral administration)	Tablet, capsule, pill, granule, powder, oral liquid	Nutrients and tonics; weak constitution; physical fatigue, during and after illnesses, anorexia, malnutrition, feverish exhaustive diseases, pregnant and nursing period (preparations not containing vitamins A and D)
15. Mineral (calcium) supplements (for oral administration)	Tablet, capsule, pill, granule, powder, oral liquid	Supplement of calcium for pregnant and nursing period, growing children, and those in middle-to-advanced ages

Source: Modified from Ref. (4).

Among the products just described, category [2(iii)] comprises the so-called medicated cosmetics (Table 2). On April 1, 1999, after much deliberation, a total of 15 categories (Table 3) (4), described in 2(viii–xi), were shifted from nonprescription medicines to quasidrugs as they had relatively mild pharmacological actions and could be sold without need for health professionals to provide information to the general public at the point of purchase. For differentiating the new entry from those "conventional" quasidrugs, they are specifically called "newly designated quasidrugs".

The term "cosmetic" means any article intended to be used by means of rubbing, sprinkling, or similar application to the human body for cleaning, beautifying, promoting attractiveness, altering the appearance of the human body, and keeping the skin and hair healthy, provided that the action of the article on the human body is mild. Such articles exclude the articles intended, besides the aforementioned purposes, for the use of drugs described earlier in categories 2 or 3, and quasidrugs (paragraph 3, Article 2 of the law).

At each stage of development, manufacture/import, distribution, and use, the prescribed regulations are put into practice, including systems of the examination for approval, manufacture/importation, distribution control, and post-marketing surveillance, respectively (2,5). As for cosmetics, the deregulation was carried out based on the government's policy to review licensing systems and ingredient labeling controls (5,6). The new regulations, effective as of April 1, 2001, supercede the Quality Standards of Cosmetics of 1967, eliminate the pre-market licensing requirement for cosmetics, and establish lists of prohibited and restricted ingredients, approved sunscreens, and preservatives, as well as new labeling requirements (7). This deregulation indicates the shift of the regulatory system to one based on the manufacturers' self-responsibility (5). As of April 1, 2001, the responsibility to ensure that any cosmetic product placed on the market is safe falls on the manufacturer (7). Similar to the requirements in the USA and the EU, the health authorities may require a manufacturer to substantiate product safety (7). The aforementioned new regulations do not apply to quasidrugs (7). Pre-market approval and licensing requirements are still in effect for quasidrugs (7). The regulatory system for the manufacture of quasidrugs is more rigorous than that for cosmetics and is more akin to that for drugs (7). At the distribution stage, however, they are treated like cosmetics (7).

COSMECEUTICALS IN JAPAN

A current definition of cosmeceuticals would cover those products "that will achieve cosmetic results by means of some degree of physiological action" (8). This product category is ranked between cosmetics and drugs. It is a well-known fact that Japan is ahead of most other countries in coping with the legal issues. A category of pseudodrugs that are what we now refer to as cosmeceuticals has already been established in the Pharmaceutical Affairs Law (9). The phrase pseudodrugs correspond to the legal category of quasidrugs. Actually, many of the topical products corresponding to the cosmeceuticals fall into the category of quasidrugs. In the Pharmaceutical Affairs Law, quasidrugs are defined as articles having "a fixed purpose of use" and "a mild action on the body" or similar articles designated by the Minister of Health, Labor, and Welfare. Their types, purpose of use, principal product form, indications, and effects are described in Tables 1–3 (2–4,10).

The manufacturers of quasidrugs are required to obtain government approvals before marketing except for some. Approval of a product under application for manufacturing (import) is contingent upon a judgment by the Ministry of Health, Labor, and Welfare regarding its adequacy as a quasidrug in view of its effectiveness, safety, and so on. It should be noted, therefore, that the examination procedures for approval as well as the data and documentation required to be submitted upon filing differ based on the indications and effects of the products (2,3). The following data must be submitted, depending on the kind of ingredients: (i) data on origin, background of discovery, use in foreign countries; (ii) data on physicochemical properties, specifications, and testing methods; (iii) data on stability; (iv) data on safety; and (v) data on indications or effects.

The scope of data actually to be attached to the application depends on the type of quasidrug: (i) new quasidrugs that obviously differ from any one of previously approved products with regard to active ingredient, usage, and dosage and/or indications or effects; (ii) quasidrugs identical with previously approved quasidrug(s); or (iii) quasidrugs that are other than those specified in the earlier two types (2,3).

For a product under application to be approved as a quasidrug, it is prerequisite that the purpose of its use is within the scope stipulated by the Pharmaceutical Affairs Law. Thus, approval of a product as a quasidrug is determined by an integrated judgment of various factors such as its ingredients, quantity (composition), indications and effects, usage and dosage, and dosage form. For example, those products whose effects are not mild and thus come under the category of poisons or deleterious drugs are not approved, even if their indications, effects, and dosage forms are within the scope of quasidrugs legislation. Likewise, products for which the purpose of use deviates from the scope of quasidrug are also not approved either, even if their effects are mild (2,3).

When viewed taking into account the essential characteristics of quasidrugs for example, it is inappropriate for products such as mouth refreshers to include any medicinal indications and effects relevant to "treatment", such as morning sickness and sterilization and disinfection of the mouth (2,3).

As a quasidrug under the law may be sold and used by any person without specific restriction, it should be a product that, in principle, can be easily and directly used by any person without involving any complex process (2,3). Generally, simplicity in handling and usage constitutes another potent factor (2,3).

COSMECEUTICALS IN THE FUTURE

Regarding cosmetic requirements, the demand for fashion has strengthened, but, at the same time, a tendency to place importance on efficacy has also emerged (11). This trend has become increasingly strong with the transition toward gerontocracy, where there is a wish to delay the biological process of aging and remain young as long as possible. However, the desire to look young and beautiful is shifting to a desire to protect the health of the skin (11).

In addition, with the increasingly sophisticated research into the skin, technology has been generating new active ingredients for antiaging skin-care products. However, some of them, such as antiwrinkle products, fall into none of the three categories—drugs, quasidrugs, or cosmetics. No existing specifications (Tables 1–3) (2–4,10) of quasidrug are suitable for such products. How, then, should those products be categorized?

In the USA, a drug is defined as "an article intended for the use in the diagnosis, mitigation, treatment or prevention of disease or intended to affect the structure or any function of the body". According to the current Federal Food, Drug and Cosmetic Act written in 1938, cosmetics are defined as "articles intended to be rubbed, poured, sprinkled, or sprayed on, introduced into, or otherwise applied to the human body or any part thereof for cleansing, beautifying, promoting attractiveness, or altering the appearance" without affecting structure or function (12–14). If, for example, a nonmedicated shampoo is designated "dandruff" shampoo, simply by virtue of the fact that it removes loose dandruff flakes as part of the cleansing process, then it would be classified as a cosmetic shampoo (13). However, a shampoo that controls dandruff flaking would be categorized as a drug, and known as "antidandruff" shampoo (13). On the other hand, an antidandruff shampoo would be regarded as a quasidrug in Japan if its action on the human body was mild.

Generally, topically applied quasidrugs are intended to mollify flaws of the skin and have a mild action on the human body, whereas drugs are intended to treat diseases (15). Therefore, hair-growing products having mild actions on male pattern baldness, which is not a disease (1), and are considered quasidrugs; on the other hand, products intended for alopecia areata, which is a kind of disease, are regarded as drugs. Aging of skin, as in wrinkling, for example, is not a disease. We should also keep in mind that "high efficacy" would not always involve "strong action". There will probably be many cosmeceutical products with mild action showing good efficacy. Accordingly, those new cosmeceutical products intended for antiaging of the skin could be categorized as quasidrugs. Legally, the Minister of Health, Labor, and Welfare can add new, novel types of product to the current list of types of quasidrug (15).

Regarding this matter, a review "... of the scope of efficacy by adding new effects, will increase incentives toward research and developments in the technological standards and quality of cosmetics" was included in the policy for promoting the Japanese cosmetic industry (11,16) published in May, 1984 by the Pharmaceutical Industry Policy Council, a consultative body of the Director of Pharmaceutical Affairs Bureau, the Ministry of Health and Welfare. The Japan Cosmetic Industry Association has set up an *ad hoc* subcommittee within its technical committee to review the scope of indications and effects of cosmetics and quasidrugs (17). We hope this effort will be successful.

REFERENCES

1. Vermeer BJ, Gilchrest BA. Cosmeceuticals: a proposal for rational definition, evaluation, and regulation. Arch Dermatol 1996; 132:337–340.

2. Editorial supervision by Pharmaceuticals and Cosmetics Division, Pharmaceutical Affairs Bureau, Ministry of Health and Welfare. Guide to Quasi-drug and Cosmetic Regulations in Japan. Tokyo: Yakuji Nippo, 1992.
3. Editorial supervision by Pharmaceuticals Affairs Assessing Group. Guide to Quasi-drug and Cosmetic Regulations in Japan. 4th ed. Tokyo: Yakuji Nippo, 2001.
4. Japan Self-Medication Industry. OTC Marketing Deregulation. PAJ Newslett 1999; Number 41:4–6.
5. Masuda M. Legislation in Japan. Handbook of Cosmetic Science and Technology. Marcel Dekker, 2001:761–767.
6. Arimoto T. The Current State of Japan's Cosmetic Regulatory System Liberalization. International Regulatory Congress, Florence, Italy, Apr. 22–23, 1998.
7. The Cosmetic, Toiletry, and Fragrance Association. CTFA International Regulatory Resource Manual. 5th ed. 2001.
8. Stimson N. Cosmeceuticals: realizing the reality of the 21st century. SÖFW J 1994; 120:631–641.
9. Kligman AM. Why cosmeceuticals? Cosmet Toiletr Mag 1993; 108:37–38.
10. Society of Japanese Pharmacopoeia. Guide to Quasi-drug and Cosmetic Regulations in Japan (Japanese ed.). 3d ed. Tokyo: Yakuji Nippo, 1996.
11. Takano K. The Trend of Cosmetic Regulations in Japan. International Information Center of Cosmetic Industries. Buenos Aires, Argentina, Oct 14–15, 1984.
12. Gilbertson WE. The Impact of the FDA's over-the-counter drug review program on the regulation of cosmetics. In: Esterin NF, ed. The Cosmetic Industry: Scientific and Regulatory Foundations. New York: Marcel Dekker, 1984:71–89.
13. Lanzet M. Innovating in a regulated environment. In: Esterin NF.ed. The Cosmetic Industry: Scientific and Regulatory Foundations. New York: Marcel Dekker, 1984:551–562.
14. Steinberg DC. Regulatory review. Cosmet Toiletr Mag 1997; 112:27–29.
15. Komiya H. Regulatory frame and problems related to quasidrug. J Jpn Cosmet Sci Soc 1991; 15:37–40.
16. Nakamura Y. Regulation and safety measures of cosmetics. J Jpn Cosmet Sci Soc 1995; 19(Suppl):164–173.
17. The Technical Committee of JCIA. Technical Report No.103. Tokyo: Japan Cosmetic Industry Association, 1997.

Index

α-Hydroxyacids. *See* AHA.
β-Hydroxyacids. *See* BHA.
β-Lipohydroxyacid, as alternative drug treatment, 250

Acne, sebum secretion in, 314, 315
Acne treatment, salicyclic acid as, 212, 213
Actinic elastosis, 336
Active ingredient, as drug identification, 616
Actives, humectants, 221
ADME studies, percutaneous, of eflornithine, 494, 495
Advanced glycation endproducts (AGE), 336
African potato, future uses of, 288
Age, variations in sebaceous gland secretion, 310
Aged dry skin, senile xerosis, 30
Aging
    effects on skin, retardation of, 620
    Hsp, 529, 530
    hyaluronan levels, 381–383
    kinetin, 409
AHA (α-hydroxyacids), 207–209, 272
    chemical structure, 208, 209
    effect on HA, 394
    effect on skin structure, 229
    in fruits, 394
    moisturizers, 226
    photoaging treatment, 272
    products, FDA review of, 635
    sources of, 208, 209
Aliphatic/alicyclic diols, for prevention of photoaging, 269
Allergen control system (ACS), for melasma, 200, 201
Allergens, pigmented cosmetic dermatitis, 198, 199
Allergic contact dermatitis (ACD), 294
All-trans-retinaldehyde (RAL), 323
All-trans-retinoic acid (RA), 323
All-trans-retinol (ROL), 323
Alternative drug treatments
    β-lipohydroxyacid, 250
    benzoyl peroxide (BPO), 249
    black tea extracts, 249
    extracts, 249, 250
    fatty acids, 250, 251
    green tea polyphenolic (GTP), 248
    hamamelis, 250
    hydroxyacids, 250
    lavender oil, 253, 254
    nitrous oxide, 257
    oatmeal, 250
    ocimum oil, 254
    oils, 253, 254
    overview, 247–258
    persimmon leaf extract, 249
    potential uses, animals, 255, 256
    potential uses, humans, 251, 252

Alternative drug treatments (*Contd.*)
  quaternium-18 bentonite, 257
  soybeans, 250
  soymilk, 250
  spearmint, 249, 250
  tea extracts, 248, 249
  vitamin C, 254, 255
  vitamin E, 254, 255
  witch hazel, hamamelis, 250
Amino acid
  basic features, 18
  decomposition sensitivity, 28
  definition of, 17
  delivery into skin, 30, 31
  derivatives, 17–34
  dissociation constant, isolectric point, 22
  optical rotation, 23–26
  skin, 18, 22, 29, 30
  solubility
    in aqueous alcohol solution, 21
    in water, 19, 20
Amino acid derivative, 31–34
  extended applications, 31–34
  N-alkylether-hydroxypropyl arginine, 33
  N-cocoylarginine ethylester, 33
  N-lauroyl lysine, 33
Anhydrous foundations, 161–163
Anthraquinone, 146
Anti-aging extracts, 95
Anti-aging treatment, dimethylaminoethanol, 365–371
Anti-inflammatory, DMAE as, 369
Antioxidant(s)
  chemical structure, 40
  environmental stressors, effects on, 51
  extracts, safety of, 92–94
  flavonoids, 63
  glutathione, 42
  lipoic acid, 70
  melatonin, 70
  photoaging, prevention of, 269
  photoprotection of skin, role in, 55, 341, 342
  as preservatives/excipents/emulsifiers, 221
  pro-oxidants, 476

  skin damage prevention, 341, 342
  thiols, 63
  topical application, 55, 74
  UVR exposure, 73
Antioxidant activity, *Emblica*, 472
Antioxidant combinations, 70, 73
  photoprotective effects of topically applied, 71, 72
Antioxidant defense enzymes, *Emblica*, 475, 476
Antioxidant defense systems skin, 37–75
Antioxidant network, activation of, 41
Arnica montana, risks of use, 288
Ascorbate (vitamin C), 39
  antioxidant properties, 39
  hydrophilic skin antioxidants, 52
  physiological levels of, 41
  prevalence in skin, 39–42
Ascorbic acid, extracts, 93
Assays, animal, for depigmentation agents, 194
Assays, human sensitization, 575
  modified Draize, 577
  repeat insult patch tests (RIPT), 575
Assays, predictive
  Buehler test, 573
  Draize test, 571, 572
  Freund's complete adjuvant test, 573
  guinea pig maximization test, 574, 575
  guinea pig sensitization tests, 571
  open epicutaneous test, 572, 573
  optimization test, 573, 574
  planning execution, 570, 571
  quantitative structure activity relationships, 571
  split adjuvant test, 574
Astaxanthin, inhibitory effect of, 343
Avocadofuran, 113
Ayurvedic herb, *Phyllanthus emblica* as, 470
Azelaic acid, depigmenting agents, 274

Back cumulative irritation test, retinyl propionate, 443, 444
  results, 447, 448
Ballistometry, photoaging analysis, 266

Balloon vine (*Cardiospermi herba*), for eczema, 286
Barium sulfate, as pigment, 150
Barrier function, of epidermis, 93, 94
Barrier protection, skin cream, 297–300
Behring's conclusion, 282
Bentonite gel, for measurement of sebum gland secretion, 308, 309
Benzoyl peroxide (BPO), as alternative drug treatment, 249
Beta carotene, as retinoid, 272
Beta hydroxy acids, as photoaging treatment, 272
Beta-sistosterone gluconate, 285
Beta-sitosterol, 282–284
BHA (β-hydroxyacids), 207, 272
Biotechnology extract, 92
Bismuth oxychloride, inorganic pearl, 151, 152
Blushers, powder, 158, 159
Botanical extracts, 89–96.
  See also Extracts.
  extraction process, 90
  origins of, 90
Brassicasterol, 281
Buehler test, predictive assays, 573
Butcher's broom, potential uses, 288

Ca^{2+}, lipids, 223
Calcium carbonate, 156
Campestrol, 281
Cancer, hyaluronan production in, 381
Capacitance conductance, photoaging analysis, 266
Cardiospermi herba (balloon vine), for eczema, 286
Carotenoids
  extracts, 93
  structure of, 342
  vitamin A, 48
Catales
  antioxidant properties, 51
  prevalence in skin, 51
CD44, as hyaluronan receptor, 384, 385
Ceramide(s)
  general structure, 103
  skin repair, effectiveness in, 106, 107
Ceramide-2 treatment, 110–112
Ceruloplasmin, as copper containing enzyme, 551
Chamber test method, 593
Chelating agents, protective creams, 300
Chelating properties, of *Emblica* antioxidant, 477, 478
Chelators, as oxidation enhancer, 476
Cholesterol sulfate, lipids and, 223
Chromium hydroxide, as pigment, 150
Chromium oxide, as pigment, 149
Cigarette paper, use with sebum gland secretion, 308, 309
Citroline (cit), 29
Classical lipstick formulations, 169, 170
Clincial panel methods, photoaging analysis, 266, 267
Collagen, effect of quenchers, 340
Collagen synthesis
  rate of, 554
  stimulation of, 122
  topical niacinimide testing results, 430
Collagen synthesis assay, topical niacinimide testing, 423
Collagenase MMP-1 inhibitory effect of *Emblica* antioxidant, 479
Color additives
  definitions of, 141, 142
  dye, 141
  extender, 142
  lake, 141
  pigment, 141
  primary/straight color, 141
  regulation of, 142–144
  toner, 142
  true pigment, 142
Color chemistry manufacture, 144, 145
Colorants, 157
  quality control of, 150, 151
  standards, 151
  test methods, 150–152
Colorimetry, photoaging analysis, 266

Condensed tannins,
    proanthocyanidins, 467
Conenzyme Q
    antioxidant properties, 45
    physiological levels, in skin, 47
    prevalence in skin, 47
    ubiquinols/ubiquinones, 45
Constitutive skin antioxidants, 39–55
    water-soluble, ascorbate, 39
Contact reactions
    epidemiology, 588, 589
    signs symptoms, 588
Contact urticaria
    animal experimental protocols,
        596, 597
    application techniques, 593
        chamber test, 593
        open test, 593
        use test, 593
    clinical test(s)
        laser-Doppler blood flowmetry,
            595, 596
        measurement of edema, 596
        measurement of erythema,
            594, 595
        quantitative methods, 594–596
        reactions, site specificity, 591
        visual scoring, 594
    human experimental protocols,
        591–594
    inhibition, 593
    irritation tests, in animals, 579, 580
    types of
        immunological contact urticaria
            (ICU), 590, 591
        nonimmunological contact urticaria,
            NICU, 589, 590
Contact urticaria syndrome. See CUS.
Copper
    absorption/transport in humans, 550
    metabolism/excretion in humans,
        550, 551
    molecular biology of, 550, 551
    molecular pharmacology,
        551, 552
Copper peptide, in skin, 549–561
Copper peptide complex, mechanism
    of, 554

Coproporphyin
    perioxidation of skin, 339
    singlet oxygen emission, 339
Corneocyte cohesion, hydroxyacid,
    effect on, 210, 211
Corneocytes
    stripped human, 102
    with TTF gel, 118
Cosmeceuticals
    advances in skin cosmetic care,
        619–622
    concept and laws
        in Europe, Japan, 6, 7
        in United States, 3–5
    definition of, 1–8, 11–13
    European definition of, 12, 615–622
    FDC definition of, 11
    growth factors in, 349–358
    Hsp in, 523–533
    in Japan, 650, 651
    topical retinols as, 322
Cosmetic allergens, pigmented cosmetic
    dermatitis, 198
Cosmetic applications
    growth factors in, 353–356
        Nouricel-MD™, 354
        TNS Recovery Complex®, 354
Cosmetic foundations, 160
Cosmetic technology, 154, 155
Cosmetic vs. drug, 620–622
    distinctions between, 630, 631
    Japan, 643–652
    legal cases, 631, 632
    legal distinction in the United States,
        625–640
Cosmetics
    color additive regulation, 141–144
    decorative, 140–182
    emulsification, level of preservatives,
        607, 608
    eye, 163
    FD&C Act, definition of, 629
    Japanese definition of, 12
    medicated, types of, in Japan, 647
    powdered, 155
Cosmetics manufacture
    emulsification, 604
    process engineering in, 603–611

Index

Cosmetics regulation
  European Union, 618, 619
  United States, 618, 619
cRBP, cytoplasmic retinol-binding protein, 442
Cream eye shadows, 166, 167
Creams
  skin barrier function, 233
  protective, 293–302
    adverse effects/contraindications, 301
    application of, 300, 301
    effects of, 294, 295
    emulsion structure, 295
    hydrating effect, 295
    mechanisms of hydration, 295, 296
    occlusion effect, 295
    special ingredients, 300
Cu^{2+} chelators, UV spectral data of, 477
CUS (contact urticaria syndrome), 587–597
  epidemiology, 588
  inhibition of, 593
  irritation tests, in animals, 579, 580
  symptoms signs, 588
Cutaneous barrier repair, 99–125
Cutaneous metabolism, retinol, 325, 326
Cytochrome c oxidase, 551
Cytokines, TNS Recovery Complex®, 354
Cytoplasmic retinol-binding protein, cRBP, 442

Dandruff. *See* Seborrheic dermatitis.
Deadly nightshade (*Dulcamara stipites*), in eczema, 286
Decomposition sensitivity, amino acids, 28
Dehydroellagitannins, 469
Depigmentation agents, 185–204
  azelaic acid, 274
  clinical evaluation of, 194–200
  ephelid, 197
  hydroquinone, 274
  melasma, effectiveness on, 189, 197
  photoaging treatment products, 274
  screening tests for, 190–194
  solar lentigo, 197

tri-luma, 274
Dermagraft™, 353
Dermal hyaluronan, 387
Derman GAG production, inhibition of, 458, 459
Dermatitis, 294
  irritant, assays, 577–582
Dermatopharmacokinetics, predictive assays, 568, 569
Dermatotoxicology, overview of, 567–582
Dermis, care of, 119–124
Desquamation, skin structure, 228–232
Dimethylaminoethanol. *See* DMAE.
Dismutases, superoxide, 49
  antioxidant properties, 50
Dispersion cosmetics, manufacture of, 608
Dissociation constant, isolectric point, in amino acids, 22
DMAE (dimethylaminoethanol), 365, 366
  anti-aging treatment, 365–371
  anti-inflammatory, 369
  biological functions, 366–368
  chemical structure, 366
  free-radical scavenger, 369
  muscarinic receptors, 368
  nicotinic receptors, 367
  pharmacological actions, 366–368
  protective creams, 300
  roles of, 369, 370
  safety of, 370, 371
  sagging skin, 370
  skin firmness, 369
Dopamine-β-monoxygenase, copper containing enzyme, 552
Draize-type tests, irritation tests, animals, 578
Drug identification, active ingredient, 616
Drug product, requirements of, 616
Drug vs. cosmetic, 620–622, 630, 631
  FD&C Act, definition of, 629
  Japan, 643–652
  legal cases, 631, 632
  legal distinction, in the United States, 625–640

Dry skin, 219–221
  causes of, 219, 220
  characteristics of, 220
  chemistry of, 221–223
  moisturizers, 220, 221
  skin irritants, 298
Dulcamara stipites (deadly nightshade), and eczema, 286
Dyes
  as color additives, 141
  natural, 147

EA (ellagic acid), 511–520
  activity
    in vitro, 516, 517
    in vivo, 517–519
  biochemical properties, 514
  clinical study results, 516–519
  effectiveness on sunburn, 515
  existence of, 514
  general properties, 514–519
  melanoma cells, 518, 519
  modes of activity, 516–519
  physicochemical properties, 514
  plants, 514
  skin whitening, in humans, 515
  treatment for skin pigmentation conditions, 515
EC (European Commission), 141
Eczema
  Cardiospermi herba (balloon vine) in, 286
  Dulcamara stipites (deadly nightshade) in, 286
  phytosterols, 286, 287
Edema scoring scale, 595
EDTA, as protective cream, 300
Eflornithine
  clinical studies for facial hair, 496–507
    Phase I, 496, 497
    Phase II and III, 497–499, 500
    results, 500–505
  delivery to hair follicles, 492–494
  hair growth inhibitor, 491, 492
  percutaneous ADME studies, pharmacokinetic studies, 494
  preclinical studies, 494

  safety of, 495, 496
  for treatment of unwanted facial hair, 489–508
Elder, potential uses, 288
Ellagic acid. *See* EA.
Ellagitannins, 467, 469
Emblica, as antioxidant, 471
  activity of, 472
  bacterial mutagenicity, 484
  chelating properties, 477, 478
  collagenase MMP-1 inhibitory effect of, 479
  defense enzymes, 475, 476
  freckle spots, 482
  hydroxy radical quenching, 472–476
  lightening normal skin color, 482
  nitrogen radical quenching, 474, 475
  safety data, 483, 484
  singlet oxygen quenching, 474
  stability of, 472
  stimulation of noncollagenic protein synthesis, 481
  stromelysin 1 (MMP-3) inhibitory effect of, 480
  superoxide anion radical quenching, 473
  UV-induced erythema, 483
Emblica officinalis, tannins of, 469
Embryonic development, hyaluronan production, 380, 381
Emollients, as dry skin treatment, 220. *See also* Moisturizers.
Emulsification
  in cosmetics manufacturing, 604
  mechanical forces in, 607, 608
    low-solubility ingredients, 608, 609
    product texture, 610
    scale-up, 610
  preservative levels, 607, 608
Emulsified foundations, 160, 161
Emulsifier levels
  decreasing, 604–607
  microfluidizer method, 604–607
Emulsifier system, stabilizing of, 606, 607
Emulsifiers
  antioxidants/preservatives/ excipients, 221

ionic, 225, 226
nonionic, 225, 226
use of in moisturizers, 224–226
Emulsion structure, of protective
  creams, 295
Endogenous, inflammatory
  disorders, 38
Enzymatic antioxidant systems, 49–51
  catales, 51
  dismutases, superoxide, 49
  enzymatic GSH, 49
Enzymatic GSH, 49
  antioxidant properties, 49
  prevalence in skin, 49, 50
Enzymatic skin antioxidants, 54, 55
Enzymes, copper containing
  ceruloplasmin, 551
  dopamine-β-monoxygenase, 552
  lysyl osidase, 551
  metallothioneins, 551
  SOD, 551
  tyrosinase, 551
Ephelid, depigmentation agents, 197
Epidermal growth factor receptor
  expression, 357
Epidermal hyaluronan, 386, 387
Epidermis
  lipids of, 93, 94
  as SC barrier, 112–119
Erythema action spectrum, 334
Erythema scoring scale, 594
Essential fatty acids, as alternative
  drug treatment, 250, 251
Essential oils, as alternative drug
  treatment, 253, 254
European Commission (EC),
  definition of cosmetics. 141
European definition of
  cosmeceuticals, 6, 7
European Economic Cosmetic
  (EEC) Directive of 1993,
  6, 11, 12
European Union, cosmetics
  regulations, 617, 618
Evaporimetry, photoaging
  analysis, 266
Evelle® supplementation
  clinical study, 538–540

  elasticity measures, 540
  results, 540–543
  roughness measures, 541
  ingredients of, 537, 538
  for skin elasticity, 538–543
Excipents/emulsifiers/antioxidants/
  preservatives, 221
Extenders, as color additives, 142
Extracellular matrix (ECM), 375
  hyaluronanin, 383
  proteins, 480, 481
Extraction process, botanicals, 90
Extracts
  antiaging, 95
  ascorbic acid, 93
  biotechnology, 92
  botanical, 89–96. *See also* Extracts.
  carotenoids, 93
  fat storage/slimming, various 94
  fish oils, 93
  flavonoids, 93
  Germanium thumbergii, 93
  lipids, various, 94
  other, as alternative drug treatment,
  249, 250
  purification of, 91, 92
  Rosmarinus (rosemary), 93
  safety of antioxidant, 92–94
    vegetable oils, 93
  selective, 91
  SOD, 93
  Syzgium aromticum, 93
  total, 91
  usage, 92
  vegetable oils, 93
Eye makeup, 163–168
Eye shadow
  cream, 166, 167
  formula, 176
  manufacturing, 176
  pressed powder, 159
Eyeliner, 167, 168
  formula, 178, 179
  manufacturing, 178, 179

Face powder, 155–158
  formula, 172–176
  loose, 157, 158

Face powder (*Contd.*)
  manufacturing, 172–176
  pressed, 158
Facial benefits study 1, retinyl
    propionate, 445, 446
  results, 450–455
Facial benefits study 2, retinyl
    propionate, 447, 448
  results, 456–458
Facial hair
  and eflornithine clinical studies,
    496–507
  methods of treatment, 490, 491
  treatment with eflornithine, 489–508
  in women, 490, 491
Facial irritation test 1, retinyl
    propionate, 444
  results, 448–450
Facial irritation test 2, retinyl
    propionate, 444, 445
  results, 456
Facial pigmentary skin disorders,
    185–190
Fat storage/slimming extracts, 94
Fats, types of, 224, 225
Fats, use in moisturizers, 224–226
Fatty chains
  saturated species, sebum
    composition, 312
  sebum composition, 311
  unsaturated species, sebum
    composition, 311
FD&C (Federal Food, Drug, and
    Cosmetic) Act
  history of, 625–629
  implementation of, 629, 630
  initial FDA action, 630, 631
  legislative history of, 627–629
    wrinkle remover cases of 1960s,
      631, 632
FDA (Food and Drug Administration),
    definition of cosmetics, 141
FDA budget, impact of regulatory
    actions, 638, 639
FDA labeling/manufacturing,
    complexities of, 638
FDA review, alpha-hydroxy acid (AHA)
    products, 635

FDA tobacco regulation, 637, 638
FDC Act of 1938, 11
Fe^{2+} chelators, UV spectral data of, 477
Federal Food, Drug, and Cosmetic Act.
    See FD&C Act.
Ferriman-Gallwey system, facial hair
    length, 498
Ferrous/ferric iron, reactive oxygen
    species, 343
Fibroblasts, as growth factor, 353
Filaggrin synthesis assay, topical
    niacinimide testing, 424
Filaggrin, 22
  NMF, 222
Fish oils, extracts, 93
Fitzpatrick Wrinkling Score, 355
Flavonoids, 63, 93
Food and Drug Administration.
    See FDA.
Food, Drug and Cosmetic Act.
    See FD&C.
Formulas, for makeup, 172–182
Foundations
  anhydrous, 161–163
  cosmetic, 160
  emulsified, 160, 161
Freckles
  as evidence of photoaging, 264
  reduction of, via *Emblica*
    antioxidant, 482
Free-radical scavenger, DMAE as, 369
Freund's complete adjuvant test,
    predictive assays, 573

GAG (glycosaminoglycans), 375
Gallo-ellagitannins, 467
Gallotannins, 467, 469
Gender, variation in sebaceous gland
    secretion, 310
Germanium thumbergii extracts, 93
GHK-Cu analogs, 552
  SPARC, 552
GHK-Cu tripeptide, 552
  clinical studies, 555–561
  digital images, 559
  immunohistological assessment, 555
  safety concerns, 559
  skin adherence, 555

Index

skin benefit results, 557
skin penetration, 554
ultrasound measurements, 559
viscoelastic properties, 558
Ginseng, potential uses, 287
Glutathione (GSH), 42, 52
    antioxidant properties, 42
    physiological levels in cutaneous tissues, 43
    prevalence in skin, 42
Gluthathione disulfide (GSSG), 42
Glycerin, in moisturizers, 226
Glycosaminoglycans, GAG, 375
Glycyl-L-histidyl-L-lysine (GHK), 552
Good manufacturing practices (GMP), 629, 630
Green tea polyphenolic (GTP)
    as alternative drug treatment, 248
Ground substance era, HA in, 375
Growth factor(s)
    in cosmeceuticals, 349–358
    in cosmetic applications, 353–356
    defined, 351
    derivations of, 353, 354
    risks associated with, 357, 358
        epidermal growth factor receptor expression, 357
    topical laser treatment, 356, 357
    topical treatment results, 355, 356
    in vitro research, 354
    in wound healing, 351–353
GSH-S-transferase (GST), 49
GSSG, and gluthathione disulfide, 42
Guaijacum, future uses, 288
Guinea pig ear swelling test, irritation tests, animals, 581
Guinea pig maximization test, GPMT, 574, 575

HA (hyaluronic acid), 374, 375
    alpha-hydroxy acids and, 394
    biology of, 377–384
    discovery of, 376
    future uses, 377
    ground substance era, 375
    hyaladherins and, 382
    mucopolysaccharide era, 376
    qualities of, 376–379
    research of, 375–377
    retinoic acid and, 394, 395
    steroids and, 395
    today's usage, 376, 377
    use in cosmetics, 395, 396
HA levels
    aging life cycle
    effect on immunity, 382
    UV exposure, 388
Hair growth, melatonin and, 416
Hamamelis (witch hazel), as alternative drug treatment, 250
Hayluronan, as skin moisturizer, 373–396
Heat shock proteins. *See* Hsp.
Heavy metals, in cosmetics, 151
High-pressure liquid chromatography (HPLC), penetration studies, 323
Hormone replacement therapy (HRT), 273
Hormones
    as photoaging treatment, 272
    rogens, 274
Horse chestnut, future uses, 288
Hsp (heat shock proteins), 523–533
    in aging, 529, 530
    cosmeceutical interest in, 527
    effects on human skin, 528–532
    future uses, 532, 533
    medical pharmaceutical usage, 526
    overview of, 524
    retinoids and, 531, 532
    skin repair process and, 526
    stress and, 523, 524, 526
    thermal tolerance, 528
    types of, 524, 525
Hsp70
    immunofluorescence of, 530, 531
    inducing of, 527
    supplying of, 527, 528
Human irritation assay, 582
Human irritation tests, 578, 579
Human sensitization assays
    modified Draize, 577
    principle features, 576
    repeat insult patch tests, RIPT, 575

Humectants, 226, 227
  moisturizers and, 226, 227
  skin structure and, 229
Hyaladherins, 382
Hyaluronan. *See also* HA.
  acute chronic inflammation, 388, 389
  in aging skin, 381–383, 387, 388
  catabolism, 390, 391
  degradation of, 391
    non-enzymatic, 391
  dermal, 387
  epidermal, 386, 387
  function of, 379–381
  intracellular, 383, 384
  oxidative stress, 393
  photoaging of skin, 388
  production of, 380
    during acute stress, 380
    during aging, 381–383
    with cancer, 381
    embryonic development, 380, 381
    during wound healing, 381
  receptors, CD44 as, 384, 385
  skin, 385, 386
  skin moisture enhancements, 394
  skin substitutes, 389
  structure of, 378, 379
  synthases, 390
  UV light, effect on, 393
Hyaluronic acid. *See* HA.
Hyaluronidase inhibitors, 391, 392
  low molecular weight, 392
  macromolecular, 391, 392
Hyaluronidases, 390, 391
Hydrated alumina, as pigment, 150
Hydration effect, of protective
    creams, 295
Hydration of skin, 221
Hydrogen peroxide, reactive oxygen
    species, 337
Hydrophilic skin antioxidants, 52, 53
  ascobate, 52
  glutathione, 52
  urate, 52
Hydroquinone, depigmenting
    agents, 274
Hydroquinone cream, 190
Hydroquinone monobenzyl, 189, 190

Hydroxy radical quenching, *Emblica* as
    antioxidant, 472, 473
Hydroxyacids, 207–214
  alternative drug treatment, 250
  biological activities, 209, 210
  corneocyte cohesion and,
      210, 211
  hypopigmenting effect, 212
  improvement skin condition,
      213, 214
  peeling caustic effects, 211, 212
  safety in using, 214
  SC functions and, 210, 211
Hydroxyl radical, reactive oxygen
    species, 337
Hydroxyzable tannins, 466
Hyluronan, conjunction with mitosis,
    379, 380
Hyperpigmentation
  of the face, 185
  hydroxyacids and, 212
  photoaging and, 265
Hyroxyacids, classification of, 209

Image analysis, of photoaging, 265
Immune system, phytosterols, effect on,
    283, 284
Immunity, HA levels, 382
Immunological contact urticaria (ICU),
    590, 591
  irritation tests, animals, 580, 581
IND (investigational new drug), 629
Indigoid, 146
Inflammatory disorders,
    endogenous, 38
Inorganic pearls, 151
  bismuthe oxychloride, 151, 152
  titanium coated micas, 152
Inorganic pigments, 147–150
Intracellular hyaluronan, 383, 384
Investigational new drug (IND), 629
Involucrin synthesis assay, topical
    niacinimide testing, 424
Ionic emulsifiers, 225, 226
Iron blue, as pigment, 149
Iron chelators
  for prevention of photoaging, 269
  skin damage prevention, 343–345

Index

Iron oxides, as pigments, 149
Irritant contact dermatitis (ICD), 294
  assays, 577–582
Irritation tests, animals, 578–582
  CUS, 579, 580
  Draize-type tests, 578
  guinea pig ear swelling test, 581
  ICU, 580, 581
  NICU, 580
  non-Draize animal studies, 578
  TMA, 581
Isolated tyrosinase inhibition test, 190
Isolectric point, amino acid,
    dissociation constant, 22
Isotretinoin, as retinoid, 271

Jambuk tree, potential uses, 288
Japan Ministry of Health Welfare,
    MHW, 141
Japanese definition, cosmeceuticals,
    6, 7, 12
Japanese quasidrugs, 643–646

Kaolin, 156
Keratin, and water, 221
Keratin synthesis assay, topical
    niacinimide testing, 424
Keratinocytes, 113–115
  epidermal lipids, 114
    clinical trials, 114–119
  niacinamide, effects on, 113
  normal human, 115, 116
  vitamin C, ascobate, 39
Ketoconazole, and seborrheic
    dermatitis, 132, 133
Kinetin, 407–411
  biology of, 408
  cell yield comparisons, 409
  chemistry of, 408
  clinical studies, 410
  effect on aging, 409
  mechanism of action, 410
Kojic acid
  clinical evaluation of, 200–204
  safety test results, 203
  toxicity of, 202

Lakes, 142, 143
  as color additive, 141
  salts, 143
Langerhans cells, UV-skin damage,
    336, 337
Lanolin, in moisturizers, 225
Laser treatment, topical growth factors,
    356, 357
Laser-Doppler blood flowmetry (LDF),
    in contact urticaria, 595, 596
Lavender oil, as alternative drug
    treatment, 253, 254
Lechithin:retinol acyltransferase
    (LRAT), 442
Levarometry, photoaging analysis, 266
LHA (lipohydroxyacid), 211
Light diffusing pigments, 154
Linoleic acid, effect on skin
    structure, 230
Lipid(s)
  classes of, 222
  composition of human, 223
    factors effecting, 233
  epidermis, barrier function
    of, 93, 94
  human, sebum composition, 310
  nonphysiological, SC hydration,
    296, 297
  physiological, SC hydration,
    296, 297
  skin hydration, 222, 223
Lipid-soluble antioxidants, 44–49
  carotenoids, vitamin A, 48
  ubiquinols, ubiquinones,
    coenzyme Q, 45
  vitamin E, 44
Lipogenesis, and skin biopsy
    samples, 425
Lipohydroxyacid, LHA, 211
Lipoic acid, 70
Lipophilic skin antioxidants, 53, 54
  ubquinol/ubiquinone, 54
  vitamin A, 54
  vitamin E, 53, 54
Liposome, lecithin base, 104
Lipstick, 168–171
  classical, 169, 170
  formula, 180, 181

Lipstick (*Contd.*)
　manufacturing, 180, 181
　solvent, 170, 171
Lysyl osidase, as copper containing enzyme, 551

Magnesium carbonate, 156
Maillard reaction, 336
Makeup, emulsion, 160, 161
Makeup formulary, 172–182
　blushers, 175, 176
　eye shadows, 176, 177
　eyeliners, 178, 179
　face powders, 172–174
　lipsticks, 180, 181
　liquid compact foundation, 174, 175
　mascaras, 177–178
　nail products, 181, 182
　pencils, 179
Makeup pencil
　formula, 179
　manufacturing, 179
Makeup technology, 154, 155
Malassezia genus, in seborrheic dermatitis, 130–132
Malassezia, treatment of, 132, 133
Manganese violet, as pigment, 149
Manufacturing, makeup, 172–182
Mascara, 163–166
　formula, 177, 178
　manufacturing, 177, 178
　water phase, 163, 164
　wax phase, 163, 164
Matrikines
　concept of, 121
　pal-KTTKS, 123
Matrix metalloprotease enzymes (MMP), 478
Membranes, phytosterols, in, 282
Mechanical force, usefulness of, 608, 609
Melanin pathway, 512
Melanogenesis inhibition, mechanism of, 191–193
　dose-dependent, 192
Melanogenesis, 511, 512
　EA, 518

Streptomycese fervents in, 192, 193
　in vitro, 194, 195
Melanoma cells, cultured with EA, 518, 519
Melasma, 186–190
　clinical tests, 195–199
　depigmentation agents and, 197
　histopathology, 187
　photographic evaluation of, 197
Melatonin, 70, 413–418
　in edible plants, 416, 417
　as food supplement, 417
　and hair growth, 416
　for UV protection, 414
Metallic soap, 156
Metallothioneins, copper-containing enzyme, 551
MHW (Ministry of Health Welfare), in Japan, 141
Mica, 156
Microfine pigments, 154
Microfluidizer method, emulsifier level reduction, 604–607
Milk thistle, risks of use, 289
Millard reaction product, flavor characteristics, 27
Minimal erythema dosis (MED), 188, 268
　melasma, 190
Minimum pigmentation dosis (MPD), 188
Minimum quaddel dosis (MQD), 189
　melasma, 190
Mitosis, hyluronan conjunction with, 379, 380
Modified Draize, human sensitization test, 577
Moisturizers, 219–236
　chemistry of, 224–227
　desquamation and, 228–232
　as dry skin treatment, 220, 221, 231
　effectiveness of, 227, 228
　as photoaging treatment, 270–272
　retinoids in, 271, 272
　and skin barrier function, 233–235
　and skin chemistry, 227, 228
　and skin structure, 228–232

AHA, 229
humectants, 229
linoleic acid, 230
N-acetylcysteine, 230
urea, 230
use on SC, 224
water, 229
Mucopolysaccharide era, HA in, 376
Muscarinic receptor, DMAE as, 368
Mushroom tyroninase, 190
Mycoplasma arthritidis, 282

N-Acetylcysteine, effect on skin structure, 230
N-Acylglutamate, introduction of, amino acid derivative, 33
NAD (nicotinamide adenine dinucleotide), 422
NADPH level assay, topical niacinimide testing, 423
NADPH levels, topical niacinimide testing results, 429, 430
Nail, acrylic hardener
  formula, 182
  manufacturing, 182
Nail, pearlescent enamel
  formula, 181
  manufacturing, 181
Nail, cream enamel
  formula, 181
  manufacturing, 181
Nail color, 171, 172
N-Alkylether-hydroxypropyl arginine, amino acid derivative, 33
NAPD, 422
Natural moisturizing factor (NMF), 222
N-Cocoylarginine ethylester PCA salt, amino acid derivative, 33
New drug application (NDA), 629
Niacinamide, 121
  in keratinocyte differentiation, 113
Niacinamide, topical
  benefits of, 421–439
  cell culture methods, 422
  collagen synthesis assay, 423
  collagen synthesis results, 430

facial benefits/study 1 and 2, 426, 427
  results, 435
facial skin tolerance results, 425, 434
filaggrin synthesis assay, 424
involucrin synthesis assay, 424
keratin synthesis assay, 424
lipogenesis skin biopsy samples, 425
materials and methods, 422
NADPH level assay, 423
NADPH level results, 429, 430
pore size measurement study, 428
Niacinamide, topical (*Contd.*)
  sebum excretion
    measurement study, 427
  pore size results, 435–438
  skin barrier evaluation, 428, 429
  skin barrier function results, 431
Nicotinamide adenine dinucleotide. *See* NAD.
Nicotinic receptors, DMAE AND, 367
Nitric oxygen, reactive oxygen species, 339, 340
Nitrogen radical quenching, *Emblica* in, 474, 475
Nitrous oxide, 257
N-lauroyl lysine, amino acid derivative, 33
Noncollagenic protein synthesis, *Emblica* antioxidant and, 481
Non-Draize animal studies, irritation tests, 578
Nonimmunological contact urticaria (NICU), 589, 590
  irritation tests, animals, 580
Noninflammatory painful response, subjective irritation, 581, 582
Nonionic emulsifiers, 225, 226
Nonphysiological lipids, and SC hydration, 296, 297
Nouricel-MD™, 354

Oatmeal, as alternative drug treatment, 250
Occlusion effect, of protective creams, 295

Ocimum oil, as alternative drug treatment, 254
Oils, fish and vegetable, 225
Oils, use in moisturizers, 224–226
Olive oil, extra virgin, risks of use, 288
Open epicutaneous test (OET), 572, 573
Open test method, 593
Optical rotation, amino acids, 23–26
Optimization test, predictive assays, 573, 574
Organic pearls, 151
Organic pigments, 145–147
  listing of, 147, 148
  stability of, 146, 147
Ornithine (Orn), 29
Ornithine decarboxylase (ODC), 491
  hair growth, 491, 492
OTC Drug Review, 632, 633
  effect on foreign markets, 635, 636
  international harmonization of, 635, 636
  warning letters, 632–635
Oxidation enhancer, chelators as, 476
Oxidative stress
  definition of, 38
  hyaluronan and, 393

Pal-KTTKS, matrikines, 121
Paresthesia, 581, 582
Pathogenesis, of photoaging, 263
PCA, moisturizers and, 226
Pearlescent pigments, 151–154
Pearls
  inorganic, 151
  organic, 151
Pencils
  materials for, 168
  product types, 168
  uses of, 168
Percutaneous absorption assays, *in vivo*, 569, 570
Percutaneous penetration assays, *in vitro*, 570
Perfluoropolyethers, protective creams, 300
Perfumes, 157
Perioxidation, with coproporphyrin, 339

Persimmon leaf extract, as alternative drug treatment, 249
Phenolic metabolism, 466
Phorbol ester, PMA and, 390
Photoaged skin
  cosmetic approaches to, 350
  pathology of, 350
Photoaging, 261–275
  analysis of, 265–267
    ballistometry, 266
    capacitance conductance, 266
    clinical methods, 266, 267
    colorimetry, 266
    evaporimetry, 266
    levarometry, 266
    twistometry, 266
    ultrasound, 265
  appearance of skin, 263–265
  color of skin, 265, 266
  history of cosmeceuticals in, 262
  hyaluronan and, 388
  image analysis, 265
  methods of study, 265–267
    clinical methods, 266, 267
    instrumentation, 265, 266
  moisturizers, 270–272
  pathogenesis of, 263
  prevention of, 267, 268
  process of, 262
  products for prevention of, 268–270
    aliphatic alicyclic diols, 269
    antioxidants, 269
    iron chelators, 269
    selenium, 270
    self tanning agents, 269
    thymidine dimmers, 269
    vitamin C, 269
    vitamin E, 270
  topical tretinoin, test results, 327–329
  treatment products, 270–274
  vitamins, 273
Photodamaged skin, GHK-Cu and, 555–561
Photographs, for evaluation of pigmentary disorders, 197

Index

Phyllanthus emblica
  as ayurvedic herb, 470
  tannins of, 469
Phyllanthus genus, 467–469
Phyllanthus tannins, 465–484
Physiological lipids, and SC hydration, 296, 297
Phytosteols, 279–289
  in cancer, 284, 285
  cholesterol-lowering foods and, 282, 283
  clinical examples of usage, 284
  eczema and, 286, 287
  future uses, 287, 288
  immune system, 283, 284
  membranes, 282
  mycoplasma arthritidis, 282
  risks in using, 288–289
  skin, 285, 286
  sources of, 281, 282
    rapeseed oil, 281
    saw palmetto, 282
    soybeans, 281
    sweet corn, 282
    wheatgerm, 282
Pigment(s)
  as color additive, 141
  inorganic, 147–150
  light-diffusing, 154
  microfine, 154
  organic, 145–147
  pearlescent, 151–154
  specialty, 152
  treated, 152–154
Pigmentary disorders, facial, types, 185–190
Pigmented cosmetic dermatitis, 197, 198
  treatment of, 198, 199
Placenta extract, skin whitening, 513
Plants, melatonin from inedible, 416, 417
PMA, as phorbol ester, 390
Polymers, 157
Pore size measurement study, topical niacinimide testing, 428
Powder products
  blushers, 158, 159
  cosmetics, 155

  face 155–158
  pressed eye shadows, 159
  quality assurance, 159
Predictive assays
  Buehler test, 573
  dermatopharmacokinetics, 568, 569
  Draize test, 571, 572
  Freund's complete adjuvant test, 573
  guinea pig maximization test, GPMT, 574, 575
  guinea pig sensitization tests, 571
  open epicutaneous test, 572, 573
  optimization test, 573, 574
  planning execution, 570, 571
  quantitative structure activity relationships, 571
  split adjuvant test, 574
Preservatives
  in face powders, 157
  reduction cosmetics, 607, 608
Primary/straight color, as color additive, 141
Proanthoyanidins, condensed tannins and, 467
Process engineering, in cosmetics manufacture, 603–611
Profilaggrin, NMF and, 222
Progesterone, melasma and, 186, 187
Proline (Pro), 29
Pro-oxidants, antioxidants as, 476
Propylene glycol, moisturizers, 226, 227
Protective creams. *See* Creams, protective.
Proteins, EMC and, 480, 481
Pseudofolliculitis treatment, salicylic acid as, 212, 213
Pumpkin seeds, medicinal uses, 284
Pycnogenol, 542, 543
  Evelle®, 542
  wound healing, 542
Pyrroridone carboxylic acid (PCA), and NMF, 22
PYSer
  inhibitory effect of, 344, 345
  synthesis of, 344

Quality control, of colorants, 150, 151
Quasidrugs
  Japan, 643–649
Quaternium-18 bentonite, 257
Quenchers, effect on collagen, 340
Quinoline, 146

RA (all-trans-retinoic acid), 323
Rapeseed oil, as source of
    phytosterols, 281
Reactive oxygen species
  astaxanthin, 343
  carotenoids, 342
  hydrogen peroxide, 337
  hydroxyl radical, 337
  iron chelators, 343, 344
  nitric oxygen, 339, 340
Reactive oxygen species (ROS), 38, 262
  scavenging of, 341–345
  singlet oxygen, 338
  skin damage, 336, 337
  superoxide anion, 337
  UV irradiation, 336–341
Receptor for HA-mediated motility
    (RHAMM), 385
Regulatory actions, impact on FDA
    budget, 638, 639
Relaxation time, T2, in human skin,
    111, 112
Repeat insult patch tests (RIPT), human
    sensitization assays, 575
Retinaldehyde (RAL), 323, 545, 546
  clinical studies results, 546
  retinoid, 272
  skin aging, 546
  topical retinoids, 545, 546
Retinoic acid receptors (RARα,
    -β, -γ), 442
Retinoic acid, effect on HA, 394, 395
Retinoid effects, assays with cutaneous
    markers, 324
Retinoid photostability, 447, 455, 446
Retinoid X receptors (RXR), 329
Retinoid(s), 120, 121
Retinoids, Hsp, 531, 532
  beta carotene, 272
  classification of, 320
  discussion of, 319–321

  isotretinoin, 271
  naturally existing, role of, 320
  photoaging treatment, 271, 272
  retinaldehyde, 272
  retinol, 271, 272
  structure of, 321
  tazarotene, 272
  topical, uses of, 321
  toxicity, 329, 330
  tretinoin, 271
Retinol, 271, 272
  cellular uptake, 324
  cutaneous metabolism, 325
  metabolism, 325, 326
  pharmacological effects, 326, 327
  retinyl propionate-acetate, testing
      results, 459–461
  testing of, 443–447
  testing results, 447–455
  uptake of, 324
  vitamin A, 322, 323
  See also Retinyl propionate, topical.
Retinol-binding protein (RBP), 324
Retinols, topical. *See* Topical retinols.
Retinyl acetate
  retinol, retinyl propionate, testing
      results, 459–461
Retinyl acetate
  testing of, 443–447
  testing results, 447–455
  See also Retinyl propionate, topical.
Retinyl palmitate, ROL palm, 323
Retinyl propionate/retinyl acetate/
    retinol, testing results, 459–461
  testing of, 443–447
    back cumulative irritation test,
        443, 444
      results, 447, 448
    facial benefits study 1, 445, 446
      results, 450–455
    facial benefits study 2, 447, 448
      results, 447, 448
    facial irritation test 1, 444
      results, 448–450
    facial irritation test 2, 444, 445
      results, 456
    human studies, 443
    stability of test materials, 443

Index

testing results, 447–455
topical, 441–461
 uses of, 442
 vs. *trans*-retinoic acid, 442
Rogenic hormones, sebaceous gland
 stimulation, 309
Rogens, hormones, 274
Rosemary (*Rosmarinus*), extracts, 93

Sagging skin, DMAE and, 370
Salicylic acid
 acne treatment, 212, 213
 corneum stratum, 210, 211
 pseudofolliculitis treatment, 212, 213
Salts, lakes, 143
Sandalwood, future uses, 288
Saturated species, sebum composition,
 fatty chains, 312
Saw palmetto
 medicinal uses, 284
 source of phytosterols, 282
SC (stratum corneum), 18, 22, 220
 bilayers of, 109, 110
 chemistry of dry, 221–223
 corneocytes in, 103
 long-term repair test results, 107
 repair of, 101–112
 short-term repair test results, 106
 signs of damage, 104–106
SC barrier
 epidermis as, 112–119
 function of, 232–235
  effects of creams, 233
  impairment, 232
  moisturizers, 233
  tested substances, 234
  water loss, 232
 schematic representation, 102
SC hydration
 physiological lipids, 296, 297
 skin creams, 294–296
Scale-up, emulsification, mechanical
 forces in, 610
Screening tests, depigmentation agents,
 190–194
Sebaceous glands
 anatomy of, 307, 308
 distribution of, 301

Seborrheic dermatitis (dandruff),
 129–133
 etiology, 130–132
 ketoconazole treatment, 132, 133
 Malassezia genus in, 130–132
 pathogenesis, 130–132
 symptoms, 129, 130
 treatment of, 132, 133
 yeasts, 130–132
 zinc pyrithione treatment, 133
Sebum, 307–315
 composition
  fatty chains, 311
  human, 310–312
  lipid class, 310
  other species, 313
  saturated species, 312
  unsaturated species, 311
 disease and, 314, 315
 excretion pore size,
  niacinimide testing, 427
  niacinimide testing results,
   435–438
 health and, 313, 314
 mammals, 313, 314
 secretion, 308
  acne, 314, 315
  age gender variation, 310
  hormonal control, 309
  measurement methods, 308, 309
   bentonite gel, 308, 309
   cigarette paper, 308, 309
   Sebutape, 308, 309
Sebutape, for measurement of sebum
 gland secretion, 308, 309
Selenium, for prevention of
 photoaging, 270
Self-tanning agents, for prevention of
 photoaging, 269
Senile xerosis, aged dry skin, 30
Singlet oxygen, reactive oxygen
 species, 338
Singlet oxygen quenching, *Emblica*
 antioxidant, 474
Skin
 amino acid delivery into, 30
 copper peptide, 549–561
 hyaluronan in, 385, 386

photodamaged, GHK-Cu, clinical
  studies, 555–561
Skin aging,
  hyaluronan in, 387, 388
  retinaldehyde, 546
Skin barrier evaluation, topical
  niacinimide testing, 428, 429
Skin barrier function, 232–235
  effects of creams, 233
  impairment, 232
  moisturizers, 233
  tested substances, 234
  topical niacinimide testing
    results, 431
  water loss, 232
Skin barrier layer components, topical
  niacinimide testing results, 431
Skin care vs. skin protection, 298
Skin cream
  barrier protection, 297–300
  barrier recovery, 297–300
  SC hydration, 294–296
Skin damage, acute, UV-induced,
  334, 335
  chronic, UV-induced, 336
Skin damage
  prevention
    antioxidants, 341, 342
    iron chelators, 343–345
    scavenging of reactive oxygen
      species, 341–345
Skin disorders, pigmentary, of the
  face, 186
Skin elasticity, Evelle® supplementation,
  538–543
Skin even-toning, 481–483
Skin firmness, DMAE, 369
Skin function
  amino acids and, 30
  integrity of, with amino acids, 30
Skin hydration, lipids, 222, 223
Skin lightening, 481–483, 513
Skin moisturizer, hayluronan as,
  373–396
Skin penetration, GHK-Cu, 554
Skin repair process, HSP, 526
Skin structure, desquamation, 228–232
Skin substitutes, uses of, 389

Skin whitening
  EA in, 515
  ingredients, 513
SOD
  copper containing enzyme, 551
  extracts, 93
  superoxide dismutase, 50
Sodium lauryl sulfate (SLS), 298
Solar lentigo, depigmentation
  agents, 197
Solubility, in cosmetics manufacture, 608
Solvent lipstick, 170, 171
Soybeans
  as alternative drug treatment, 250
  as source of phytosterols, 281
Soymilk, as alternative drug
  treatment, 250
SPARC, GHK-Cu analogs, 552
Spearmint, as alternative drug
  treatment, 249, 250
Split adjuvant test, predictive
  assays, 574
Squalene, in sebaceous glands, 310
Standardized black tea extracts, SBTE, as
  alternative drug treatment, 249
Stanols, 280
  chemical structure of, 280
Starch, 156
Stargrass root, future uses of, 288
Steroids
  HA and, 395
Sterols, skin, 285, 286
  animal, plants, 281
  chemical structure of, 280
  defined, 279
  plant, 279–281
Stigmasterol, 281
Stinging nettle, medicinal uses, 284
Stomelysin 1 (MMP-3)
      inhibitory effect of
  Emblica antioxidant, 480
Stratum corneum. *See* SC.
Streptomycese fervents, melanogenesis,
  192, 193
Stress
  effect on health, 523, 524
  Hsp and, 526
  hyaluronan production, 380

Subjective irritation, noninflammatory painful response, 581, 582
Sun damage and skin appearance, 263, 264
Sunburn, 335
Sunscreens and photoaging prevention, 268, 269
Superoxide anion, reactive oxygen species, 337
Superoxide anion radical quenching, *Emblica* antioxidant, 473
Superoxide dismutases
  prevalence in skin, 50
  SOD, 50
Sweet corn, as source of phytosterols, 282
Syzygium aromaticum, extracts, 93

T2 relaxation time, human skin, 111, 112
Talc, 155
Tannery agents, protective creams, 300
Tannins, 466
  classes of, 469
  hydrolyzable, 466
    ellagitannins, 467
    gallo-ellagitannins, 467
    gallotannins, 467
  occurrence of, 469
  Phyllanthus as source of, 467–469
Tazarotene, as retinoid, 272
Tea extracts, as alternative treatment, 248, 249
Tensides, 298
  as skin irritants, 298
Teratogenicity, 329
Test methods
  chamber test, 593
  open test, 593
  use test, 593
Thiols, 63
Thymidine dimmers, for prevention of photoaging, 269
Tissue inhibitory metalloprotease-1 (TIMP-1), 479
Titanium coated micas, inorganic pearls, 152
Titanium dioxide, as pigment, 148

TNS Recovery Complex®,
  cytokines, 354
  growth factor, 354
Tobacco, regulation by FDA, 637, 638
Toner, as color additive, 142
Topical applications
  vitamin C, 63
  vitamin E derivatives, 55, 62
Topical niacinamide, benefits of, 438, 439
Topical retinoids, 319–330
  absorption, 323, 324
  cosmeceuticals, 322
  cutaneous metabolism, 323
  historical background, 322
  penetration, 323, 324
  uses of, 321
Topical retinyl propionate, 441–461
Toxicity, oral, 29
TransCyte™, 353
Transepidermal water loss (TEWL), 104, 266
Trans-retinoic acid (t-RA), 442
Trans-retinoic acid, vs. retinyl propionate, 442
Treated pigments, 152–154
Tretinoin
  photoaged skin, 350
  photoaging, test results, 327–329
  retinoid, 271
  topical (all-*trans*-retinoic acid), 327–329
Triarylmethane, 146
Triglycerides
  moisturizers, 225
  sebaceous glands, 310
Tri-luma, depigmenting agents, 274
Trimellitic anhydride-sensitive mouse assay, TMA, irritation tests, animals, 581
True pigment, as color additive, 142
Twistometry, photoaging analysis, 266
Tyrosinase, 512
  copper containing enzyme, 551
  inhibition, 190, 191, 194
Tyrosine, synthesis of
  melanin from, 512

Ubiquinol/ubiquinone
  coenzyme Q, 45
  lipophilic skin antioxidants, 54
  physiological levels in skin, 47
Ultramarines, as pigments, 149
Ultrasound, photoaging analysis, 265
Ultraviolet. See UV.
United States cosmetics regulations, 617, 618
Unsaturated species, sebum composition, fatty chains, 311
Urate
  antioxidant properties, 44
  hydrophilic skin antioxidants, 52
  prevalence in skin, 44
Urea
  effect on skin structure, 230
  moisturizers, 226
Urocanic acid (UA), 30
Use test method, 593
UV absorber, 30
UV care, 333–345
UV exposure
  exogenous, 38
  HA levels, 388
UV light, effect on hyaluronan, 393
UV protection, melatonin, 414
UV rays
  minimum erythema dose (MED), 334
  Cu^{2+} chelators, 477
  Fe^{2+} chelators, 477
UV stress, Hsp, 528
UV-induced
  erythema, reduction of, Emblica antioxidant, 483
  ROS, on epidermal hyaluronan, 118
    histologic changes, 335
    Langerhans cells, 336, 337
    skin damage, acute, 334, 335
    skin damage, chronic, 336
    skin pigmentation, EA in, 515
UV-A/UV-B/UV-C, 333, 334

VANIQ™, 491, 495
Vegetable oils, extracts, as antioxidants, 93

Vitamin A
  antioxidant properties, 48
  carotenoids, 48
  lipophilic skin antioxidants, 54
  prevalence in skin, 48
  retinol, 322, 323
Vitamin C
  as alternative drug treatment, 254, 255
  ascobate, ketalactone, 39
  photoprotective effects of topically applied, 64–69
  prevention of photoaging, 269
  skin whitening, 512
  topical applications, 63
Vitamin E
  derivatives, topical application, 55, 62
  alternative drug treatment, 254, 255
  prevention of photoaging, 270
  lipophilic skin antioxidants, lip-solubles, 44
  photoprotective effects of topically applied, 56–61
  prevalence in skin, 45
Vitamin(s), as photoaging treatment, 272
VPS grading system, 454–459

Water
  in skin hydration, 221
  in skin structure, 229
Water loss
  effect on skin barrier function, 232
  SC, 232
Water-soluble antioxidants, ascorbate, 39
Wax esters, sebaceous glands, 310
Wheat germ, as source of phytosterols, 282
Witch hazel, hamamelis, as alternative drug treatment, 250
Wound healing
  four phases of, 351, 352
  growth factors, 351, 353
  hyaluronan production, 381

Wrinkle remover cases of 1960s, legislation, 631, 632

Xanthenes, 146

Yeast, seborrheic dermatitis, 130–132

Zinc, lipids, 223
Zinc oxide
 as pigment, 148, 149
 protective creams, 300
Zinc pyrithione, treatment of seborrheic dermatitis, 133